BSAVA Manual of Canine and Feline Musculoskeletal Disorders:
A Practical Guide to Lameness and Joint Disease
second edition

Editors:

Gareth Arthurs
PGCertMedEd MA VetMB CertVR CertSAS DipSAS(Orth) FHEA FRCVS
Arthurs Orthopaedics and University College Dublin
Veterinary Hospital, Belfield, Dublin 4, Ireland

Gordon Brown
BVM&S CertSAO DipSAS(Orth) MRCVS
Grove Referrals,
Holt Road, Fakenham, Norfolk, NR21 8JG, UK

Rob Pettitt
BVSc PGCertLTHE DipSAS(Orth) SFHEA FRCVS
Small Animal Teaching Hospital, Institute of Veterinary Science,
University of Liverpool, Leahurst Campus,
Chester High Road, Neston CH64 7TE, UK

Published by:

British Small Animal Veterinary Association
Woodrow House, 1 Telford Way,
Waterwells Business Park, Quedgeley,
Gloucester GL2 2AB

A Company Limited by Guarantee in England
Registered Company No. 2837793
Registered as a Charity

Copyright © 2018 BSAVA

All rights reserved. No part of this publication may be reproduced, stored in a retrieval system, or transmitted, in form or by any means, electronic, mechanical, photocopying, recording or otherwise without prior written permission of the copyright holder.

The colour illustrations in this book (excluding 4.1, 12.2, 12.5, 12.6, 12.10, 12.13, 12.14, 12.20, 21.42a and 24.31) were drawn by S.J. Elmhurst BA Hons (www.livingart.org.uk) and are printed with her permission

The drawings in figures 12.2, 12.5, 12.6, 12.10, 12.13, 12.14 and 12.20 were created by Allison L. Wright, MS, CMI, Athens, Georgia, USA

Figures 4.1, 21.42a and 24.31 were designed and drawn by Vicki Martin Design and are printed with their permission

A catalogue record for this book is available from the British Library.

ISBN 978 1 905319 69 5

The publishers, editors and contributors cannot take responsibility for information provided on dosages and methods of application of drugs mentioned or referred to in this publication. Details of this kind must be verified in each case by individual users from up to date literature published by the manufacturers or suppliers of those drugs. Veterinary surgeons are reminded that in each case they must follow all appropriate national legislation and regulations (for example, in the United Kingdom, the prescribing cascade) from time to time in force.

Printed in India by Imprint Digital
Printed on ECF paper made from sustainable forests

Save 15% off the digital version of this manual. By purchasing this print edition we are pleased to offer you a reduced price on online access at www.bsavalibrary.com
Enter offer code 15MSD286 on checkout

Please note the discount only applies to a purchase of the full online version of the *BSAVA Manual of Canine and Feline Musculoskeletal Disorders: A Practical Guide to Lameness and Joint Disease, 2nd edition* via **www.bsavalibrary.com**. The discount will be taken off the BSAVA member price or full price, depending on your member status. The discount code is for a single purchase of the online version and is for your personal use only. If you do not already have a login for the BSAVA website you will need to register in order to make a purchase.

4345PUBS18

Titles in the BSAVA Manuals series

For further information on these and all BSAVA publications, please visit our website: **www.bsava.com**

Contents

Operative Techniques: grading system

The editors have graded each of the OT surgical procedures by complexity to help the reader understand whether the procedure is one that they should consider attempting.

/ This technique can be achieved by surgeons with limited orthopaedic skill and experience.

// This technique requires moderate experience and skill.

/// This is an advanced technique.

Contributors

Ralph Abercromby
BVMS CertSAO MRCVS
Anderson Abercromby Veterinary Referrals,
1870 Building, Jayes Park Courtyard,
Forest Green Road, Ockley, Dorking RH5 5RR, UK

Briony Alderson
BVSc CertVA DipECVAA MRCVS
Small Animal Teaching Hospital,
Institute of Veterinary Science, University of Liverpool,
Leahurst Campus, Chester High Road,
Neston CH64 7TE, UK

Angus Anderson
BVetMed PhD DipSAS(Orth) FRCVS
Anderson Abercromby Veterinary Referrals,
1870 Building, Jayes Park Courtyard,
Forest Green Road, Ockley, Dorking RH5 5RR, UK

Gareth Arthurs
PGCertMedEd MA VetMB CertVR CertSAS DipSAS(Orth) FHEA FRCVS
Arthurs Orthopaedics & University College Dublin
Veterinary Hospital, Belfield, Dublin 4, Ireland

Nicholas J. Bacon
MA VetMB CertVR CertSAS DipECVS DipACVS FRCVS
Fitzpatrick Referrals - Oncology and Soft Tissue,
Surrey Research Park, 70 Priestley Road,
Guildford GU2 7AJ, UK

School of Veterinary Medicine,
VSM Building, University of Surrey,
Daphne Jackson Road, Guildford GU2 7AL, UK

Richard Barrett Jolley
BSc(Hons) DPhil(Oxon) FHEA FBPhS FPhysiol
Institute of Ageing and Chronic Disease,
University of Liverpool, William Henry Duncan Building,
6 West Derby Street, Liverpool L7 8TX, UK

Brian Beale
DVM DipACVS
Gulf Coast Veterinary Specialists,
1030 Wirt Road, Houston, TX 77055, USA

Sebastien Behr
DVM(Hons) DipECVN MRCVS
Willows Veterinary Centre & Referral Service,
Highlands Road, Shirley, Solihull B90 4NH, UK

Gordon Brown
BVM&S CertSAO DipSAS(Orth) MRCVS
Grove Referrals,
Holt Road, Fakenham, Norfolk NR21 8JG, UK

Neil Burton
BVSc CertSAS DipSAS(Orth) PGCert(HE) FHEA MRCVS
Wear Referrals,
Veterinary Hospital, Bradbury,
Stockton-on-Tees TS21 2ES, UK

Steve Butterworth
MA VetMB CertAcct CertVR DipSAO MRCVS
Weighbridge Referral Centre,
Kemys Way, Llansamlet,
Swansea SA6 8QF, UK

Stephen Clarke
BVMS DipSAS(Orth) DipECVS MRCVS
Willows Veterinary Centre & Referral Service,
Highlands Road, Shirley, Solihull B90 4NH, UK

Dylan Clements
BSc BVSc PhD DipSAS(Orth) DipECVS FHEA FRCVS
Royal (Dick) School of Veterinary Studies and
Roslin Institute, Easter Bush, Roslin,
Midlothian EH25 9RG, UK

Louise Dale
RVN A1 Assessor VTS(Anaesthesia and Analgesia)
Small Animal Teaching Hospital,
Institute of Veterinary Science, University of Liverpool,
Leahurst Campus, Chester High Road,
Neston CH64 7TE, UK

Mike Farrell
BVetMed CertVA CertSAS DipECVS MRCVS
Davies Veterinary Specialists,
Manor Farm Business Park, Higham Gobion,
Hitchin SG5 3HR, UK

Toby J. Gemmill
BVSc MVM DipSAS(Orth) DipECVS MRCVS
Willows Veterinary Centre & Referral Service,
Highlands Road, Shirley,
Solihull B90 4NH, UK

Mike Guilliard
MA VetMB CertSAO FRCVS
Mike Guilliard Orthopaedics Limited,
Anvil Cottage, Wrinehill Road, Wybunbury,
Nantwich, Cheshire CW5 7NU, UK

Don Hulse
DVM DipACVS DipECVS
Texas A&M University,
400 Bizzell St, College Station,
TX 77843, USA

John Innes
BVSc PhD CertVR DipSAS(Orth) FRCVS
Chester Gates Veterinary Specialists,
Units E&F, Telford Court, Gates Lane,
Chestergates Road, Chester, Cheshire CH1 6LT, UK

Sorrel Langley-Hobbs
MA BVetMed DipSAS(Orth) DipECVS FHEA MRCVS
Bristol Veterinary School,
University of Bristol, Langford House,
Langford, Bristol BS40 5DU, UK

John Lapish
BSc BVetMed MRCVS
94 Union Road,
Sheffield S11 9EJ, UK

Rebecca Lewis
BSc(Hons) PhD FHEA
School of Veterinary Medicine,
VSM Building, University of Surrey,
Daphne Jackson Road, Guildford GU2 7AL, UK

Thomas W. Maddox
BVSc PhD PGCertHE CertVDI DipECVDI FHEA MRCVS
Small Animal Teaching Hospital,
Institute of Veterinary Science, University of Liverpool,
Leahurst Campus, Chester High Road,
Neston CH64 7TE, UK

Andy Moores
BVSc DipSAS(Orth) DipECVS FRCVS
Anderson Moores Veterinary Specialists Ltd,
The Granary, Bunstead Barns, Poles Lane,
Hursley, Winchester, Hampshire SO21 2LL, UK

Bill Oxley
MA VetMB DipSAS(Orth) MRCVS
Willows Veterinary Centre & Referral Service,
Highlands Road, Shirley, Solihull B90 4NH, UK

Rob Pettitt
BVSc PGCertLTHE DipSAS(Orth) SFHEA FRCVS
Small Animal Teaching Hospital,
Institute of Veterinary Science, University of Liverpool,
Leahurst Campus, Chester High Road,
Neston CH64 7TE, UK

Jonathan Pink
BSc BVetMed CertSAS DipECVS MRCVS
Willows Veterinary Centre & Referral Service,
Highlands Road, Shirley, Solihull B90 4NH, UK

Simona Tiziana Radaelli
PhD DipECVN MRCVS
Neurology CPD Ltd,
Solihull, UK

Geoff Robins
BVetMed FACVSc
Australia

Simon Roch
BVSc CertSAS DipSAS(Orth) MRCVS
Kentdale Veterinary Orthopaedics Ltd,
Moss End Business Village, Crooklands LA7 7NU, UK

Bernadette Van Ryssen
DVM PhD
Department of Medical Imaging and Small Animal
Orthopedics, Ghent University,
Salisburylaan 133, 9820 Merelbeke, Belgium

Harry Scott
BVSc CertSAD FRSB DipSAS(Orth) DipECVN DipECVSMR CCRP FRCVS
Southern Counties Veterinary Specialists,
6, Forest Corner Farm, Hangersley,
Ringwood BH24 3JW, UK

Emma Scurrell
BVSc DipACVP MRCVS
Cytopath Ltd,
Ledbury, Herefordshire HR8 2EY, UK

G. Diane Shelton
DVM PhD DipACVIM
Comparative Neuromuscular Laboratory,
University of California, San Diego,
9500 Gilman Drive, La Jolla, CA 92093, USA

David Strong
BVMS CertAVP MRCVS
ROAR-Surgical Ltd, UK

Foreword

I am delighted to write the Foreword for this new edition of the *BSAVA Manual of Canine and Feline Musculoskeletal Disorders: A Practical Guide to Lameness and Joint disease*. This manual has its roots in the *Manual of Small Animal Arthology*, first published by BSAVA in 1994, of which I was co-editor with Robert Collinson.

The reason for tracing this manual's genealogy is that it highlights the tremendous progress that has been made in small animal orthopaedics in the past quarter of a century. In its first version there were just four paragraphs devoted to arthroscopy and two sentences to describe MRI, one of which stated it was prohibitively expensive for routine imaging and likely to remain largely a research tool. How things have changed!

Advanced diagnostic imaging, including CT, MRI and arthroscopy now enables us to diagnose conditions that were, at best, little more than figments of our imagination 25 years ago. Instrumentation and implant technology have improved beyond our wildest dreams allowing the successful management of conditions that were previously difficult, if not impossible, to treat. There is also a much greater awareness of the scientific merit of publications – I hesitate to use the phrase evidence-based medicine – so it is a pleasure to see the limitations of studies pointed out by the contributors, allowing the reader to assess the relative strength of apparently conflicting findings.

The editors are to be commended for producing a manual that is of excellent scientific quality whilst being practical in nature. They have chosen a team of contributors from academia and referral practice who are acknowledged leaders in their field and whose enthusiasm for the subject is clear to see. I congratulate all those involved on an excellent publication.

John E. F. Houlton MA VetMB DVR DipSAO DipECVS MRCVS

Preface

Welcome to the second edition of the *BSAVA Manual of Canine and Feline Musculoskeletal Disorders*. This manual is the second reincarnation of the original *BSAVA Manual of Small Animal Arthrology*, published in 1994 and builds on the success of the first edition of the *BSAVA Manual of Canine and Feline Musculoskeletal Disorders* that was published in 2006. This edition has been written in a style to complement its other manuals in the BSAVA series with as little overlap as possible. Where necessary, however, clear cross-referencing to other BSAVA manuals, such as *Canine and Feline Fracture Repair and Management*, *Neurology*, *Oncology*, as well as titles covering diagnostic imaging and small animal medicine is provided.

Given the considerable evolution of the diagnosis, understanding and treatment options for many disorders, this second edition has been extensively rewritten. The remit from the outset was to start from the beginning, reorganize and rewrite all chapters. We have made every effort to include all advances relevant to clinical practice. Examples include the investigation of lameness including use of force plates and kinematics, provision of detail on the current understanding of elbow dysplasia and the wide array of available treatment options, the inclusion of physiotherapy and rehabilitation, detail on diagnostic and surgical arthroscopy and a basic understanding of three-dimensional imaging, such as CT and MRI. We include, for completeness, discussion of new, advanced surgical techniques such as tibial osteotomies for cranial cruciate ligament disease, cementless total hip replacement for hip dysplasia and replacement of the trochlear sulcus for patellar luxation, together with guidance on the level of training and experience that is necessary to achieve consistently good results.

Each chapter has been developed and refined by both the authors and editors during the course of this project, and we hope and believe the result of this painstaking process is an excellent manual that will be fit for another 10 years.

The manual is divided into four principle sections:

- Lameness investigation
- Musculoskeletal disorders
- Principles of orthopaedic surgery
- Management of specific disorders, ordered by individual joints.

The joint specific chapters follow a common theme: they comprise a main section and then, where relevant, Imaging and Operative Techniques sections follow. Maintaining the clear, no-nonsense, easy-to-pick-up-and-read style of the BSAVA manuals has been at the forefront of our minds during writing and editing, and we have included as many informative, quick reference images, figures and tables as possible to complement the text.

We, as editors, feel privileged to have worked with such a broad range of talented authors whose combined international skills, knowledge and experience is impressive and very difficult to match. It has truly been a privilege to work with such a team of inspiring veterinary surgeons with expertise in various fields and we are confident that the talent of each individual shines through their chapter.

We have learnt that editing a manual is no easy task. The honest truth is that had we known what was involved at the beginning, we would have likely taken much more persuasion to accept the task! The journey has been hard, and at times a little painful, but we have each learnt so much and are grateful to each other's professional, courteous and supportive collegiate work; the clear and positive channels of communication have been invaluable.

We are very grateful to the excellent publishing team at BSAVA Woodrow House for all the hard work and everything they have done to make sure this project has reached its destination.

We extend our heartfelt thanks for the excellent medical illustrations provided by Samantha Elmhurst, and her tireless willingness to consider an improved redraw of an already very good drawing with a view to achieving our joint aim of maximum clarity and accuracy of purpose. Thank you so much Sam, we have never met you in person, but we feel we now know you well!

Finally, the contributions that authors and editors alike have made are only possible in work done extracted from precious personal time. Quality time otherwise spent with family and friends has been sacrificed. This we wholeheartedly acknowledge; we are grateful and apologise to those with whom we should have spent more time. Now, finally, after 5 years of effort, we can all return to a more normal life hopeful in the knowledge that you, dear fellow veterinary surgeon or nurse reader, can enjoy referring to this book whenever you are faced with a musculoskeletal conundrum.

Gareth Arthurs
Gordon Brown
Rob Pettitt
August 2018

Chapter 1

Normal locomotion

Neil Burton and Gordon Brown

Normal quadruped locomotion requires the combined and coordinated efforts of the central nervous, musculoskeletal and neuromuscular systems to produce efficient and fluid movement. The pattern of limb and whole body movements that an animal uses repetitively during locomotion is known as its gait. Lameness is an altered gait that results in diminished locomotor function. It is essential that the clinician recognizes and understands normal gait patterns so that the presence, extent and potential significance of abnormality can be appreciated.

> 'It seems to me that one cannot fairly judge lameness, in any species, unless one is familiar with the normal gait of the patient undergoing a diagnostic examination. There is still a lot that we do not know nor understand about the gaits of our canine patients.'
> Geoff Sumner-Smith (2011)

In individual animals, significant variation in normal gait is seen according to their age, size, conformation, training, and their health and fitness status.

- Puppies have learnt to walk well by 2–3 weeks of age, but during later locomotor development the larger breeds in particular can appear awkward, gangly and apparently poorly coordinated until approaching skeletal maturity.
- Dogs with relatively short backs and relatively long legs (described in common parlance as 'short-coupled') risk interference between their thoracic and pelvic limb pairs during locomotion and to avoid this they may alter their gait to pace or to 'crab-run' where the trunk is slightly angled relative to the direction of movement (so that when viewed from behind the hindlimbs do not follow the same track as the forelimbs).
- Broad-chested dogs cannot track narrowly with their thoracic limbs which compromises their efficiency at faster gaits.
- Small breed dogs exhibit greater variation in normal gaits and need to use faster gaits more frequently to enable them to 'keep up' over the same distance in the same time.

In spite of these variations, gaits can usually be identified as an expression of one of five basic types – walk, trot, pace, canter and gallop. The characteristics and within-type variations of these gaits are summarized in Figure 1.1.

Gaits are described as symmetrical (walk, pace and trot) when the movements of the left and right limb patterns mirror each other and the intervals between footfalls are almost evenly spaced. In asymmetrical gaits (canter and gallop), limb movements on one side do not mirror the other and footfalls are unevenly spaced. One full cycle (a stride) is divided into a stance phase (braking, support then propulsion) and a swing phase.

The normal canine centre of mass or centre of gravity (COG) is located just caudal to the thoracic limbs so that 60% of the dog's weight is borne by the thoracic limbs and 40% by the pelvic limbs. The COG can be shifted cranially by lowering the head and neck, and caudally by raising the head. Moving the head to the side shifts the COG laterally. The tail also contributes to longitudinal and lateral shifts in the COG, depending on its length and mass. Walking involves the generation of propulsive energy by the skeletal muscles and a cyclical exchange of gravitational potential energy with the kinetic energy of the centre of mass. Forward motion is generally initiated by one pelvic limb, which shifts the COG cranially and towards the contralateral thoracic limb that in turn reaches cranially to support the moving mass. At slow gaits (walk) the COG rhythmically oscillates between left and right and the trunk, head and tail swing from side to side to maintain equilibrium. At rapid gaits, forward momentum and inertia are increased and there is less lateral oscillation. As speed increases, fewer limbs provide simultaneous support and the paws impact and 'track' the ground nearer the median plane to maintain balance during forward movement.

The pelvic limbs are designed for propulsive activity that accounts for approximately 70% of their stance time, with 30% of stance time in braking. They are relatively long, angular and heavily muscled and they connect directly to the vertebral column via the coxofemoral and sacroiliac joints. Push-off forces are generated by the pelvic limbs and assisted by epaxial muscle contraction; they propel the animal forwards and elevate the COG. Elevation of the COG is necessary to extend the duration of forward motion that is temporally limited by the pull of gravity. The thoracic limbs then act to support and absorb some of this gravitational potential and kinetic energy during the early (braking and support) stance phase.

The thoracic limbs are designed primarily for braking, support and directional changes. Approximately 60% of stance time is in braking and 40% in propulsion. Relative to the pelvic limbs, they are shorter and straighter and connected to the trunk by fibromuscular attachments; they have no direct bony articulation. They provide upward

Gait	Gait description	Paw-strike sequence	Limb sequence
Walk	• Four beat gait • Duration of stance phase exceeds that of swing phase for each limb • Bodyweight is supported alternately by two and three limbs, providing maximum weight-bearing stability • The neck and head are lowered during thoracic limb swing phase, and raised during its stance/support phase • The trunk undulates both laterally and vertically, with the tail and head swinging towards the side being supported • It is the slowest and least tiring gait		Each limb steps sequentially (lift, swing, support, thrust) in the order: • LP, LT, RP, RT • Pelvic limb is placed just ahead of where thoracic limb had been placed prior to lifting off
Trot	• Two beat gait • The pelvic limb of the diagonal pair impacts very slightly earlier than the thoracic limb (but they appear to impact simultaneously) • The pelvic limb provides propulsion in upward and forward directions • The trunk is held rigidly and oscillates only vertically, while the neck and head are fixed in an upright position • In a fast trot, there is a suspension phase between each diagonal pair of limbs impacting the ground • The trot is an efficient ground-covering gait		Right and left diagonal limbs alternate in supporting weight: • LT and RP • RT and LP • The pelvic limb is placed on to the spot where the thoracic limb on the same side had been located prior to lifting off
Pace	• Two beat gait • There is usually a short period of suspension between the left limbs impacting the ground and the right limbs, particularly at increased speed • It is an ungainly, energy inefficient gait; it is difficult to change speed or turn • The pace is a normal puppy gait • Dogs generally pace because of fatigue, obesity, and lack of fitness or physical weakness • Dogs that have problems with limb interference may find it easier to pace than to crab-run		Ipsilateral limbs are used alternately to support weight: • LP and LT • RP and RT
Canter	• Three beat gait • One thoracic limb leads; the leading limb is the one that is not part of the diagonal pair (lifts off just before suspension). It bears weight for a longer period of time than the other thoracic limb • When moving in a circular path, the dog nearly always leads with the thoracic limb closest to the centre of the circle because the contralateral pelvic limb shifts the animal's centre of gravity laterally (towards the centre of the circle) as well as forwards • On a straight path, a dog will normally change the leading limb to alleviate fatigue or to prepare to turn	Left-lead canter	The sequence of limb impact on the ground is in the pattern 1–2–1: a pelvic limb, then a diagonal pair, then a thoracic limb, followed by a suspension phase at faster speeds Left-lead canter: • RP, LP and RT, then LT Right-lead canter: • RP, LP and LT then RT
Gallop	• Each pelvic and thoracic limb lands slightly ahead of the contralateral limb • In transverse and rotatory gallop, a suspension period follows lifting of the second-impacting (leading) thoracic limb • In rotatory gallop, there is a second suspension period after lifting of the second-impacting pelvic limb (the leap suspension phase) • The dog gains stride length (and thus speed) by means of sagittal trunk flexion; the abdominal muscles bring the pelvis forwards enabling the pelvic limb paws to impact far ahead of the spot where the thoracic limb paws had impacted the ground • Extension of the trunk during propulsion by the pelvic limbs produces a leap that enables the thoracic limbs to impact far ahead of their static anatomical reach • Epaxial and hamstring muscles support the bodyweight and elevate the body's centre of gravity during the leap suspension phase	Rotatory gallop Transverse gallop	The rotatory gallop is a four beat, double suspension gait used at higher speeds. The pattern of limb impact rotates: • RP and LP • Suspension • LT and RT • Suspension The transverse gallop is a four beat, single suspension gait used at lower speed. Thoracic and pelvic limbs impact in the same order: • LP and RP • LT and RT • Suspension

1.1 Characteristics of the five main canine gait patterns. LP = left pelvic limb; LT = left thoracic limb; RP = right pelvic limb; RT = right thoracic limb.

propulsion but contribute to forward propulsion only when retracting in contact with the ground while forward of the COG or if the animal is pulling a load that shifts the COG caudally. During support, the thoracic limbs in particular act as struts with the movement of the body acting as an inverted pendulum, conserving the energy expended in elevating the trunk to counteract gravity. The weight of the falling trunk during limb braking stretches limb muscles and ligaments, converting gravitational potential energy to elastic strain energy (Figure 1.2). This then rebounds as kinetic energy and assists in elevating the trunk once again as the COG passes forward of the weight-bearing limb. The coordinated efforts of the central nervous, musculo-skeletal and neuromuscular systems allow locomotion to proceed in effect by repetitively throwing the COG forwards and then catching it.

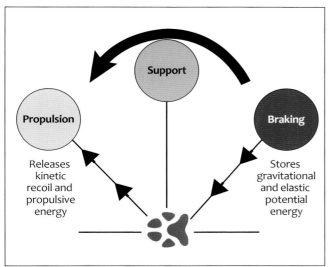

1.2 The spring-loaded inverted pendulum model of repetitive limb movement during the stance phase, illustrating cyclical generation and partial recycling of energy during movement.

In dogs, up to 70% of the mechanical energy required to lift and accelerate the COG is recovered via this spring-loaded, inverted pendulum mechanism. Cats are less energy-efficient during locomotion due to reduced vertical oscillation and a different footfall pattern (Bishop et al., 2008).

Speed ranges for the different gaits of dogs and cats overlap to an extent, so a number of gaits may be possible at a given speed with the trot having the largest speed range. In the slower symmetrical gaits, increasing speed is achieved as a result of reduced cycle time (increased cycle frequency) and increased stride length. A threshold is then reached where the animal must adopt an asymmetrical gait pattern in order to move faster. A combination of the introduction of one or more suspension phases when no paw is in contact with the ground and increased stride length as a result of sagittal flexion of the spine allows for more rapid locomotion.

In the cat, development of locomotor skills is rapid and by 6 weeks of age kittens are capable of adopting all adult gaits. Cats are capable of moving very precisely using diagonal or pacing gaits. Unlike dogs, which indirectly register (i.e. the ipsilateral pelvic limb paw drops slightly behind and to the side of where the thoracic limb paw struck), cats directly register, with each pelvic limb paw placed almost directly in the print of the corresponding thoracic limb paw. The distribution of load between the thoracic and pelvic limbs is slightly more even than in

dogs (Romans et al., 2004). Cats frequently accelerate through the trot into a bounding type gallop (where the thoracic limb and pelvic limb pairs touch down simultaneously), with the canter being less frequently used. Overland, cats' observed speed when walking or at a moderate trot varies between 0.6 and 1.5 m/s (Blaszczyk and Loeb, 1993), which overlaps considerably with that of dogs. To cover the same distance, cats, with their relatively short stride length, will take more strides per unit time than dogs. When hunting or anxious (e.g. while being observed in the consulting room), cats adopt an energy-inefficient, stealthy walk with slow deliberate movements, the limbs highly flexed and the COG close to the ground (Bishop et al., 2008). The cat's combination of rapid short strides during upright gaits and the adoption of a stealthy walk can make visual assessment of subtle abnormal gait (lameness) challenging.

Gait analysis

Gait analysis is the quantitative evaluation of musculo-skeletal function (DeCamp, 1997); it can be either subjective or objective. While objective gait analysis in the veterinary field is a relatively new development, the desire for the characterization of animal gait dates as far back as 350 bc in Aristotle's *De Motu Animalium* (On the Gait of Animals).

Subjective assessment

Subjective assessment of gait, which is based on visual observation of severity of lameness, can be recorded using a numerical rating scale (NRS) or a visual analogue score (VAS) (Figure 1.3). The NRS offers numerical categories, which may have a descriptive term attached, to best describe a patient's lameness, whereas VAS is a continuous scale over which lameness is scored on a line between two extremes of the variable. VAS appears marginally more sensitive at classifying lameness than

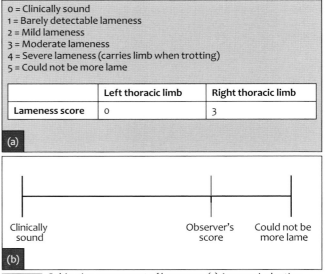

0 = Clinically sound
1 = Barely detectable lameness
2 = Mild lameness
3 = Moderate lameness
4 = Severe lameness (carries limb when trotting)
5 = Could not be more lame

	Left thoracic limb	Right thoracic limb
Lameness score	0	3

(a)

Clinically sound   Observer's score   Could not be more lame

(b)

1.3 Subjective assessment of lameness. (a) A numerical rating scale (NRS) offers numerical categories, which may have a descriptive term attached, to best describe a patient's lameness. (b) A visual analogue score (VAS) is a continuous scale; degree of lameness is scored on a line between two extremes of the variable.
(a Modified from Quinn et al., 2007)

NRS but both systems do little to control intra- or inter-observer variation; thus ambiguity in the description of a gait abnormality may persist with this approach. Several studies have suggested that when compared with quantitative gait analysis, observers cannot reliably discriminate abnormal from normal or the severity of lameness that may be present (Evans *et al.*, 2003; Burton *et al.*, 2009).

Objective analysis

Animal locomotion can be objectively defined by the use of kinetics, paw pressure analysis (Weigel *et al.*, 2005) and kinematics. Kinetic and kinematic data can be used to define normal gait (Allen *et al.*, 1994), interbreed variation in gait (Colborne *et al.*, 2005) and lameness (Budsberg, 2001), as well as the response to therapeutic agents (Horstman *et al.*, 2004), surgery (Burton *et al.*, 2011) and rehabilitation (Marsolais *et al.*, 2002).

Kinetic analysis

Kinetic analysis can be defined as the measurement of ground reaction forces (GRFs) during locomotion, including magnitude, direction and location. Kinetic analysis is performed using force platforms that consist of a load cell through which the load borne by a limb during the stance phase can be resolved into three component forces: F_x (mediolateral), F_y (craniocaudal) and F_z (vertical) (Figure 1.4). Of these forces, vertical ground reaction force (F_z) is the dominant vector and is most directly correlated with axial loading of the limb. F_y force can be subdivided into propulsion and braking force and F_x into side-to-side movement (Budsberg *et al.*, 1987). Kinetic data can be collected with the patient either walking or trotting; the effectiveness of evaluating GRFs at both of these gaits has been validated (Evans *et al.*, 2003). As a rule, subtle lameness is more evident during kinetic analysis at a trot rather than a walk as higher GRFs are generated at this gait. During objective kinetic gait analysis, lame dogs may not trot consistently due to pain; this results in a failure to collect data if the foot is not placed on the force platform. As a result, these data are not available for use in comparative studies of lame dogs, which can lead to study bias towards less lame dogs (Evans *et al.*, 2003). Analysis of moderate to severe lameness is best undertaken at a walk.

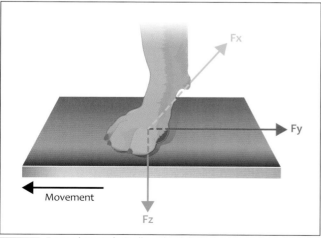

1.4 Force plate analysis allows load during stance to be resolved into three component forces: F_x (mediolateral), F_y (craniocaudal) and F_z (vertical). Of these forces, GRF (F_z) is the dominant vector.

Ground reaction force (GRF) data can be displayed and assessed graphically (Figure 1.5). Normal thoracic limb GRF curves are of greater magnitude than those of the pelvic limb, reflecting the 60:40 distribution of bodyweight in the thoracic and pelvic limbs (Off and Matis, 1997). Parameters such as peak vertical force (PVF), stance time, total force (defined as the area under the curve), rate of change of force (defined as tangent to the curve) and falling slope (rate of unloading of the limb) can be defined. A combination of both PVF and falling slope are suggested as optimal for discriminating sound and lame dogs following cruciate ligament surgery (Evans *et al.*, 2005). Multiple strikes of each limb on the force platform allow average GRF to be calculated for each limb. While kinetic analysis permits a global assessment of limb load, lameness cannot readily be localized to a component part of a limb based on these data alone, as information on the angular excursion and moments generated by each limb segment is absent. However, serial data collection can allow quantification of how GRFs change as a function of time and hence if lameness is improved or worsened. In cases of bilateral disease, compensatory gaits may involve shifting of forces cranially or caudally to offload them from the affected legs, resulting in increased forces through the unaffected limbs.

Pressure-sensitive mats allow quantification of the centre of pressure, but differ from force plate platforms, in that they do not directly measure the applied force vector, horizontal or shear components of the applied force. They can, however, be used to capture data on static weight-bearing across all four limbs, as well as on multiple limb strikes from the patient on a single pass.

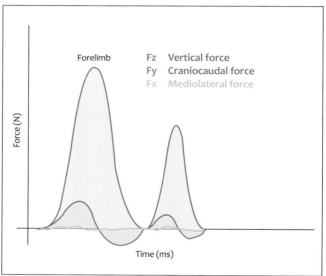

1.5 Kinetic data can be assessed graphically when force (Newtons) is plotted as a function of time (milliseconds) as shown in this diagram illustrating a single forelimb and hindlimb step. GRF (F_z) is the dominant vector and is most directly correlated with axial loading of the limb. Forelimb curves are greater in magnitude than those for the hindlimb, reflecting the respective 60%:40% distribution of bodyweight.

Kinematic analysis

Kinematic analysis can be defined as the measurement of angular displacement of joints, stride length and velocity. Historically, traditional video cameras were used to capture the gait of an animal and sequential freeze-frame analysis permitted joint angles through stance and swing to be calculated. However, this is a labour-intensive and time-consuming process and only permits assessment of kinematic variables in a single plane. This technique has been superseded by the use of retro-reflective markers attached to the skin overlying the centres of rotation of the joints (Figure 1.6). Multiple infrared cameras sample light reflected from these markers at high frequency (typically 200 Hz for a dog walking or trotting). Cameras can be spatially calibrated prior to the onset of data capture, such that data are sampled three-dimensionally (Figure 1.7). Thus, individual joint flexion/extension, angular velocity, peri-articular force (joint moment), adduction/abduction and internal/external rotation can be mapped simultaneously.

Morphometric data either from cadaver studies or, more recently, utilizing computed tomographic data combined with regression equations, can be used to quantify the volume, mass, centre of mass and radius of gyration of each segment of the canine thoracic and pelvic limb. By defining the limb as a system of linked segments, these data can be combined with kinetic and kinematic data to yield the angle, moment and power contributions of each limb segment across the joints through an inverse dynamics approach (see Figure 1.6bc). Inverse dynamics allows the timing of muscle contraction to be calculated as well as the determination of concentric or eccentric contraction. In addition, by summating the moments about each joint, the total support moment can be derived for a limb. This can then be compared to the contralateral limb as a ratio or a symmetry index. Inverse dynamics have revealed specific gait compensations affecting the elbow in dogs with medial coronoid process disease (Burton et al., 2008) and in stifle and hock in dogs predisposed to and suffering from cranial cruciate ligament disease.

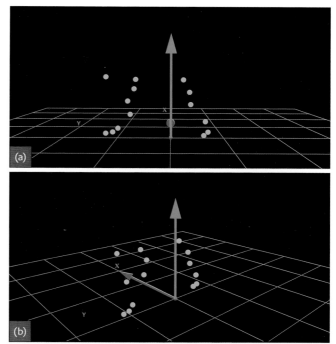

1.7 Kinematic data are collected via multiple spatially calibrated infrared cameras sampling reflected light. Data can be sampled either (a) two-dimensionally or (b) three-dimensionally. The blue arrow denotes the plane of F_z and the red arrow denotes the plane of F_x. The green dots denote the position of retroreflective markers affixed to the skin overlying the bony prominences of the thoracic limb (seven markers) and pelvic limb (six markers) as well as one affixed to the neck to denote head position.

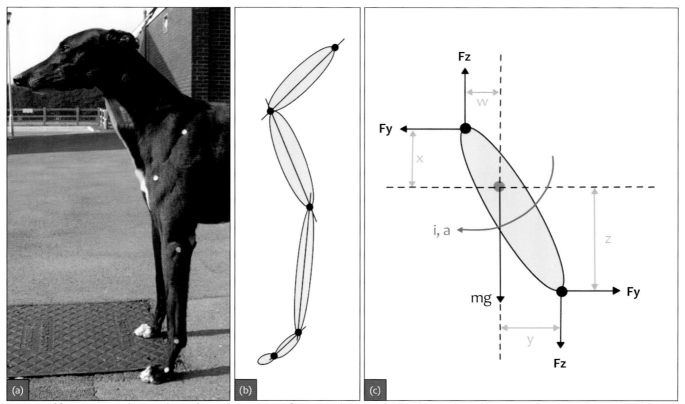

1.6 (a) Kinematic analysis can be performed using retroreflective markers attached to skin overlying the centres of rotation of the joints; the reflected light is detected by infrared cameras. (b) Mathematically, the limb can be represented as a linked segment model. (c) Cadaveric data can be applied to each limb segment model to define the volume, centre of mass (red dot), weight (mass x gravity; mg), joint reaction forces (F_z, F_y), moment arms (w, x, y, z), inertia (i) and angular acceleration (a). These data, when combined with kinetic and kinematic data, can be used to define the angular, moment and power contributions of each segment within the limb.

While gait analysis is a powerful tool for quantitative assessment of gait, such modelling is not without limitation as several important assumptions are made from the data. These include the following:

- Joint centres are modelled as a single joint. This is appropriate when assessing simple hinge joints such as the elbow, but carpal and stifle joints are more complex as the joint's centre of rotation is variable though the range of motion
- Segments are rigid and do not deform during movement. However, the skin moves and thus may not overlie the centre of rotation during motion
- The velocity of the patient affects stance time, angular excursions of joints, joint moment and power amplitudes (Colborne et al., 2006). Thus, power amplitude can reduce with increased lameness, or with reduced velocity of the patient
- 'Handedness' or limb dominance may exist in sound dogs, predisposing to larger GRFs for that limb as a consequence (Colborne, 2008).

The availability and use of objective measurement in orthopaedic practice is limited; when available, it usually involves kinetic analysis. It is important to understand that subjective clinical gait examination and the analysis of GRFs do not represent the same thing (Voss et al., 2007). Whereas limb and whole body motion is observed subjectively during gait observation, kinetic gait analysis only accounts for limb loading; some dogs that are subjectively lame can have normal GRFs. Kinematic analysis in conjunction with kinetic analysis will better characterize overall gait but such detailed analysis is time-consuming and only available in a few centres.

Summary

In summary, it is essential that clinicians dealing with the investigation of lameness have an understanding of normal gait and an awareness of the techniques and the limitations of both subjective and objective gait analysis. In clinical practice, subjective analysis is used by the vast majority of clinicians and is an essential and satisfactory diagnostic and monitoring tool. Inter- and intra-observer variations are accepted limitations but, with increasing experience, intra-observer variation is reduced. Inter-observer variation can be minimized by adopting agreed scales between clinicians to categorize lameness or by ensuring, where possible, that re-examination of lameness cases is undertaken by the same clinician.

References and further reading

Allen K, DeCamp CE, Braden TD and Bahns M (1994) Kinematic gait analysis of the trot in healthy mixed breed dogs. *Veterinary and Comparative Orthopaedics and Traumatology* **7**, 148–153

Bishop KL, Pai AK and Schmitt D (2008) Whole body mechanics of stealthy walking in cats. *PLoS One* **3**, e3808

Blaszczyk J and Loeb GE (1993) Why cats pace on the treadmill. *Physiology and Behaviour* **53**, 501–507

Budsberg SC (2001) Long-term temporal evaluation of ground reaction forces during development of experimentally induced osteoarthritis in dogs. *American Journal of Veterinary Research* **62**, 1207–1211

Budsberg SC, Verstraete MC and Soutas-Little RW (1987) Force-plate analysis of walking gait in the healthy dog. *American Journal of Veterinary Research* **48**, 915–918

Burton NJ, Dobney JA, Owen MR et al. (2008) Joint angle, moment and power compensations in dogs with fragmented medial coronoid process. *Veterinary and Comparative Orthopaedics and Traumatology* **21**, 110–118

Burton NJ, Owen MR, Colborne G et al. (2009) Can owners and clinicians assess outcome in dogs with fragmented medial coronoid process? *Veterinary and Comparative Orthopaedics and Traumatology* **22**, 183–189

Burton NJ, Owen MR, Kirk LS et al. (2011) Conservative versus arthroscopic management for medial coronoid process disease in dogs: a prospective gait evaluation. *Veterinary Surgery* **40**, 972–980

Colborne GR (2008) Are sound dogs mechanically symmetric at trot? No, actually. *Veterinary and Comparative Orthopaedics and Traumatology* **21**, 294–301

Colborne GR, Innes JF, Comerford EJ et al. (2005). Distribution of power across the hindlimb joints in Labrador Retrievers and Greyhounds. *American Journal of Veterinary Research* **66**, 1563–1571

Colborne GR, Walker AM, Tattersall AJ et al. (2006) Effect of trotting velocity on work patterns of the hindlimbs of Greyhounds. *American Journal of Veterinary Research* **67**, 1293–1298

DeCamp CE (1997) Kinetic and kinematic gait analysis and the assessment of lameness in the dog. *Veterinary Clinics of North America: Small Animal Practice* **27**, 825–840

Evans R, Gordon W and Conzemius M (2003) Effect of velocity on ground reaction forces in dogs with lameness attributable to tearing of the cranial cruciate ligament. *American Journal of Veterinary Research* **64**, 1479–1481

Evans R, Horstman C and Conzemius M (2005) Accuracy and optimization of force platform gait analysis in Labradors with cranial cruciate disease evaluated at a walking gait. *Veterinary Surgery* **34**, 445–449

Horstman CL, Conzemius MG, Evans R et al. (2004) Assessing the efficacy of perioperative oral carprofen after cranial cruciate surgery using non-invasive, objective pressure platform gait analysis. *Veterinary Surgery* **33**, 286–292

Marsolais GS, Dvorak G and Conzemius MG (2002) Effects of postoperative rehabilitation on limb function after cranial cruciate ligament repair in dogs. *Journal of the American Veterinary Medical Association* **220**, 1325–1330

Off W and Matis U (1997) Gait analysis in dogs. *Tierärztliche Praxis* **25**, 8–14 (German)

Quinn MM, Keuler NS, Lu Y et al. (2007) Evaluation of agreement between numerical rating scales, visual analogue scoring scales, and force plate gait analysis in dogs. *Veterinary Surgery* **36**, 360–367

Romans CW, Conzemius MG, Horstman CL et al. (2004) Use of pressure platform gait analysis in cats with and without bilateral onchectomy. *American Journal of Veterinary Research* **65**, 1497–1501

Voss K, Imhof J, Kaestner S et al. (2007) Force plate gait analysis at the walk and trot in dogs with low-grade hindlimb lameness. *Veterinary and Comparative Orthopaedics and Traumatology* **20**, 299–304

Waxman AS, Robinson DA, Evans RB et al. (2008) Relationship between objective and subjective assessment of limb function in normal dogs with an experimentally induced lameness. *Veterinary Surgery* **37**, 241–246

Weigel JP, Arnold G, Hicks DA et al. (2005) Biomechanics of rehabilitation. *Veterinary Clinics of North American Small Animal Practice* **35**, 1255–1285

Chapter 2

Lameness examination

Harry Scott

Lameness can be defined as diminished function that makes movement, especially locomotion, difficult or impossible. It includes stiffness when moving and difficulty jumping or rising. A gait abnormality is a deviation from the normal pattern of locomotion for a given individual and may or may not involve diminished function. An altered gait is conventionally considered to be a manifestation of lameness and the clinician therefore requires a working knowledge of the expected normal gait pattern for the patient in question before any deviation from normal can be detected (see Chapter 1).

Lameness is usually the result of dysfunction of a limb or limbs and is most commonly the result of an orthopaedic disorder. Orthopaedic lameness can be divided into those conditions that are painful and those where limb movement is restricted but pain-free (mechanical lameness). Examples of mechanical lameness include fibrotic myopathies of the gracilis or infraspinatus muscles and lameness following arthrodesis of a joint such as the carpus or tarsus.

Lameness may also occur as a consequence of neurological disease. Neurological causes of lameness and gait abnormality may be subdivided into those that are associated with paresis (weakness or reduced ability to generate gait) and/or ataxia (incoordination), and those that cause lameness with no detectable motor (paretic) or sensory (ataxic) neurological deficits. In the absence of detectable deficits, neurological lameness results from pain associated with a nerve root or nerve lesion; differentiation from orthopaedic causes of lameness in these cases can be challenging. To complicate matters it is not unusual for orthopaedic and neurological causes of lameness to co-exist (for example in animals with fractures and concurrent nerve injury). Furthermore, a number of bilateral orthopaedic disorders may present acutely as apparent weakness and be misinterpreted as paresis. Examples include some individuals with cruciate deficiency or cases of bilateral calcaneal tendon or tibial tuberosity avulsions. Key signs of neurological causes of lameness are listed in Figure 2.1. It is worth noting that general proprioceptive ataxia and upper motor neuron paresis almost always occur together and clinically it is unnecessary to recognize the separate signs of these two systems. Neurological causes of lameness are discussed further in Chapter 12.

Sign	Description
Ataxia	Incoordinated gait as a consequence of general proprioceptive ataxia (the three forms of ataxia are general proprioceptive, vestibular and cerebellar)
Lower motor neuron (peripheral) flaccid paresis	Reduced ability to support weight resulting in a shortened stride length
Upper motor neuron (central) spastic paresis	Reduced ability to generate gait resulting in an increased stride length
Hypermetria	Type of ataxia in which the limb is flexed excessively during the protraction phase of gait
Hypometria	Type of ataxia in which the limb is flexed less than normal during the protraction phase of gait
Dysmetria	Type of ataxia in which there is an inability to properly direct or limit limb movement; it may describe a combination of hypermetria and hypometria
Disconnected gait	Thoracic and pelvic limbs move at different rates
Unprovoked pain	Vocalization – a common sign of nerve root impingement or entrapment (nerve root signature)
Nerve root signature	Lameness associated with nerve root compression in which the limb is held either intermittently or constantly in a flexed position high off the ground
Kyphosis	A common sign of back pain (kyphosis can also be a consequence of weight redistribution away from the pelvic limbs)
Low head carriage	A common sign of neck pain
Stumbling or falling	A common sign of ataxia

2.1 Key signs associated with neurological causes of lameness.

Lameness diagnosis

A thorough, methodical and problem-based approach to lameness diagnosis is recommended and summarized, alongside an alternative approach, in Figure 2.2; a general overview of the process is presented as an algorithm in Figure 2.3.

History

History-taking comprises gathering of background information (Figure 2.4) and specific questioning (Figure 2.5) relevant to the presenting complaint. It is time-consuming and requires patience to unravel all of the relevant information. The history invariably provides vital clues as to the aetiology of the lameness and it is frequently possible to compile a provisional mental list of differential diagnoses purely on the basis of the background information and history. History-taking is an acquired skill that is refined with

experience. In taking a full and comprehensive history, the clinician should start with general questions and progress to more specific questions relevant to the key concerns of the client. Leading questions should be avoided since it is a natural tendency for clients to say what they think that the clinician wants to hear and this information may be unintentionally inaccurate or misleading.

The client should be questioned to ascertain the precise nature of the presenting complaint including which limb the client thinks the patient is lame on and whether the lameness ever appears to shift to another limb. This may seem obvious but there is frequently confusion about which limb the patient is lame on especially when assessing thoracic limb lameness. In all cases, the clinician should subsequently observe the animal's gait and confirm which limb(s) is/are involved. The client should be asked to describe the lameness and how it manifests itself, for example through head-nodding, skipping, difficulty rising or reduced exercise tolerance. Client observations of their

Approach to diagnosis	Methodology	Advantages	Disadvantages
Differential diagnosis			
A problem-oriented approach that entails a general clinical, brief neurological and detailed orthopaedic examination and consideration of all available data to define and list the key problem(s)	• Problems are listed, together with their potential aetiologies, to produce a list of potential/differential diagnoses • A diagnostic plan is formulated to confirm or eliminate each differential diagnosis starting with the most likely. Investigations are chosen in order of preference on the basis of those that are least invasive and/or expensive but are predicted to have the greatest diagnostic yield • Treatment is instigated on the basis of the results (in some cases immediate treatment may be initiated pending the results of outstanding tests). Treatment can then be reviewed in the light of subsequent information. In cases where it has not been possible to achieve a specific diagnosis, a therapeutic trial may be initiated • The patient's progress is monitored and the plan is then modified accordingly	• Logical thought processes are promoted by considering all possible aetiologies for each problem • Rarely fails to achieve a definitive diagnosis even in cases with lameness of unusual or obscure aetiology • Concurrent disease is not missed	• Time-consuming (examination requires at least 30–45 minutes if performed properly) • May not be applicable if there are cost constraints
Pattern recognition			
Previous experience is used to recognize a pattern of characteristics typical for a particular condition	• An attempt is made to localize the seat of lameness and subsequently a tentative diagnosis is made based on the old adage that common things occur commonly • The clinician's experience enables him or her to recognize the condition and perform appropriate tests to confirm the diagnosis if indicated	• Useful where there are cost and time constraints. Initial examination can be performed in a 10–15 minute consultation • This is a commonly used screening method in many cases where diseases are relatively obvious • Can at times be reasonably accurate because certain signs are associated with certain diseases or conditions	• This method will often succeed but the success rate is dependent on the experience of the clinician and for atypical or obscure causes of lameness it will fail • Significant concurrent disease may be missed
Shotgun approach			
	• The whole limb or limbs are investigated using all available diagnostic tests. Resort may be made to this method particularly in cases where it has not been possible to localize the source of lameness	None	• Risk that either nothing will be found or there will be a number of findings of unknown significance – some or all of which may be incidental • Inevitably involves unnecessary tests and/or treatments that are a waste of time, effort and money and often fail to achieve a diagnosis

2.2 Approaches to lameness investigation.

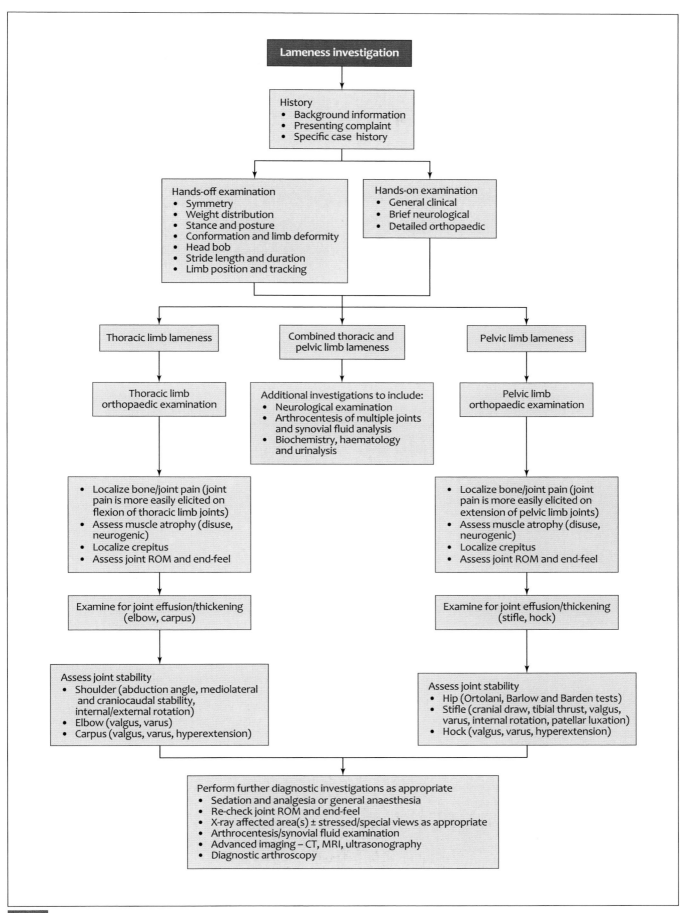

2.3 Algorithm for lameness investigation. CT = computed tomography; MRI = magnetic resonance imaging; ROM = range of movement.

Information	Relevance
Signalment	Breed, age and sex association in many conditions
Weight/body condition	Underweight – appropriate diet or co-existent illness? Overweight – confounding effect on lameness and recovery
Diet	Quality of diet; quantity/frequency of feeding, especially in growing animals. Appropriate for individual concerned?
Duration of ownership	Past history of trauma, pre-existing or recurrent conditions
Vaccination status	General background information. Rarely of direct relevance to development of orthopaedic disease
Intended use (pet or working dog)	Intended level of function anticipated post injury; owner's expectations
Previous illness or injury	Recurrent conditions; summation effect of new on old injuries
Exercise regimen	Level of fitness and activity in respect to mechanism of injury Rehabilitation/owner's expectations of recovery
For immature animals – health of siblings	Hereditary component for many developmental joint diseases
Travel history or country of origin if imported	Potentially widens the differential diagnosis list

2.4 Key background information to be obtained when taking a history.

- Which limb does the owner think the animal is lame on?
- Is the animal ever lame on any other limb(s)?
- When did the lameness start?
- How severe is the lameness?
- Did the lameness start suddenly or was it insidious?
- How long has the animal been lame?
- Has there been any response to previous drug therapy?
- Was the onset of lameness associated with a traumatic event?
- Does the lameness fluctuate in severity?
- Is the lameness worse after exercise?
- Does the lameness improve with rest?
- Is the lameness worse during exercise?
- Is the lameness worse first thing in the morning?
- Is the lameness worse on hard or irregular surfaces?

For cats, additional information should be elicited by questioning about lifestyle changes such as elimination outside the litter tray, changes in attitude, activity level and ability to jump.

2.5 Key questions to consider when taking a history.

pet should not be ignored as they are usually accurate; it is their interpretation of these observations that is frequently flawed. On occasions a video of the patient can be helpful especially if the lameness is intermittent or exacerbated by, or associated with, significant exercise.

Having a standard, logical approach to history-taking for lameness cases minimizes the risk of key questions (see Figure 2.5), and therefore answers being omitted. Identifying a pattern (Figure 2.6) to the lameness can help to narrow the list of differential diagnoses.

Specific client questionnaires (clinical metrology instruments) have been designed in an attempt to assess pain, physical function and quality of life. Such tools are used for research purposes to evaluate a treatment or intervention, but can also be used for clinical patient management to assess the progression of lameness and disability over time. Examples include the Liverpool Osteoarthritis in Dogs (LOAD), Helsinki Chronic Pain Index (HCPI) and the Canine Brief Pain Inventory (CBPI) questionnaires.

- Dogs with osteoarthritis will usually have chronic lameness of insidious onset that waxes and wanes and is worse in the morning and after rest that has followed a period of exercise (i.e. 'lameness after rest after exercise' or LARAX). Lameness often improves as the dog warms up; this may take several minutes or just a few steps.
- Infection is usually acute to subacute, progressive and associated with severe lameness, for example in the case of a cat bite abscess or septic arthritis.
- A peracute or acute onset of non-progressive lameness is more typical of bone fracture or joint luxation; there is usually a history of obvious trauma unless the patient has suffered an unobserved traumatic incident. Unobserved trauma is a common occurrence in outdoor cats and is easily confused with lameness resulting from infection.
- If there is a lesion of the pads or paw, there is usually a history of moderate to severe lameness that is worse on hard or irregular surfaces and improves or resolves on soft or smooth surfaces. An example would be a corn of the digital pad.
- With muscle, tendon and ligament disorders such as biceps tendon injuries or partial cranial cruciate ligament rupture, lameness frequently gets worse during exercise and improves with rest.

2.6 Examples of lameness patterns.

Feline osteoarthritis is a common disease, the significance of which is now better appreciated. In contrast to the situation in the dog, lameness is not the predominant clinical sign. Lifestyle changes, such as reduced activity, weight loss, changes in attitude, inability to jump, urination and defaecation outside the litter tray and other non-specific signs are much more common and questions to the animal owner should be directed appropriately (Lascelles et al., 2012).

Hands-off examination

Much information can be gleaned from this part of the examination and it also has the benefit of allowing the patient to relax before being submitted to a potentially uncomfortable physical examination. Hands-off examination can be subdivided into two distinct components – observation in the consulting room and gait analysis.

Observation in the consulting room

- Dogs should be observed as they enter the consulting room for evidence of lameness. Cats are more difficult to examine but once the room is secure they can be encouraged to move freely on the floor. Observe the animal's behaviour as it moves around the room: how it walks, sits, lies down and how it moves between these positions. Cats, when stressed, frequently adopt a stealthy, crouched gait making assessment challenging.
- Look to see if the patient stands symmetrically on all four limbs. Additionally, observe for evidence of weight redistribution away from the affected limb(s) resulting, for example, in kyphosis in dogs with severe bilateral hip dysplasia or bilateral cranial cruciate ligament (CCL) disease. Dogs with unilateral lameness may stand with the digits less splayed or, if lameness is more severe, with only the digital pads contacting the floor (toe-touching lameness).
- Observe whether the patient stands, sits, and lies down normally and can rise from these positions without struggling. Dogs with stifle pain will often display a positive sit test: due to a reluctance to fully flex the joint, rather than sitting squarely on the haunches the dog will sit with the affected stifle partially extended and the limb out to the side. Other features of lameness may

include shifting from one limb to another, reluctance to stand up, holding the limb at an abnormal angle or in an unusual position, muscle tremors in the affected limb and intermittently holding the limb off the ground.

- Conformation and limb deformity should also be assessed although there is wide variation between dog breeds. Certain conformations can be associated with specific conditions, for example bow-legged (genu varum) dogs with medial patellar luxation and knock-kneed (genu valgum) dogs with lateral patellar luxation. In addition, moderate to severe muscle atrophy may be visible in non-obese dogs with a short hair coat.
- Unprovoked crying or yelping should raise the index of suspicion for a neurological aetiology and a full neurological examination should be performed. In animals with nerve root signature (see Figure 2.1) there may, however, be no detectable neurological deficits.

Gait analysis

Gait analysis is the study of the pattern or sequence of limb and body movements used for locomotion. While the ability to conduct detailed objective analysis of kinetic and kinematic parameters may be available in some referral centres and research institutions, in practice gait assessment is usually limited to subjective observation.

Once the patient's posture and stance have been observed at rest, all dogs with subtle, mild or moderate lameness should be examined in motion. There is little value in performing gait analysis of a patient with severe or non-weight-bearing lameness and it is clearly contraindicated for animals with major traumatic injuries. Gait observation should preferably be performed when the patient is not receiving any anti-inflammatory or analgesic medication that may mask the lameness. Gait observation can either be performed indoors if there is a long wide corridor available or outdoors on an even surface away from traffic and distraction. The dog should be led on a short leash for a distance of about 15 metres directly away from and then towards the clinician to allow gait observation in both directions. To fully assess the gait, it is often also useful to walk alongside the dog or have it walked past the observer. If neurological dysfunction is suspected, it is useful to have the owner turn the dog in circles in both directions to detect weakness or incoordination. For small dogs whose legs move very quickly and for all dogs with subtle lameness, it can be useful to take a video of the lameness so that it can be replayed in slow motion. Dogs should be examined walking, trotting or pacing, and running if necessary. An assistant may be required if the client is unable to do this.

Identifying the lame limb can be difficult if the lameness is subtle or mild and particularly when bilateral. Thoracic limb lameness tends to be more challenging than pelvic limb lameness. Abnormalities of gait that may be observed are summarized in Figure 2.7.

- **Walking:** initial evaluation should be performed at a slow controlled pace so that the movement of each limb can be observed individually. Thoracic limb lameness is best observed as the dog walks towards you, and pelvic limb lameness as the dog walks away from you.
- **Trotting:** mild lameness that may not be detectable when the dog is walking, will become more apparent when the animal is made to trot as more force is placed on the limbs at greater velocity. The trot is also the only gait in which thoracic and pelvic limbs are never assisted in weight-bearing by the contralateral limb.

- **Head nod:** head nodding occurs as the dog attempts to reduce the forces acting through a painful thoracic limb. The head is raised when the lame limb is weight-bearing and lowered (nodded) when the sound limb is weight-bearing (down is sound). It should be noted that head nodding could also be a feature of pelvic limb lameness, but to a lesser extent. For pelvic limb lameness, the head will nod down when the affected limb contacts the ground as more weight is transferred to the forequarters.
- **Stride length and duration:** lameness if asymmetrical usually presents as a short stride length and reduced stance time on the affected limb and a long stride length and increased stance time on the contralateral limb. Other features include a stiff and stilted gait as a result of reduced joint excursion in the affected limb(s).
- **Limb tracking:** tracking refers to the position of the limbs under the body. When a dog is trotting the thoracic and pelvic limbs should be straight and should converge on a centre point under the dog's body. Look for limbs crossing the centre line, circumduction of limbs, symmetry of limb tracking and wide-based thoracic or pelvic limbs. Some breeds, particularly herding dogs, have pelvic limbs that are 'cow-hocked' with internally rotated tarsi and externally rotated feet as a normal part of their conformation.
- **Symmetry:** other features to look for are flexion and extension of individual joints, circumduction and abnormal limb placement. Bunny-hopping may be seen in dogs with bilateral pelvic limb lameness, and is often associated with hip pain as the dog uses both limbs simultaneously in an attempt to reduce hip extension.

2.7 Gait analysis signs.

However, diagonal thoracic and pelvic limbs strike the ground simultaneously and so differentiation between thoracic and pelvic limb lameness may be more difficult.

- **Pacing:** pacing is similar to the trot except that ipsilateral rather than diagonal thoracic and pelvic limbs strike the ground simultaneously. The limb joints are moved through a smaller range of motion and there is more side-to-side motion of the body; as a consequence the gait appears stiff and stilted compared to the trot. The pace is a normal gait for some large heavily muscled breeds of dog. Because joint excursion is reduced, some dogs may also use it preferentially with musculoskeletal disorders, such as osteoarthritis and spinal pain.
- **Running:** this is rarely practical or productive in the clinical setting. If the dog is only lame at high speed, then the owner should be asked to provide a video.

If at the time of examination no lameness or gait abnormality is detected or lameness is very subtle, intermittent or waxing and waning, it may be better to defer further investigations and repeat the examination in a few weeks' time.

Following gait evaluation at a walk and trot, a subjective assessment of the grade of lameness should be made. The author uses a five-point numerical rating scale outlined in Figure 2.8. A record of the grade of lameness is useful for comparison between cases and for monitoring

Grade	Description
0 (none)	No lameness is observed
1 (mild)	Lameness is subtle and only consistently observed at a trot
2 (mild to moderate)	Mild lameness is present at a walk and is worse at a trot
3 (moderate)	Obvious lameness is present at both gaits
4 (moderate to severe)	Obvious lameness is present at both gaits and may be intermittently non-weight-bearing
5 (severe)	Lameness is non-weight-bearing most or all of the time

2.8 Grading of lameness using a numerical rating scale.

changes over time. Some clinicians use a 10-point system and others use a verbally descriptive scale, i.e. no, mild, moderate, severe, or non-weight-bearing lameness.

Following the hands-off examination the clinician should know which limb(s) is/are affected and to what degree locomotor function is impaired. Taken together with the information from the history and signalment, this should suggest to the clinician some of the more likely potential differential diagnoses.

Hands-on examination
General clinical examination

The first part of the hands-on examination should be a general clinical examination. Large- and medium-sized dogs are best examined on the floor where they will be more relaxed. Small dogs and cats can be examined on the floor but it is often more convenient for the clinician to place the animal on a raised surface such as a table with a non-slip surface. General clinical examination is undertaken to make an assessment of general health and identify concurrent disease or injury that may be related directly or indirectly to the lameness. There is, for example, a high incidence of thoracic injury in animals that have suffered fracture or luxation as a result of a road traffic accident, which could be overlooked to the detriment of the patient's welfare in favour of the more obvious, but non-life-threatening orthopaedic injury. Findings from the clinical examination will ultimately determine the animal's suitability for sedation, anaesthesia or a particular treatment option.

Routine neurological assessment of lameness

A brief neurological examination is performed as a routine and extended to a full examination if neurological involvement is suggested from the history, gait analysis, general clinical examination or on finding an abnormal response to postural reaction and segmental reflex testing. The most useful postural reaction is the animal's ability to hop laterally on a limb. The other test that is commonly performed is paw replacement. In this test the animal is supported and the dorsal surface of the paw is placed on the ground. Delay or absence of an immediate return of the palmar or plantar surface of the paw to the ground is abnormal. No individual test can distinguish conscious general proprioception from unconscious (cerebellar) general proprioception and, although in common usage, it is incorrect to use the clinical term conscious proprioception. Postural reactions test the integrity of many components of the peripheral and central nervous system and may be abnormal before there is any detectable abnormality in the gait. They are, therefore, sensitive indicators of pathology in any part of the nervous system that is involved with limb movement; on their own they are not useful for lesion localization.

In the pelvic limb the patellar reflex is the most reliable tendon reflex. In the thoracic limb there are no completely reliable tendon reflexes and the only dependable segmental reflex is the withdrawal reflex. To test the patellar reflex, hold the stifle in partial flexion and strike the straight patellar ligament with a patellar hammer or any blunt instrument. Brisk extension of the stifle joint is a normal response. Ideally the reflex should be assessed with the animal standing and in both left and right lateral recumbency as sometimes it may be absent in one position and not the other. In dogs older than 10 years, one or both patellar reflexes may be absent

with no other neurological signs present. Withdrawal reflexes are evaluated in the pelvic and thoracic limbs by compressing the skin at the base of the third phalanx of a digit or the interdigital web using digital pressure or tissue forceps. A normal response is prompt withdrawal of the limb with flexion of the carpus, elbow and shoulder in the thoracic limb and the hock, stifle and hip joints in the pelvic limb. Nociception can also be tested by increasing the compression to make the stimulus sufficiently noxious to elicit a conscious response. It is important to check the withdrawal reflexes at the end of the examination because the noxious stimulus may upset the patient making further handling difficult. For further information see Chapter 12 or the BSAVA Manual of Canine and Feline Neurology.

Orthopaedic examination

The purpose of the hands-on examination, areas of which are illustrated in Figure 2.9, is to refine the problem list and thus narrow the list of differential diagnoses by localizing the affected area(s). It may be possible to arrive at a definitive diagnosis based on palpation and manipulation alone, for example with certain fractures or luxations, or by performing manoeuvres that are specific for individual conditions such as cranial draw or tibial compression tests for CCL rupture.

The key to a successful orthopaedic examination is to be methodical and thorough. Painful areas should always be examined last to avoid losing the patient's cooperation. It is tempting to examine only the affected limb, but it is important to examine the whole patient so that nothing relevant is missed. The examination can be performed quickly if it is done in a consistent and systematic fashion so that nothing is omitted.

Most dogs will allow a full orthopaedic examination when they are fully conscious. Dogs are examined standing but some patients, especially giant breeds, may prefer to lie down. It is important to allow the animal to assume a position in which it is comfortable, relaxed and cooperative and the clinician should alter their approach to accommodate this. A comprehensive examination may not be possible if the dog is very nervous, tense, aggressive or in too much pain. Cats are notoriously uncooperative and can be difficult to examine but will usually tolerate at least a limited orthopaedic examination, especially if handled patiently and gently. In some cases it may be necessary to complete the orthopaedic assessment following sedation or general anaesthesia. This is often combined with further diagnostic tests such as radiography.

Pain is defined as an unpleasant sensory and emotional experience associated with actual or potential tissue damage. Pain is a subjective phenomenon and it is therefore not possible to accurately measure it objectively. The clinician needs to look for evidence that a manoeuvre induces a repeatably demonstrable outward expression of the presence of pain on palpation or manipulation, such as turning to look at the affected part, attempting to move away, withdrawal of the affected limb or, in more extreme cases, attempting to bite the examiner. More subtle signs include cessation of panting, lip-licking, fidgeting and pupillary dilation. Vocalization is surprisingly uncommon unless pain is severe and/or neurogenic in origin. Allowance should be made for the temperament of the patient. At one end of the spectrum some patients will appear to be painful wherever they are touched, whereas at the other extreme some patients are so stoical that they do not show any overt signs of pain.

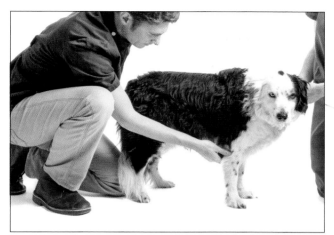

In weight-bearing stance, palpation of elbow effusions is performed by running the fingers or thumb caudally from the lateral epicondyle where a fluid distension of the joint capsule may be felt. Periarticular thickening may also be apparent in chronic conditions of the elbow.

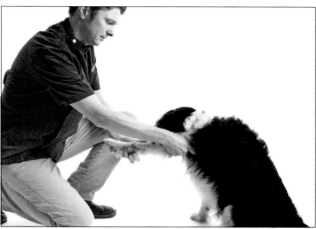

Individual joint manipulation to evaluate the presence of an abnormal range of motion (increased or decreased) and to assess any associated resentment. Note that manipulation of certain joints (such as the elbow) may also cause manipulation of neighbouring joints (such as the shoulder) and pathology may be bilateral.

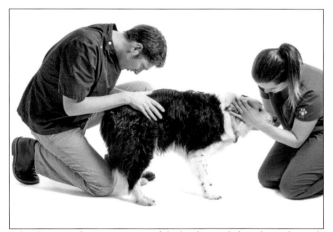

Palpation to evaluate symmetry of the lumbar and gluteal muscles and detect pain foci. Other muscle groups that should be routinely palpated include the hamstring, quadriceps and gastrocnemius muscles.

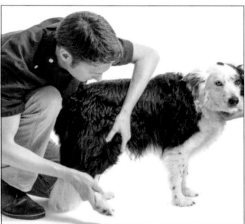

The cranial tibial thrust manoeuvre can be performed with the dog standing or lying down and is a frequently performed, specific test for the diagnosis of CCL disease.

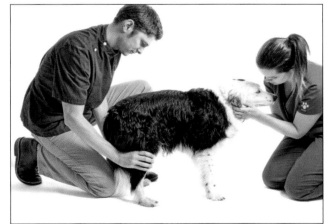

Palpation of the stifles and hocks may provide information regarding the presence of effusions (particularly during standing) or periarticular thickening. Stifle effusions may be palpated as a fluid bulge medial and lateral to the straight patellar ligament.

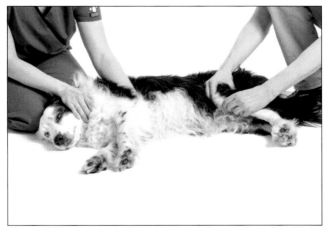

The cranial draw test may also be used to confirm craniocaudal stifle instability in cases with CCL disease. Manipulation of the stifle with the patient in this position may also be used to evaluate for the presence of collateral or caudal cruciate ligament ruptures.

2.9 Elements of the hands-on orthopaedic examination.

Palpation

The clinician should start with the thoracic limbs if the patient has pelvic limb lameness, and *vice versa*. The author prefers to palpate the limbs from proximal to distal, palpating the contralateral limb simultaneously and comparing for similarities and differences. Palpation is useful to detect evidence of muscle atrophy, thickening, swelling and joint effusion. The clinician should be familiar with major anatomical landmarks and reference may be made to standard texts and to anatomical skeletal models. The contralateral limb serves as a normal control unless the condition is bilateral.

Palpation of musculature can provide information about the use of a limb over time. Disuse (or more commonly, reduced use) muscle atrophy will produce a palpable reduction in the muscle mass within a few weeks and is most easily appreciated adjacent to a bony prominence such as the spine of the scapula. A more objective assessment of muscle atrophy can be obtained by measuring limb circumference with a Gulick tape measure (Figure 2.10). Muscle atrophy that is rapid and severe is more likely to have a neurogenic origin and should prompt a full neurological examination. Muscles that are most vulnerable to disuse atrophy are muscles that maintain standing, support bodyweight and cross a single joint, such as the quadriceps group. Muscles that are least vulnerable to atrophy are flexor muscles that cross more than one joint, such as the hamstrings. Muscle mass is slow to recover and apparently normal animals may show atrophy for several months following resolution of lameness. Gentle palpation of muscles and other soft tissue structures should be performed to check for evidence of pain, heat, swelling, thickening, discontinuity or abnormal or irregular texture.

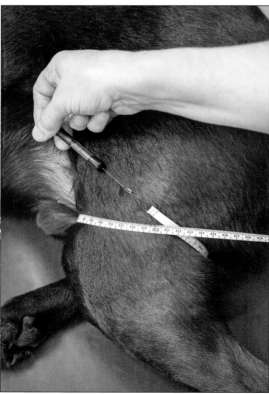

2.10 The use of the Gulick tape measure to assess upper thigh circumference. It is spring-loaded to a fixed tension and allows accurate, comparable and repeatable measurements.

Palpation of bones is used to establish the position and relative spatial relationship of normal bony landmarks that may be altered if there is deformity, fracture or luxation. An attempt should be made to differentiate pain on bone palpation from surrounding soft tissue or adjacent joint pain. Marked diaphyseal bone pain, for example, in juvenile medium and large-breed dogs, especially the German Shepherd Dog, is suggestive of panosteitis.

Manipulation

The next step is a more detailed examination of the limbs, including manipulation of joints. It is important that joint manipulation is undertaken sympathetically, as forced manipulation in either flexion or extension will elicit a pain response. The author prefers to start this part of the examination distally and work proximally. Joints should be put through their full range of motion (ROM) in all planes using the contralateral limb as a control, but bearing in mind the possibility of bilateral conditions. Joint ROM can be measured objectively using a goniometer and this can be useful to assess changes over time. As a point of reference, the normal ROM for Labrador Retrievers assessed by goniometry is given in Figure 2.11, but it is variable to an extent between breeds. In dogs, reduced ROM occurs with osteoarthritis but Lascelles *et al.* (2012) found that in cats, radiographically confirmed osteoarthritis cannot be predicted with certainty using palpation or goniometry.

Joint	Joint motion	Normal range of motion in degrees
Carpus	Flexion	32
	Extension	196
Elbow	Flexion	36
	Extension	166
Shoulder	Flexion	57
	Extension	165
Tarsus	Flexion	38
	Extension	165
Stifle	Flexion	41
	Extension	162
Hip	Flexion	50
	Extension	162

2.11 Median range of joint motion in Labrador Retrievers measured by goniometry. (Note that the straight position is 180 degrees.)

The term 'end-feel' is the subjectively assessed sensation imparted to the examiner's hands at the end of the range of joint motion. Slowly applying moderate pressure at the end of the range of movement and noting the character of resistance should be used to assess end-feel. The author's interpretation of end-feel is outlined in Figure 2.12. Some joints will be painful through their normal ROM, whereas with others pain may only be elicited by stressing the joint at the end of the normal range either in flexion or extension. An equivocal pain response should be repeatable to ensure that it is genuine and comparison should be made with the contralateral joint and other normal joints. Joints should also be tested for abnormal motion such as rotation, and medial and lateral instability in joints where these types of motion are not normally expected. In addition to pain, other indications of joint disease include reduced ROM and crepitus.

Crepitus is a palpable or audible conflict of either bone (usually) or soft tissues as they move relative to each other. Marked crepitus following trauma usually indicates fracture

End-feel	Sensation	Interpretation
Bony/hard/unyielding	Bone approximates bone resulting in an abrupt stop	Always pathological May be indicative of extensive periarticular osteophytosis
Capsular/firm	A firm but slightly yielding sensation associated with tension in the joint capsule	Normal for many joints, e.g. carpal extension Abnormal if associated with reduced range of motion Pathological capsular end-feel is usually firmer than normal capsular end-feel
Soft tissue approximation	Motion is halted by compression of soft tissues or fluid resulting in a reduction in range of motion with a soft end-feel	Normal for some joint, e.g. stifle flexion Abnormal if it occurs too early in the range of motion or in a joint normally having a capsular end-feel May be seen in joints with substantial effusion or periarticular oedema
Empty/painful	Resistance is not felt because the patient resists full range of joint motion	Joint pain is always pathological

2.12 Variation in end-feel of joints.

whereas a somewhat subtler crepitus may be associated with subluxation or luxation. Fracture should not be ruled out on the basis of an absence of crepitus. Crepitus is also a feature of chronic joint disease, particularly where there are extensive osteophytes and cartilage erosion with exposure of subchondral bone. Crepitus is easily referred along a bone so care should be taken to move only one joint at a time. Apparent crepitus is a normal feature following arthrotomy and the placement of monofilament suture material. Pain-free audible clicking of joints when manipulated is a normal feature and does not necessarily indicate joint pathology.

Examination of the thoracic limb

Thoracic limb lameness is less common than pelvic limb lameness and can be more challenging both to diagnose and to treat. It accounts for approximately 25% of all cases of lameness in the author's referral practice. A list of the main differential diagnoses for thoracic limb lameness is provided in Figure 2.13 and additional details of the investigation (and management) of specific conditions are to be found in the relevant individual chapters.

The distal limb

The same physical examination is appropriate for both the thoracic and pelvic limbs distal to the carpometacarpal and tarsometatarsal joints. The limited soft tissue covering of the distal limb facilitates examination so that any swelling, thickening, deformity or abnormal joint posture is more easily appreciated. Thickening of the interphalangeal and metacarpophalangeal joints is not uncommon in older dogs as a result of previous injury or osteoarthritis and may be an incidental finding. The potential significance of a lesion should be assessed by applying digital pressure (deep palpation) over the area and, if the lesion involves a joint, by manipulation to check for a pain response.

The pads, claws and interdigital webbing should be inspected for pyoderma, lacerations, foreign bodies, claw injuries and infections that can all cause relatively severe lameness. The pads of predisposed breeds (Greyhounds and other sight hounds) should be inspected very carefully for the presence of a corn. Corns can be subtle but typically affect the main weight-bearing (third and fourth) digital pads of the thoracic limb. The ROM of the distal and proximal interphalangeal joints and the metacarpophalangeal joints (MCPJ) should each be assessed individually. Reduced flexion is common, especially in the MCPJ of older dogs, but is of no significance unless it is associated with pain. The integrity of the collateral ligaments of these

joints should be assessed with the joint extended so that the ligaments are under tension, otherwise there will be a false impression of joint subluxation. The paired palmar sesamoid bones of the metacarpophalangeal joints (particularly sesamoid bones 2 and 7 in breeds predisposed to sesamoid disease such as Rottweilers) and the single dorsal sesamoid bones should be palpated for evidence of pain, swelling or excessive movement. Confirmation that a sesamoid is painful can usually be obtained by simultaneously hyperextending the joint and applying digital pressure over the bone.

Carpus

The carpus functions as a hinge joint. There is limited soft tissue cover; therefore any swelling or thickening is easily appreciated. The accessory carpal bone is a prominent landmark on the palmar aspect, with the insertion of the flexor carpi ulnaris tendon palpable on the proximal margin. Synovial effusion is readily palpated on the dorsal aspect of the joint. Firm swelling on the medial aspect of the antebrachiocarpal joint together with pain on flexion of the carpus are suggestive of stenosing tenosynovitis of the abductor pollicis longus tendon or medial collateral ligament sprain. Mild bilaterally symmetrical valgus is part of the dog's normal conformation and is exaggerated in chondrodystrophic breeds; excessive valgus or varus deformity should be noted. Bilateral carpal varus secondary to chronic sprain of the lateral collateral ligament complex is common in mature Dobermanns.

The normal carpus and digits should flex so that the digital pads contact the caudal surface of the antebrachium. Forced full flexion of the carpus should be avoided, as it is invariably painful. Carpal extension in dogs beyond approximately 200 degrees is considered abnormal and may indicate hyperextension injury. Collateral ligament integrity should be checked with the joint in extension by medially and laterally stressing the carpus. Medial and lateral movement is greater in young dogs and in cats and should not be diagnosed as instability unless excessive. Isolated collateral ligament injury is rare but when it does occur, the medial collateral ligament is usually affected.

Antebrachium

Prominent bony landmarks that should be palpated distally are the ulnar and radial styloid processes on the lateral and medial aspects respectively. Proximally the caudal ulna and olecranon are the major bony landmarks. Almost the entire radius and ulna can be palpated, with the exception of the radial head and proximal metaphysis, which are covered by muscle bellies and are palpable only

Location	Skeletally immature	Frequency	Skeletally mature	Frequency
Distal limb and paw	Sesamoid dysplasia/ fragmentation	+	Corn Foreign body DJD of MCPJ Trauma • (Sub)luxation • Laceration Hypertrophic pulmonary osteopathy	+++ + ++ + ++ +
Carpus	Flexural deformity	+	Hyperextension Carpal varus Incomplete ossification of radial carpal bone Ligamentous injury – usually medial, rarely lateral or dorsal Accessory carpal bone displacement Abductor pollicis longus tendinopathy	++ + + + + +
Antebrachium	Growth disturbance Congenital deformity Retained cartilaginous core Metaphyseal osteopathy Panosteitis	++ + + + ++	Hypertrophic pulmonary osteopathy	+
Elbow	Elbow dysplasia Medial coronoid disease OCD Ununited anconeal process Incongruity IOHC Congenital luxation (Type I and II)	+++ +++ ++ ++ ++ ++ +	Flexor enthesopathy Humeral intracondylar fissure Avulsion extensor carpi radialis origin Late development of clinical signs associated with elbow dysplasia, especially medial coronoid pathology	+ ++ + ++
Brachium	Panosteitis	++	Triceps tendon avulsion / rupture	+
Shoulder and scapula	OCD Congenital luxation Shoulder dysplasia Incomplete ossification of caudal glenoid	++ + + +	Dorsal luxation scapula Teres minor myopathy Biceps tendinopathy/rupture Shoulder instability/subluxation Traumatic luxation Infraspinatus bursal ossification Infraspinatus/supraspinatus contracture Supraspinatus tendinopathy/ mineralization Incomplete ossification of caudal glenoid	+ + + + + + + + +
Any thoracic/ pelvic limb bone	Congenital anomaly Panosteitis Fracture Bone cyst	+ +++ +++ +	Fracture Neoplasia Osteomyelitis Panosteitis	+++ ++ + +
Any thoracic/ pelvic limb joint	Congenital anomaly Developmental dysplasia	+ +++	Osteoarthritis Septic arthritis Immune-mediated arthropathy (Sub)luxation Articular fracture Neoplasia	+++ ++ + ++ ++ +

2.13 Differential diagnoses for thoracic limb lameness. + = rare; ++ = seen with some regularity; +++ = common; DJD = degenerative joint disease; IOHC = incomplete ossification of the humeral condyle; MCPJ = metacarpophalangeal joint; OCD = osteochondritis dissecans.

on the lateral aspect. The radius and ulna cross in the dorsal plane from proximal to distal; the proximal ulna is situated caudomedially and the distal ulna is lateral. The extensor muscles of the carpus and digits are palpable on the craniolateral antebrachium and the flexor muscles of the carpus and digits are palpable on the caudomedial antebrachium. The antebrachium of the dog has a limited ability to pronate and supinate, unlike the cat, in which the extent of pronation and supination is intermediate between that of the dog and human.

Elbow

The elbow is a complex hinge joint. The bony landmarks of the elbow that should be palpated are the lateral and medial epicondyles of the humerus and the olecranon of the ulna. The normal elbow should flex so that the cranial surface of the antebrachium contacts the cranial aspect

of the brachium but flexion may be reduced in dogs that are heavily muscled. The elbow is a common site of lameness, largely because of the high prevalence of developmental elbow disease in medium and large-breed dogs. The condition is occasionally seen in smaller breeds. Elbow dysplasia is an umbrella term for a collection of clinical diseases that manifest usually as a mild to moderate lameness in young dogs. Lameness is often bilateral and may appear to shift from one limb to the other. If signs are bilaterally symmetrical, lameness may be difficult to recognize, and because these dogs are young they may remain very active despite the pathology. Dogs with disease affecting the medial compartment of the elbow frequently stand with the elbows adducted and the antebrachium externally rotated. In an attempt to reduce movement of the elbow joint, affected dogs adopt a characteristic paddling gait in which they flip the front feet forwards.

Synovial effusion is best appreciated when the dog is weight-bearing by palpating the area between the lateral epicondyle and the olecranon, through the anconeus muscle. In short-coated breeds, a marked effusion may be evident to the naked eye. It is not possible to determine the nature of intra-articular pathology from clinical examination alone, but in dogs with medial coronoid disease evidence of focal pain can often be elicited by palpation directly over the medial coronoid process immediately distal to the medial epicondyle. In young dogs with elbow dysplasia, the range of joint motion is often within normal limits but there may be resentment to full flexion, especially if combined with external rotation (supination) of the antebrachium and flexion of the carpus to 90 degrees. In dogs of the predisposed spaniel breeds, pain on performing this manoeuvre, on elbow extension and additionally on digital compression across the humeral condyle, is suggestive of humeral intracondylar fissure. Young dogs with an ununited anconeal process often appear more painful on elbow extension. Reduced elbow extension is seen less frequently than reduced flexion in dogs with elbow pathology but is easier to appreciate on manipulation. In older dogs with elbow dysplasia the examination findings are typical of osteoarthritis with palpable joint thickening, crepitus and reduced range of joint motion.

Brachium

The distal humerus is readily palpated. Major distal bony landmarks include the single humeral condyle, the lateral (extensor) epicondyle and the larger medial (flexor) epicondyle. Lesions affecting the distal humerus, such as condylar fractures and intracondylar fissure, are common causes of lameness in spaniel breeds. In the midshaft region of the humerus the diaphysis and the large muscles overlying the bone should be palpated for abnormalities. Proximally the humerus is palpable and the bone should be assessed for evidence of pain, swelling, thickening or change of texture. The proximal humerus is a common site of neoplasia in predisposed breeds.

Shoulder joint and scapula

The shoulder is an enarthrodial (shallow ball and socket) joint. Prominent bony landmarks that should be palpated are the acromion, the greater tubercle, the intertubercular groove, the scapular spine and the supraspinatus and infraspinatus muscles cranial and caudal to the spine of the scapula respectively. The distance between the acromion and greater tubercle should be evaluated and compared to the contralateral limb. Loss of the normal spatial relationship occurs if the shoulder is luxated.

Synovial effusion and joint thickening cannot be appreciated because palpation of the joint is hindered by the surrounding musculature. Interpretation of shoulder manipulation is challenging; evaluation of shoulder joint stability is contentious and it is frequently difficult to definitively locate a focus of pain. Atrophy affecting the supraspinatus and infraspinatus muscles is readily apparent as the spine of the scapula becomes more prominent but this finding is not specific for diseases of the shoulder joint. It is not uncommon, on the basis of observation of a dog's gait, for a dog to be presented by the owner for 'shoulder lameness'. There is, however, no characteristic gait that typifies lameness localized to this joint with the exception of that associated with fibrotic myopathy of the infraspinatus muscle (see Chapter 18). The temptation to use the shoulder joint as a scapegoat for undiagnosed lameness should be avoided.

The shoulder is capable of wide excursive movement in all directions although its primary movements during ambulation are flexion and extension. The bony anatomy of the shoulder joint is inherently unstable and the joint relies heavily on the surrounding support structures to provide dynamic stability. It is lesions of these surrounding structures that are commonly the underlying cause of lameness especially in mature dogs. Reduced ROM of the shoulder is difficult to detect unless the scapula is held in a fixed position because of the mobility of the scapula on the body wall. Shoulder pain on manipulation can be difficult to differentiate from elbow pain as it is not possible to fully extend the shoulder without extending the elbow. It is, however, possible to manipulate the elbow without concurrent movement of the shoulder joint and therefore prior assessment of the elbow is recommended.

There is no clinical test that is 100% specific or sensitive for pathology of the intact biceps tendon; however, full flexion of the shoulder joint with the elbow joint in extension places the biceps tendon under tension and a pain response is suggestive of pathology. Digital pressure on the tendon in the region of the intertubercular groove just medial to the greater tubercle can enhance this response (Bruce *et al.*, 2000). The clinician should be aware that pain associated with this test might simply be an indication of cranial shoulder pathology. The manoeuvre also places tension on the biceps brachii and brachialis muscles that insert just distal to the medial coronoid process in an area formerly known as the ulnar tuberosity. It forces the medial coronoid process against the radial head, which may cause pain in dogs with medial coronoid disease. Increased flexion of the shoulder allowing the elbow to be raised above the level of the axial skeleton when performing this test indicates complete rupture of the biceps tendon.

A more reliable indicator of shoulder pathology is the abduction test, which usually elicits pain when there is injury to the medial supporting structures (medial glenohumeral ligament and subscapularis). It is also claimed that medial instability can be evaluated by measuring the abduction angle (Cook *et al.*, 2005) although this is not universally accepted (Devitt *et al.*, 2007). Normal abduction angles are in the region of 30 degrees. An increase in the angle compared with the contralateral limb may occur when there is incompetence of the medial supporting structures. However, an increase in the abduction angle can also be a non-specific finding when there is shoulder muscle atrophy from any cause. Abduction angles greater than 45–50 degrees are more likely to be significant. Comparison should always be made with the contralateral shoulder, even pressure must be exerted on both shoulders, the shoulder must be in an extended position and the examiner should be aware that pathology might be bilateral.

Examination of the pelvic limb

Pelvic limb lameness is more common than thoracic limb lameness in dogs, largely as a result of the prevalence of both CCL disease and hip dysplasia. In the author's referral practice, pelvic limb lameness accounts for approximately 75% of all lameness cases seen. A list of the main differential diagnoses for pelvic limb lameness is provided in Figure 2.14. Additional details of investigation (and management) of specific conditions affecting the pelvic limb are to be found in the relevant individual chapters.

Location	Skeletally immature	Frequency	Skeletally mature	Frequency
Distal limb and paw	Sesamoid dysplasia/fragmentation	+	Corn Foreign body Trauma • (Sub)luxation • Laceration Hypertrophic pulmonary osteopathy	++ + + ++ +
Tarsus	OCD	++	Shear injuries Proximal intertarsal subluxation Intertarsal/tarsometatarsal subluxation Achilles tendon • Avulsion • Laceration • Tendinopathy DDF tendinopathy Displacement SDF Late onset lameness associated with OCD	++ ++ + + + ++ + + +
Crus	Pes varus Metaphyseal osteopathy	+ +	Hypertrophic pulmonary osteopathy	+
Stifle	Femoral condylar OCD Patellar luxation Tibial tuberosity avulsion	+ ++ ++	CCL degeneration CCL-associated meniscal injury Patellar luxation (medial) Patellar luxation (lateral) Patellar tendon rupture / laceration Collateral ligament rupture Stifle luxation Displacement of long digital extensor tendon	+++ ++ ++ + + + + +
Thigh	Quadriceps contracture	+	Fibrotic myopathy • Gracilis • Semimembranosus Iliopsoas strain Avulsion of the tendon • Origin gastrocnemius • Origin popliteus	 + + + + +
Hip and pelvis	Avascular necrosis of femoral head Hip dysplasia Slipped capital physis	++ +++ +	Heterotopic osteochondrofibrosis Hip osteoarthritis Hip luxation	+ ++ ++

2.14 Differential diagnoses for pelvic limb lameness. + = rare; ++ = seen with some regularity; +++ = common. CCL = cranial crucial ligament; DDF = deep digital flexor; OCD = osteochondritis dissecans; SDF = superficial digital flexor.

Tarsus

The tarsus, or hock, is the collective and inclusive term for the bones and joints between the tarsocrural joint and the tarsometatarsal joints. The tarsus consists of seven tarsal bones and their articulations with each other. The tarsocrural joint is responsible for 85% of the movement of the tarsus and functions as a constrained hinge joint. The major palpable landmarks are the calcaneus, the common calcaneal tendon and the medial and lateral malleoli. The limited soft tissue covering in the region facilitates examination. Swelling, thickening, hyperextension, deviation and deformity are readily appreciated. Full flexion of the hock is not possible without simultaneous passive stifle flexion and *vice versa* because there are muscles that cross both joints. If the hock is able to flex with the stifle extended, this indicates severe strain injury or rupture of the common calcaneal tendon.

Synovial effusion of the tarsocrural joint is evaluated by palpating one of the four out-pouches of the joint capsule that are positioned dorsolaterally, dorsomedially, plantarolaterally and plantaromedially. In most dog breeds, with the stifle flexed the normal tarsus should flex so that the dorsal surface of the metatarsus almost touches the cranial aspect of the crus. The tendon of the deep digital flexor muscle runs caudal to the tibia and medial to the calcaneus. If there is pathology of the synovial sheath of the deep digital flexor tendon (which communicates with the tarsocrural joint), pain and distension of the sheath can be appreciated by palpation caudomedial to the distal tibia,

cranial to the common calcaneal tendon. Reduced tarsal flexion is generally a sensitive indicator of joint pathology whereas extension is usually maintained.

In the dog, medial and collateral ligament integrity should be checked with the joint in both extension (long collateral ligaments) and flexion (short collateral ligaments) by abduction and adduction of the pes relative to the tibia. Cats only have short collateral ligaments and do not have long collateral ligaments spanning the whole tarsus. The feline tarsocrural joint has a greater ROM in the transverse plane (especially varus) and this should not be confused with instability. Palpation of the common calcaneal tendon is best performed during weight-bearing. Swelling, thickening, and pain on palpation of the distal tendon and its insertion on the tuber calcanei may indicate tendinopathy or partial rupture. Marked hyperflexion of the talocrural joint will be observed during loading if there is complete rupture, but will be more subtle with a characteristic (clumping) flexion of the digits noted (Figure 2.15) if the superficial digital flexor tendon remains intact. Hyperextension of the proximal intertarsal joint resulting from rupture of the plantar ligaments and plantar fibrocartilage will give a similar appearance, although in this case the calcaneus will be maintained in a proximal position by the intact Achilles tendon. Lateral luxation of the superficial digital flexor tendon from the calcaneus is occasionally seen in certain breeds, most notably the Shetland Sheepdog, and is diagnosed by the finding of local swelling and by palpation of the tendon as it slips in and out of its normal location over the lateral process of the tuber calcanei.

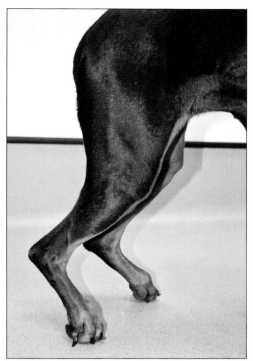

2.15 Digital clumping is observed in cases of partial calcaneal tendon failure where the superficial digital flexor tendon remains intact. Area shaved for ultrasound examination.

Crus

Prominent bony landmarks that should be palpated distally are the distal tibia and fibula including the lateral and medial malleoli. The fibula can only be palpated for a short distance adjacent to its lateral malleolus, whereas the cranial and medial aspects of the tibia can be palpated along its entire length. Proximal landmarks include the cranial tibial muscle on the proximolateral aspect of the tibia and the tibial tuberosity cranially. The combined medial and lateral bellies of the gastrocnemius muscle can be palpated caudal to the proximal tibia and should be followed distally to the insertion of the common calcaneal tendon on the tuber calcanei, checking for swelling, thickening or discontinuity.

Stifle

The stifle is a complex hinge joint. The main structures of the stifle extensor mechanism should be palpated on the cranial aspect of the joint. These are the patella, the tibial tuberosity and the patellar tendon. Additional bony landmarks that should be palpable (unless the patient is obese) include the medial femoral condyle and the area of the medial fabella just caudoproximal to it and, on the lateral aspect from distal to proximal, the fibular head, the lateral femoral condyle and the area of the lateral fabella.

Synovial effusion occurs as an early feature in dogs with intra-articular stifle pathology and can readily be appreciated by palpating either side of the patellar ligament. Effusion results in loss of the small concave depression normally palpable on either side of the patellar ligament and associated loss of contour of the margins of the patellar ligament.

Flexion and extension may be painful and the presence of an audible and/or palpable click is suggestive of medial meniscal tearing or detachment. Chronic cranial cruciate ligament instability results in medial fibrosis and thickening

of the joint, which can be palpated as a medial buttress on the proximal aspect of the tibia. In these cases osteophytes will generally prevent clear palpation of the distinct femoral condyles. There will be preferential atrophy of the quadriceps muscle group. The medial and lateral collateral ligaments should be checked with the stifle in extension by abduction and adduction of the crus respectively.

Medial patellar luxation is a common cause of a 'skipping/hopping' type intermittent lameness especially in small-breed dogs. The stability of the patella is evaluated by palpation, starting with the stifle in full extension and then slowly flexing the joint. If the patella is stable through a normal ROM, placing first lateral and then medial pressure on the patella as the stifle is slowly flexed and extended should further test stability. Patellar stability can also be tested by external and internal rotation of the tibia with the stifle joint in partial flexion, but not all patients will tolerate this while conscious. There may be crepitus in more longstanding cases as a result of retropatellar cartilage erosion and corresponding loss of cartilage on the adjacent trochlear ridge. The degree of subluxation or luxation of the patella is normally graded on an increasing scale of severity from I to IV (see Chapter 23).

If a dog is reluctant to sit squarely on its haunches and instead sits with one pelvic limb consistently extended outwards, this is described as a positive sit test (Figure 2.16). It indicates a reluctance to fully flex the stifle and is commonly observed with CCL disease. Confirmation of loss of integrity of the CCL is obtained by performing the cranial draw and tibial compression tests that assess craniocaudal stifle stability. Both stifles should be compared, although bilateral disease is common with this condition. The tests should be performed carefully as both false-positive and false-negative results can occur. Apparent slight craniocaudal instability resulting from a degree of inward rotation of the tibia during testing is a normal finding; although it is increased if there is CCL insufficiency, it should not be confused with cranial draw. Similarly, in young dogs there is a normal degree of craniocaudal laxity which can be differentiated from cranial draw on the basis of the well defined end point as the normal ligament becomes taut. The integrity of the caudal cruciate ligament should be checked at the same time by performing a caudal draw as rarely this may be ruptured, either in isolation or as a component of a multiple ligament injury.

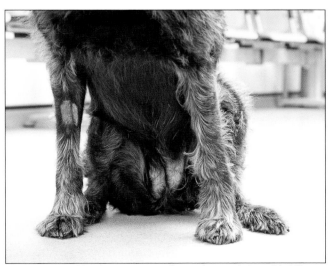

2.16 A positive sit test, commonly seen in association with CCL disease, is a non-specific finding in dogs with stifle pathology that causes discomfort on flexion.

The tibial compression test is usually well tolerated in the conscious standing or recumbent patient even in cats and large-breed dogs. The cranial draw test is more reliably performed under sedation or anaesthesia with the patient in lateral recumbency. It is important to perform the draw test in both flexion and extension in order to fully assess the ligament. Both tests require practice to perform them correctly and it is worth practising these techniques on normal animals. False-negative tests may be seen in early cases when there is only partial rupture of the CCL, or in some chronic cases where there is extensive periarticular fibrosis that contributes to stifle stability (see Chapter 23).

Thigh

The femur is palpable proximally and distally but is not palpable over the mid-diaphysis because of the large overlying muscle masses on all sides. These include the quadriceps group cranially, the biceps femoris and tensor fascia lata laterally, the adductors medially and the hamstring muscle group caudally. The muscles should be palpated individually for abnormalities, which are rare, and for muscle atrophy, which usually reflects reduced use associated with pelvic limb lameness.

Hip

The hip is a spheroidal (ball and socket) joint with a wide range of joint motion. The hip should be pain-free through a normal range of joint motion. If there is hip joint pathology, pain is more readily appreciated on extension and abduction of the joint. Chronic lameness with pain on hip extension in immature small-breed dogs is commonly caused by avascular necrosis of the femoral head (Legg–Calvé–Perthes disease). The hip cannot be fully extended without simultaneous passive extension of the stifle, which increases patellofemoral contact pressure, and may cause pain in animals with stifle pathology. Thus it is important to initially examine the stifle and rule out stifle pathology in animals with apparent pain on hip extension. A false-positive response to hip extension can also be seen in patients with lumbosacral disease because extending the hip also results in extension of the lumbosacral joint. However, dogs with lumbosacral disease do not generally resent abduction of the hip joint.

Severe hip laxity in immature dogs with hip dysplasia can sometimes be appreciated during manipulation when the joint is felt to subluxate and then reduce spontaneously. The Barden hip lift and Ortolani tests (see Chapter 22) can be used to provide a more objective assessment of hip laxity but these manoeuvres are painful and should not be performed in the conscious patient. In older dogs with chronic osteoarthritis and extensive periarticular fibrosis, hip joint extension may be extremely limited.

Iliopsoas muscle strain (groin strain) is increasingly being recognized in very active dogs and is characterized by variable lameness with circumduction of the limb and reduced performance. Pain can be elicited on direct palpation of the muscle group as it passes along the cranioventral border of the ilium to insert on the lesser trochanter of the femur, and by combined extension and internal rotation or abduction of the hip joint.

Pelvis

The gluteal muscles cranial and dorsal to the hip joint should be palpated for asymmetry, which occurs with chronic pelvic limb lameness. The major anatomical landmarks that should be palpated in the pelvic region are the ischiatic tuberosity, the greater trochanter of the femur and the cranial dorsal iliac spine. The relative positions of these three landmarks make the shape of an inverted triangle. Loss of this spatial relationship occurs if there is pelvic fracture or hip luxation.

Further investigation

Following the clinical and orthopaedic examination, further investigation is often needed to establish a definitive diagnosis. Diagnostic investigations are mentioned briefly here but are covered in greater detail in the relevant sections of the manual (see Chapters 3, 4, 15 and the relevant anatomical regional chapters).

Examination under sedation or anaesthesia

While it is important to generate as much information as possible from examination of the conscious patient, examination under sedation or anaesthesia is the preferred method of assessing and confirming joint instability. It may also be indicated in fractious or uncooperative patients or when the patient is too painful to examine conscious and when manoeuvres are being performed (e.g. Barden and Ortolani tests) which are painful even for dogs with normal joints.

Imaging

Radiography remains the imaging modality of choice because of its affordability, availability and familiarity. Orthogonal views of all areas of interest identified by orthopaedic examination should be obtained. Particular attention should be paid to correct positioning to achieve films of diagnostic quality; oblique views of joints or bones are rarely helpful and are often confusing.

Ultrasonography is useful in the investigation of soft tissue injuries, for example tendinopathies. However, the technique requires the use of specialized equipment and considerable operator experience and expertise.

Nuclear scintigraphy is used primarily in patients with obscure lameness to localize the lesion by identifying increased rates of bone remodelling. However, the availability of nuclear scintigraphy is limited and there are health and safety implications associated with its use.

Advanced imaging by computed tomography (CT) and magnetic resonance imaging (MRI) is becoming increasingly available in veterinary practice. CT is particularly useful for investigation of bone pathology and MRI for soft tissue injuries. There is, however, considerable overlap between the two modalities. Advanced imaging is not a shortcut to diagnosis and candidates should be selected with care following appropriate clinical evaluation and lameness localization. These techniques are expensive and if used inappropriately on a diagnostic 'fishing trip' may simply demonstrate (potentially multiple) pathologies of unknown significance.

Detailed discussion of imaging for orthopaedic disease is provided in Chapter 3.

Synoviocentesis

Evaluation of joint fluid (see Chapter 4) is an under-employed technique in the investigation of joint disease. It is particularly useful where there is multiple joint involvement and in the differentiation between inflammatory (infectious or immune-mediated) and degenerative causes of joint disease.

Diagnostic local anaesthesia

Intra-articular injection of local anaesthetic under sedation followed, on recovery, by repeat gait analysis and orthopaedic examination has long been suggested as a way of localizing lameness to a specific joint. Although the author has not found the technique to be helpful, several recent studies have shown promising results, in particular (but not exclusively) with lameness resulting from elbow and shoulder pathology. In one study of 90 dogs with unilateral elbow lameness (subsequently confirmed by CT and arthroscopy to have medial coronoid disease), 87% of dogs showed temporary improvement in lameness and confirmed clinical localization after intra-articular injection of the local anaesthetic mepivicaine (Van Vynckt *et al.*, 2012). A false-negative result was observed in 13% of dogs. In interpreting this test, a significant improvement in lameness in response to the intra-articular injection is required to confirm a positive result. As such it is most useful in dogs with moderate to severe lameness.

Biopsy

Biopsy of bone or synovial membrane (see Chapter 4) may be indicated in the further investigation of pathology affecting bone or joints respectively.

Arthroscopy

Arthroscopy (see Chapter 15) is performed as both a diagnostic and a therapeutic modality and has greatly reduced the need for open arthrotomy. Arthroscopy is particularly useful in the investigation and/or treatment of pathology affecting the shoulder, elbow and stifle joints. It requires expensive equipment, experience and expertise and is usually best performed at a specialist referral centre.

References and further reading

Arthurs G (2011) Orthopaedic examination of the dog: 1 Thoracic limb. *In Practice* **33**, 126–133

Arthurs G (2011) Orthopaedic examination of the dog: 2 Pelvic limb. *In Practice* **33**, 172–179

Bruce WJ, Burbidge HM, Bray JP and Broome CJ (2000) Bicipital tendinitis and tenosynovitis in the dog: a study of 15 cases. *New Zealand Veterinary Journal* **48**, 44–52

Cogar SM, Cook CR, Curry SL, Grandis A and Cook JL (2008) Prospective evaluation of techniques for differentiating shoulder pathology as a source of forelimb lameness in medium and large breed dogs. *Veterinary Surgery* **37**, 132–141

Cook JL, Renfro DC, Tomlinson JL and Sorenson JE (2005) Measurement of angles of abduction for diagnosis of shoulder instability in dogs using goniometry and digital image analysis. *Veterinary Surgery* **34**, 463–468

Devitt CM, Neely MR and Vanvechten BJ (2007) Relationship of physical examination test of shoulder instability to arthroscopic findings in dogs. *Veterinary Surgery* **36**, 661–668

Jaegger G, Marcellin-Little DJ and Levine D (2002) Reliability of goniometry in Labrador Retrievers. *American Journal of Veterinary Research* **63**, 979–986

Lascelles BD, Dong YH, Marcellin-Little DJ *et al.* (2012) Relationship of orthopaedic examination, goniometric measurements, and radiographic signs of degenerative joint disease in cats. *BMC Veterinary Research* **8**, 10

Platt S and Olby N (2013). *BSAVA Manual of Canine and Feline Neurology, 4th edn.* BSAVA Publications, Gloucester

Scott HW and Witte PG (2011) Investigation of lameness in dogs: 1 Forelimb. *In Practice* **33**, 20–27

Van Vynckt D, Verhoeven G, Saunders J *et al.* (2012) Diagnostic intra-articular anaesthesia of the elbow in dogs with medial coronoid disease. *Veterinary and Comparative Orthopaedics and Traumatology* **2**, 307–313

Witte PG and Scott HW (2011) Investigation of lameness in dogs: 2 Hindlimb. *In Practice* **33**, 58–66

Chapter 3

Imaging

Thomas W. Maddox

Diagnostic imaging is considered an integral part of the work-up of most animals that present with evidence of a musculoskeletal disorder. When performed correctly and using the most appropriate modality, imaging, should significantly reduce the differential diagnoses for a case and can often allow a specific diagnosis to be made.

All of the diagnostic imaging modalities available to veterinary practitioners have a role to play in imaging musculoskeletal cases, but radiography, as the most widely available and arguably the easiest to perform, remains the mainstay of imaging of musculoskeletal disease. Computed tomography (CT) is increasingly being used, particularly for conditions affecting bones, while ultrasonography, magnetic resonance imaging (MRI) and scintigraphy (nuclear medicine) are all able to provide additional specific and complementary information. Some of the most common reasons for imaging a musculoskeletal case are detailed in Figure 3.1.

- Acute or chronic lameness
- Skeletal or joint pain
- Fracture confirmation, characterization and post-reduction assessment
- Monitoring fracture or osteotomy healing
- Assessment of joint luxation/subluxation and stability
- Evaluation of swelling centred on bones/joints
- Monitoring of/screening for inherited musculoskeletal disease
- Metabolic bone disease
- Neoplastic or systemic disease with skeletal or joint involvement

3.1 Indications for musculoskeletal imaging.

The imaging examination

Imaging examinations may be viewed as diagnostic tests, the results of which must always be interpreted in conjunction with the findings of the clinical examination, the pertinent history and other diagnostic tests. Based on the evaluation of the patient's history, gait evaluation and orthopaedic examination (see Chapters 1 and 2), a list of differential diagnoses is initially formulated. An imaging study is then performed to help confirm the diagnosis or at least narrow the list of differential diagnoses.

The diagnostic value that imaging can bring to case management is dependent on four key aspects:

- Determination of the correct anatomical region to image

- Selection of the most appropriate modality (or modalities)
- Performance of a technically competent imaging examination
- Accurate interpretation of the results of the study undertaken.

Errors can be introduced at any stage in this process and may result in a compromised examination at best and a misdiagnosis at worst. With the increasing availability of advanced imaging modalities, the selection of the most appropriate modality is no longer as straightforward as it was previously. However, it remains true that most conditions are at least detectable on high quality plain radiographs, even if they cannot always be fully characterized. It is rarely incorrect to consider radiographs as the initial 'screening' modality. Conversely, immediately performing an MRI (except in some cases of neurological disease following appropriate neurolocalization) could prove unnecessarily expensive, and occasionally embarrassing. The greater sensitivity of modalities such as MRI and CT can also result in identification of additional lesions of uncertain clinical significance. These may or may not need to be further investigated or considered depending on the circumstances of the case. The basic principles and indications for all of the imaging modalities are considered in the following sections.

Radiography

The advent of digital radiography (DR) detection systems has had a significant impact on imaging of the musculoskeletal system. Although the process of obtaining radiographs and principles of interpretation remain the same as with conventional film-screen radiography, there are important differences that merit consideration, particularly with respect to the artefacts encountered.

Generation of the primary X-ray beam is the same regardless of the technique used, and indeed most X-ray generators are equally suitable for either digital or conventional radiography:

- A tungsten filament is heated to produce a cloud of electrons that are then accelerated across a vacuum in an X-ray tube by a potential difference or voltage (kV) to collide with an anode target (Figure 3.2)

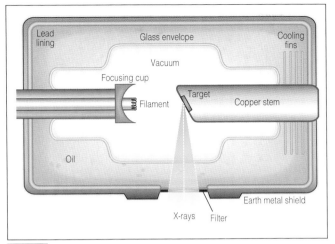

3.2 A simple (stationary or fixed anode) X-ray tube.

- Rapid deceleration and atomic interactions on collision result in the production of X-ray photons that exit the tube through a glass window as the primary X-ray beam
- The primary beam is then attenuated (absorbed, scattered and transmitted) as it passes through the patient according to the thickness, physical density and effective atomic number of the structures and tissues it encounters.

The methods by which the attenuated primary beam (latent image) received by the imaging receptor is detected and then recorded constitute the main difference between digital and conventional radiography.

Conventional radiography

With film-screen radiography, a polyester film base covered with an emulsion of gelatin with suspended silver bromide particles is used to record the latent image. Silver bromide particles are sensitive to both X-ray and visible light photons, which cause a small alteration in their chemical structure. This structural alteration means that when the film is chemically processed and developed, the silver bromide molecules become visible as black silver grains; regions of the film exposed to X-rays are thereby darkened.

The blackening of film by X-ray photons is a very inefficient process and film is much more sensitive to visible light. Consequently, most radiographic cassettes incorporate phosphorescent screens. These screens emit light when stimulated by X-ray photons, increasing the efficiency of the process and meaning that most of the blackening seen on the film is actually caused primarily by visible light and not directly by X-rays.

Film-screen radiography has been in use for over 100 years and as such has probably been refined to the peak of its development. It is a mistake to assume that digital techniques have superseded film-screen radiographs in terms of image quality; indeed the spatial resolution of mammography films still exceeds that possible with digital systems (although a lower contrast resolution negates this advantage to some degree). The benefits of digital imaging lie in the flexibility of the format, elimination of need for chemical development, ease of storage (archiving) and the wide exposure latitude.

Digital radiography

Digital radiography systems can be divided into two categories; namely computed radiography (CR), which uses a photosensitive phosphor plate to record the latent image, and direct digital radiography (DDR), which produces a digital image without the need for any processing steps. In both cases the output is essentially identical.

Computed radiography

Superficially, CR systems appear to resemble conventional film-screen radiography in that they comprise cassettes of varying sizes that require processing to generate a viewable image. However, instead of undergoing chemical photographic development, the imaging plate inside the cassette is read by a laser. The plate consists of a photostimulable phosphor which, rather than immediately emitting light upon X-ray exposure (like a conventional radiographic screen), captures the latent image. When placed inside a plate reader, a helium–neon laser scanned over the plate provides a small amount of energy to stimulate the delayed release of light, which is collected by a light guide and then amplified and digitized. The plate is then automatically erased by exposure to a very bright white light.

Direct digital radiography

There are several different types of DDR systems (Figure 3.3). The main practical difference compared with CR is that an image is generated almost immediately without the need to place a cassette into a reader (indeed there usually are no cassettes).

The terminology used creates potential for confusion between direct conversion and direct readout. The former relates to direct conversion to electrical signals at the imaging plate level, while the latter concerns the direct transfer of image data from the plate to the computer. All DDR systems are so called because they have direct readout to the computer (regardless of how the X-ray photons are converted to electrical data), while CR systems require a reader.

Regardless of the exact equipment used, the output of all digital radiographic systems is truly digital data collected into a computer file. Standardization efforts between systems manufacturers in the 1990s led to the development of the Digital Imaging and Communication in Medicine (DICOM) standard, which means that the files concerned can be communicated readily and without a loss in quality. DICOM files are also tagged with information regarding the patient, equipment used and area imaged which is essentially impossible to alter and hence such information must be entered carefully and correctly when initiating the study. DICOM images can be either displayed on a monitor (soft copy) or printed on transparent film and viewed on a light box (hard copy).

The printing of all forms of digital imaging studies negates many of the inherent advantages of digital imaging (including image manipulation and easy archiving). Accordingly, an archive system needs to be in place to allow for the storage, accessing and viewing of the images. Such systems are known as Picture Archival and Communications Systems (PACS) and are distinct from standalone DICOM viewing software systems such as OsiriX (Pixmeo, Geneva, Switzerland) or eFilm (Merge Healthcare, Chicago, IL). DICOM viewers allow the image files to be reviewed and manipulated, but still require connection to a PACS to search and access the imaging files. Many PACS will incorporate their own inbuilt DICOM viewing software.

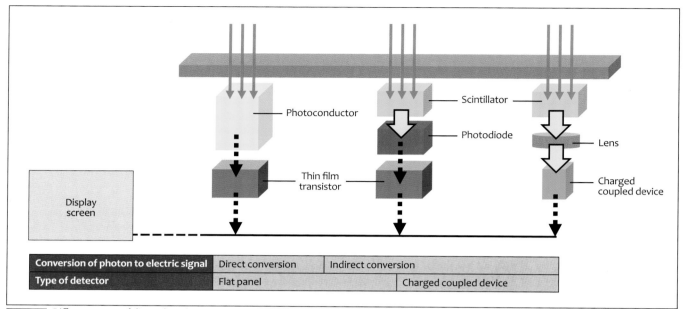

Conversion of photon to electric signal	Direct conversion	Indirect conversion	
Type of detector	Flat panel		Charged coupled device

3.3 Different types of direct digital radiography systems. Flat panel detectors either directly or indirectly convert X-rays into electric signals; direct detectors use a photodetector to immediately transform X-rays (red arrows) to electric signals (dotted arrows), while indirect detectors use a scintillator to convert X-rays to visible light (yellow arrows) that is then transformed to an electrical charge by a photodiode. Charged coupled devices (CCD) also use scintillators to convert X-rays to light, which is then focused on to the CCD chip via a lens and converted to an electrical charge.

In addition to the obvious benefits provided by an image file that can be easily manipulated, a significant advantage for all forms of DR over conventional film, is the ability to tolerate a wide range of exposures. For film the dynamic range or latitude for which it can accurately display a range of exposures is narrow and sigmoidal (S-shaped). This means film can be easily over- or under-exposed; this may even occur on the same image if regions of the body with significant differences in thickness are radiographed. Digital radiographic systems have a much wider dynamic range, which is also more linear (Figure 3.4) and so visible effects of incorrect exposure are rarely seen. Additionally, image contrast and brightness can be altered after acquisition, in order to better evaluate

bony or soft tissue structures. This, however, does not mean that correct technique is irrelevant; incorrect exposure can still result in artefacts and not all images can be rescued by alteration of post-acquisition processing.

Radiographic technique

Most musculoskeletal radiography utilizes a vertical primary X-ray beam and a simple tabletop technique. The use of a radiographic grid is required for tissue thickness greater than 10 cm. 'Lateral' views are obtained with the target limb lowermost and next to the cassette (i.e. mediolateral rather than lateromedial). Craniocaudal or caudocranial views are obtained depending on the exact region being radiographed and the operator's preference. Pre-exposure labeling with appropriate left/right markers is imperative and routine addition of such positional labels during processing should be avoided. Radiographs obtained for surgical planning should include markers of a known size to allow correction of radiographic magnification.

Occasionally horizontal beam radiography may be of value when conventional positioning is difficult. However, this must only be used if the radiography room has been designed with this in mind; there are obvious radiation safety concerns regarding the direction of the primary beam on to a wall without sufficient attenuating properties and the permission of the relevant authority must be sought. Further details of specific radiographic procedures (including special views) are described in the chapters relating to the joints concerned.

Routine views
Orthogonal views

Radiographs are a two-dimensional view of a three-dimensional structure and full characterization of a lesion cannot be achieved without comparing the appearance on at least two views obtained at right angles to one another. Such

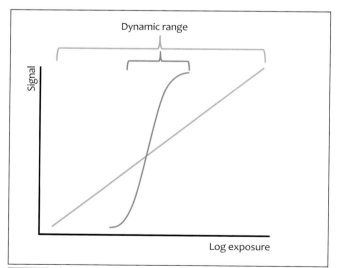

3.4 Characteristic curves for digital and conventional radiography systems showing their performance over a range of exposures. The curve for conventional film-screen radiography (red) is narrow and sigmoidal, with only the central part being linear. This results in a narrow dynamic range. The equivalent plot for digital systems (blue) is a straight line over a much larger range, meaning that digital systems can display a wider range of exposures correctly (wide dynamic range).

orthogonal views are considered a prerequisite for radiographing most body regions and musculoskeletal structures are no exception. Some lesions will be poorly detectable, or occasionally completely invisible, on a single view (Figure 3.5).

Contralateral limbs

It is often prudent to obtain radiographs of the contralateral limb, sometimes to act as a control to compare with the clinically affected limb, or for implant sizing or precontouring purposes in some fracture repairs. Additionally, in cases of suspected likely bilateral disease, images of the contralateral limb should be acquired routinely as part of the full diagnostic work-up.

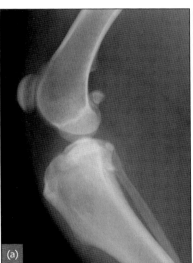

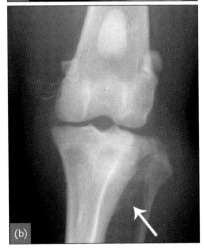

3.5 (a) Mediolateral and (b) caudocranial views of the stifle of a dog. The mediolateral view shows few abnormalities aside from a likely joint effusion. However, the caudocranial view shows focal soft tissue swelling around the head of the fibula and ill defined amorphous periosteal reaction (arrowed) in the proximal interosseus space between the tibia and fibula. There is cortical lysis of the proximal lateral tibia and subtle lysis of the fibular head. Histopathology confirmed an osteosarcoma.

Additional views

These include simple oblique views such as 45-degree plantaromedial–dorsolateral oblique and plantarolateral–dorsomedial oblique views of the tarsus, or tangential ('skyline') views such as the cranioproximal–craniodistal view of the intertubercular groove of the humerus (Figure 3.6). Also included are flexed views of joints such as the elbow or tarsus (Figure 3.7) and 'splayed toe' mediolateral views of the digits. Further details of area-specific views are included in the relevant joint chapters; the increasing use of cross-sectional imaging means they are less commonly utilized.

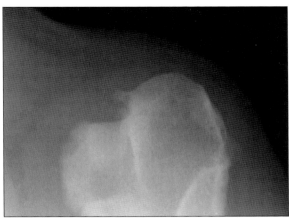

3.6 Cranioproximal–craniodistal view of the intertubercular groove of the proximal humerus of a dog, which shows irregular osteophyte formation on the medial aspect of the greater tubercle. Further faint mineralization is visible just proximal to the bicipital groove suggestive of mineralization within/adjacent to the biceps tendon. The groove itself is increased in opacity indicating sclerosis and osteophytosis.

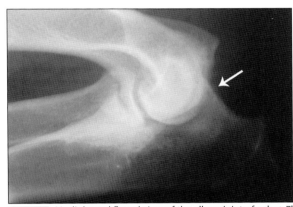

3.7 Mediolateral flexed view of the elbow joint of a dog. Flexing the joint means that the anconeal process can be viewed unobstructed by the medial supracondylar crest: in this case, subtle osteophytosis (arrowed) along the border of the anconeal process is now evident.

Stress radiography

The application of opposing forces to differing parts of the skeletal system during radiographic examination is termed stress radiography. The forces involved are often shearing forces, but distraction and rotation forces can also be employed (Figure 3.8). These techniques are probably underutilized but can be invaluable in documenting joint instability, especially for known or suspected traumatic joint injury. For the purposes of radiation safety it is important that forces are applied through the use of tapes, ties and sandbags and not through personnel being present during radiographic exposure.

Stress radiographs are often employed to demonstrate medial and/or lateral instability associated with failure of collateral support. However, it can sometimes be necessary to assess dorsopalmar/plantar or craniocaudal stability, for example in cases of carpal hyperextension injury.

There are few published values for the degree of joint deviation that can be considered normal, and the huge variation seen in small animal patients reduces the usefulness of such values. Gross instability is not normally

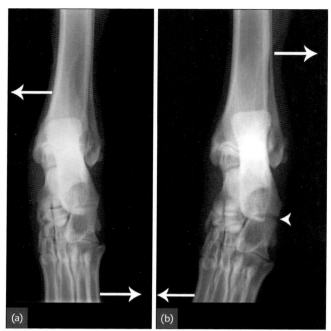

3.8 Stress radiography to demonstrate instability in a tarsus with multiple injuries, including a comminuted central bone fracture. Rope ties are used to apply shearing force proximal and distal to the tarsus in the direction of the arrows. (a) Stressing the medial aspect of the joint results in no significant change, but (b) stressing the lateral aspect results in widening of the calcaneoquartal joint (arrowhead) and indicates either damage to the collateral ligament or instability due to the collapse of the central tarsal bone buttress as a result of fracture.

difficult to recognize and is normally associated with soft tissue swelling and limb dysfunction. However, in less definitive cases, comparison with stressed views of the contralateral joint can be useful. Care should be taken here to ensure that subject positioning and the magnitude of distractive force applied are comparable. When using the contralateral joint as an internal control, it should be remembered that pathology can be present bilaterally. This is less likely with traumatic injuries, but conditions such as degenerative carpal hyperextension might be expected to show bilateral changes and interpretation should be made with reference to the clinical picture.

Contrast radiography

Contrast agents are substances employed during imaging examinations to enhance or increase the visible contrast of structures or fluids within the body. When used during radiographic examinations, these substances can be either positive or negative agents and create radiographic contrast by having a considerably different physical density or effective atomic number to the surrounding tissues. Negative contrast agents are primarily gases (of very low density) and are not generally employed in musculo-skeletal imaging. Positive contrast agents include high atomic number substances such as iodine and barium. Only iodine-based media are suitable for musculoskeletal imaging. Specific uses include myelography, arthrography, angiography/lymphangiography and sinography.

Myelography

The injection of non-ionic, low osmolar iodinated contrast media into the subarachnoid space at either the cisterna magna or via lumbar injection at L5–L6 or L6–L7 was the standard of care in spinal imaging until cross-sectional

imaging became more widely available. With an experienced operator, myelography can delineate a variety of extradural, intradural–extramedullary and some intra-medullary lesions.

Consideration of the characteristics and site of the lesion, the clinical history and signalment of the patient will often allow a diagnosis to be made, but little diagnostic information is provided on the nature of intramedullary lesions. Myelography has the advantage that a sample of cerebrospinal fluid is obtained for analysis during the procedure. However, it is an invasive procedure that can be associated with complications resulting in patient morbidity and also technical complications leading to a non-diagnostic study. CT myelography typically uses lower volumes of contrast and allows lesions to be characterized in multiple planes.

Arthrography

Theoretically, contrast media can be instilled into any joint space to better define intra-articular structures, articular surfaces and bursal extensions. Practically, it is rarely used in joints other than the shoulder joint where it can allow delineation of osteochondrosis lesions and pathology involving the biceps tendon and tendon sheath, although even here its use has been largely superseded by other imaging techniques. Further details of this procedure are included in the chapter on the shoulder. Joint puncture sites for arthrography are the same as those used for synovial fluid sampling (see Chapter 4).

Angiography/lymphangiography

The use of radiographic angiography studies to determine vascular flow and vessel patency has been largely super-seded by ultrasonography, CT and, to some extent, MRI. Lymphangiography is still occasionally employed to assess diffuse limb swelling and can also be conducted as part of a CT examination. The simplest technique for this procedure when imaging limbs is to inject a small volume (1–2 ml) of 200–300 mg iodine/ml into the interdigital subcutis between the pads and then acquire a series of images of the limb proximal to the injection site 1–3 minutes after completion of the injection.

Sinography

Contrast is instilled into a draining tract in an attempt to identify the origin of the tract or delineate a causal agent such as a foreign body. The increased use of the cross-sectional imaging modalities has meant that this technique is no longer frequently performed.

Other body regions

In addition to radiographic examination of the contra-lateral joint or limb, it may be appropriate to examine other body regions. Where a lesion of the musculoskeletal system has been identified that is potentially neoplastic, the abdomen and thorax should be evaluated for evidence of metastatic disease (Figure 3.9). The documentation of metastatic lesions can increase confidence in a diagnosis of neoplasia for the suspect lesion as well as being a requirement of the staging process.

In cases involving significant trauma, imaging of the thorax and/or abdomen is indicated to evaluate for radiographic signs consistent with the presence of con-current injuries such as pulmonary contusions, pneumo/haemothorax, haemoabdomen or evidence of urinary tract trauma.

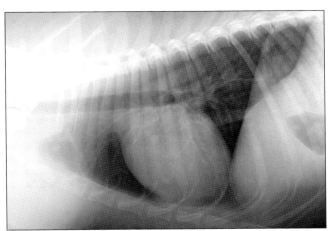

3.9 Left lateral recumbent view of the thorax of the same dog as in Figure 3.5. Several small pulmonary soft tissue nodules are apparent (most obvious superimposed over the cardiac silhouette); three views of the thorax were obtained and nodules seen on all of them. The finding of pulmonary nodules is significant for the staging of the dog's disease, and they also increase diagnostic certainty for the stifle lesion being neoplastic.

Sometimes the identification of specific musculoskeletal disease in one region should prompt radiography of other bones or joints. For example, identification of erosive changes in one or more joints should prompt imaging of other joints to evaluate for an erosive polyarthritis.

Where conformational malalignment is suspected or known to play a role in the development or management of orthopaedic conditions (for example, distal femoral varus or valgal deformities in medium to large-breed dogs with patella instability) then the radiographic examination should be extended to give full limb views including the joints proximal and distal to the area of interest. Alternatively CT evaluation is undertaken allowing an easier and more complete three-dimensional evaluation of deformities.

Optimizing image quality

Regardless of whether digital or conventional radiography is used, there are a number of simple rules that should be followed to ensure that the images produced are of optimal quality. These are summarized in Figure 3.10.

Aim	Procedure
Eliminate motion artefact	Adequate sedation/anaesthesia Use of sandbags and ties
Increase contrast	Collimate tightly to reduce scatter formation Use low kV technique to reduce scatter reaching film/imaging plate Use grid to reduce scatter reaching film/imaging plate
Reduce penumbra/increase sharpness	Use small focal spot of X-ray tube (if available) Use fine detail film-screen combinations or imaging plates (if available)
Reduce geometric distortion	Centre over area of interest (especially if a joint) Ensure critical structures are parallel to imaging plate/cassette
Use correct exposure factors	Produce and use exposure chart Critically evaluate exposure as part of radiographic assessment and reject if inadequate

3.10 Actions that can be taken to improve radiographic quality.

Positioning aids, particularly ties, are essential for musculoskeletal imaging and a variety of sizes and types should be available (Figure 3.11). Grids reduce the level of scatter radiation and are seldom required in musculoskeletal imaging of the mid to distal limb, as the tissue thickness of the regions being radiographed rarely exceeds the 10 cm limit for when a grid would be beneficial. Grids are routinely used in radiography of thicker regions such as the pelvis, spine and sometimes the shoulder. Close collimation for these regions is also important to maximize image quality.

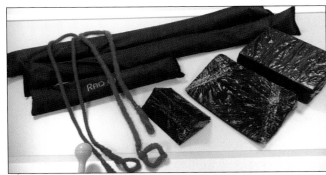

3.11 Examples of radiographic positioning aids. Shown are sandbags of various sizes, radiolucent foam wedges and blocks (plastic-covered) and ties.

Development and processing errors

A full discussion of the problems created by incorrect development is beyond the scope of this text, and in any case these are less common with well maintained automated processors and largely eliminated by the use of digital systems. Underdevelopment can result in a very light appearing image (including the area surrounding the patient but within the primary beam) and can be caused by the processor running too fast, at too low a temperature or using exhausted developing chemicals. Overdevelopment leads to a very dark film (including unexposed areas under metallic markers) and results from extended development times or too high a temperature. Light fogging (from faulty cassettes or poor dark room conditions) will also darken the radiographic film. Browning can be seen with films that are inadequately washed or fixed.

Artefacts specific to digital radiography

With digital systems it is imperative that appropriate radiographic technique is still observed; basic faults in technique such as patient malpositioning, motion artefact and double exposures are all still possible. Furthermore, while digital systems are far more tolerant of minor variations in exposure, significant over- or underexposure will compromise images.

There are also a number of artefacts specific to DR that can degrade image quality (Drost *et al.*, 2008). Some of these are considered below.

Under/overexposure

When the image detector does not receive enough X-ray input this simple lack of information results in a grainy or mottled image with a low level of signal to noise (as opposed to film-screen systems where an image would be barely visible). Digital systems compensate to produce a moderately acceptable image, but image quality is still degraded and this is particularly apparent when it is enlarged (Figure 3.12).

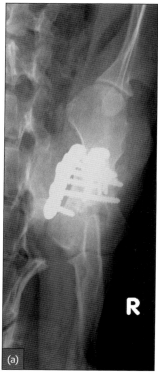

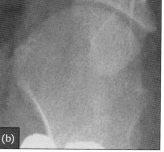

3.12 (a) A significantly underexposed digital radiograph (obtained with CR system). The image shows a moderately mottled or grainy appearance. (b) This becomes more obvious when the image is enlarged.

The wide latitude of digital systems means that over-exposure is rare. Overexposure can be better tolerated as in this situation there is no lack of information reaching the detector. However, ultimately the receptor system will become saturated and result in an image that appears very flat with little contrast.

Incorrect exposure cannot easily be assessed by inspecting the image and as such, manufacturers have had to develop a method to communicate exposure information to the user. This usually takes the form of a value known as the exposure index, which is a numerical value indicating the degree of exposure (Figure 3.13). The manufacturer will specify a range of values that this index should fall within, in order to optimize image quality and ensure that the patient is not receiving an unnecessarily high radiation dose.

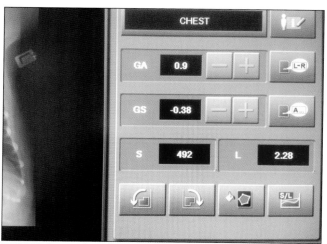

3.13 Screen shot of a computed radiography reader console. This manufacturer terms the exposure index the 'S value'. The S value of 492 indicates that the radiograph is correctly exposed according to the system manufacturer's guidelines.

Look-up table errors

The unprocessed raw data produced by a digital system cannot be viewed in any meaningful sense and has to be converted to an image, which can then be displayed. This conversion is achieved through the use of look-up tables; these are essentially curves detailing how bright a pixel on a monitor should be displayed for a given amount of detector excitation. Differing look-up tables can be applied in different situations and are part of the so-called processing algorithms used for various body regions. Applying an inappropriate look-up table can result in information being lost from an image, such as the 'clipping' of soft tissues from the margins of a body part (Figure 3.14).

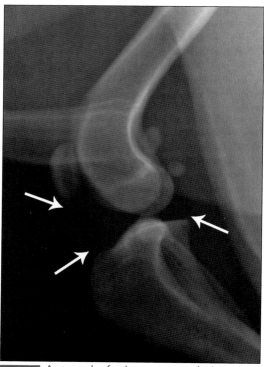

3.14 An example of an image converted using an inappropriate look-up table. The soft tissues around the stifle (arrowed) have been clipped from the image and cannot be evaluated.

Collimation

Although appropriate collimation can be easily simulated by cropping a digital image, adequate collimation is still vitally important. Aside from improving image contrast and reducing the dose of scattered radiation, digital systems rely on some form of collimation in order to process the image correctly. If there is inadequate collimation then the system determines that the radiograph is overexposed and makes the image too light (Figure 3.15). Alternatively, the system will attempt to apply automatic collimation and incorrectly 'black out' regions of the image. Manually applying appropriate collimation during image processing usually allows the correct image to be displayed.

Foreign material within the system

This is only likely to be seen in CR, as direct digital systems are sealed with no cassette or film being removed for processing. Foreign material on the CR imaging plate creates a similar artefact to that seen with material inside a conventional film cassette; in both cases photons are blocked, creating focal white marks on the image.

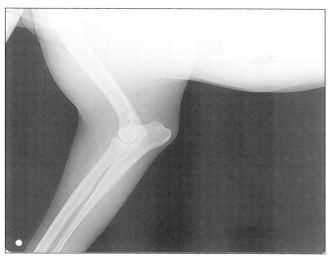

3.15 Inadequate collimation has resulted in this radiograph being incorrectly processed by the system, creating a very light image with little contrast.

However, this artefact is still relatively uncommon in most CR systems (as the process is automated within the plate reader), compared with conventional film processing which involves a degree of manual handling. Dirt on the CR reader system's light guide will create fine white lines across the image.

Double exposure

Double exposure can occur with any radiography system when a detector is inadvertently exposed prior to obtaining the desired image. It can also occur if a CR plate is not fully erased by the plate reader. When a double exposure is made with a conventional film-screen system the resultant image is usually very dark; however, the wide latitude of CR systems means that the two images are displayed normally and merely superimposed (Figure 3.16).

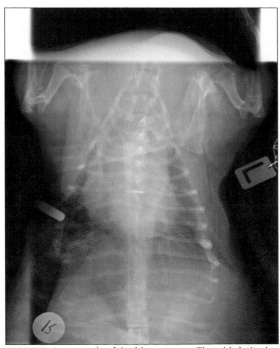

3.16 An example of double exposure. The wide latitude means that both images are displayed normally, resulting in a potentially confusing radiograph until the error is recognized.

Moiré artefact

This artefact is seen as alternating light and dark bands across the image when viewed on a display monitor. It is caused when a static (non-oscillating) grid is used with a digital (CR or DDR) system. It occurs due to the creation of a cross-interference pattern between the lines of the grid and those of the display monitor (Figure 3.17). Use of a moving grid (Potter–Bucky) or if this is not available then one with a very high grid-line frequency (greater than 70 lines/cm) will eliminate this artefact.

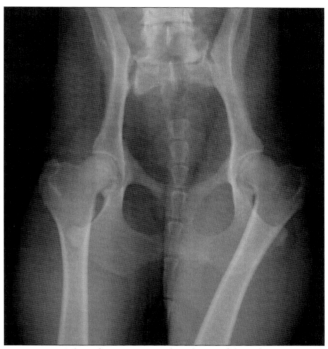

3.17 Moiré artefact on a ventrodorsal view of the pelvis. Alternating light and dark bands are present across the image when a static radiographic grid of low frequency is used. Use of a moving grid will eliminate this artefact.

Überschwinger artefact

This artefact, also known as the rebound artefact, is the result of an image processing error (usually an excessively edge-enhancing processing algorithm). It manifests itself as a radiolucent region around the edges of strongly radiopaque structures (Figure 3.18). Aside from being aesthetically displeasing, it can also be diagnostically confusing as it often creates a radiolucent halo around orthopaedic implants, potentially simulating the appearance of implant loosening or low-grade associated infection. Close inspection often reveals that the halo also affects adjacent soft tissues and is uniformly present around the entirety of the implant/implants, which would be unlikely in situations of actual implant loosening. Adjustment of the processing algorithm can minimize the effect of this artefact.

Summary

Radiography in all its forms is a relatively inexpensive, fast, high spatial resolution imaging modality. Its fundamental drawback is its poor contrast resolution; specifically the inability to distinguish between all types of soft tissue (except fat) and even to distinguish between soft tissue and fluid. As such, it lends itself well to imaging of osseous pathology but soft tissue changes are comparatively poorly characterized. Additionally, the inherent limitation of its

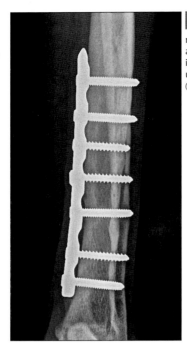

3.18 Überschwinger artefact. A subtle radiolucent halo is present around many of the screws used in the repair of this radius and ulna fracture.
(Courtesy of Gareth Arthurs)

two-dimensional nature introduces a degree of ambiguity to almost all lesions seen, which can be only partly resolved by taking orthogonal/multiple views. All the subsequent imaging modalities have been developed at least in part to try to overcome some of these limitations.

Cross-sectional imaging

Computed tomography

A CT unit consists of a scanning gantry, sliding patient table, associated hardware and an operator console. The gantry is a ring-shaped structure containing a rotating X-ray tube head and a detector array, through which the patient moves during the examination (Figure 3.19).

Basic principles

The basic principles of CT can be summarized as follows:

- As the tube and detector rotate around the patient, a series of wedge-shaped projections are taken at up to 1000 incremental projection angles around the patient (Figure 3.20)
- This is repeated multiple times as the patient travels through the gantry, either sequentially as a series of separate slices or continuously as a volumetric helix (in spiral or helical CT)
- As the amount of X-ray attenuation by the patient has been recorded by the detector at each projection angle, the average attenuation of each volume element (voxel) in that particular section of the patient can be calculated (by iterative processes or filtered back projection)
- This gives each voxel a value (in units known as Hounsfield units (HU)) directly related to how much it has attenuated the X-ray beam
- Hounsfield units are related to the X-ray attenuation of pure water, so that water has a value of 0.0 HU, fat is −50 HU, bone is >100 HU and air is −1000 HU.
- The Hounsfield units of each voxel can be displayed on a greyscale monitor as pixels of varying brightness.

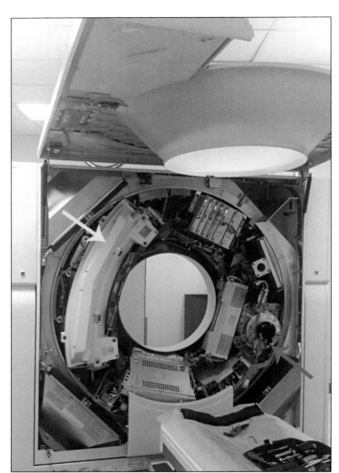

3.19 The interior of a 4-slice CT gantry (open for servicing). The X-ray tube head (red arrow) is clearly visible, with the detector array (yellow arrow) arranged exactly opposite.

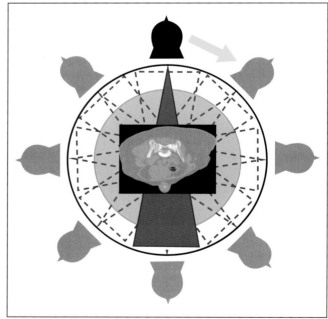

3.20 Rotation of the X-ray tube around the patient. For simplicity the number of projection positions has been reduced to eight; in reality up to 1000 projections may be obtained. For each projection, a wedge-shaped primary X-ray beam passes through the patient and is recorded by the opposing detector. The circular region where all of these projections overlap is termed the scan field of view. Body parts outside the scan field of view will not be correctly imaged.

Single slice CT detectors only record one slice at a time, but multislice detectors can record anything from 2 to over 100 slices at a time. Previously, CT has required the patient to be anaesthetized in order to limit motion artefact as the patient moves through the gantry. However, the advent of multislice/multidector technology has significantly reduced scan times (to less than 10 seconds in some cases), and their increasing use in the veterinary sector means that CT examination is possible in only lightly sedated patients.

The ability to reconstruct images with differing processing algorithms of various levels of spatial frequency, slice thickness and contrast allows images to be optimized to display specific tissues ('soft tissue algorithm and window level/width' or 'bone algorithm and window level/width'). For most musculoskeletal imaging, bone algorithms are necessarily required, but soft tissue reconstructions are still valuable (Figure 3.21).

Images can also be reconstructed in multiple planes (multiplanar reconstruction (MPR)), often allowing a better appreciation of the extent of lesions (Figure 3.22). Volume or surface rendering techniques can be used to construct three-dimensional representations of structures; these are not often required from a diagnostic standpoint, but are useful in enhancing understanding of pathology, or for surgical planning purposes (Figure 3.23).

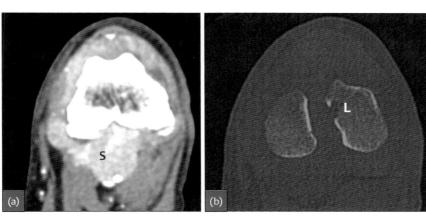

3.21 (a) Soft tissue and (b) bone transverse reconstructions of the stifle of a dog with a periarticular histiocytic sarcoma. The bone reconstruction is useful for demonstrating subtle cortical destruction and bone lysis (L) of the lateral femoral condyle and the soft tissue reconstruction highlights the large soft tissue mass present (S).

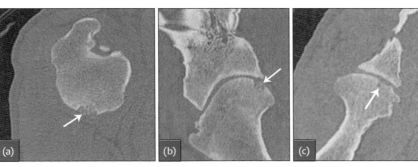

3.22 Multiplanar reconstructions (MPR) in the (a) transverse, (b) sagittal and (c) dorsal planes of the shoulder of a dog with a caudal humeral head osteochondrosis lesion. The lesion (arrowed) is relatively difficult to detect in the dorsal plane, but clearly visualized in the sagittal and transverse planes.

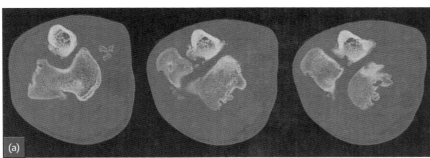

3.23 (a) Representative transverse images and (b) three-dimensional surface renderings of the bones of the elbow of a dog with severe joint incongruency (the levels of the transverse images are indicated by the dotted lines). There is abnormal morphology of the humeral condyle and moderate lateral subluxation of the radial head. Extensive secondary osteophyte formation is evident. Although the reconstruction is not necessary for the diagnosis, appreciation of the morphological changes is much easier with a three-dimensional representation. The levels of the transverse images 1–3 in (b) relate to the images from left to right in (a).

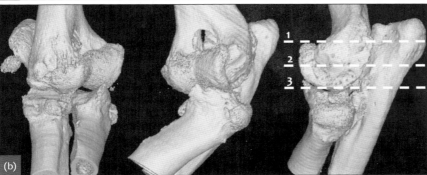

Indications

As CT utilizes X-ray transmission through the patient to construct images, it follows that conditions likely to be clearly represented on radiographs are well imaged by this modality. However, the tomographic (slice-based) nature of CT removes superimposition. Furthermore, post-acquisition computer processing and reconstruction frequently means that subtle, ambiguous or even unde-tected findings on radiographs are well depicted. The understanding of complex lesions can also be consider-ably enhanced. In particular CT is well suited to character-izing osseous abnormalities of complex three-dimensional structures such as the skull and pelvis (Figure 3.24), although its increased soft tissue resolution compared with radiography means that imaging of soft tissue path-ology can also be rewarding.

CT is used with increasing frequency in the diagnosis of elbow disease, particularly pathology involving the medial coronoid process and for humeral intracondylar fissure (HIF), previously termed incomplete ossification of the humeral condyle (IOHC) (Carrera *et al.*, 2008; Groth *et al.*, 2009). The advantages of the use of CT for imaging these conditions are clear when the location of likely lesions is considered. The region of the medial coronoid is not well depicted on conventional radiographs (Figure 3.25) and in order to clearly depict a humeral intracon-dylar fissure the primary X-ray beam needs to be aligned nearly parallel with the fissure (Figure 3.26). In both cases oblique radiographic views can be attempted (the 15-degree craniolateral–caudomedial oblique for medial coronoid pathology and the 15-degree craniomedial–caudolateral for IOHC), but some superimposition of other structures will remain (particularly of the olecranon in the case of the IOHC oblique view). The cross-sectional nature of CT means that both lesions are very clearly visible on transverse images obtained with this modality.

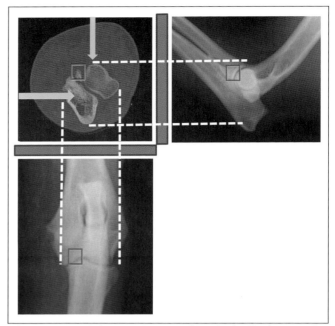

3.25 The medial coronoid process of the ulna (red box) is not well visualized on standard mediolateral and craniocaudal radiographs of the elbow due to superimposition (yellow arrows represent the direction of the primary X-ray beam for these views). A lack of superimposition means that the fragmented coronoid is easily visualized on a transverse CT image of the elbow.

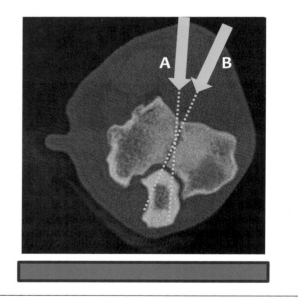

3.26 A transverse CT image demonstrating why a humeral intracondylar fissure is not well represented on a standard craniocaudal radiograph of the elbow; the primary X-ray beam (A) is not parallel to the fissure. An oblique view (B) will better depict the fissure, but some superimposition of the olecranon will still remain on the radiograph.

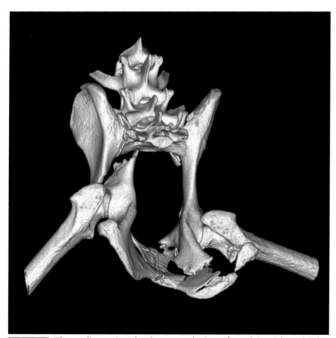

3.24 Three-dimensional volume rendering of a pelvis with multiple comminuted fractures. Characterization of the fractures in complex structures such as the pelvis is enhanced by the three-dimensional reconstruction.

Contrast CT

The computed tomographic imaging of purely osseous disease is unlikely to be significantly enhanced by the administration of intravenous or systemic contrast material; however, soft tissue lesions are frequently better observed by their pattern of contrast uptake. This is espe-cially true for neoplastic disease, and even neoplastic lesions of bone (for example primary bone tumours or metastatic neoplasia) will show an appreciable degree of contrast enhancement.

CT arthrography has been employed in the investigation of some musculoskeletal diseases, principally those affecting the scapulohumeral joint and stifle (Tivers *et al.*, 2009).

Magnetic resonance imaging

In contrast to the other modalities, which involve passing some sort of sound wave or X-ray beam into the patient and recording either what passes through or is reflected back, MRI works on entirely different principles. In MRI the signal recorded is actually generated by the patient itself, through a complex combination of manipulation of strong magnetic fields and radiofrequency pulses. The technique makes use of the fact that most biological tissues contain an abundance of protons (hydrogen atom nuclei). These protons all generate tiny individual magnetic fields, which under normal circumstances are randomly oriented and cancel one another out.

Basic principles

The basic principles of MRI can be summarized as follows:

- The patient is placed inside a powerful magnet with a magnetic field that is aligned longitudinally with the bore of the MRI machine
- The strong external magnetic field results in alignment of the tiny individual magnetic fields generated by the billions of protons within the patient's tissues, creating a so-called net magnetization vector in the longitudinal direction
- A perpendicular radiofrequency pulse applied at a specific (resonating) frequency tilts the net magnetization vector away from longitudinal towards a transverse orientation
- The transverse orientation of the net magnetization vector produces a small but recordable radiofrequency signal
- When the applied radiofrequency pulse ceases the net magnetization vector slowly returns to longitudinal alignment (relaxes) and the small signal quickly decays
- The initial strength and subsequent rate of decay of the signal largely depends on specific characteristics of the tissue in which the protons are located (known as the T1 and T2 relaxation times of the tissue)
- The manipulation of the frequency of radiofrequency pulses and timing of signal recording is used to emphasise (weight) T1 or T2 properties of tissues and generate high tissue contrast
- Slices within the patient are selected and spatially encoded by varying the magnetic field to allow construction of images (in any plane of orientation).

MRI offers similar advantages to CT; its cross-sectional nature means that superimposition of body structures is not a concern. Multiplanar reconstruction is possible for sequences that acquire a volume of data and other non-volumetric sequences can be acquired in multiple planes (typically transverse, sagittal and dorsal/frontal) (Figure 3.27).

The basic T1- or T2-weighted sequences are supplemented by a large number of variations, which can result in the suppression of fat (short tau inversion recovery (STIR)) or fluid (fluid-attenuated inversion recovery (FLAIR)) or accentuate other properties of tissues. The necessary

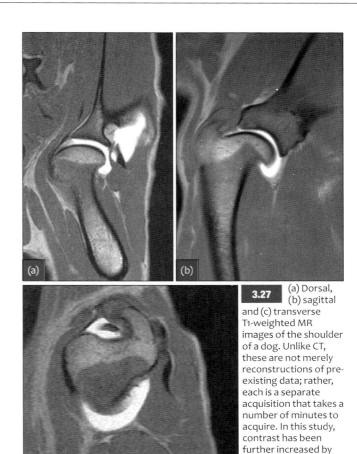

3.27 (a) Dorsal, (b) sagittal and (c) transverse T1-weighted MR images of the shoulder of a dog. Unlike CT, these are not merely reconstructions of pre-existing data; rather, each is a separate acquisition that takes a number of minutes to acquire. In this study, contrast has been further increased by the injection of a gadolinium-based contrast medium into the shoulder joint.

acquisition of multiple sequences results in prolonged scan times and general anaesthesia is a prerequisite for MRI in animals.

Indications

Without doubt the prime advantage of MRI lies in its superior soft tissue resolution which far exceeds that of the other modalities, with only ultrasonography being remotely comparable. This makes it ideally suited to imaging of conditions affecting muscles and nervous tissue. Bone can also be well imaged, although the spatial resolution is mildly inferior to that achieved by CT.

MRI excels in the imaging of the central nervous system and therefore musculoskeletal conditions with a suspected neurological aetiology are best imaged with this modality, as are myopathies (either inflammatory or neurogenic). In situations where soft tissue pathologies are common or suspected, such as the shoulder joint, MRI can be a useful technique. The shoulder and stifle are the joints that are currently most often evaluated with MRI (Schaefer *et al.*, 2010). Although reasonable broad agreement has been found between abnormalities identified on shoulder MRI and surgical findings, there were still some discrepancies in the exact pathology identified, particularly with respect to the supraspinatus tendon (Murphy *et al.*, 2008). The use of MR arthography may improve the visualization of the important structures of the shoulder region (Schaefer *et al.*, 2010), but clinical studies validating its use are currently lacking. Obtaining high quality images can be more difficult for smaller joints and unfamiliarity with the normal MRI appearance can make interpretation challenging.

Ultrasonography

Ultrasonography uses the production and reflection of ultra-high frequency (>1MHz) sound waves to generate an image. There is no involvement of ionizing radiation.

Basic principles

The basic principles of ultrasonograhy can be summarized as follows:

- A beam of sound waves is generated by the ultrasound probe by the high frequency deformation of a piezoelectric crystal as it is subjected to an alternating electrical current
- The sound waves travel into the patient until they encounter an interface and are reflected back to the probe as an echo
- The probe also acts as a receiver; reflected (echo) sound waves are able to deform the piezoelectric crystal and produce a voltage (signal)
- This signal is converted into an image by displaying the depth of the reflected interface and the strength of the returning echo as its brightness
- The process is continually repeated, building a real-time image that is constantly updated.

Indications

Ultrasonography is comparatively underutilized in the investigation of musculoskeletal problems in small animals, but with a skilled and experienced operator it can provide much additional information. However, it would be rare for it be used as the sole imaging modality and it is probably best thought of as an adjunct to radiography or other forms of advanced imaging. Additionally, the difficulty of evaluating static images after acquisition represents a significant limitation.

With ultrasonography, only the external surface of bone is visible as the soundwaves are unable to adequately penetrate normal cortex and therefore most osseous lesions are not well characterized. However, lesions causing defects in the cortical surface such as primary and meta-static bone tumours and severe osteomyelitis can be imaged more successfully, and bone surface pathology such as periosteal reaction and osteophyte formation can be evaluated.

Ultrasonography does allow excellent assessment of soft tissue lesions and is particularly well suited for the evaluation of muscle and tendon injuries. Its usefulness in periarticular pathology of the shoulder has been estab-lished, allowing assessment of the supraspinatus, infra-spinatus and biceps brachii musculotendinous structures (Figure 3.28). It is considered superior to arthrography for evaluation of the biceps tendon and sheath (Bruce *et al.*, 2000). Similarly, its value for investigating pathology of the common calcaneal tendon is well recognized (Lamb and Duvernois 2005; Caine *et al.*, 2009). Ultrasound eval-uation in expert hands has also proved useful in the examination of the menisci of the stifle when assessing for pathology of the medial meniscus, but is more limited for evaluation of the cruciate ligaments (Gnudi and Bertoni 2001; Mahn *et al.*, 2005).

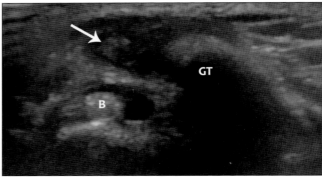

3.28 Transverse ultrasonographic image of the proximal humeral region. The biceps tendon (B) can be identified in transverse section surrounded by a moderate anechoic tendon sheath effusion. There is a heterogeneous, predominantly hypoechoic region with a small focus of mineralization (arrowed) adjacent to the greater tubercle (GT), representing tendinopathy of the supraspinatus tendon insertion.

Scintigraphy

Scintigraphy (or nuclear medicine) uses a radiopharma-ceutical agent to identify a system or physiological process within the body. The radionuclide most often used is technetium 99m (TC99m), and in musculoskeletal imaging this is usually coupled with either methylene diphosphonate (MDP) or hydroxymethylene diphospho-nate (HDP).

Basic principles

The basic principles of scintigraphy can be summarized as follows:

- The radiopharmaceutical agent is carefully injected intravenously, in accordance with appropriate radiation safety protocols
- It localizes to the soft tissues 5–20 minutes post-injection and to the skeletal system after approximately 2 hours
- The location of the agent within the body is identified as the radioactive isotope decays with the emission of gamma photons with energy of 140 keV
- Gamma photons are detected by a large sodium iodide crystal coupled to a series of photomultiplier tubes in a device called a gamma camera.

The principle advantage of scintigraphy lies in its ability to provide functional information, as it gives evidence about underlying physiological processes. This is opposed to the anatomical imaging of radiography, MRI or CT, where essentially only structural changes are seen. Its main dis-advantage is that, while it is sensitive in identifying areas of pathology, the changes seen are often non-specific and supplementary imaging is often required.

Indications

Like ultrasonography, nuclear medicine is probably under-utilized in small animal musculoskeletal imaging, but its popularity in the investigation of lameness in equine patients illustrates how useful it can be in certain cases. The standard gamma cameras used in equine centres can easily be used for small animal patients by lowering them to the ground and imaging the patient on the head of the camera. Limited availability and the difficulties of manag-ing a radioactive patient are likely reasons for why it has not been more widely used.

It is most often used in cases of occult lameness where a source of pain is difficult to localize, or where conventional imaging has been unrewarding (Schwarz *et al.*, 2004). It can also be of value in determining if potentially incidental findings should be considered as a potential cause of lameness (Figure 3.29).

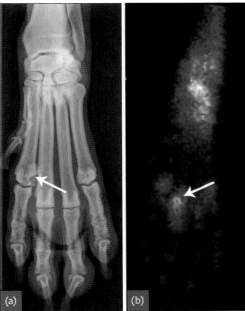
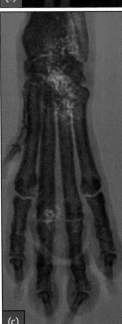

3.29 (a) Dorsopalmar radiograph of the manus showing multipartite/fragmented sesamoids of the metacarpophalangeal joint of the second digit (arrowed). This is a potential cause of lameness in some dogs. (b) The scintigraphic image of the corresponding region shows a region of increased uptake of radiopharmaceutical agent in the third digit (arrowed). (c) Fusion of the two images using appropriate software shows the increased activity to be related to the metacarpophalangeal joint of the third digit, indicating the sesamoid changes are unlikely to be significant in this case. The significance of the apparent increased uptake is in part interpreted by comparison with images from the contralateral limb, but the clinician needs to be aware of the possibility of bilateral pathology.

Principles of interpretation

Detailed discussion of the principles of interpretation for all of the diagnostic imaging modalities are beyond the scope of this chapter and only radiological interpretation will be considered in depth. Radiography represents the most widely used modality and most musculoskeletal cases will be radiographed at some stage of their work-up. However, interpretation of all imaging modalities is inherently similar (Figure 3.30).

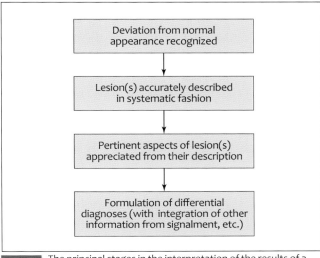

3.30 The principal stages in the interpretation of the results of a diagnostic imaging study.

Interpretation of musculoskeletal radiographs can be challenging; the large degree of normal variation that exists and the sometimes subtle changes that can result from many conditions mean that detection of significant abnormalities is often difficult. Even if a formal radiographic report is not generated, adoption of a systematic approach to the examination and evaluation of the images is recommended. Additionally, there is no substitute for familiarity with the region being examined and consultation with examples of normal radiographic anatomy (be that the patient's contralateral limb, another patient's radiographs or a radiographic atlas) is useful.

Viewing radiographs

Radiographic images, either on display monitors or viewing boxes, are best viewed in an environment with low ambient lighting and as free as possible from distraction. The use of multiple monitors or light boxes is useful, especially for viewing series of orthopaedic studies. If monitors are used they should be of full diagnostic quality; the image display and resolution of most conventional computer displays is not sufficient to be used for accurate interpretation of radiographs in particular.

There are several schemes that have been formulated to aid the reading of radiographs. Some of these advocate a geometric search pattern, starting from the outside of the image and working centrally or *vice versa*. Others suggest a system-based approach, considering all the visible organ systems and checking these for abnormalities (Figure 3.31); alternatively a checklist in the form of a mnemonic (ABCDE) can be followed (Figure 3.32).

Organ	Aspects to consider
Joints	• Alignment • Joint space width • Osteophytes/enthesophytes • Subchondral bone (lysis/sclerosis)
Bone	• Periosteum/endosteum • Cortex • Medulla
Soft tissue	• Muscles • Fascial planes • Skin surfaces

3.31 Example of a system-based approach for reviewing musculoskeletal radiographs.

Area	Aspects to consider
A: alignment	• Evidence of fractures/loss of cortex • Alignment of joints • Abnormal morphology of long bones
B: bones	• Opacity (general and focal) • Corticomedullary distinction • Trabecular pattern
C: cartilage	• Joint effusion • Subchondral sclerosis • Joint space width • Vacuum phenomenon
D: devices	• Positioning of orthopaedic implants • Implant loosening/failure/associated osteomyelitis
E: everything else	• Soft tissue changes (swelling/atrophy/opacity)

3.32 A mnemonic for reviewing musculoskeletal radiographs. Note cartilage is not radiographically distinguishable under normal circumstances, but is used as a proxy for 'joint' as 'ABJDE' would be a poor mnemonic.

Although they vary in nature, the ultimate purpose of all of these approaches is similar; to ensure that the reader critically examines all the visible structures in the radiograph being considered. The exact method used is not critical, but it is important that a systematic approach is adopted and, once developed, that this approach is applied consistently.

Reporting radiographs

Only once a radiograph has been fully evaluated can it then be interpreted, either mentally or through the formulation of a radiographic report. A typical, formal report has up to seven sections (Figure 3.33). Even if there is no requirement to generate an actual report, appreciating similar aspects when assessing radiographs can help to develop a methodical approach.

Characterization of any lesion appreciated on a radiograph is best achieved by the consideration of five fundamental aspects of its radiographic appearance, often called radiographic or Röntgen signs (Figure 3.34).

It should be apparent that if all recognized lesions are considered in terms of these signs, then no significant aspect will be missed. Perhaps more importantly, consideration of these aspects is crucial in determining a list of plausible differential diagnoses for the lesion identified (Figure 3.35).

The concept of radiographic opacity is a basic one, but fundamental to radiological interpretation. Radiopacity is essentially a function of effective atomic number and physical density (Figure 3.36). Common misconceptions include failure to appreciate that fat has a distinct (lesser) radiopacity to soft tissue and a mistaken belief that soft tissue and fluid have differing radiographic opacities when they are actually indistinguishable (Figure 3.37).

Report section	Considerations	Comments
Patient identification	Identify the species, age, sex, and breed/type	Even if these are known, careful re-evaluation of them should influence the list of differential diagnoses
Radiographs examined	List the regions, views, contrast studies (and dates if serial radiographs)	This ensures that no studies are unevaluated and may highlight missing images
Radiographic quality	Consider patient positioning, centring, collimation, exposure, labelling and artefacts	Significant deficiencies in quality may hamper diagnosis or create a misdiagnosis
Radiological description	Description of all observed abnormalities in terms of their radiographic signs	This should be restricted to descriptive terms and not interpretative (i.e. a 'region of radiolucency' not a 'region of osteolysis')
Conclusion	Succinct summary of key finding(s)	As above
Radiological diagnosis	List the diagnosis or differential diagnoses for all significant findings	Differential diagnoses should be prioritized with most likely listed first based on radiological findings AND signalment
Recommendations	For repeat/serial radiographs, radiographs of other regions, use of other modalities, performance of further diagnostic tests, surgery	Emphasizes the role of imaging in overall case management

3.33 The main components of a radiological report.

Radiographic (Röntgen) sign	Consideration	Relevant musculoskeletal examples
Size	The size of a specific lesion or changes in the size of a structure	A 35 x 25 mm region of radiolucency within the distal radius A reduction in ulnar length due to premature closure of the distal ulnar physis
Shape	The overall shape of a lesion and also the shape of its margins and its definition	A well defined, smoothly marginated circular radiolucency in the proximal tibia representing a bone tunnel A poorly defined, irregularly shaped, focal region of radiolucency due to an osteosarcoma
Position	The anatomical location of a lesion or the displacement of a structure from its normal position	Mineralization adjacent to the greater tubercle in a supraspinatus tendinopathy Distal displacement of the medial fabella in a gastrocnemius avulsion
Opacity	In terms of the five basic radiographic opacities, i.e. gas, fat, soft tissue/fluid, bone and metal	A focal region of intramedullary sclerosis in panosteitis Gas lucency in the soft tissues in postsurgical emphysema
Number	The number of lesions identified or a variation from the normal number of structures present	Three focal radiolucencies within the ilial wing Additional digits in polydactyly

3.34 The five radiographic or Röntgen signs that must be considered when evaluating an identified lesion on a radiograph.

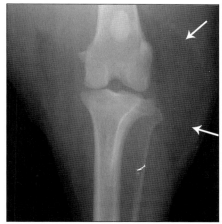

3.35 Caudocranial radiograph of a dog with a palpable swelling adjacent to the stifle. This swelling can be identified radiographically (delineated by the arrows). An accurate characterization of the lesion in terms of its radiographic signs would read as follows: 'There is a single large (20 x 60 mm) smoothly marginated and well defined, oval-shaped, mass of fat opacity present in the soft tissues lateral to the stifle joint. No changes are seen in the adjacent bones'. Correct identification of the lesion as being of fat opacity, with non-aggressive characteristics, means that the appropriate differential diagnosis of a benign lipoma is quickly achieved.

Radiographic appearance	Effective atomic number (Z)	Approximate density (g/cm³)	Tissue/material
Black (radiolucent)	7.8	0.001	Gas (air)
Dark grey	6.5	0.92	Fat
Mid grey	7.5 7.6	1.00 1.04	Fluid Soft tissue
Light grey/white	12.3	1.65	Mineral (bone)
Bright white (radiopaque)	High	High	Metallic

3.36 The five radiographic opacities are gas, fat, fluid/soft tissue, mineral and metallic. The reason for their relative radiopacities is related to their physical density and effective atomic number.

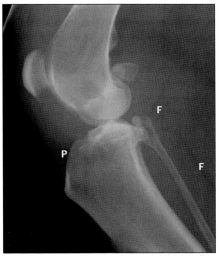

3.37 Mediolateral radiograph of the stifle of a dog. There is severe cranial displacement and compression of the infrapatellar fat pad (P) and caudal displacement of the fascial planes (F) of the caudal musculature. Fat radiopacity allows identification of the infrapatellar fat pad and fascial planes and detection of an increase in synovial mass (likely joint effusion). However, the inability to distinguish soft tissue from fluid limits the definitive conclusion that this represents joint effusion and in fact this was a synovial tumour. Subtle lysis of the distal patella can be appreciated.

Although the radiographic opacities are presented as five discrete categories, the thickness of the tissue concerned is also influential. A large thickness of soft tissue will have a similar apparent opacity to a small thickness of bone. Similarly, bone surrounded by only a small amount of soft tissue due to muscle atrophy may appear less radiopaque than equivalent bone covered with a normal amount of soft tissue.

Interpretation of findings

In many cases the initial assessment must be whether the radiographic appearance represents deviation from normal. While comparison to the contralateral joint is often useful, bilateral disease should always be considered, particularly for developmental and degenerative conditions such as elbow dysplasia, osteochondrosis, cranial cruciate ligament disease or degeneration of the plantar tarsal ligaments. Traumatic conditions are more likely to be asymmetrical and indeed, comparison with the contralateral joint is a fundamental part of the assessment of some conditions such as tibial tuberosity avulsion (Figure 3.38). Although physeal closure times have been established (Figure 3.39), there exists such a wide variation that comparative films are particularly useful when the skeleton is immature.

Once significant changes in the tissues and/or structures seen on musculoskeletal radiographs have been identified, differential diagnoses need to be considered for the lesions.

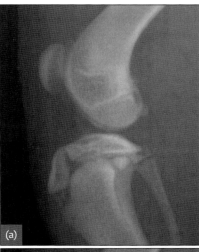
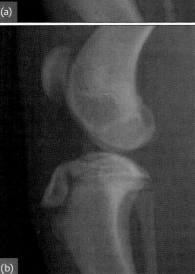

3.38 Mediolateral radiographs of the (a) right and (b) left stifles of a dog. There is an avulsion of the tibial tuberosity of the right stifle and very mild proximal displacement of the tibial tuberosity can be seen. However, establishing the diagnosis is easier when comparison is made with the normal left stifle (the possibility of bilateral disease should be considered). This dog also has a Salter–Harris Type II fracture and minor displacement of the proximal tibial physis as well as a greenstick fracture of the fibula.

Bone	Location of physis/ ossification centre	Approximate age of closure/fusion
Scapula	Supraglenoid tubercle	4–7 months
Humerus	Greater tubercle Proximal physis Medial epicondyle Lateral and medial parts of condyle	4 months 10–13 months 6 months 6–9 weeks
Radius	Proximal physis Distal physis	5–11 months 6–12 months
Ulna	Olecranon Anconeal process Distal physis	5–10 months 3–5 months 6–12 months
Carpal bones	Accessory carpal	2–5 months
Metacarpals/ metatarsals	Proximal metacarpals/ metatarsals 1 Distal metacarpals/ metatarsals 2–5	6 months 5–7 months
Phalanges	Proximal	4–6 months
Pelvis	Acetabulum Iliac crest Tuber ischii	4–6 months 12–24 months 8–10 months
Femur	Neck Greater trochanter Lesser trochanter Distal physis	6–11 months 6–10 months 8–13 months 6–11 months
Tibia	Medial and lateral condyles Tibial tuberosity Proximal physis Distal physis Medial malleolus	6 weeks 6–8 months 6–12 months 5–11 months 5 months
Fibula	Proximal physis Lateral malleolus	6–12 months 5–11 months
Calcaneus	Tuber calcis	3–8 months

3.39 Approximate age of closure for the major physes of dogs visible on radiographs.
(Data from Sumner-Smith, 1966; Morgan, 1981; Dennis, 2010)

Radiographic signs	Change	Consideration relating to musculoskeletal disease
Size	Increased	More diffuse: • Cellulitis, inflammation More focal: • Neoplasia • Joint effusion (if intra-articular) • Ligamentous injury
	Decreased	• Muscle atrophy (disuse/ neurogenic)
Opacity	Gas	• Postsurgical emphysema • Open fractures • Cellulitis with gas-producing organisms (uncommon) • Penetrating wounds • Foreign bodies (wood) may contain fine linear gas opacities
	Fat	• Lipoma/liposarcoma
	Radiopaque material	• Foreign body • Dystrophic mineralization (of tendons) • Debris on coat

3.40 Potential causes for changes seen in the soft tissues of musculoskeletal radiographs.

Soft tissues

Soft tissue changes can easily be overlooked in musculo-skeletal radiology but, frequently, alterations in soft tissue size, or occasionally opacity, can inform understanding of the pathological process. Occasionally the changes may highlight a previously unconsidered region and allow identification of a subtle lesion. Considerations for radiographically visible changes in soft tissues are summarized in Figure 3.40.

Joints

Joints are often the focus of evaluation when musculo-skeletal radiographs are examined, sometimes to the exclusion of other pathology. Joint pathology is common and can frequently result in lameness; however, incidental findings are also common and particularly seen in older animals. With the exception of bone, all the important components of joints (cartilage, joint fluid, joint capsule/ synovium, menisci) are of soft tissue opacity and so cannot be reliably differentiated in most circumstances. The use of contrast media can help to delineate some of these structures and some joints (for example the stifle) have a degree of natural contrast afforded by surrounding fat.

Joint effusions are generally only visible in the stifle, tarsus and carpus, and only in the stifle can this reliably be differentiated from extracapsular swelling. Radiographic findings that may be potentially misleading include:

- Joint space width: should always be interpreted with caution in non-weight-bearing radiographs. While gross alterations (such as subchondral bone directly in contact or markedly asymmetrical width across a joint) are usually genuine findings, artefactual changes are common. Poor patient positioning (especially for the stifle and shoulder joints) and inappropriate centring are common causes
- Irregular articular margins: are a feature of normal endochondral ossification and so may be detected in juvenile joints, particularly the femoral condyles, for several months after birth
- Periarticular mineralization: can have a variety of causes (Mahoney and Lamb, 1996), many of which are normal (specifically various sesamoids and secondary ossification centres) and some of which have questionable clinical significance (mineralizing tendinopathies). Further details of these are given in Figure 3.41.

Bones

Bone as a tissue has only a limited response to disease: essentially it can be produced or destroyed. Most bone pathology is manifested as some combination of these processes, skewed more towards one or the other. Approximately 30–50% of mineral content has to be lost from bone before this can be appreciated radiographically, and this will typically take 7–10 days from the onset of insult.

The pattern and distribution of bone lesions is important. Focal bone loss (often but not exclusively osteolysis) has very different causes to more diffuse or generalized loss (often termed osteopenia). Furthermore, the specific pattern of focal lysis exhibited is often associated with varying biological behaviour (Figure 3.42). The number of bones involved and the location of the changes within the bone can also influence the differential diagnoses that should be considered (Figure 3.43).

Mineralization	Joint location	Comments/details
Accessory ossification centres (NA)	Shoulder	Caudal glenoid rim Caudal glenoid rim avulsion (I or CS)
	Scapula	Distal acromion
Osteochondral[a] fragments (CS)	Shoulder/elbow/stifle/tarsus	Osteochondritis dissecans
	Elbow	Fragmented medial coronoid process
Osteoarthritis (I or CS)	General	
Articular fractures (CS)	General	
Ununited ossification centres (usually CS)	Elbow	Ununited anconeal process
Ligament avulsions (CS)	General	Collateral ligaments
	Stifle	Insertion/Origin of cranial cruciate Origin of long digital extensor
Soft tissue mineralization	General	Synovial osteochondromatosis (usually CS) Myositis ossificans (usually CS) Calcinosis circumscripta (I or CS)
	Hip	Heterotopic osteochondrofibrosis (von Willebrand's disease) (usually CS)
	Stifle	Meniscal mineralization (I or CS)
Mineralizing tendinopathies (I or CS)	Shoulder	Biceps tendon origin Infraspinatus insertion Supraspinatus insertion
	Elbow	Flexor origins
	Proximal femur	Gluteal insertion (greater trochanter) Iliopsoas insertion (lesser trochanter)
	Stifle	Gastrocnemius origin
	Calcaneus	Calcaneal tendon insertion
Sesamoids (NA)	Shoulder	Clavicle (brachiocephalic muscle)
	Elbow	Tendon of origin of supinator
	Carpus	Abductor pollicis longus
	Stifle	Patella (quadriceps femoris) Fabellae (lateral and medial) Gastrocnemius Popliteal (popliteus muscle)
	Tarsus	Lateral tarsal tarsometatarsal bone
		Intra-articular tarsometatarsal bone
	Metacarpo/metatarsophalangeal joint	Single dorsal (extensor tendons)
		Paired palmar/plantar (interosseus muscles)
	General (I or CS)	Bipartite/fractured/fragmented

3.41 Periarticular mineralized bodies include normal anatomical features (NA), incidental findings (I) and clinically significant pathology (CS). [a]Osteochondral describes the structure, not the aetiology, of pathology.

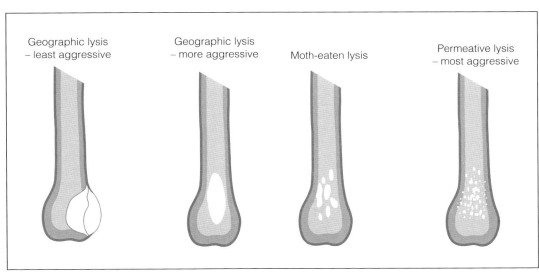

3.42 Types of focal bone destruction (lysis) seen on radiographs.

Distribution	Potential causes
Generalized (throughout skeleton)	Metabolic, congenital disease (hyperparathyroidism, hypo- and hypervitaminosis D, hypervitaminosis A (cats), mucopolysaccharidosis)
Polyostotic (multiple bones in same limb or throughout skeleton)	Disuse atrophy Multiple myeloma, lymphoma Metastatic neoplasia (more often diaphyseal) Osteomyelitis (haematogenous) Osteomyelitis (secondary to septic arthritis) Invasive soft tissue tumour (synovial if near joint)
Monostotic (multiple lesions single bone)	Metastatic neoplasia Osteomyelitis (haematogenous)
Monostotic (single lesion)	Bone cysts (rare, non-aggressive appearance) Primary bone tumour (often metaphyseal) Osteomyelitis (penetrating wound, surgery) Invasive soft tissue tumour

3.43 Distribution and potential causes of bone loss.

Increased bone opacity is often termed sclerosis. It may simply reflect an increased thickness of the bone surface but can often be seen in subchondral or peri-articular regions in association with degenerative joint disease. Other causes of polyostotic increases in bone opacity include panosteitis, metaphyseal osteopathy, bone infarction and metastatic neoplasia.

Bone production will often take the form of a periosteal reaction and the type of change seen can give information on the biological behaviour of the underlying process (Figure 3.44). Integrating all of this information (pattern of lysis, periosteal reaction and distribution of lesions) can assist in formulating appropriate differential diagnoses for identified lesions (Figures 3.45 and 3.46).

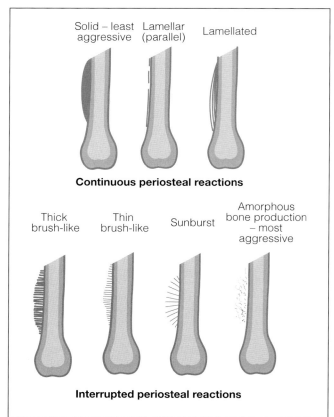

Solid – least aggressive Lamellar (parallel) Lamellated

Continuous periosteal reactions

Thick brush-like   Thin brush-like   Sunburst   Amorphous bone production – most aggressive

Interrupted periosteal reactions

3.44 Periosteal reactions from those considered least to most aggressive.

Feature	Appearance in aggressive disease	Appearance in benign disease
Lesion location	Predilection sites for primary bone neoplasia are metaphyseal regions (distal radius/ulna, proximal humerus, distal femur, proximal and distal tibia)	No typical location but metabolic disease will affect multiple bones
Pattern of lysis	Moth-eaten to permeative	Geographic if present
Cortical involvement	Likely destruction	Rarely destroyed, occasionally thinned if expansile lesions
Periosteal new bone	Interrupted patterns with poorly defined margins	Continuous with well defined margins
Zone of transition (from abnormal to normal bone)	Long and poorly defined	Short and well defined
Soft tissue swelling associated with lesion	Usually severe and focal	Mild and more diffuse
Rate of progression (on sequential radiographs)	Rapid	Slow

3.45 Features useful for differentiating benign and aggressive bone lesions. Note that benign and aggressive do not refer to benign and malignant neoplasia; osteomyelitis can have an aggressive radiographic appearance (particularly fungal causes). Mixed lesions should be categorized according to their most aggressive feature.

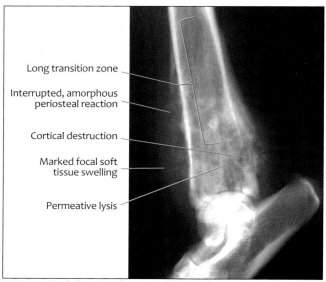

Long transition zone

Interrupted, amorphous periosteal reaction

Cortical destruction

Marked focal soft tissue swelling

Permeative lysis

3.46 Mediolateral radiograph of the distal crus of a dog. The lesion shows all the signs of aggressive bone disease listed in Figure 3.45. Additionally, the lesion is monostotic and its location (distal tibial metaphysis) is a predilection site for primary bone tumours. The final diagnosis was osteosarcoma.

Accurate detection of lesions, along with the precise evaluation and assessment of the significance of any identified findings, is fundamental to radiological interpretation. The information provided by other imaging modalities (if used and appropriate) is often complementary, and the successful integration of this information is vital to the effective use of diagnostic imaging in the management of musculoskeletal cases.

References and further reading

Bruce WJ, Burbidge HM, Bray JP *et al.* (2000) Bicipital tendinitis and tenosynovitis in the dog: A study of 15 cases. *New Zealand Veterinary Journal* **48**, 44–52

Caine A, Agthe P, Posch B *et al.* (2009) Sonography of the soft tissue structures of the canine tarsus. *Veterinary Radiology and Ultrasound* **50**, 304–308

Carrera I, Hammond GJC and Sullivan M (2008) Computed tomographic features of incomplete ossification of the canine humeral condyle. *Veterinary Surgery* **37**, 226–231

Dennis R (2010) Skeletal system: general. In: *Handbook of Small Animal Radiological Differential Diagnosis*, pp. 1–37. Elsevier Ltd, Churchill Livingston, Edinburgh

Drost WT, Reese DJ and Hornof WJ (2008) Digital radiography artifacts. *Veterinary Radiology and Ultrasound* **49**, S48–S56

Gnudi G and Bertoni G (2001) Echographic examination of the stifle joint affected by cranial cruciate ligament rupture in the dog. *Veterinary Radiology and Ultrasound* **42**, 266–270

Groth AM, Benigni L, Moores AP *et al.* (2009) Spectrum of computed tomographic findings in 58 canine elbows with fragmentation of the medial coronoid process. *Journal of Small Animal Practice* **50**, 15–22

Lamb CR and Duvernois A (2005) Ultrasonographic anatomy of the normal canine calcaneal tendon. *Veterinary Radiology and Ultrasound* **46**, 326–330

Lo WY and Puchalski SM (2008) Digital image processing. *Veterinary Radiology and Ultrasound* **49(1)**, S42–S47

Mahn MM, Cook JL and Balke MT (2005) Arthroscopic verification of ultrasonographic diagnosis of meniscal pathology in dogs. *Veterinary Surgery* **34**, 318–323

Mahoney PN and Lamb CR (1996) Articular, periarticular and juxta-articular calcified bodies in the dog and cat: A radiologic review. *Veterinary Radiology and Ultrasound* **37**, 3–19

Morgan JP (1981) *Radiology of Skeletal Disease – Principles of Diagnosis in the Dog.* Iowa State University Press, Ames, Iowa

Murphy SE, Ballegeer EA, Forrest LJ and Schaefer SL (2008) Magnetic resonance imaging findings in dogs with confirmed shoulder pathology. *Veterinary Surgery* **37**, 631–638

Schaefer SL, Baumel CA, Gerbig JR *et al.* (2010) Direct magnetic resonance arthrography of the canine shoulder. *Veterinary Radiology and Ultrasound* **51**, 391–396

Schwarz T, Johnson VS, Voute L *et al.* (2004) Bone scintigraphy in the investigation of occult lameness in the dog. *Journal of Small Animal Practice* **45**, 232–237

Sumner-Smith G (1966) Observations on epiphyseal fusion in the canine appendicular skeleton. *Journal of Small Animal Practice* **7**, 303–311

Tivers MS, Mahoney PN, Baines EA *et al.* (2009) Diagnostic accuracy of positive contrast computed tomography arthrography for the detection of injuries to the medial meniscus in dogs with naturally occurring cranial cruciate ligament insufficiency. *Journal of Small Animal Practice* **50**, 324–332

Widmer WR (2008) Acquisition hardware for digital imaging. *Veterinary Radiology and Ultrasound* **49**, S2–S8

Chapter 4

Sampling and laboratory investigation

Emma Scurrell and Gareth Arthurs

Synovial fluid collection and analysis

Collection of synovial fluid

Synovial fluid collection by arthrocentesis (a joint tap) and its subsequent analysis is one of the most frequently performed and arguably most underutilized diagnostic tests in small animal orthopaedics. Synovial fluid analysis is primarily used to investigate and differentiate between septic arthritis, immune-mediated joint disease, osteoarthritis (degenerative joint disease) and the normal joint (see Chapter 5).

Patient restraint

Synovial fluid collection should be undertaken with the patient sedated or anaesthetized to avoid discomfort and prevent inadvertent movement at a critical moment. Arthrocentesis is usually part of a wider investigation and any planned imaging studies can be undertaken during the same period of sedation or anaesthesia.

Preparation

Prior to sampling, an area of skin over the joint (approximately 5 x 5 cm) is clipped, cleaned and aseptically prepared. Sterile gloves should be worn following aseptic hand preparation.

Needles

Synovial fluid is viscous and therefore a relatively wide-bore needle should be used to maximize fluid flow through the needle. A 21 G, 2.5 cm (1 inch) needle is used for most joints. A 23 G, 1.25 cm (0.5 inch) needle may be used for small joints, e.g. most cat joints and the carpi and tarsi of small dogs. A 19 G, 3.75–5.0 cm (1.5–2 inch) needle may be needed for the elbow, stifle and particularly the shoulder joint in medium to large-breed dogs. The use of the shortest needle of adequate length gives better hand control for joint penetration.

Syringe

A larger syringe produces more negative pressure, but may be more difficult to operate in a controlled fashion while trying to accurately control needle position in a very small joint. A 2 ml syringe is used for small joints and a 5 ml syringe for larger joints. The needle should be held still and gentle negative pressure applied to the syringe to aspirate synovial fluid. The pressure should be released before withdrawing the needle.

Sampling sites

Representative joints are chosen based on the clinical signs and the suspected underlying pathology. If osteoarthritis or septic arthritis is suspected, then just the affected joint is aspirated. If immune-mediated joint disease is suspected then multiple (a minimum of four) joints are aspirated. It is usual to aspirate the small joints of the distal limbs, i.e. tarsi and carpi, as the disease is usually most severe in these joints.

Positioning

The patient is positioned to allow an approach to the most easily accessible aspect of the joint and avoid neurovascular structures. The limb and joint are held steadily in a position that allows introduction of the hypodermic needle directly into the centre of the joint with minimal capsular trauma and without striking cartilage or bone. Good technique minimizes pain associated with the procedure and reduces the risk of iatrogenic haemorrhage and minor cartilage damage. Access points for joints are illustrated in Figure 4.1.

Carpus

The carpus comprises the antebrachiocarpal (ABC), intercarpal and carpometacarpal joints; the latter two communicate. The ABC joint is the high motion joint and is used for arthrocentesis. The patient is placed in dorsal or lateral recumbency and the carpus is flexed; this opens the dorsal aspect of the ABC joint, which can be palpated as a depression between the distal radius and the carpal bones. A needle is introduced perpendicular to the skin surface, ideally between the carpal extensor tendons, but these can be difficult to identify.

Elbow

The elbow joint can be accessed through caudomedial, caudolateral or distomedial approaches. The authors believe the distomedial approach is the simplest and least likely to cause intra-articular damage. For the distomedial and caudomedial approaches, the patient is placed in

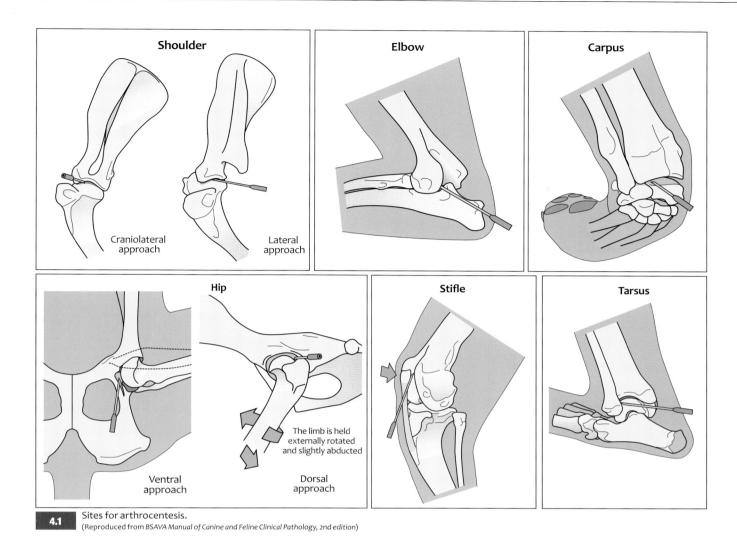

4.1 Sites for arthrocentesis.
(Reproduced from BSAVA Manual of Canine and Feline Clinical Pathology, 2nd edition)

lateral recumbency with the target limb lowermost. The elbow is held in a neutral position. For the distomedial approach, the needle is introduced 1–2 cm distal to the medial epicondyle and is directed proximally at an angle of about 45 degrees, in between the medial condyle of the humerus and the ulna. For the caudomedial approach, the needle is introduced caudal to the elbow at a point level with the medial epicondyle and directed approximately 30 degrees cranially and laterally, again in between the medial condyle and the ulna. For the caudolateral approach, the technique is the same as for the caudomedial approach, except that the patient is positioned in lateral recumbency with the target limb uppermost, and the joint is approached from the caudolateral aspect.

Shoulder

The shoulder can be approached by a craniolateral or lateral approach; the latter is arguably more straightforward. The patient is placed in lateral recumbency with the target limb uppermost. The shoulder is held in a neutral position. For the lateral approach, the acromion of the scapula is palpated, the needle inserted 1–2 cm immediately distal to it and directed medially and 30 degrees proximally. Traction can be applied to the distal limb to open the shoulder joint. The shoulder is a relatively deep joint and the needle will need to be inserted to a depth of between 1–5 cm depending on patient size. For the craniolateral approach, the needle is directed into

the cranial aspect of the joint proximal to the greater tubercle. The needle is directed caudally and medially by about 40 degrees.

Tarsus

The tarsus (tibiotarsal or talocrural joint) is one of the hardest joints to successfully aspirate, particularly if there is no effusion. The tarsus may be approached from the plantarolateral, plantaromedial, dorsomedial and dorsolateral aspects. The patient is best placed in dorsal recumbency for cranial access, sternal recumbency for caudal access, or lateral recumbency for medial or lateral access. The malleoli are palpated and the joint flexed and extended; the joint capsule may be felt bulging under the skin, particularly if digital pressure is applied to the opposite side of the joint; this can help with accurate needle placement. The needle is placed just axial to the malleoli, on the cranial or caudal aspects.

Stifle

The stifle is probably the most frequently aspirated joint; often as part of the investigation to confirm the degenerative nature of the arthropathy accompanying cranial cruciate ligament failure, or to investigate for septic arthritis as a complication of surgery. The patient is placed in dorsal recumbency with the limb extended caudally; this gives access to the cranial aspect of the stifle. The stifle is flexed, the patellar ligament is palpated and the needle introduced medial or lateral to it and directed into the centre of the joint but not so far as to encroach on the cruciate ligaments. Alternatively, the needle may be introduced just lateral to the patellar ligament with the joint partially flexed. Digital pressure is applied to the medial aspect and the needle directed proximally and adjacent to the lateral trochlear ridge of the femur.

Hip

The patient is placed in lateral recumbency with the affected limb uppermost. The femur is externally rotated and may be slightly adducted. The greater trochanter is palpated and the needle is introduced just cranial and dorsal to it and directed into the joint at a neutral to slightly cranial angle. Needle penetration caudal to the greater trochanter risks iatrogenic sciatic nerve injury and is to be avoided. Alternatively, and less commonly, the hip may be accessed by a ventral approach with the patient in dorsal recumbency. The femur is abducted and the pectineus muscle is palpated; its origin at the iliopectineal eminence of the pelvis is at the cranioventral aspect of the acetabular fossa. The hip joint is accessed just caudo-medial to that point with the needle inserted and directed 45 degrees dorsocranially.

Interphalangeal and metacarpophalangeal/ metatarsophalangeal joints

The patient is placed in dorsal recumbency as these joints are best approached from the dorsal aspect immediately medial or lateral to the extensor tendons. The centre of the joint can be identified by palpation and flexion/extension. The joint is flexed and a small needle is directed into the centre of the joint. These joints are difficult to aspirate synovial fluid from, unless effused and, frequently, only a small volume (needle hub) is aspirated.

Submitting synovial fluid to the laboratory

- **Direct smears of synovial fluid:** compression (squash, 'crush-prep') smears made immediately at the time of sampling are often the most informative (Figure 4.2a). If the synovial fluid is of poor viscosity, using a 'blood smear' technique may be possible (Figure 4.2b). As with all fluid samples, rapid air drying of the smears (a hair dryer on low heat can be useful) will help prevent interpretative error due to cell shrinkage; e.g. neutrophils can become shrunken, dark and rounded and mistaken for small lymphocytes by the unsuspecting clinician (Figure 4.3). These slides are preferably then submitted unstained. It is also important that the smears are made at the time of sampling to avoid *in vitro* changes, including cell degeneration. The appearance of artefactual vacuolation in macrophages seen as an *in vitro* change may be confused with the cytoplasmic vacuolation seen in macrophages in osteoarthritis. In addition, macrophages and neutrophils remain active for some time after the fluid has been collected and, in the presence of iatrogenic blood contamination, macrophages can phagocytose red cells giving a false impression of a pre-existing haemarthrosis. Evidence of erythrophagia in fresh smears confirms the presence of a true haemarthrosis.
- **EDTA (ethylenediaminetetraacetic acid) tube (1 ml):** the remaining synovial fluid can be submitted in an EDTA tube to perform protein estimation and nucleated

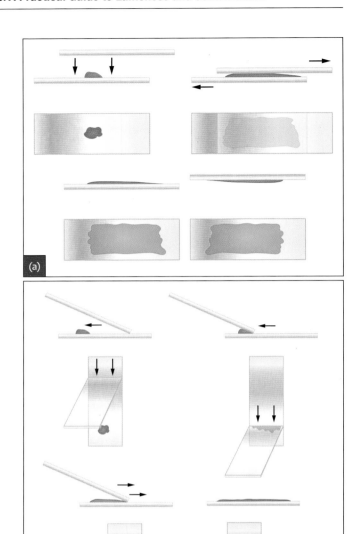

4.2 Routine techniques for the preparation of a synovial fluid smear. (a) 'Crush-prep' technique. (b) 'Blood smear' technique, which may be useful for synovial fluid with poor viscosity.

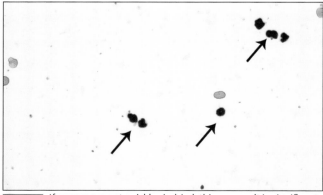

4.3 If smears are not quickly air dried, this can result in significant drying artefact and loss of cell detail. These are neutrophils (arrowed) in which drying artefact has resulted in cell shrinkage; such dark, rounded up cells may be mistaken for lymphocytes. (Wright–Giemsa stain, original magnification X400)

cell counts. Note that EDTA will interfere with both microbiology and the mucin clot test.

- **Blood culture medium:** if septic arthritis is suspected, a fresh blood culture bottle should be used (Figure 4.4): the sealing cap is removed and the rubber surface swabbed with spirit. A fresh sterile needle attached to the syringe containing the sampled fluid is inserted through the rubber cap into the bottle; negative pressure is usually present in the bottle and can vigorously aspirate the contents of the syringe. Where only very small samples are obtained, culture medium may be aspirated into the syringe before being gently 'injected' back into the bottle, maximizing the sample harvest.
- **Transport swab:** if blood culture medium is not available, a standard culture and sensitivity transport swab (e.g. with Amies transport medium) can be used, but more false-negative results are likely.
- **Heparin tube:** for the mucin clot test (rarely performed).

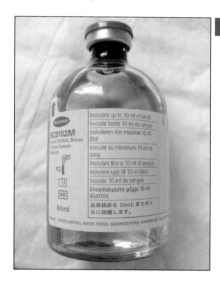

4.4 A blood culture medium bottle.

Note: where sample volume is limited, the suspected disease process should dictate what the most important tests are for that patient. For example, if sepsis were suspected the most important tests would include at least one direct smear of the synovial fluid for cytology and submission of remaining fluid for culture and sensitivity.

Whatever the sample being submitted to the laboratory, the clinician should add the signalment and pertinent case details to the submission form to assist interpretation of the findings.

Evaluation of synovial fluid
Gross examination

Examination of synovial fluid with the naked eye to observe its volume, colour, turbidity and viscosity is the first useful step. The volume of synovial fluid can be increased or decreased in disease and is often best judged using clinical experience. Normal synovial fluid is clear, colourless to pale yellow and viscous; the viscosity is attributable to its high hyaluronic acid (mucin) content. The most common reason for discolouration is haemorrhage, which results in a sample that ranges from red to yellow-orange (xanthochromia, due to haemoglobin breakdown). Distinction between true haemarthrosis and iatrogenic blood contamination is best done at the time of

sampling. True haemarthrosis typically results in a uniformly red sample at the time of sampling, whereas in the case of iatrogenic haemorrhage, the synovial fluid sample may initially be clear and then streaks of blood are seen in the synovial fluid. Increased nucleated cell counts and protein levels will result in a turbid sample. Viscosity is assessed subjectively when the synovial fluid is expelled from the needle on to the slide, or when it is suspended between the thumb and forefinger. In both scenarios, the synovial fluid should form a strand of 2.5–5 cm before it breaks. A decrease in viscosity is due to the enzymatic digestion of the glycosaminoglycan; this indicates joint disease is present but it is not aetiologically specific. Finally, it is important to communicate these findings with the pathologist, particularly if only air-dried smears are submitted.

Protein concentration

Protein concentration can be measured using biochemical techniques but it is usually measured by refractometry. Normal synovial fluid usually has a protein level of less than 25 g/l. Because normal synovial fluid does not contain clotting factors (including fibrinogen), it does not clot *in vitro*. If left to stand undisturbed, however, the synovial fluid may gel – this is referred to as thixotropism and is distinguished from clotting by gentling shaking the sample, thereby restoring its fluid state. Inflamed joints typically have increased protein levels and if true clotting does occur *in vitro*, it indicates haemorrhage and/or protein exudation into the joint.

Mucin clot test

This is a test performed to assess the degree of polymerization of hyaluronic acid (mucin) in synovial fluid. The viscosity of synovial fluid is attributed to its hyaluronic acid content and hence normal joints produce a good mucin clot with this test. EDTA breaks down hyaluronic acid and interferes with this test so heparin is preferred as an anticoagulant. The test essentially involves addition of 2.0–5.0% acetic acid to the synovial fluid. In normal joints, precipitation of the hyaluronate results in the formation of a firm clot, indicating good mucin content and quality. The quality of the clot typically deteriorates in inflamed joints (e.g. immune-mediated polyarthritis or septic arthritis) or with acute haemarthrosis. Good clot formation may still occur in some cases of degenerative joint disease. The additional information is unlikely to change the diagnosis and this test is rarely performed.

Total nucleated cell counts

A total nucleated cell count (TNCC) is typically performed in a laboratory using a haemocytometer or an electronic cell counter. Adding hyaluronidase to the synovial fluid may be required to reduce viscosity and cell clumping so that the cell count is accurate. If there is insufficient sample available, the nucleated cell count may be estimated by examining a direct preparation: in normal synovial fluid, there are usually 2–3 nucleated cells per 400X field (using a X40 lens objective) in the body of the smear. Visual estimates are, however, open to error, particularly if the thickness of the smear varies and there is cell clumping. In general, an overestimation of cellularity is likely using this method. The number of nucleated cells varies between the different joints in the same animal but as a rule of thumb, most normal joints have a TNCC of less than 3000/μl.

Synovial fluid cytology

This is often the most informative test. A practical classification scheme of cytological findings includes normal synovial fluid, haemarthrosis, degenerative arthropathy or inflammatory arthropathy (Figure 4.5). It is worth noting, however, that there may be some overlap in cytological findings between these different categories. Good communication between the clinician and the pathologist is vital because ultimately, the interpretation of the cytological findings requires knowledge of the clinical history, imaging findings and other relevant information.

Smears of synovial fluid commonly have a granular pink proteinaceous background (Figure 4.6), not to be confused with bacteria. If sufficient cell numbers are present, the cells tend to line up in rows, a phenomenon known as 'windrowing' (Figure 4.7) that indicates normal viscosity. The main nucleated cell types that are described in synovial fluid include neutrophils, lymphocytes and large mononuclear cells. Large mononuclear cells include cells derived from blood monocytes, macrophages and synovial membrane cells. It is often not possible to distinguish between these cells and it is also of no practical importance to do so. When evaluating smears it is important to identify whether an increase in neutrophils is present (normally <5% of the population) and to pay careful attention to the morphology of the large mononuclear cells.

Haemarthrosis: Normal synovial fluid should contain very few, if any, erythrocytes. If a significant number of erythrocytes are present, this could indicate true haemarthrosis (e.g. trauma, secondary to inflammation or a coagulopathy) or iatrogenic haemorrhage. The best indicators of pre-existing haemorrhage include erythrophagia in a smear made immediately following sampling, and the presence of blood breakdown pigments (e.g. haemosiderin and haematoidin) in macrophages (Figure 4.8). A significant amount of iatrogenic haemorrhage can be problematic because leucocytes from the circulation enter the sample and can make evaluation for active inflammation difficult. Knowledge of the circulating leucocyte counts can be helpful in these cases and necessitates submission of a concurrent blood sample to the laboratory.

Degenerative arthropathies: The nucleated cell count is normal or mildly increased. The dominant cell type consists of large mononuclear cells, more than 10% of which contain expanded vacuolated cytoplasm with or without pink granular material (Figure 4.9). Bouts of mild active inflammation characterized by mildly increased numbers of neutrophils and low-grade haemorrhage may be seen in some cases.

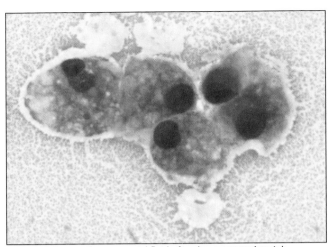

4.6 Smears from synovial fluid often have a granular pink proteinaceous background. The cells are vacuolated mononuclear cells consistent with macrophages from a joint with degenerative joint disease. (Wright–Giemsa stain, original magnification X400)

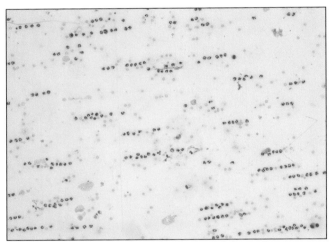

4.7 Inflammatory arthropathy. Neutrophils line up in rows indicating normal viscosity of the sample, a phenomenon known as 'windrowing'. (Wright–Giemsa stain, original magnification X200)

Inflammatory arthropathies: These can be divided into infectious and non-infectious causes. In both cases there is usually a moderate to marked increase in neutrophils (Figure 4.10). Distinction between a septic and non-infectious inflammatory arthropathy is often not possible by cytology alone. It is common not to identify bacteria in

Condition	Colour	Viscosity	TNCC	Cell type
Normal	Colourless to straw-coloured	Good	<3000 cells/µl	Mononuclear: >90% Neutrophils: <10% (and typically <5%)
Haemarthrosis	Uniformly bloody	Decreased	2500–3000 cells/µl	Mononuclear: normal to mildly increased Neutrophils: similar to that of the circulation or mildly increased
Degenerative arthropathy	As normal	Usually good but can be decreased	Usually normal or mildly increased <5000 cells/µl	Mononuclear: >90%; macrophages are vacuolated Neutrophils: <10%
Inflammatory arthropathy (infectious or immune-mediated)	Turbid and may be bloody	Variable but usually decreased	Typically markedly increased 15,000–250,000 cells/µl	Mononuclear: 5–25% Neutrophils: 75–95%

4.5 Cytological characteristics of synovial fluid. TNCC = total nucleated cell count.

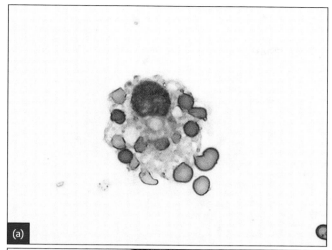

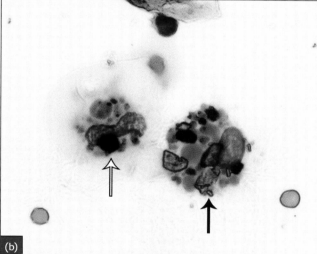

4.8 (a) A macrophage containing phagocytosed erythrocytes (erythrophagia). This can be pathological or can occur *in vitro*, in samples with iatrogenic haemorrhage. (Wright–Giemsa stain, original magnification X1000) (b) Joint with chronic haemarthrosis. Two macrophages contain intracytoplasmic haemoglobin breakdown products that include haemosiderin (dark green pigment, white arrow) and haematoidin (bright yellow pigment, black arrow). (Wright–Giemsa stain, original magnification X1000)

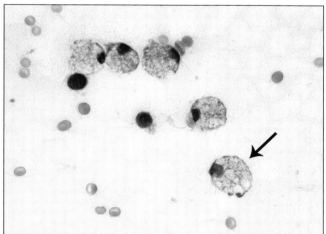

4.9 Arrow indicates a large mononuclear cell consistent with a macrophage that contains expanded vacuolated cytoplasm in a joint with degenerative joint disease. (Wright–Giemsa stain, original magnification X400)

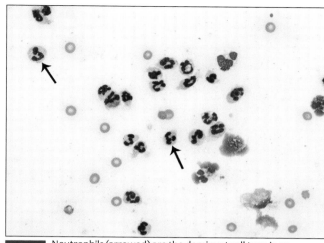

4.10 Neutrophils (arrowed) are the dominant cell type in an inflammatory arthropathy of either infectious or non-infectious aetiology. (Wright–Giemsa stain, original magnification X400)

septic synovial fluid; although the presence of karyolytic degenerative changes in neutrophils may raise the suspicion for infection, the absence of such change does not rule out sepsis.

- **Infectious arthropathies:** agents that may be involved in an infectious arthropathy (in which live microorganisms are present within the joint) include bacteria (Figure 4.11), Mycoplasmas, rickettsiae (e.g. *Ehrlichia canis*), spirochaetes (e.g. *Borrelia burgdoferi*), protozoa (e.g. *Leishmania donovani*), fungi and, rarely, viral agents (e.g. feline calicivirus in kittens). The most common causes of infectious arthritis, however, are bacterial and the most common isolates include *Staphylococcus* and *Streptococcus* spp. Other isolates may include *Escherichia coli*, *Pasturella*, *Erysipelothrix*, *Salmonella*, *Pseudomonas*, *Corynebacterium*, *Brucella* and various anaerobes.

Mycoplasmas are the smallest free-living microorganisms and the spiral-shaped *Borrelia* organisms are often very few in number, making their detection by routine microscopy highly improbable. The *Ehrlichia* morula within neutrophils and the amastigotes of *Leishmania* within macrophages in synovial fluid have been reported in dogs, but, again, this is not common.

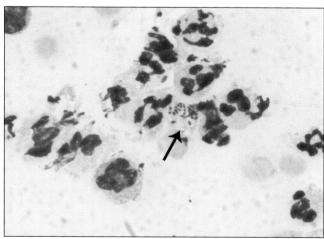

4.11 Synovial fluid from a septic joint. Intracytoplasmic bacteria are identified within the degenerate neutrophils (arrowed). (Wright–Giemsa stain, original magnification X400)

Joint infection usually affects a single joint and rarely multiple joints, depending on the underlying cause and route of infection. Surgical site infection is the commonest cause of joint sepsis. Trauma and subsequent haemarthrosis and/or pre-existing joint disease (e.g. degenerative joint disease) may predispose a single joint to haematogenous bacterial infection. When septic arthritis is associated with a bacterial endocarditis or umbilical infection, it has the potential to affect multiple joints. Certain tetracycline-responsive infections (e.g. *B. burgdorferi* and *Mycoplasma* spp.) can also cause a neutrophilic polyarthritis. Haematological and biochemical findings in septic arthritis may be normal or there may be an inflammatory leukogram, elevated serum alkaline phosphatase, hypoalbuminaemia, hypoglycaemia and thrombocytopenia.

- **Non-infectious inflammatory arthropathies:** immune-mediated arthropathies are typically shifting in nature and involve multiple joints. Even if only one joint is clinically involved, the sampling of multiple joints is indicated as it may confirm polyarthritis. As with infectious arthropathies, there is a significant increase in neutrophils but the neutrophilic component may decrease with chronicity. They are classified according to whether they are erosive or non-erosive in nature and to whether there is a known or suspected inciting cause (see Chapter 6). The detection of lupus erythematosus cells in dogs with the autoimmune disease systemic lupus erythematosus (SLE) is mentioned in most texts, but, in the authors' experience, this is a rare finding.

Joint-related neoplasia

Involvement of the joint space by a primary synovial neoplasm or by direct extension into the joint from the surrounding tissues or via metastatic spread (e.g. lymphoma, carcinoma) can occur. In general, the diagnosis of neoplasia from synovial fluid evaluation is unlikely. If a mass lesion is present, direct sampling of the mass will be more rewarding (Figure 4.12) than submitting only synovial fluid for examination. Occasionally, the synovium can be incidentally sampled during arthrocentesis and these clumps of cells should not be misinterpreted as a neoplastic process (Figure 4.13).

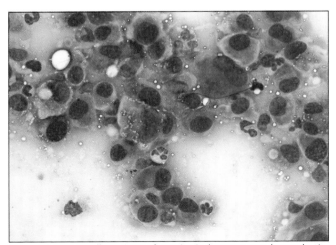

4.12 Fine-needle aspirate of a periarticular mass reveals neoplastic cells typical of a histiocytic sarcoma. (Wright–Giemsa stain, original magnification X400)

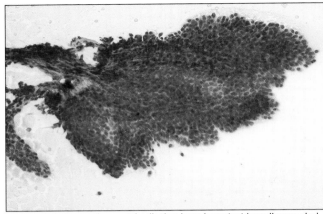

4.13 A clump of synovial cells that have been incidentally sampled during arthrocentesis. This must not be misinterpreted as being neoplastic. (Wright–Giemsa stain, original magnification X400)

Synovial fluid microbiology

When significant neutrophilic inflammation is present and infection is suspected, bacterial culture is often used to identify the agent responsible and to assist in distinguishing between an infectious and a sterile immune-mediated aetiology. However, it is very important to be aware that a negative culture does not preclude diagnosis of sepsis. In some cases where infection is suspected, a negative result may reflect infection with an anaerobe that is difficult to grow. Positive culture is more likely with samples submitted in blood culture medium. Culture of synovial membrane biopsies can also be performed. It is important to realize that there are some bacteria that will simply not be identified using routine aerobic culture techniques. These include *Mycoplasma* spp., *Borrelia* spp. and *Mycobacteria* spp.

Mycoplasmal arthritis: This is an uncommon cause of neutrophilic polyarthritis in dogs and cats (e.g. *Mycoplasma felis*) and the culture of *Mycoplasma* spp. requires specialized media and techniques (species-specific diagnostic antisera). Polymerase chain reaction (PCR) may aid with the identification of *Mycoplasma* spp.

Borrelia burgdorferi (Lyme disease): Arthritis in dogs caused by the tick-transmitted Gram-negative spirochaete *B. burgdorferi*, can be difficult to diagnose. Acute infections are characterized by a neutrophilic arthritis/polyarthritis that with chronicity goes on to manifest as a non-specific lymphoplasmacytic synovitis. Low spirochaete density and the low sensitivity of microscopy make direct observation of these organisms in synovial fluid unlikely.

> Serology is the test of choice for diagnosis. This is because identification of the organism itself (e.g. by PCR, culture or direct visualization) is difficult, not widely available and can be expensive (see below). Laboratory results should always be interpreted with other corroborative evidence of Lyme disease, namely known tick exposure, consistent clinical signs and response to treatment

- **Serology:** the presence of a positive antibody titre supports exposure to the spirochaete but does not indicate that the dog's clinical signs are definitely caused by the organism. In fact, many seropositive dogs do not become clinically ill with Lyme disease. The timing of serology is important, as serology in the early stage of infection can be negative. Under experimental conditions, antibody levels reached a maximum 90–180 days post tick exposure (Straubinger, 2000). IgM antibodies against *Borrelia* spp. are produced 1–2 weeks post infection and remain elevated for up to 2 months. IgG-ELISA positive titres are positive within 4–6 weeks, peak at 3 months and can last 1–2 years post exposure. More recently, qualitative and quantitative ELISA tests detecting antibodies directed against the C6 peptide of the organism have become commercially available. These C6 antibody tests are able to differentiate naturally infected from vaccinated dogs and the antibody response can be detected 3–5 weeks after experimental infection (reviewed in Wagner *et al.*, 2012).

- **Culture:** this is the most definitive test but special media are required, the low number of organisms makes it difficult and it can take several weeks. Collagen-rich tissue, e.g. skin or synovium, is the sample of choice for culture. Culture of blood, urine, cerebrospinal fluid or synovial fluid is generally unrewarding. Under experimental conditions, culture performed using a skin biopsy sample was positive in the first 3 months post tick exposure. By the fourth month, only 50% of the skin biopsies were positive and after antibiotic treatment, none of the biopsies were positive (Straubinger, 2000).
- **PCR:** the usefulness of PCR for detecting *B. burgdoferi* in canine synovial fluid is currently not certain. In humans, it is a sensitive test for detecting *B. burgdoferi* DNA when clinical signs are present. False-negatives have been reported, however, in experimentally infected dogs with active joint inflammation (Susta *et al.*, 2012). If PCR is to be performed for diagnosis in chronically infected or treated dogs, a skin or synovial membrane biopsy sample should be submitted, rather than blood or synovial fluid. In reality, however, the DNA of *B. burgdoferi* is rarely detected in the tissues of naturally infected dogs, particularly if formalin-fixed tissue is used as opposed to fresh tissue. Under experimental conditions, only 1.6% of blood samples were positive for *B. burgdoferi* using PCR (Straubinger, 2000).

Mycobacterial synovitis: This is generally uncommon in companion animals in the UK but may be seen in cats. Feline tuberculosis joint infection has been reported (Lalor *et al.*, 2017). Identification of acid-fast bacilli, either in synovial fluid or in a synovial biopsy sample, is very useful to confirm the presence of a mycobacterial infection, but this does not allow identification of the causative species and, in the authors' experience, the number of organisms present can be very low. Fresh tissue culture is ideal but it requires a specialized laboratory, can take up to 2–3 months and will not always yield a positive result. It may be possible to confirm mycobacterial infection and whether or not the organism is a member of the tuberculosis complex by using PCR. Fresh tissue is preferred for PCR as the risk of a false-negative is increased with formalin-fixed tissue, especially if very low numbers of organisms are present. An interferon-gamma (IFNγ) test for the ante-mortem testing of tuberculosis in cats can be performed using heparinized blood (Rhodes *et al.*, 2011).

Mycology: If fungal infection is suspected, a standard transport swab (normally with Amies transport medium) can be submitted or tissue samples can be placed in a sterile container and wrapped in a sterile saline-soaked swab to prevent desiccation.

Serological analysis
Serology
When evaluating the musculoskeletal system, there are some serum biochemical parameters that can be useful, but they are not stand-alone diagnostic tests and must be interpreted in the light of the clinical presentation and other diagnostic tests.

Alkaline phosphatase
Increased osteoblastic activity causes an increase in alkaline phosphatase (ALP) in dogs and cats, e.g. hyperparathyroidism, bone tumours, healing fractures, canine panosteitis and craniomandibular osteopathy. Note that the bone isoenzyme level of ALP can be much higher in young animals in the first 6–9 months of life (up to six times the normal limit in some cases).

Calcium, parathyroid hormone, PTHrp and Vitamin D
Multiple factors can alter serum calcium and, therefore, it must be evaluated in conjunction with serum albumin, phosphorus, urea (BUN) and creatinine concentrations. Calcium is usually measured and reported as total calcium, which predominantly includes ionized calcium (iCa) and protein-bound calcium. However, it is only the ionized calcium that is biologically active in bone formation, neuromuscular activity and clotting. Total serum calcium concentrations need to be adjusted for alterations in plasma protein (particularly albumin): e.g. if the dog is hypoalbuminaemic, the protein-bound fraction of calcium will decrease and therefore the total calcium will also decrease; however, the iCa concentration is not affected. Falsely elevated serum calcium levels can occur with lipaemia. Falsely decreased serum calcium levels can occur with prolonged sample storage and/or the use of calcium-binding anticoagulants, e.g. citrate, EDTA and oxalate. Formulas do exist to estimate the percentage of calcium bound to plasma proteins but these are fairly crude in comparison to direct measurement of the iCa concentration. Measurement of iCa is possible at specialist laboratories and is usually performed in conjunction with **parathyroid hormone (PTH)** measurement to help distinguish between primary hyperparathyroidism, parathyroid suppression, primary hypoparathyroidism and secondary hyperparathyroidism. Where PTH and iCa levels suggest parathyroid-independent hypercalcaemia, it is possible to measure **parathyroid hormone-related peptide (PTHrP)**, a hormone produced by a variety of malignant tumours (see below). Finally, it is possible to measure two forms of **vitamin D**: 25-hydroxyvitamin D (25(OH)D) and 1,25-dihydroxyvitamin D (calcitriol). The level of 25(OH)D is a good marker of vitamin D status and may be valuable when investigating hyper- and hypocalcaemia with respect to vitamin D toxicity and deficiency. Sample collection and the correct transport conditions are critical for accurate analysis of iCa, PTH and vitamin D metabolites; hence, laboratory guidelines need to be referred to before sample collection.

With respect to the musculoskeletal system, hypercalcaemia may be seen in conjunction with osteomyelitis, uncommonly with a primary destructive bone tumour (e.g. osteosarcoma), metastases to bone (e.g. carcinoma) and more commonly as a paraneoplastic syndrome (pseudohyperparathyroidism), (e.g. anal sac adenocarcinoma, adenocarcinomas at other sites, multiple myeloma and lymphoma). Mild hypocalcaemia can occur in cases of renal and nutritional hyperparathyroidism, resulting in fibrous osteodystrophy.

Creatine kinase, lactate dehydrogenase and aspartate aminotransferase

These are the enzymes that increase with skeletal muscle damage. Lactate dehydrogenase (LDH) and aspartate aminotransferase (AST) are not muscle-specific and, therefore, must not be interpreted in isolation. Creatine kinase (CK) is the most specific but is also the most short-lived. CK rises rapidly after muscle damage and peaks at about 6–12 hours. It reduces to normal within 2 days unless the muscle damage is persistent. In chronic myopathies where myonecrosis is no longer present, CK levels may be normal or only very mildly elevated. LDH takes several days to reach its peak level and several weeks to return to normal. AST peaks after 12–24 hours and remains elevated for 5–6 days. Note that CK levels are approximately double in young dogs less than 6 months old compared with mature dogs.

Potassium

Massive skeletal muscle damage or necrosis can cause hyperkalaemia because the potassium within skeletal muscle fibres is released into the circulation.

Myoglobin

Rhabdomyolysis (e.g. secondary to ischaemia, trauma or toxaemia) results in a release of myoglobin into the circulation and, if a certain concentration is exceeded, surplus myoglobin is excreted in the urine (myoglobinuria). Note that commercial urine strip tests will not differentiate between myoglobin and haemoglobin. In such cases, it can be useful to spin down a blood sample taken from the same patient (spin it down immediately after collection to avoid haemolysis): because myoglobin does not pigment the plasma, if the plasma is discoloured pink/red, it indicates that the discolouration of the urine is likely due to the presence of haemoglobin.

Immunology

Rheumatoid factor

This is a non-specific autoantibody (usually of the IgM type) that is present at low levels in normal healthy dogs and can be increased in a wide variety of inflammatory, infectious (e.g. pyometra) or neoplastic diseases. Measurement of rheumatoid factor (RF) within the serum, and/or synovial fluid, can be performed when investigating a case of polyarthritis as one of the criteria to distinguish an immune-mediated arthritis from other types of arthritis. It is not, however, a specific indicator of rheumatoid arthritis; there can be significant variation between individual dogs and false-negatives can occur. It has limited practical use in differentiating types of inflammatory joint disease, or influencing treatment.

Anti-nuclear antibodies

These are autoantibodies against nuclear components, including DNA and histones. Anti-nuclear antibody (ANA) tests can be used to support a diagnosis of SLE where at least one major clinical sign of the disease is present, but it is important to realize that positive results can be seen in a variety of infectious and non-immune-mediated diseases. For example, dogs that do not have SLE may have elevated titres for both RF and ANA. Interpretation of ANA measurement in conjunction with the clinical presentation is always important.

Synovial membrane and periarticular tissue biopsy

Synovial membrane biopsies are not routinely performed but may be indicated in the investigation of inflammatory joint disease, synovial neoplasia, in rare conditions, such as villonodular synovitis, and to obtain tissue for culture. Biopsies are performed under sterile operating conditions, either arthroscopically or by conventional arthrotomy. Conventionally, an approach is made to the joint until the joint capsule is exposed and a small section of joint capsule is excised (approximately 10 x 5 mm) by sharp dissection (usually a No. 11 blade). Care is taken to handle tissue gently so as to minimize crush-induced artefact. The sample is placed in 10% neutral-buffered formalin for histopathology. The specimen can be fixed to a piece of board (e.g. wood from a tongue depressor) using 25 G needles at either end, with the synovial surface facing up to prevent curling and aid orientation. Larger samples are likely to be more representative and diagnostic; this is particularly important when trying to rule out the presence of a neoplastic process. Malignant neoplasms are commonly associated with extensive necrosis and the pathologist relies on the presence of at least some viable tissue to make the diagnosis (Figure 4.14). Some tumours, particularly histiocytic sarcomas, often contain a significant inflammatory component; hence multiple biopsy samples are ideal to avoid 'false-negative' results. If infection is suspected then a second sample should be taken and submitted for culture and sensitivity. This is placed in a sterile container with a sterile saline-soaked swab to prevent desiccation, or in transport medium. If there is a high clinical index of suspicion for mycobacterial infection (see the section on mycobacterial synovitis above), the biopsy samples of affected synovial tissue can be divided into three to four parts: one part can be formalin fixed for histopathology and the remaining fresh tissue parts can be frozen down in separate pots, should PCR and/or culture be required.

It is important to realize that histopathology of the synovium in inflammatory conditions is often not aetiologically specific and, in many instances, evaluation of the synovial fluid will be more informative. In acute joint

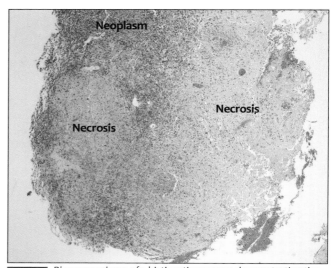

4.14 Biopsy specimen of a histiocytic sarcoma demonstrating the extensive necrosis often present in malignant tumours. The larger the biopsy specimen, the more likely it is to be diagnostic. (Haematoxylin and eosin stain, original magnification X40)

sepsis, a significant exudate may be present in the joint space but the synovium itself may only reveal acute oedema and hyperaemia with minimal inflammatory infiltrate. In less acute or chronic cases, the synovium commonly contains a lymphoplasmacytic infiltrate accompanied by synovial villous hyperplasia without a significant neutrophilic inflammatory component because neutrophils typically exude into the joint space (Figure 4.15). The lymphoplasmacytic infiltrate is not aetiologically specific and simply reflects chronic antigenic stimulation (Figure 4.16). A similar infiltrate can be found in the synovium of joints with chronic sterile/immune-mediated arthritis or degenerative joint disease.

Pannus comprises fibrovascular and histiocytic tissue that extends from the synovium and spreads over the articular cartilage, resulting in its destruction. It typically presents as a velvety membrane coating the cartilage surface. The main differential diagnoses for pannus include rheumatoid arthritis and chronic infectious fibrinous arthritis.

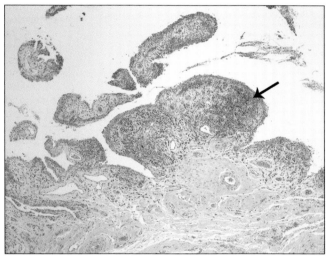

4.15 Biopsy specimen of synovium: there is a lymphoplasmacytic to lymphonodular infiltrate (arrowed) accompanied by synovial villous hyperplasia. (Haematoxylin and eosin stain, original magnification X40)

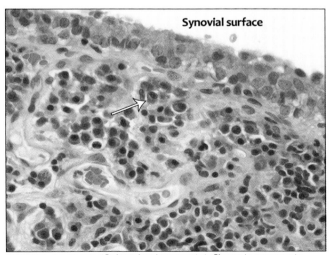

Synovial surface

4.16 A non-specific lymphoplasmacytic infiltrate is common in most inflammatory arthropathies. The arrow points to a plasma cell. (Haematoxylin and eosin stain, original magnification X400)

Bone biopsy

General considerations

Bone biopsy may be indicated to investigate structural pathology and is required to confirm definitively a diagnosis of bone neoplasia or osteomyelitis; rarely, bone biopsy may be used to investigate other bone pathology. If, however, a dog has an advanced destructive bone lesion affecting a limb and the owner is only willing to pursue amputation, then biopsy specimens from the lesion, or preferably the lesion in its entirety, can be submitted to the pathologist post amputation.

If limb-sparing surgery is a possible treatment option (e.g. an osteolytic lesion in the distal radius of a dog), the biopsy approach must be coordinated with the surgical plan so that the biopsy tract and the immediate surrounding tissue are removed *en bloc* with the diseased bone. It is reported in human patients that bone sarcomas can recur locally from tumour seeding along biopsy tracts but that fine-needle aspirates using a 22–25 G needle do not pose a significant risk of seeding (Errani *et al.*, 2013).

Technique

The main methods to biopsy a bone lesion include fine-needle aspiration (FNA), needle/core biopsy and open biopsy. In the authors' experience, FNA and core biopsy are sufficiently accurate and carry a reduced risk of complications and decreased cost. FNA and needle biopsy are complementary techniques and are often performed together, although good quality fine-needle aspirates alone can be definitive. More information on the subtype of tumour is likely to be achieved with a core biopsy.

A bone biopsy is a painful procedure that should be performed under general anaesthesia, with sterile preparation of the biopsy site. Sterile preparation can be regional, as the biopsy sample is taken by limited incision or percutaneous penetration of the skin. The area of bone to be biopsied is carefully planned from diagnostic imaging, i.e. computed tomography (CT) or radiographs. Placement of the biopsy needle is important to maximize diagnostic success. For example, the vast majority of primary bone sarcomas arise within the medullary cavity and extend outwards through the cortex. Their presence results in reactive periosteal and endosteal bone formation. The aim is to biopsy the area of osteolysis to maximize the chance of a diagnosis. To avoid false-negatives by biopsying just the reactive bone, the needle should extend well into the lesion (Figure 4.17). If possible, multiple biopsy specimens should be taken to maximize the chance of achieving a diagnosis.

Core biopsy samples may be obtained using a bone trephine (e.g. Michele 3–5 mm) or more commonly an 8–11 G Jamshidi™ needle or similar (Figure 4.18). Jamshidi™ needles are not as robust and are not ideal for very dense bony lesions. To perform a core biopsy, a stab incision is made through the skin using a No. 11 blade (Figure 4.19) and a bone biopsy needle, such as a Jamshidi™ needle, is introduced into the bone (Figure 4.20). The needle is driven through the bone; it is hard work to drive the biopsy needle through normal bone, but pathological bone is usually softer. Once the Jamshidi™ needle has gone through the bone, it is withdrawn. The stilette is used to extract the biopsy sample from the Jamshidi™ needle. Note that the sample is pushed backwards from the needle tip and out of the handle (Figure 4.21). This prevents deformation of the sample if the end of the needle becomes deformed. Figure 4.22 shows a good quality core biopsy specimen, confirming an osteosarcoma with typical production of osteoid.

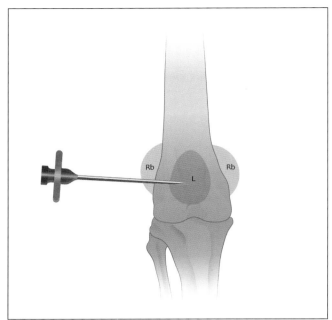

4.17 Correct placement of the needle is important to maximize the chance of a diagnosis. Reactive periosteal and endosteal bone needs to be avoided. L = lesion; Rb = reactive bone.
(Redrawn after Simon Scurrell)

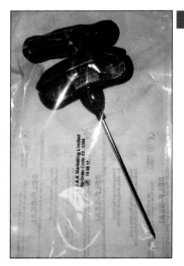

4.18 A Jamshidi™ needle.

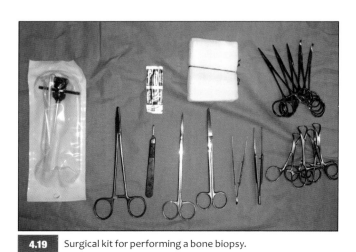

4.19 Surgical kit for performing a bone biopsy.

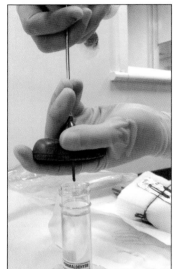

4.20 Performing a bone biopsy using a Jamshidi™ needle.

4.21 The core biopsy specimen is ejected in reverse through the handle.

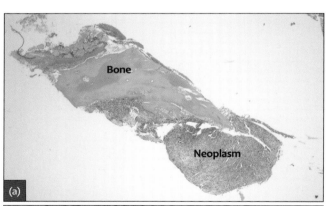

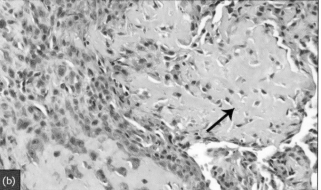

4.22 (a) Good quality trucut biopsy of an osteolytic lesion. (Haematoxylin and eosin stain, original magnification X20) (b) Osteosarcoma. The neoplastic cells are producing osteoid (arrowed), the hallmark of an osteosarcoma. (Haematoxylin and eosin stain, original magnification X200)

Bone biopsy can be a challenging procedure; if the correct area of bone is not sampled, a non-representative sample is acquired that does not achieve a representative diagnosis, which can lead to misdiagnosis. Correct biopsy location can be confirmed using fluoroscopic guidance or by taking post-biopsy radiographs showing the biopsy tracts. Rarely, if the bone is already very weak, further weakening through biopsy can result in bone fracture, either at the time of biopsy or during weight-bearing post biopsy

The use of ultrasound-guided FNA to produce direct smears for cytology has been described with a reported sensitivity of 97% (Britt *et al.*, 2007). However, an earlier report warned of the potential dangers of false-negative results achieved by FNA and that tissue core biopsy with analysis is essential if results are non-diagnostic (Samii *et al.*, 1999). In general, if the lesion is 'soft' enough, FNA may well be sufficient to confirm the presence of a malignancy. There is an erroneous perception that sarcomas do not exfoliate well, but using a 22–23 G needle and applying vacuum while moving the needle tip within the lesion frequently yields a diagnostic cell harvest (Figure 4.23). The FNA of 'hard lesions' should be performed after a core biopsy sample has been obtained.

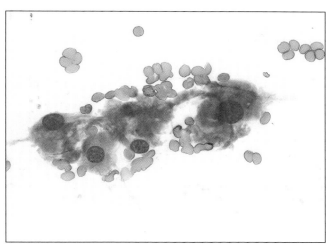

4.23 Fine-needle aspirate of an osteosarcoma. The neoplastic cells are interspersed with bright pink matrix, consistent with osteoid. (Wright–Giemsa stain, original magnification X400)

Submitting bone biopsy samples

For histopathology, samples should be fixed in 10% neutral-buffered formalin; a tissue:fixative ratio of at least 1:10 and up to 1:20 is recommended. For culture and sensitivity, the sample should be submitted in a transport swab, in a saline-moistened sterile swab within a sterile pot or in a blood culture bottle. It is very important that the specimen is accompanied by case signalment, history, clinical findings and a working clinical diagnosis.

A team approach is paramount when it comes to bone pathology, since close cooperation between the clinician and pathologist helps ensure the correct diagnosis is made. Signalment, history and clinical information together with relevant imaging findings are often suggestive of the nature of the pathology (see Chapter 11) and should be available to the pathologist. The pathologist should also be informed if there has been a previous infection or fracture at the site of biopsy.

Muscle biopsy

Muscle biopsies are rarely performed, but may be required in the diagnostic work-up of neuromuscular disease. Muscle biopsy sample processing is a very specific procedure; the laboratory and histopathologist that will analyse the sample should be contacted prior to obtaining samples to check on specific storage and transport requirements. Depending on the type of muscle pathology suspected, fresh or fresh-frozen samples might be required, with samples couriered urgently to the laboratory on ice. For the diagnosis of inflammatory or neoplastic disease, however, fixation with formalin for routine diagnostic histopathology should suffice. Acquiring the muscle biopsy sample is relatively straightforward; a standard surgical approach is made to the muscle and a small linear section (10 x 5 x 5 mm) is excised by sharp dissection (No. 11 blade) with care to induce minimal iatrogenic damage (see Chapter 10).

Additional diagnostic techniques

For the majority of cases, microscopic examination of routine sections stained with haematoxylin and eosin will be sufficient to achieve a diagnosis. The most common additional diagnostic techniques include special stains, immunohistochemistry and PCR. Special stains are used to identify suspected pathogens or demonstrate specific cell components or products. For example, Gomori methenamine silver or periodic acid–Schiff stains highlight fungal walls that are rich in polysaccharides. Other commonly used special stains for pathogens include the Gram stain for bacteria and the acid-fast Ziehl–Neelsen stain for mycobacteria (Figure 4.24).

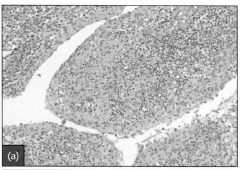

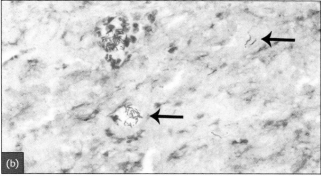

4.24 (a) A biopsy sample taken from the thickened synovium of a stifle joint in a cat reveals granulomatous inflammation. Mycobacterial infection is a very important differential diagnosis in such a case and an acid-fast stain is required to screen for the bacteria. (Haematoxylin and eosin stain, original magnification X100) (b) A Ziehl–Neelsen stain confirms the presence of acid-fast bacilli (arrowed), typical of *Mycobacterium* spp. (Haematoxylin and eosin stain, original magnification X400)

Immunohistochemistry is used to demonstrate antigen(s) within tissue sections using specific antibodies. This antigen–antibody binding complex is then visualized using a coloured histochemical reaction. Indications for immunohistochemistry include immunophenotyping and predicting prognosis in neoplasia (Figure 4.25), further characterizing cellular infiltrates and identifying pathogens.

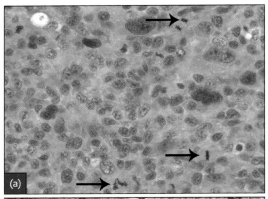

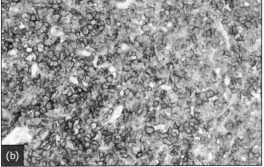

4.25 (a) A biopsy sample taken from a periarticular mass in a dog indicates a malignant neoplasm, consistent with a histiocytic sarcoma. The arrows indicate mitotic figures. Immunohistochemistry can then be performed to support the diagnosis. (Haematoxylin and eosin stain, original magnification X400) (b) Immunohistochemistry for the leucocyte antigen CD18 is performed and immunopositivity is indicated by the brown staining. This together with the haematoxylin and eosin findings, is typical of a histiocytic sarcoma. (Haematoxylin and eosin stain, original magnification X200)

PCR is a technique used to amplify a DNA sequence. Its many applications include further characterization of neoplasms, detection of genetic mutations and pathogens. PCR cannot distinguish active infection from residual DNA.

References and further reading

Britt T, Clifford C, Barger A et al. (2007) Diagnosing appendicular osteosarcoma with ultrasound-guided fine-needle aspiration: 36 cases. Journal of Small Animal Practice 48, 145–150

Clements DN (2006) Arthrocentesis and synovial fluid analysis in dogs and cats. In Practice 28, 256–262

Errani C, Traina F, Perna F et al. (2013) Review article: Current concepts in the biopsy of musculoskeletal tumours. The Scientific World Journal 5, 1–7

Gogna A, Peh WCG and Munk PL (2008) Image-guided musculoskeletal biopsy. Radiology Clinics of North America 46, 455–473

Greene C and Bennett D (2012) Musculoskeletal Infections. In: Infectious Diseases of the Dog and Cat, 4th edn, ed. C Greene, pp. 908–911. Elsevier Saunders, Missouri

Lalor SM, Clarke S, Pink J, Parry A, Scurrel E et al. (2017) Tuberculosis joint infections in four domestic cats. Journal of Feline Medicine and Surgery Open Reports 1–8

Macwilliams PS and Friedrichs KR (2003) Laboratory evaluation and interpretation of synovial fluid. Veterinary Clinics of North America: Small Animal Practice 33, 153–178

Montgomery RD, Long IR Jr, Milton JL, DiPinto MN and Hunt J (1989) Comparison of aerobic culture, synovial membrane biopsy, and blood culture medium in detection of canine bacterial arthritis. Veterinary Surgery 18, 300–303

Parry BW (1999) Synovial Fluid. In: Diagnostic Cytology and Hematology of the Dog and Cat, 2nd edn, ed. RL Cowell, RD Tyler and JH Meinkoth, pp. 104–119. Mosby Inc., St Louis

Rhodes SG, Gun-Moore DA, Boschiroli ML et al. (2011) Comparative study of IFN and antibody tests for feline tuberculosis. Veterinary Immunology and Immunopathology 144, 1–2

Samii VF, Nyland TG, Werner LL and Baker TW (1999) Ultrasound-guided fine-needle aspiration biopsy of bone lesions: a preliminary report. Veterinary Radiology and Ultrasound 40, 82–86

Straubinger RK (2000) PCR-based quantification of Borrelia burgdoferi organisms in canine tissues over a 500-day post infection period. Journal of Clinical Microbiology 38, 2191–2199

Susta L, Uhl EW, Grosenbaugh DA et al. (2012) Synovial lesions in experimental canine Lyme borreliosis. Veterinary Pathology 49, 453–461

Villiers E and Blackwood L (2005) BSAVA Manual of Canine and Feline Clinical Pathology, 2nd edn. BSAVA Publications, Gloucester

Wagner B, Freer H, Rollins A et al. (2012) Antibodies to Borrelia burgdorferi OspA, OspC, OspF, and C6 antigens as markers for early and late infection in dogs. Clinical and Vaccine Immunology 19, 527–535

Chapter 5

The normal joint

Richard Barrett Jolley and Rebecca Lewis

Common anatomical features of joints

Where adjacent bones meet, there is typically a synovial joint or diathrosis (Figure 5.1). While canine and feline joints may appear to be anatomically dissimilar, in functional terms they share numerous common features, including cartilage-covered bone ends, a joint space filled with synovial fluid, a thick membrane encasing the joint and a series of associated ligaments and tendons.

The epiphyses of the bones are coated with hyaline (articular) cartilage and encapsulated by the synovial membrane, which secretes synovial fluid into the joint space, enabling almost frictionless movement. The synovial membrane is itself surrounded by, and fused with, a thicker membrane called the fibrous capsule which in some joints can thicken to form the capsular ligaments, in contrast to extracapsular ligaments that are distinct from the joint capsule. Ligaments stabilize the joint and help restrict any abnormal range of movement. Additional cartilaginous structures called menisci are found between the two opposing cartilage surfaces in some joints. These structures have multiple roles, the most important of which are to stabilize the joint and absorb some of the shock of movement. The subchondral zones of the epiphyses are adapted to interact biochemically with the articular cartilage. Movement of the joint is facilitated by the action of muscles which merge into tendons before crossing the joint to insert on bone. In some joints, the tendon of a muscle originates within the joint. A small fluid-filled structure known as the bursa may be present between the tendon and the bone, reducing friction during movement. Within some joints, a fat pad is present to aid distribution of synovial fluid.

Joint innervation

Joints lack motor innervation but, with the exception of cartilage, most joint tissues are densely innervated with sensory neurons, allowing the animal to detect joint movement, position and pain. Sensory nerves innervate both mechanically activated receptors (mechanoreceptors) and, of particular interest to the clinician, pain receptors (nociceptors). In the adjacent muscles, mechanosensitive muscle spindles are important for control of muscle reflexes and resting muscle tone. In addition, a range of proprioceptive neurons innervate joint mechanoreceptors (Figure 5.2) and project through spinal cord ascending tracts to the brain, providing positional information (Figure 5.3). Integrity of all these neurons is important for normal function of joints; loss of sensory innervation will lead to joint instability and ultimately, joint damage. Indeed, muscle weakness has been shown to be a predictor of the onset of osteoarthritis (Roos et al., 2011). Many afferent neurons that innervate joints are typical nociceptors, expressing the peptide neurotransmitters calcitonin gene related peptide

5.1 Overview of typical synovial joint structure using the example of the stifle. The stifle has intra-articular cruciate ligaments and menisci; these structures are not common to all joints.

Receptor	Morphology	Stimulus detected	Distribution
Pacinian corpuscles	Cylindrical	Compression	Ligaments Menisci
Ruffini endings	Globular	Stretch	Joint capsule Ligaments Menisci
Golgi receptors	Fusiform	Excessive force	Tendons Joint capsule Ligaments Menisci

5.2 Mechanoreceptors associated with normal joints. (Data from the cat knee joint, Freeman and Wyke, 1967)

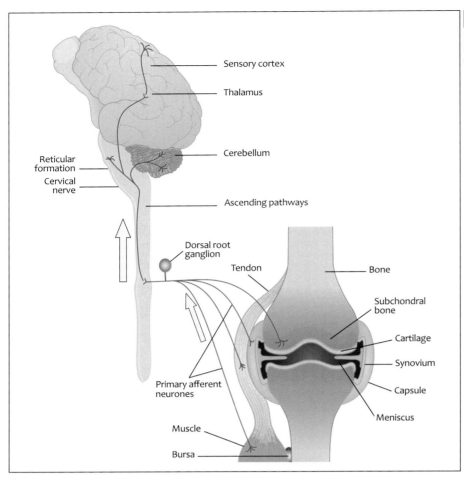

5.3 Anatomical structures and sensory innervation of a schematic joint. The joint is richly innervated with primary afferent (sensory) nerves detecting movement, position (proprioception) and pain (nociception).

and substance P (SP) (Schaible *et al.*, 2009). These neurons are thin, unmyelinated C fibres and thinly myelinated Aδ fibres and, thus, conduct slowly. Most parts of the joint have nociceptive innervation, including ligaments, meniscus, subchondral bone and synovium (Figure 5.3). Although cartilage itself is usually aneural, under certain circumstances it does contain nociceptive neurons (Mapp and Walsh, 2012); this could be during a transient developmental stage before the tertiary structure of the joint is fully formed or the result of joint damage and remodelling. The normal joint, thus, generates pain in response to excessive movement or loading, but joint damage will lead to local inflammation and sensitization of neurons and reduce the threshold for generation of such pain.

Cartilage

There are two types of cartilage present in joints: fibrocartilage and hyaline cartilage. The main differences between these types are location and structure. Hyaline cartilage (from *hyalos*, the Greek for glassy) forms the articular cartilage, and is found covering the subchondral bone within the joint, where it provides a protective, load-absorbing, low-friction surface for articulation of joints (Figure 5.4); it is highly glossy in appearance and contains very fine type II collagen fibres. In contrast, fibrocartilage is found in the meniscus, between intervertebral discs of the spine and where ligaments connect to bones; it contains type I as well as type II collagen. Of all the joint structures, probably the best understood is the articular cartilage.

Articular cartilage

Articular cartilage consists of a low-friction extracellular matrix (ECM) that comprises about 70% water and 20% structural proteins as well as various enzymes. Within this structure are spaces (lacunae) containing cells called chondrocytes (Figures 5.4 and 5.5). Cartilage is frequently described as having distinct regions according to the depth of the tissue, termed the superficial, middle and deep zones (Figure 5.4). The superficial zone is the furthest away from the bone and accounts for 10–20% of the cartilage; the middle zone accounts for up to 60%, while the deep zone accounts for up to 30%. The overall thickness of cartilage is different between joints and within different areas of the joint, and relates to the size of the animal and the load-bearing of the joint. For example, feline femoral articular cartilage is approximately 0.2 mm thick, whereas in a medium-sized dog it could be up to 1 mm thick.

The chondrocytes maintain the cartilage by establishing a balance between replacing degraded macromolecules and increasing synthesis in response to injury. In return, the ECM protects the chondrocytes from mechanical stress placed on the joint. There is a relatively high ECM to cell volume ratio and in general, the larger the animal, the lower the chondrocyte density. In the case of canine and feline femoral cartilage, chondrocyte density is 10 and 20% respectively by volume (Stockwell, 1971). The ability of articular cartilage to withstand pressure and maintain a smooth lubricated surface is vital for smooth articulation of joints. Since cartilage lacks a capillary network, it is hypoxic and acidic compared to most other tissues. The extremely high

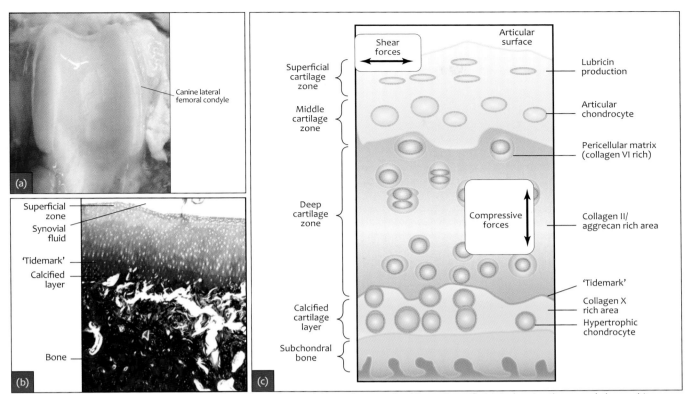

5.4 Normal cartilage. (a) Exposed femoral trochlear sulcus and ridges of a young healthy canine stifle joint, showing the normal glossy white appearance of articular hyaline cartilage. (b) Histological section of healthy cartilage, showing cartilage zones, 'tidemark', calcified layer and the subchondral bone (Masson tricolour stain). (c) Schematic diagram showing the layers of cartilage.
(b, Courtesy of Drs Simon Tew and Mandy Peffers)

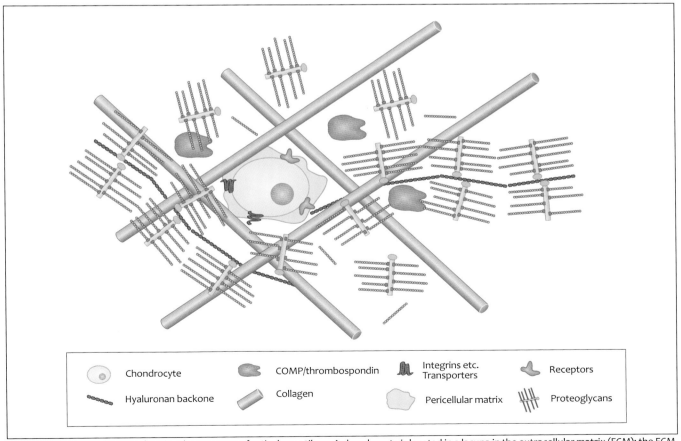

5.5 Schematic diagram showing the structure of articular cartilage. A chondrocyte is located in a lacuna in the extracellular matrix (ECM); the ECM contains negatively charged proteoglycan chains and type II collagen fibres. COMP = cartilage oligomeric matrix protein.

protein content also creates a condition of increased osmotic potential compared to other tissues. This draws water into cartilage and maintains its turgor.

Chondrocytes

Chondrocytes are the only resident cells of cartilage; they synthesize all structural components of the ECM, the constituent enzymes of cartilage, and produce a range of soluble local mediators, such as ATP, nitric oxide, growth factors and cytokines.

The morphology of chondrocytes varies according to the region of cartilage in which they lie. Superficially, they are small and flattened, becoming more ovoid in shape when situated in the middle zone. In the deep zone they may form short columns of larger, round cells. A fourth layer of cartilage is present at the interface between cartilage and bone, also known as the calcified zone. Very few chondrocytes are found in this region. The interface between the calcified and non-calcified cartilage zones is termed the 'tidemark' and is clearly visible histologically (see Figure 5.4b).

Despite their enclosure within the lacunae of cartilage, chondrocytes are subject to compressive loads and are deformed by normal activity and weight-bearing by joints. They express membrane proteins, which detect physical activity and change their metabolism in response to these mechanical stimuli. Chondrocyte metabolic activity is, therefore, directly related to the type of mechanical load placed on the cartilage; generally, moderate cyclical loading stimulates maximal proteoglycan production. Inactivity of joints may lead to accelerated thinning of cartilage. The mechanotransduction pathway is not fully understood, but is believed to involve a number of ion channels, membrane transporters and adhesion molecules, such as integrins (Lewis *et al.*, 2011; Figure 5.6).

Cells in all tissues need to communicate with each other and with the rest of the body as a part of normal homeostasis. Chondrocytes achieve this in two ways: firstly, by the secretion of soluble mediators that diffuse into the synovial fluid, and secondly by dendritic projections to neighbouring chondrocytes that enable direct intercellular communication via gap junction (cx43) channels (Mayan *et al.*, 2013). Gap junction-mediated intercellular communication is a common feature of normal mammalian joint tissues, including meniscus (Hellio Le Graverand *et al.*, 2001), intervertebral disc (Errington *et al.*, 1998), ligament and tendon (Benjamin and Ralphs, 1997).

Protein chemistry of cartilage extracellular matrix

The ECM is made up of a collagen fibre meshwork and negatively charged proteoglycans, which attract positively charged ions (cations), such as Ca^{2+} and Na^+.

Proteoglycans contribute to cartilage rigidity, stability and durability during compression and consist of a core protein covalently bound to glycosaminoglycan (GAG) disaccharide moieties (Figure 5.7a). Water is attracted to the carboxyl and sulphate groups of these molecules. Since each GAG is negatively charged, they repel each other, creating a well organized mesh network within which water molecules become immobilized. The major proteoglycan of cartilage is aggrecan, which consists of a core protein linked to chondroitin and keratan sulphate GAG moieties. This macromolecule is, in turn, linked to long chains of hyaluronate GAG polysaccharide polymers forming massive

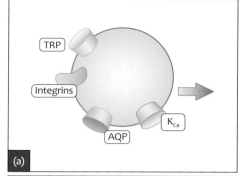

(a)

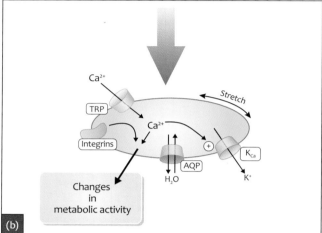

(b)

5.6 Mechanical activity changes the metabolic activity of chondrocytes, by mechanisms that are not yet well understood. (a) Resting chondrocyte. (b) Membrane stretch activates a number of membrane proteins, including integrins and transient receptor potential channels. Together these mobilize intracellular calcium and change the metabolic activity of the chondrocyte. Simultaneously, a sequence of events, including activation of potassium channels and water permeation through aquaporin channels, allows chondrocytes to decrease their physical size and prevent the cell membrane from rupturing. AQP = aquaporin (water) channels; K_{Ca} = calcium-activated potassium channels; TRP = transient receptor potential channels.
(Lewis *et al.*, 2011)

and highly complex proteoglycans (Figure 5.7bc). The ECM also contains a number of other similar proteoglycans (Figure 5.8) and other important glycoproteins, such as the 524 kDa cartilage oligomeric matrix protein (COMP) or thrombospondin, which is a useful marker of cartilage turnover. For healthy cartilage, the turnover of proteoglycans and collagens is very slow with half-lives of months, or even many years in the case of collagen (Maroudas *et al.*, 1992).

Cartilage tensile strength (resistance to stretch) is afforded by collagen, of which there are a number of different types. Types II, IX and XI form a tensile fibril network within cartilage, supporting the proteoglycans. Type VI collagens are localized adjacent to chondrocytes (the pericellular matrix) and may be involved in attachment of the chondrocyte to the ECM. In the superficial zone of cartilage, collagen can account for up to 65% of tissue content. Figure 5.9 illustrates the distribution of collagen found in joint ECM. There are a number of proteins which physically connect the ECM to the surface of chondrocytes. Anchorin CII, the integrins and the hyaluronate receptor (also known as chondrocyte cell surface marker CD44) anchor the cell to the matrix, but also allow for direct signalling between the ECM and the chondrocyte.

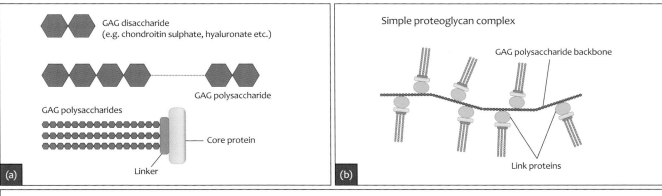

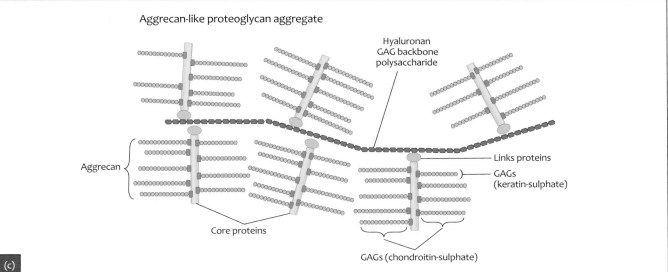

5.7 Proteoglycans of cartilage extracellular matrix. (a) Glycosaminoglycans (GAGs) are largely composed of disaccharides, such as chondroitin sulphate or hyaluronate. These disaccharides are linked together to form polysaccharides. These combine with a core protein to form a proteoglycan. (b) Several proteoglycans can combine together, linked by a hyaluronan 'backbone'. (c) Many GAGs, linked by core proteins, can join together to form aggrecan aggregates, one type of proteoglycan.

Proteoglycan	Core protein: approximate MW (kDa) (canine gene) [location]	GAG Components	Number of GAGs	Location	Notes
Aggrecan	210 (ACAN) [Chr 3:52.00–52.03 Mb]	Chondroitin sulphate Keratan sulphate	~130	Throughout (especially deep zone cartilage)	Forms huge protein complexes with long chains of the GAG hyaluronan (see Figure 5.5)
Decorin	40 (DCN) [Chr 15:31.83–31.88 Mb]	Chondroitin sulphate Dermatan sulphate	1	Outer pericellular	Binds to TGF-β
Biglycan	40 (BGN) [Chr X:121.33–121.34 Mb]	Chondroitin sulphate Dermatan sulphate	2	Outer pericellular	Also known as proteoglycan-I (PG-I)[a] Binds to collagen type II
Syndecan-1	32 (SDC1) [Chr 17:15.22–15.24 Mb]	Chondroitin sulphate Heparan sulphate	1–3	Chondrocyte surface membrane	Cell adhesion; receptor for growth factors including FGF
Lubricin	200 (PRG4) [Chr 7:19.36–19.38 Mb]	Keratan and chondroitin sulphate structurally related GAGs	Many	Especially superficial zone of cartilage Synovial fluid	Also found in canine tendon, ligament, meniscus and muscle[b] Also known as proteoglycan 4[c]
Asporin	40 (ASPN) [Chr 1:98.88–98.91 Mb]	Similar to decorin/biglycan[d]	–	Overlaps with decorin/biglycan	May inhibit TGF-β
(Not a protein/proteoglycan)		Hyaluronic acid	Thousands	–	Unsulphated GAG in cartilage/synovial fluid Long chains can reach >1000 kDa

5.8 Proteoglycans of extracellular matrix. Note that the extracellular matrix also contains a number of other important chondrocyte-synthesized protein components which are neither proteoglycan nor collagen, such as the matrilins (1 and 3) and COMP, together with many enzymes and endogenous enzyme inhibitors. COMP = cartilage oligomeric matrix protein; FGF = fibroblast growth factor; GAG = glycosaminoglycan; MW = molecular weight; TGF = transforming growth factor.
(Data from [a] Fisher et al., 1989; [b] Sun et al., 2006; [c] Swann et al., 1981; [d] Lorenzo et al., 2001).

Collagen type	Gene (α-chain stoichiometry)	Typical joint tissue location	Notes
I	COL1A1, COL1A2 (2 x α1, 1 x α2)	Tendons, ligaments and menisci	Fibril-forming
II	COL2A1 (3 x α1)	Throughout articular cartilage. Also found in menisci and intervertebral disc ECM	Fibril-forming
VI	COL6A1, COL6A2, COL6A3, COL6A5	Pericellular cartilage	–
IX	COL9A1, COL9A2, COL9A3	Articular cartilage (non-pericellular)	Associates with type II and XI fibrils A 'FACIT' collagen; a type of collagen that is also a type of proteoglycan
X	COL10A1	Hypertrophic/mineralizing zones of cartilage	
XI	COL11A1, COL11A2 (1 x α1, 1 x α2)	Throughout articular cartilage	Fibril-forming (with type II)

5.9 Distribution of collagen types found in joint extracellular matrix (ECM).

Enzyme content

A large number of protein-cleaving enzymes are found in cartilage ECM. The chief enzymatic constituents are the matrix metalloproteinases or metalloproteases (MMPs), 'a disintegrin and metalloproteinase' (ADAM) and 'a disintegrin and metalloproteinase with thrombospondin motifs' (ADAMTS). Cartilage contains many different types of MMPs (Figure 5.10). There is also a series of endogenous enzyme inhibitor proteins which are termed 'tissue inhibitors of metalloproteinases' (TIMPs). The presence of an appropriate balance of enzymes and enzyme inhibitors is critical to the preservation of normal cartilage, although the complex interactions between these are still the subject of intense research.

Enzymes of cartilage also frequently have a signalling role, cleaving inactive membrane receptors which then enter an active state. This is especially true of the serine proteinases, which are also found in synovial membranes and fluid. Some of these activate the proteinase-activated receptors (PARs). If such enzymes diffuse to the vicinity of nociceptive nerve endings, they will sensitize those nerves to painful stimuli.

Cartilage mediators, growth factors, hormones and cytokines

Chondrocytes are a rich source of diffusible extracellular mediators; mediators can also diffuse into the cartilage from the subchondral bone or from the synovial fluid. These mediators can induce changes in chondrocyte activity, such as inducing or protecting from apoptosis (programmed cell death or 'shrink' death) or increasing production of ECM components. Typical mediators identified in the normal cartilage include cytokines, such as interleukin-1β (IL1-β) or growth/differentiation factors, such as fibroblast growth factor-2 (FGF-2) or FGF-18. The specific role of each of these mediators in normal cartilage homeostasis is not known, but the balance of their activities is likely to be critical for prolonged healthy joint function. For example, IL-1β will induce cell death in chondrocytes, whereas FGF-18 is thought to promote production of chondrocytes (Davidson et al., 2005), so-called 'chondrogenesis'. The concentrations of these mediators are likely to change dramatically with the onset of joint disease.

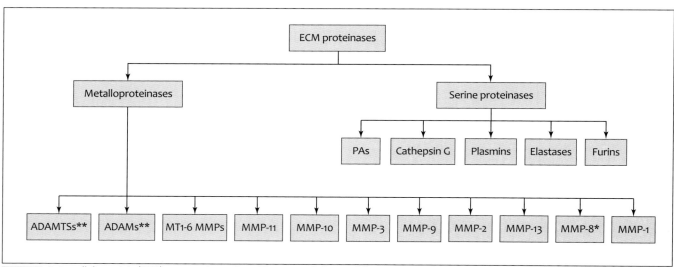

5.10 Extracellular matrix (ECM) enzymes in cartilage. The correct balance of the enzymes and of their endogenous inhibitors is crucial for healthy cartilage homeostasis. Change in their expression would lead to, and result from, cartilage degeneration. ADAM = a disintegrin and metalloproteinase; ADAMTS = a disintegrin and metalloproteinase with thrombospondin motifs; MMP = matrix metalloproteinase; MT = membrane type; PAs = plasminogen activators; *MMP8 is also known as collagenase 2; **25 ADAM genes, 19 ADAMTS genes.

Hypertrophic chondrocytes of cartilage

Hypertrophic chondrocytes are remarkably large cells which participate in endochondral ossification; resting chondrocytes become proliferative, then greatly enlarged (hypertrophy) before finally dying (apoptosis), leaving a scaffold for the invasion of osteoclasts and the formation of extracellular bone matrix (Figure 5.11). There are many biochemical differences between resting and hypertrophic chondrocytes, but one key change is a switch from production of type II collagen to type X collagen. These processes are particularly rapid during fetal development, but continue postnatally until closure of the physes. Hypertrophic chondrocytes are not normally found in mature articular cartilage. It has been suggested that an inappropriate switch of chondrocytes in the articular cartilage to a hypertrophic-like phenotype may contribute to some arthritic disease states.

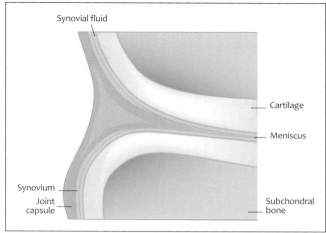

5.12 The meniscus of a stifle joint, located around the edges of the articular cartilage. In the stifle, the peripheral aspect of the medial meniscus is continuous with the joint capsule, while the lateral meniscus is a separate structure. The meniscus is wedge-shaped when viewed in this cross-section.

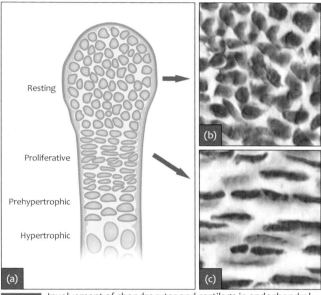

5.11 Involvement of chondrocytes and cartilage in endochondral ossification at joints. (a) The chondrocytes in articular cartilage are described as 'resting' and are sparsely distributed. Moving towards the subchondral bone, they are organized in a columnar distribution and are called proliferative. Chondrocytes in the next layer are then termed prehypertrophic, while those closest to the subchondral bone are hypertrophic and greatly enlarged. (b) Resting and (c) proliferative chondrocytes from cartilage as indicated by the arrows (stained with haematoxylin and eosin).
(b–c, Reproduced with permission from Li and Dudley, 2009)

Meniscus

Certain joints, such as the stifle and temporomandibular joint, contain menisci (singular 'meniscus'). These are fibrocartilaginous structures that provide considerable stability and distribute the load from the rounded bone ends to a relatively larger tissue surface area of the joint. The menisci additionally provide important shock absorbance to the joint. Damage to the menisci will lead to osteoarthritis.

In the stifle, the peripheral aspect of the medial meniscus is continuous with the joint capsule, while the lateral meniscus is a separate structure, without attachments to the joint capsule. Crescenic rather than circular, they are wedge-shaped when viewed in cross-section (Figure 5.12). The ends of the menisci form ligaments that attach to the adjacent bone. In the stifle, the medial and lateral menisci are attached to the tibia through cranial and

caudal meniscotibial ligaments and cranially the intermeniscal ligament links the two. Caudally, the lateral meniscus also has an attachment to the femur via the meniscofemoral ligament.

The outer thirds of the menisci, like the joint capsule, contain capillaries and nerve endings, but neither of these are present at the thinnest and most central parts, where nutrition is derived from diffusion or from cyclical pumping of nutrients from the joint fluid during loading. Nerve endings within the menisci are used to aid proprioception; nociceptors are also present. The biochemical composition of the menisci is similar to (but distinct from) that of other cartilage, namely water, proteoglycan aggregates and collagen (types I and II). Menisci have particularly high tensile strength and resistance to shear stress, which is maintained by a greater degree of collagen type II organization than is seen in articular cartilage (Figure 5.13). It is the orientation of these collagen fibres that enables the menisci to absorb shock; as the joint is loaded, the circumferentially oriented collagen fibres elongate and the meniscus extrudes peripherally from the joint. This is

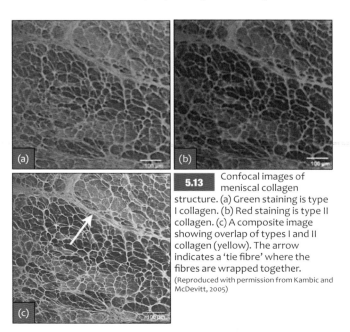

5.13 Confocal images of meniscal collagen structure. (a) Green staining is type I collagen. (b) Red staining is type II collagen. (c) A composite image showing overlap of types I and II collagen (yellow). The arrow indicates a 'tie fibre' where the fibres are wrapped together.
(Reproduced with permission from Kambic and McDevitt, 2005)

referred to as a hoop stress; the force derived from this hoop stress is able to restrain the menisci as it extrudes. The specific distribution of proteoglycans within the meniscus depends on the region of the meniscus; the inner third is approximately 8% proteoglycan, whereas the outer third is only 2% (Englund et al., 2012).

Synovium and synovial fluid

The capsule of synovial joints is vascular, innervated and contains two major layers: an outer fibrous layer, which arises as a continuation of the periosteum and an inner more cellular layer known as the synovial membrane. The synovial membrane produces synovial fluid which provides lubrication, cushions joint impact and nourishes the cartilage.

The synovial membrane itself can be subdivided into two layers: the innermost layer immediately adjacent to the joint space (the synovial intima) and an outer, more supportive layer, which is termed the subintima. Both layers contain blood vessels; however, lymphatics are largely restricted to the subintima. Of the two layers, the inner layer is more cellular and produces the synovial fluid, whereas the outer layer is rich in collagen and provides greater physical support (Figure 5.14). The cells of the synovial membrane are known as synoviocytes, of which there are two types: the macrophage-like type A and the more fibroblast-like, secretory type B, which produce the synovial fluid. In the normal joint, the synovial membrane also contains mast cells (in most species); when inflamed the membrane also becomes infiltrated by white blood cells. The synovial fluid itself is a protein-rich ultra-filtrate of plasma containing both hyaluronic acid (the unsulphated polysaccharide GAG) and lubricin. Just as cyclical loading stimulates metabolic changes in chondrocytes, it also stimulates production and turnover of synovial fluid (Ingram et al., 2008). Mediators can diffuse between the synovial membrane, fluid and articular cartilage (Allan, 1998).

Subchondral bone

The subchondral bone is a thin layer of bone immediately beneath the calcified layer of cartilage (see Figure 5.4) and is classed as a joint tissue. The irregular surface between the calcified cartilage and the subchondral bone allows for transformation of shear forces during compression. Normal subchondral bone attenuates about 30% of the load through the joint, in comparison to the 1–3% that is attenuated by cartilage. The subchondral bone contains Haversian canals which are aligned parallel to the cartilage and contain both blood vessels and unmyelinated nerve fibres (typical of pain-sensing neurons). The vascularized area of subchondral bone is called the articular vascular plexus. It is this vascularization of the subchondral bone that allows constant remodelling of the joint in response to loading and unloading. Below the subchondral bone is the trabecular bone. Despite the separation of subchondral bone from articular cartilage by the calcified layer of cartilage, there is biochemical communication between the two tissues. The subchondral bone is becoming of increasing interest to clinicians and scientists, since pathological changes to it occur with the onset of osteoarthritis.

Ligaments and tendons

Ligaments attach bone to bone, whereas tendons attach muscle to bone. Despite this functional difference, the tissues are similar, both being type I collagen-rich connective tissues. Both are essential for joint stability and healthy joint function. While neither tissue heals quickly, Amiel et al. (1984) argue that ligaments are more metabolically active than tendons, with larger cell nuclei and more DNA. Ligaments also contain slightly more proteoglycan and less total collagen, but with relatively more type III collagen.

Ligaments are important for constrained joint movement and stability within a normal range, whereas tendons

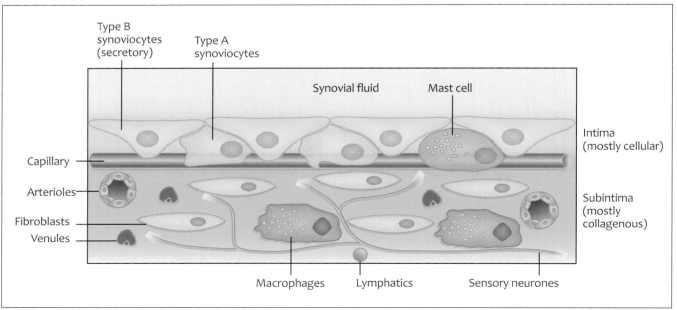

5.14 Several cell types are found in the synovium. The type B synoviocytes primarily produce the synovial fluid, but several cell types are involved with immune functions and blood vessels. Nerve endings are present within the synovium and could be activated by painful stimulation.

facilitate movement. Most joints have a number of ligaments that each prevents excessive movement in a given plane, e.g. medial collateral ligaments prevent valgus (outward) movement and lateral collateral ligaments prevent varus (inward) movement. In the stifle joint, the cranial and caudal cruciate ligaments prevent craniocaudal translation of the tibia and femur relative to each other. In addition, the cranial cruciate ligament resists internal rotation of the tibia relative to the femur and hyperextension of the stifle joint. Ligaments and tendons are both prone to injury; as they are viscoelastic tissues, they are more resistant to slow application of a given force than to rapid application of force (the tissue has time to absorb the energy and the physical shape changes to accommodate) (Hildebrand et al., 2004). Damage or loss to joint ligaments will result in instability and the development of osteoarthritis.

Biochemical similarities with cartilage are clear; all three tissues are hypocellular, containing about 10% cells (in mature tissue) with high (70%+) water content, and constituent cells communicate via gap junctions rather than neurons. The primary tensile protein is collagen (type I in ligaments and tendons, type II in cartilage). The internal organization of ligaments and tendons consists of fascicles: longitudinal groups of collagen fibres separated by septae and enveloped in a thin connective tissue sheath, known as the endoligament or endotendon (Figure 5.15). These in turn contain fibre bundles, within which are sub-fascicles. Sub-fascicles consist of collagen fibrils, made up of collagen macromolecules. All of these molecules within the tendon are grouped longitudinally, running in parallel to one another. This arrangement gives the ligaments and tendons their strength. Ligaments and tendons also contain high concentrations of the proteoglycans decorin, elastin and fibronectin.

While cartilage is avascular (i.e. contains no blood vessels), tendons and ligaments have few blood vessels. Unlike cartilage, both ligaments and tendons contain nerve endings including those for proprioception (detection of joint position and movement). The elastin molecules within tendons are critical for an important tendon function: energy storage and release. As an animal's foot hits the ground, the body decelerates, causing kinetic energy to be stored as strain energy in the tendons. The elastic recoil of tendons, as the foot leaves the ground, causes this energy to be converted back to kinetic energy. Elastin makes up the elastic fibres of ligaments and tendons, which enables the tendons to act as these biological 'springs'. Levels of elastin in the tendons can vary between species, particularly with ageing, and this can affect recovery after injury.

References and further reading

Allan DA (1998) Structure and physiology of joints and their relationship to repetitive strain injuries. *Clinical orthopaedics and related research* **351**, 32–38

Amiel D, Frank C, Harwood F, Fronek J and Akeson W (1984) Tendons and ligaments: a morphological and biochemical comparison. *Journal of Orthopaedic Research* **1**, 257–265

Benjamin M and Ralphs JR (1997) Tendons and ligaments – an overview. *Histology and Histopathology* **12**, 1135–1144

Davidson D, Blanc A, Filion D et al. (2005) Fibroblast growth factor (FGF) 18 signals through FGF receptor 3 to promote chondrogenesis. *Journal of Biological Chemistry* **280**, 20509–20515

Englund M, Roemer FW, Hayashi D, Crema MD and Guermazi A (2012) Meniscus pathology, osteoarthritis and the treatment controversy. *Nature Reviews Rheumatology* **8**, 412–419

Errington RJ, Puustjarvi K, White IR, Roberts S and Urban JP (1998) Characterisation of cytoplasm-filled processes in cells of the intervertebral disc. *Journal of Anatomy* **192**, 369–378

Fisher LW, Termine JD and Young MF (1989) Deduced protein sequence of bone small proteoglycan I (biglycan) shows homology with proteoglycan II (decorin) and several nonconnective tissue proteins in a variety of species. *Journal of Biological Chemistry* **264**, 4571–4576

Freeman MA and Wyke B (1967) The innervation of the knee joint. An anatomical and histological study in the cat. *Journal of Anatomy* **101**, 505–532

Hellio Le Graverand MP, Ou Y, Schield-Yee T et al. (2001) The cells of the rabbit meniscus: their arrangement, interrelationship, morphological variations and cytoarchitecture. *Journal of Anatomy* **198**, 525–535

Hildebrand KA, Frank CB and Hart DA (2004) Gene intervention in ligament and tendon: current status, challenges, future directions. *Gene Therapy* **11**, 368–378

Ingram KR, Wann AK, Angel CK, Coleman PJ and Levick JR (2008) Cyclic movement stimulates hyaluronan secretion into the synovial cavity of rabbit joints. *Journal of Physiology* **586**, 1715–1729

Kambic HE and McDevitt CA (2005) Spatial organization of types I and II collagen in the canine meniscus. *Journal of Orthopaedic Research* **23**, 142–149

Lewis R, Feetham CH and Barrett-Jolley R (2011) Cell Volume Regulation in Chondrocytes. *Cellular Physiology and Biochemistry* **28**, 1111–1122

Li Y and Dudley AT (2009) Noncanonical frizzled signaling regulates cell polarity of growth plate chondrocytes. *Development* **136**, 1083–1092

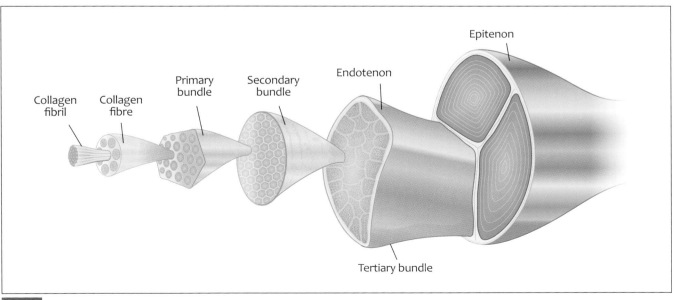

5.15 Structure of a tendon, showing the internal organization of collagen.

Collagen fibril | Collagen fibre | Primary bundle | Secondary bundle | Endotenon | Epitenon | Tertiary bundle

Lorenzo P, Aspberg A, Onnerfjord P *et al.* (2001) Identification and characterization of asporin. a novel member of the leucine-rich repeat protein family closely related to decorin and biglycan. *Journal of Biological Chemistry* **276**, 12201–12211

Mapp PI and Walsh DA (2012) Mechanisms and targets of angiogenesis and nerve growth in osteoarthritis. *Nature Reviews Rheumatology* **8**, 390–398

Maroudas A, Palla G and Gilav E (1992) Racemization of aspartic acid in human articular cartilage. *Connective Tissue Research* **28**, 161–169

Mayan MD, Carpintero-Fernandez P, Gago-Fuentes R *et al.* (2013) Human articular chondrocytes express multiple gap junction proteins: differential expression of connexins in normal and osteoarthritic cartilage. *American Journal of Pathology* **182**, 1337–1346

Roos EM, Herzog W, Block JA and Bennell KL (2011) Muscle weakness, afferent sensory dysfunction and exercise in knee osteoarthritis. *Nature Reviews Rheumatology* **7**, 57–63

Schaible H-G, Richter F, Ebersberger A *et al.* (2009) Joint pain. *Experimental Brain Research* **196**, 153–162

Stockwell RA (1971) Cell density, cell size and cartilage thickness in adult mammalian articular cartilage. *Journal of Anatomy* **108**, 411–421

Sun Y, Berger EJ, Zhao C *et al.* (2006) Mapping lubricin in canine musculo-skeletal tissues. *Connective Tissue Research* **47**, 215–221

Swann DA, Slayter HS and Silver FH (1981) The molecular structure of lubricating glycoprotein-I, the boundary lubricant for articular cartilage. *Journal of Biological Chemistry* **256**, 5921–5925

Chapter 6

Arthritis

Ralph Abercromby, John Innes and Dylan Clements

Arthritis is a broad term used to describe any condition affecting a synovial joint. Any abnormality of a synovial joint will cause inflammation to a greater or lesser extent and hence can be said to cause 'arthritis'. Thus there are many causes of arthritis and many of these initiating factors (e.g. ligament rupture, osteochondrosis) are dealt with elsewhere in this manual. For the purposes of this manual, the term 'arthritis' is used to bring together the diagnosis and management of the disease processes involved in three main categories of joint disease: osteoarthritis, immune-mediated polyarthritis and infective arthritis.

Arthritis can be subdivided as shown in Figure 6.1. Traditionally, arthritis is subdivided into 'inflammatory' and 'non-inflammatory' (or 'degenerative') subtypes. Of course, this subdivision describes the *relative* degree of inflammation in these disease processes because all forms of arthritis involve inflammation to some extent.

Classification systems are helpful to structure a diagnostic and therapeutic approach, but it should be remembered that there are many pathogenic processes that are common to all forms of arthritis, although the relative importance of these different processes and the rate at which these progress, may differ.

Infective arthritis

Infective arthritis is an inflammatory arthropathy caused by an infective organism. It may be debilitating and have severe consequences. Definitive diagnosis requires identification or culture of the organism. Empirically, however, differential diagnoses would include inflammatory arthritides that, on the basis of clinical signs and findings, are considered likely to be the result of an infective organism, but for which a specific organism cannot be identified. A wide variety of organisms, including Mycoplasmas, viruses, bacteria, *Chlamydia*, fungi and protozoans, have been reported to cause infective arthritis, but in the UK the vast majority of cases are bacterial in origin.

> When reviewing published clinical material on septic (bacterial) arthritis, it should be noted that the vast majority relates to small series or individual cases, is retrospective and lacks control groups. This, in part, may explain inconsistencies between reports

Bacterial arthritis

Joint infection can occur haematogenously, by direct penetration (surgery, open wound, penetrating foreign body) or by extension from local infection (osteomyelitis, soft tissue infection). A wide variety of bacteria are implicated, but the most commonly isolated organisms in the dog are *Staphylococcus pseudintermedius*, *Staphylococcus aureus* and beta-haemolytic streptococci. In the cat, commonly isolated bacteria include *Pasteurella multocida* and *Bacteroides* spp., reflecting the oral flora and the prevalence of cat bites as a cause.

Haematogenous spread and surgical infections account for the vast majority of cases. Bennett and Taylor (1988) reported most cases were haematogenous in origin, while Marchevsky and Read (1999) reported that stifle surgery was the main risk factor. Clements *et al.* (2005) identified that 17 of 32 cases (56%) had previous articular surgery and 14 of 32 cases had no previous surgery. Total joint replacements can also become infected (Figure 6.2).

Non-inflammatory arthritis

• Osteoarthritis
  • Idiopathic (primary)
  • Secondary
• Traumatic arthritis
• Coagulopathic arthritis

Inflammatory arthritis

• Immune-mediated arthritis
  • Erosive
    – Rheumatoid arthritis
    – Periosteal proliferative polyarthritis
  • Non-erosive
    – Idiopathic: type I (idiopathic), type II (reactive), type III (gastrointestinal disease), type IV (neoplasia)
    – Systemic lupus erythematosus
    – Drug reactions
    – Breed-associated immune-mediated polyarthritis (IMPA)
• Infective arthritis
• Bacterial
• Borrelial
• Protozoal
• Mycoplasmal
• Fungal
• Mycobacterial
• Crystal-induced arthritis
  • Hydroxypatite
  • Calcium pyrophosphate (pseudogout)
  • Sodium urate (gout)

6.1 Classification of canine and feline arthritis.

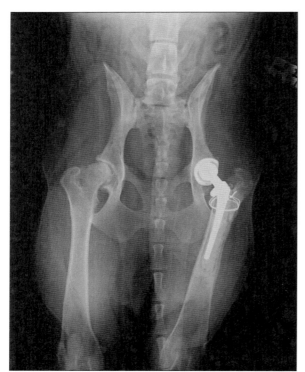

6.2 Total hip replacement with meticillin-resistant *Staphylococcus aureus* (MRSA) infection affecting the femoral component. The continuous radiolucent zone at the femoral cement–bone interface indicates implant loosening. This case was successfully managed with the extraction of the implants, application of a gentamicin-impregnated collagen preparation (Collatemp EG) within the femoral canal and systemic antibiotics.

The incidence is low, affecting about 1% of primary cemented hip replacements, but is higher with revision surgery (Dyce and Olmstead, 2002).

Infective arthritis related to non-surgical articular wounds is reported (Clarke and Ferguson, 2012), but is uncommon. Where previous surgery is not a predisposing factor, pre-existing joint disease (degenerative or inflammatory) is typically present in dogs (Clements *et al.*, 2005) and humans (Kaandorp *et al.*, 1997). Only rarely is a separate focus of primary infection identified (e.g. in the skin, bladder, prostate, kidneys, gastrointestinal tract, lungs, gingivae or anal glands).

Pathogenesis

Within the joint, the loop configuration of the blood supply to the synovial villi, and the highly vascular, areolar connective tissue, which lacks a limiting basement membrane, may assist the localization of systemic infection to the synovium. The resultant host immune response results in marked local inflammation. Synovial phagocytes and migrating polymorphonuclear leucocytes (PMNs, neutrophils) kill and engulf intra-articular bacteria during a complex interaction involving proinflammatory cytokines, proteolytic enzymes and exo/endotoxins. The synovium and the synovial fluid become hypercellular, predominantly with PMNs, and as a result the synovial fluid becomes rich in proteolytic enzymes released from PMNs, macrophages and synovial cells, leading to synovial, cartilage and bone necrosis. High levels of inflammatory mediators, such as tumour necrosis factor (TNF) and interleukins, rapidly deplete the local supply of proteinase inhibitors and rapid cartilage destruction ensues.

Experimentally, glycosaminoglycans are lost before collagen. The breakdown of supporting cartilage matrix reduces collagen fibril support, and joint motion causes mechanical damage. For cartilage to be preserved, aggressive measures must be taken before matrix breakdown occurs. Experimentally, even if antibiotics are administered within 24 hours, cartilage proteoglycan loss is not prevented although collagen loss is reduced (Mathews *et al.*, 2010).

Granulation tissue and synovial abscesses can result in articular cartilage and bone erosion in a fashion similar to that seen with pannus. Subchondral bone is weakened and direct pressure necrosis of the cartilage may result from joint effusion.

Synovial fluid is typically free of blood clotting factors, but in infective arthritis, fibrin deposits are formed, which limit the normal exchange of cartilage metabolites and nutrients with synovial fluid, further contributing to the inflammatory cycle and permanent joint damage.

The severity of articular cartilage damage is variable and depends on the number, type and virulence of the organism, the extent to which they multiply and both the local and general immune status of the patient.

Typically, only one joint is affected (monoarthropathy). Several joints (poly/pauci/oligo arthritis) can, however, be affected by systemically borne infective organisms in the immune incompetent neonate or immunosuppressed patient. Immature infective polyarthritis (puppy/kitten) is uncommon but when present is usually secondary to omphalophlebitis, mammary or uterine infections of the bitch/queen or a streptococcal pharyngitis. In the adult, polyarthritis may be encountered secondary to septicaemia, such as that accompanying bacterial endocarditis. Bacterial polyarthritis is significantly less common than septic arthritis affecting only a single joint.

Clinical presentation

Medium- and large-breed dogs are more likely to suffer septic arthritis than small- or toy-breeds, perhaps due to the former's larger joint surface areas or prevalence for conditions such as cruciate disease and elbow dysplasia that predispose to degenerative joint disease and/or orthopaedic surgery, both of which are risk factors for septic arthritis.

Male dogs are affected more frequently than female. In two of the larger case series (Bennett and Taylor, 1988; Clements *et al.*, 2005) the ratio was approximately 2:1. Whereas immune-mediated disease appears preferentially to affect smaller distal joints, bacterial infective arthritis, especially when associated with surgery, affects the larger joints (stifle, elbow, hock, hip). Clements *et al.*, (2005) identified that stifles and, to a slightly lesser degree, elbows were the most commonly infected joints. This, however, reflected the high frequency of surgeries on these joints; when the rate of infection relative to surgery numbers on each joint was examined, hocks were affected most commonly (stifle 1.7%, elbow 1.5%, hock 2.7%). The interval between surgery and clinical signs of infection varies considerably (days to years). Clinical onset may be acute or, less commonly, chronic in onset. Signs may include localized heat and swelling, erythema or abnormal appearance of the joint, visible/palpable joint effusion, local lymphadenopathy and perhaps pain on joint manipulation (Figure 6.3). Sinus formation and discharge may be present. Pyrexia is not a consistent finding and its absence does not preclude infection. A minority of cases exhibit signs of systemic disease, such as a heart murmur accompanying bacterial endocarditis. A few will be depressed or recumbent, some sufficiently so that neurological disease

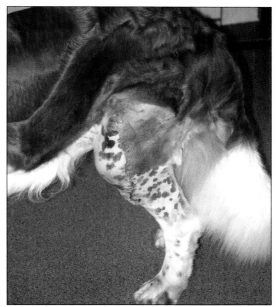

6.3 Infected stifle joint following surgery for cranial cruciate ligament disease. The region around and cranial to the left stifle exhibits swelling, erythema and discharge.

is considered initially as a differential diagnosis. Joint instability (i.e. cruciate rupture or joint luxation/subluxation) can result from inflammatory damage to supporting tissues.

Diagnosis

Early definitive diagnosis is essential to limit irreversible intra-articular changes. This will allow appropriate management and prevent inappropriate medication with immuno-suppressive drugs where the arthropathy is mistakenly assumed to be immune-mediated rather than septic.

Diagnosis and differentiation from other arthritides are based on a combination of history, physical findings, radiographic interpretation and laboratory analysis (Figure 6.4). While clinical findings may support a presumptive diagnosis

Step 1: History and clinical signs
The history and clinical signs reveal:
- A single affected joint
- Previous surgery or pre-existing degenerative joint disease in the affected joint
- The presence of swelling of the limb ± distal oedema
- Acute onset (often, but not always)
- Patient is systemically unwell and pyrexic (often, but not always)

Step 2: Smear test
The smear test performed on a synovial fluid sample reveals it to be highly cellular with a predominately neutrophil population

Step 3: Automated cell count
The automated cell count performed on a synovial fluid sample reveals:
- Neutrophil count at least 15×10^9/l and usually $>50 \times 10^9$/l
- Neutrophil distribution at least 75% and usually >90%

Outcome: Very high suspicion of septic arthritis – institute therapy unless there is a good reason not to begin treatment

Step 4: Identification of degenerative neutrophils in synovial fluid sample

Step 5: Culture and sensitivity testing
Culture and sensitivity testing of a synovial fluid sample results in positive identification of the causative organism

Outcome: Definitive diagnosis confirmed (unless cytology does not support the diagnosis, in which case a false-positive culture and sensitivity result should be considered)

6.4 Simple step-by-step approach to the diagnosis of synovial sepsis.

of infective arthritis, definitive diagnosis demands identification of a dramatically increased cell count with a very high proportion of neutrophils and, ideally, a positive culture of the organism, although the latter is not always possible.

It is very important to realize that a negative culture and sensitivity result does NOT exclude an infected joint. It simply means that bacteria were not grown, i.e. there is a high chance of a false-negative result. Similarly for degenerate neutrophils, they are often not seen. The most important test for bacterial arthritis is a high index of clinical suspicion plus a very high neutrophil count in the joint fluid

Imaging: Radiographic signs depend on the stage of disease and organism involved (Figures 6.5 to 6.8). They are not specifically diagnostic for infective arthritis, demonstrating only secondary changes such as joint effusion, associated soft tissue thickening, displacement of soft tissues and fascial planes, and osteophytosis. Subchondral erosion can develop within 10–14 days (dependent on organism present) and, if present, indicates articular cartilage damage and associated poor prognosis. Non-erosive septic arthritis is more common than erosive.

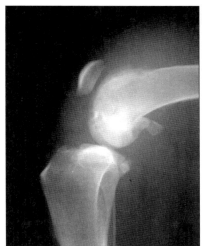

6.5 Mediolateral view of the stifle of a dog with septic arthritis showing considerable soft tissue swelling/joint effusion and moderate degenerative joint disease.

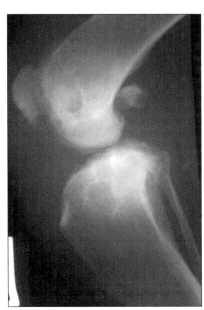

6.6 Mediolateral view of the stifle of a dog with septic arthritis following surgery for cranial cruciate rupture managed with an intra-articular graft and bone tunnels. The radiograph shows considerable soft tissue thickening/joint effusion, moderate subchondral bone erosion and widening of the bone tunnels.

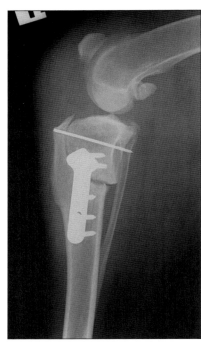

6.7 Mediolateral view of the stifle of a dog with septic arthritis following tibial plateau levelling osteotomy surgery for cranial cruciate ligament rupture. The radiograph shows moderate soft tissue thickening/joint effusion, including in the region of the patellar tendon, and subtle periosteal new bone on the cranial aspect of the tibial tuberosity (intra-articular and extra-articular changes).

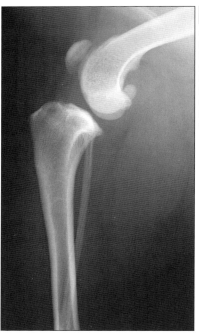

6.8 Mediolateral view of the stifle of a dog with septic arthritis and cranial cruciate ligament rupture. The radiograph shows moderate to marked soft tissue thickening/joint effusion without significant skeletal degenerative changes.

Plain radiographs provide a baseline assessment and may indicate the presence or absence of contiguous osteomyelitis or, in the immature patient, epiphyseal and physeal involvement. Serial radiography allows assessment of progression of disease, particularly with respect to the bone. Articular cartilage changes cannot be assessed using non-weight-bearing radiographs unless the destruction is so severe that it has progressed to subchondral bone remodelling and erosion. Arthroscopy is a much better tool to assess articular cartilage damage.

Rarely, further imaging such as computed tomography (CT) (Buttin *et al.*, 2013), magnetic resonance imaging (MRI), scintigraphy (Stern *et al.*, 2007) or ultrasonography (Brisson *et al.*, 2004) may be considered appropriate, especially if a radiolucent foreign body is being sought.

Haematology and biochemistry: Haematology and biochemistry tests are neither diagnostic nor consistent. Results observed can include neutrophilia, low-grade anaemia, mild thrombocytopenia, increased erythrocyte sedimentation rate, elevated liver enzymes, hyperglobulinaemia, hypoglycaemia and low titres of anti-nuclear antibody and rheumatoid factor (Bennett and Taylor, 1988). As these are non-specific results for septic arthritis, such tests are not indicated in the majority of patients unless there is a clinical concern of systemic involvement or other disease.

Synovial fluid examination: Synovial fluid assessment is the most important diagnostic procedure in the investigation of septic arthritis (see also Chapter 4). The essential feature of septic arthritis is neutrophilic inflammation, occasionally but not always accompanied by evidence of intracellular bacteria. The differential diagnoses for synovial neutrophilic inflammation are immune-mediated joint disease, which is normally a polyarthropathy (i.e. affects multiple joints), and septic arthritis, which is normally a monoarthropathy (i.e. affects a single joint).

Fluid from infected joints is typically inflammatory in nature with an increased volume, turbidity, elevated protein (frequently clotting on exposure to air due to the presence of fibrin) and a poor mucin clot (Figures 6.9 and 6.10). The white cell count will be elevated, the predominant cell generally being the neutrophil. Cell numbers are typically in excess of 40×10^9 cells/litre. In acute cases cell numbers may exceed 200×10^9/l, but in low-grade disease may be $<10 \times 10^9$/l. PMNs (neutrophils) usually exceed 90% of white blood cells but can be as low as 25% (compared to a normal joint where they typically comprise less than 5%).

Illustration of how fluid cell counts are expressed differently according to units of fluid volume used. In each example the absolute cell count is exactly the same:
- Litre (l): cell count = 7.4×10^9 cells/litre
- Millilitres (ml): cell count = 7.4×10^6 cells/ml
- Microlitres (µl): cell count = 7.4×10^3 cells/µl

Gross appearance
- Increased volume
- Increased turbidity
- Reduced viscosity
- Increased protein
- Poor mucin clot

Microscopic appearance
- Elevated white cell count
- Peripheral cell polymorphonuclear leucocytes (neutrophils)
- Degenerative neutrophils (occasional)
- Intracellular/extracellular bacteria (occasional)

6.9 A quick reference guide to the gross and microscopic features of septic arthritis/infected joint fluid.

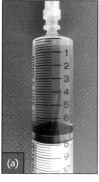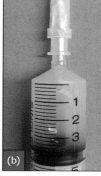

6.10 (a) Synovial fluid from a stifle with degenerative joint disease. Note that the fluid is slightly yellow and transparent. (b) Synovial fluid from a septic stifle. Note that the fluid is discoloured, cloudy and opaque.

While an obvious increase is usually evident, relative and absolute neutrophil counts can each overlap with ranges found in non-infected (immune-mediated) inflammatory disease. Neutrophils may, but do not necessarily, exhibit degenerative and toxic changes such as pyknotic nuclei, degranulation and cell rupture. Intracellular or extracellular bacteria are pathognomonic but are uncommonly seen (Figure 6.11).

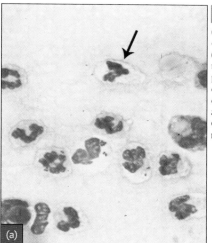

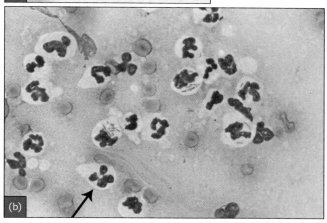

6.11 Synovial fluid showing (a) intracellular bacterial cocci (arrowed) and (b) intracellular bacterial rods (arrowed). The presence of these organisms confirms the diagnosis of septic arthritis. (Wright–Giemsa stain, original magnification X1000)

Bacteriology: Synovial fluid should be cultured in all cases where septic arthritis is suspected or is a potential differential diagnosis. Positive culture confirms a diagnosis of septic arthritis, but a false-negative may occur in as many as 50% of cases when synovial fluid is cultured directly (Montgomery *et al.*, 1989; Clements *et al.*, 2005). Incubation of infected fluid in blood culture medium (Figure 6.12) prior to culture reduces the false-negative rate (Montgomery *et al.*, 1989). In *in vivo* experiments, Montgomery reported a false-negative culture rate of 33% for synovial membrane, 44% for synovial fluid, and 0% of fluid post 24-hour incubation in blood culture medium. Culture of synovium appears no more likely to produce positive culture than that of fluid, is more invasive and is, therefore, rarely justified.

Though prior administration of antibiotics may limit successful culture, Clements *et al.* (2005) found no relationship between previous antimicrobial administration and culture result of synovial fluid, or the identification of bacteria on a synovial fluid smear.

Aseptic technique, i.e. skin clip and preparation, sterile gloves, changing of needles between sampling and injection into growth medium, must be followed to

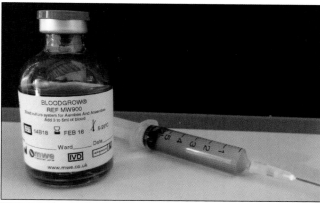

6.12 Blood culture medium used to culture synovial fluid. This is the best technique to minimize the likelihood of a false-negative result.

limit iatrogenic contamination, both of the joint and of the sampled tissue, that could otherwise lead to a septic arthritis or a false-positive culture and sensitivity result respectively (Figure 6.13, see Chapter 4).

Polymerase chain reaction (PCR) has been used to identify bacterial DNA but appears no more helpful than culture (Jalava *et al.*, 2001). Interpretation can also be difficult, with a positive result perhaps reflecting material from a single circulating bacterium, possibly present due to joint inflammation but not representing an active joint infection (Muir *et al.*, 2007).

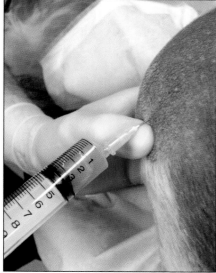

6.13 Aseptic synovial arthrocentesis technique. The skin should be prepared and normal standards of surgical asepsis observed to prevent the introduction of infection. A sterile technique should be used and sterile gloves worn. Surgical drapes could also be considered.

Treatment

A wide variety of treatment options has been reported but the evidence base is limited, and restricted to retrospective studies only.

Systemic antibiotic therapy is a feature of all treatment regimens. Adjunct methods that may be considered include joint aspiration, joint irrigation, arthroscopic synovectomy, open arthrotomy and debridement/lavage, and local antibiotic delivery systems.

In the absence of a positive culture result but where there is the suspicion of septic arthritis, treatment is begun with a broad-spectrum antibiotic (such as co-amoxiclav or cefalexin) and subsequently modified depending on culture results and response to treatment. Intravenous therapy is often begun for speed of delivery but replaced soon with oral medication. Duration of therapy is typically for an extended period, usually a minimum of 6 weeks, and should be continued at least until cell numbers and morphology have reduced to within the normal range (or within the 'normal' range for any pre-existing joint disease, such as osteoarthritis).

In the uncommon case of a probable septic arthritis, i.e. borderline cytology results and negative culture, and where mono-articular immune-mediated arthropathy is an alternative differential diagnosis, if there has been no or limited response to antibiotic and non-steroidal anti-inflammatory drugs (NSAIDs) treatment, the case should be reviewed, synovial fluid analysis repeated and corticosteroid therapy may be carefully instigated. Corticosteroids may also be considered for the case where infection has been resolved satisfactorily but clinical signs and synovial fluid assessment suggest a continued non-infective/immune-based arthritis.

The need for surgery or joint irrigation in the absence of a penetrating wound or infected implant is controversial. In one series of 32 cases (Clements et al., 2005), no difference was found between the eight cases treated with antibiotics alone and the 24 cases treated surgically (arthrotomy, arthroscopically and/or needle lavage). Where foreign material is present (foreign body, implant, non-absorbable or long-lasting suture material), it is advisable to remove the potential nidus of infection so long as it is safe to do so. Unless an alternative is available, orthopaedic implants may have to be retained in the presence of infection until deemed redundant, e.g. bone healing and remodelling are complete. Where there is an unsatisfactory response to medical management, surgery/irrigation may be indicated.

Joint irrigation can be performed with a copious volume of sterile isotonic fluid (e.g. Hartmann's solution) via two large bore needles (to allow egress of blood and fibrin clots) in different, ideally distant, regions of the joint (Figure 6.14).

Arthroscopy allows simultaneous examination of articular structures (arguably better than with arthrotomy), irrigation of the joint and may also allow removal of foreign material. However, restrictive periarticular fibrosis and severe proliferative synovitis may render arthroscopy difficult. Synovectomy, manual or with a power shaver, is not routinely performed as it is not supported currently by clinical evidence. It is difficult to recommend open arthrotomy with placement of indwelling drains (Figure 6.15) due to the increase in tissue trauma, increase in patient care requirements, and difficulty of maintaining sterility of the

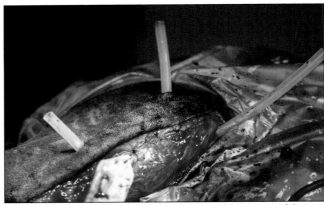

6.15 Surgical debridement and placement of drains. Use of drains requires considerable care and attention. Sterility of the drains post surgery must be assured and ensured.

drains postoperatively, unless arthroscopy is unavailable, implants require removal or fibrin clots prevent successful irrigation via needles.

Local, slow release, antibiotic delivery systems may be indicated, for instance where culture and sensitivity suggest use of an antibiotic with a toxicity profile precluding long-term systemic use. Such carriers are most commonly used in the face of multiresistant organisms, such as meticillin-resistant *Staphylococcus aureus* (MRSA). Non-biodegradable, e.g. antibiotic-impregnated polymethylmethacrylate beads (Figure 6.16), and biodegradable, e.g. antibiotic-impregnated collagen 'sponge' (Figure 6.17) carriers have been reported in small animal veterinary practice (Brown and Bennett, 1988; Owen et al., 2004). The non-absorbable beads have the disadvantage of being more bulky and requiring an additional surgical procedure for removal.

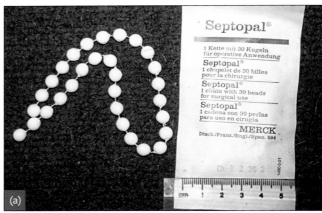

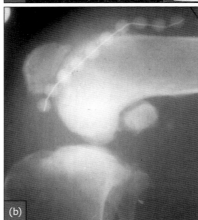

6.16 (a) Gentamicin-impregnated polymethylmethacrylate (PMME) beads are commercially available. Each bead contains 7.5 mg of gentamicin sulphate. Kits are available to make similar beads at the time of surgery. (b) Mediolateral view of the stifle of a dog with septic arthritis being treated with surgically implanted gentamicin-impregnated PMME beads. The beads require removal once the infection has resolved.

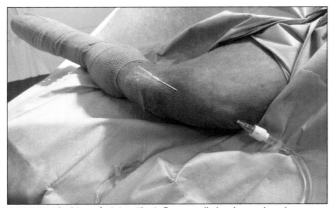

6.14 Flushing of a joint. The inflow needle has been placed proximolateral to the patella and the egress needle is distomedial.

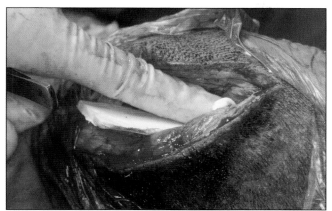

6.17 Gentamicin-impregnated collagen sponge being inserted into an infected stifle joint. The collagen is broken down and resorbed within 1–7 weeks following implantation and therefore does not require surgical removal.
(Courtesy of Dr M Owen)

Prognosis

With appropriate therapy, considerable clinical improvement is typically seen within 24 to 48 hours. Regular repeat synovial fluid analysis (cell numbers, types and morphology) should be performed to monitor progress and antibiotics continued until results are within normal limits, or consistent with pre-existing osteoarthritis. Repeat culture and sensitivity should be performed if joint fluid indicates a failure of response or a deterioration in signs. Antibiotic therapy is continued until after cell numbers/differential counts have returned to normal and typically for a minimum of 4–6 weeks. The author [RA] typically repeats cytology at 2 and then 4–6 weeks after beginning therapy and continues antibiotics for 2 weeks after apparent resolution of active infection. Frequency of arthrocentesis and duration of antimicrobial administration must, however, depend on signs and progress.

Anti-inflammatory drugs, controlled physiotherapy and nutraceuticals may assist recovery but outcome is variable. There may be a trend for poorer outcomes associated with heavier patients, longer duration of lameness, and higher synovial fluid nucleated cell count at presentation (Clements et al., 2005).

Other types of infective arthritis

Borrelia

The tick-borne spirochaete *Borrelia burgdorferi* can cause multisystemic inflammatory disease, including arthritis, in humans and animals. It is passed between vertebrate hosts by tick vectors (nymph or adult). In the UK the most common vector is *Ixodes ricinus* (sheep tick) but *B. burgdorferi* has been isolated from other ticks too. Though the first documented case of Lyme disease in the UK was reported in 1990, PCR studies on historic samples show its presence in UK ticks dates at least from the late 1800s.

Serum titres of antibodies to *Borrelia burgdorferi* exhibit national and regional variation and about 95% of seropositive dogs will remain asymptomatic. Though cats exhibit similar levels of seroconversion (4.8% of UK cats), clinical signs are apparently absent or rare (May et al., 2008).

A reddish rash can be seen for the first week or so after tick attachment. The classic 'bull's eye' expanding erythematous skin lesion (erythema chronicum migrans) of human Lyme disease is not seen in dogs. More commonly,

signs are of acute pyrexia, lethargy and shifting lameness with swollen joints associated with an inflammatory, non-erosive arthritis. Other signs seen less commonly include protein-losing nephropathy, arrhythmia secondary to myocarditis and neurological signs.

Clinical signs are typically not pathognomonic and laboratory tests are divided between those that demonstrate presence of the organism and antibody tests reflecting exposure. Demonstration of the organism by culture, cytology or PCR assay can be difficult, results being slightly higher from tissue samples (synovium or bite region) than from blood or synovial fluid. A positive PCR test does not prove the presence of live, active organism. Similarly, given the prevalence of asymptomatic seropositive animals and the possibility of cross-reaction, a positive test alone does not prove the organism as the cause of signs, although a clinical case is unlikely to be serologically negative. A four-fold increase in IgG antibody titres is strongly supportive but can take several weeks to occur. PCR tests, especially those with primers to plasmid DNA, are more sensitive.

A presumptive diagnosis of Lyme disease should include (Littman et al., 2006):

* Evidence of exposure to *B. burgdorferi*
* Clinical signs consistent with Lyme disease
* Consideration of other differential diagnoses
* Response to treatment.

Doxycycline is the drug of choice in adults, though other antimicrobials are effective. In growing animals an alternative, perhaps amoxicillin, should be used. Clinical response is often seen within 48 hours and treatment continued typically for at least 4 weeks though this may not prevent persistence. Persistence of infection in the dog appears shorter than in humans (Goossens et al., 2001).

Chronic immune-mediated non-erosive polyarthritis (type II) may persist secondarily despite antimicrobial therapy.

Vaccination for Lyme disease is available in both Europe and the USA but is considered a non-core vaccine and its use is controversial, generally being used in dogs in high risk geographical areas with a high risk of exposure (e.g. outdoor or hunting dogs).

Protozoal arthritis

Infection with the protozoan *Leishmania*, spread by the sand fly, can cause a serious and potentially fatal prolific systemic disease of the reticuloendothelial system, including synovium. Endemic regions include Mediterranean Europe (*Leishmania infantum*), Africa, Asia and America (South, Central and southern states of the USA). Cases in temperate regions, including the UK, generally result from travel to, or importation from, infected regions. However, there have been cases in the UK involving dogs that have not travelled (Hillman and Shaw, 2010).

Whether or not infected animals develop disease depends on their immune status. In endemic regions, 60–70% are infected but only 10% develop disease.

Clinical signs are varied and include lethargy, wasting, lymphadenopathy, pyrexia, splenomegaly and dermatitis. Most cases develop cutaneous signs and a variable minority exhibit stiffness, lameness and arthritis which can be monoarthritic, oligo(pauci)arthritic or polyarthritic in nature (Spreng, 1993; McConkey et al., 2002; Sbrana et al., 2014) and can be erosive (Wolshrijn et al., 1996) or non-erosive. Disease may be a granulomatous reaction to the presence of the organism within the joint or a type III hypersensitivity reaction with deposition of immune complexes.

Diagnosis is suspected on clinical signs, consistent history of travel or potential exposure and the presence of inflammatory joint changes, and confirmed definitively on direct cytological observation of parasitic amastigotes in synovial fluid or lymph node aspirates, or positive serology/PCR tests. Amastigotes are not observed in all cases and blood tests lack 100% sensitivity and specificity.

Treatment with meglumine antimoniate or miltefosine (neither licensed for use in the UK) in combination with allopurinol can result in improvement or stabilization of signs in many, but not all, patients. Renal function requires monitoring and relapse is possible.

Public health implications must be considered, given the zoonotic nature of leishmaniasis and the risk of persistently infected/carrier status.

A canine vaccination against *Leishmania* (CaniLeish, Virbac) has recently been brought to the UK market and perhaps may be considered to complement other preventative measures including use of antiparasitic collars or 'spot-ons' and keeping animals in at dawn and dusk when sand flies are most active.

Rickettsial arthritis

Infection with the obligate intracellular tick-borne Gram-negative bacteria of the genera *Ehrlichia* and *Anaplasma* causes disease in wild and domesticated animals and in humans in many areas of the world. Dogs, like people, are incidental hosts infected through the bite of an infected nymphal or adult *Ixodes* tick vector. The geographical distribution of *Ehrlichia* spp. and *Anaplasma* spp. closely follows that of the tick vectors responsible for transmission. Infected dogs in the UK are likely to have been abroad or been in contact with dogs that have; however, since 2013, there have been reports of ehrlichiosis in dogs that have not travelled abroad (Wilson *et al.*, 2013). Cats may be seropositive for infection but feline clinical disease is uncommon.

In dogs, a non-erosive arthritis can result from infection (Stockham *et al.*, 1986; Cowell *et al.*, 1988) but signs are typically non-specific, such as pyrexia, lethargy, weight loss, blood dyscrasia, haemorrhage and lymphadenopathy.

Acute and chronic (delayed clinical signs) forms of the disease are reported. Synovial fluid from affected joints shows signs of inflammation, and radiographic changes reflect the non-specific soft tissue changes of effusion and periarticular swelling.

Ehrlichia morulae may be visible in Giemsa-stained blood smears (Stockham *et al.*, 1992) and in 1–2% of synovial fluid PMNs (Cowell *et al.*, 1988). Serology (indirect fluorescent antibody (IFA) and enzyme-linked immunosorbent assays (ELISA)) tests and PCR tests are available to assist diagnosis but, depending on the test, laboratory and organism, cross-reaction, false-positives and false-negatives may occur.

Ehrlichia spp. and *Anaplasma* spp. in dogs and cats are sensitive to doxycycline (10 mg/kg daily for 28 days is currently recommended) and the response of polyarthritis to treatment is good, although a carrier state may persist and recrudescence of disease may occur. Neurological abnormalities and fatalities can result from the more systemic disease manifestations.

Most *Ehrlichia* spp. and *Anaplasma* spp. that infect pets are zoonotic agents, infecting people in the same way as animals, via the bite of an infected tick. Prevention of infection in each is by tick control/prevention of tick bite. Though pets are not considered a source of human infection, direct transmission between animals and humans with contaminated blood or tissue is possible.

Mycoplasma arthritis

Mycoplasma spp. are normal commensal inhabitants of feline and canine conjunctival membranes, respiratory passages and urogenital tracts but can cause clinical signs. Joint infection is rare. Two *Mycoplasma* species (*M. felis*, *M. gateae*) have been implicated as having pathological significance in the cat (Moise *et al.*, 1983; Hooper *et al.*, 1985; Zeugswetter *et al.*, 2007). In the dog, *M. spumans* (Barton *et al.*, 1985) and *M. edwardii* (Stenske *et al.*, 2005) have been cultured from cases of polyarthritis. Feline polyarthritis has been associated with immune deficiency/suppression (Hooper *et al.*, 1985; Bonilla *et al.*, 1997) and monoarthritis with possible trauma (Liehmann *et al.*, 2006).

Radiographic signs are typically non-specific and non-erosive, although erosive arthritis has been associated with *M. gateae* in the cat. Joint fluid is typically turbid and inflammatory in appearance. Organisms can be demonstrated with Giemsa, Wright's or Leishman stains and can be cultured. *Mycoplasma* are sensitive to a variety of antimicrobials including fluoroquinolones, macrolides, tetracycline, lincomycin, clindamycin and aminoglycosides. Treatment for an extended period appears necessary.

Bacterial L-forms

Bacterial L-forms are cell wall deficient bacteria that can, in culture, revert to their parent cell wall state. Their formation is facilitated by the use of cell wall damaging antimicrobials and host immune responses. They are difficult to culture or demonstrate with light microscopy but can be identified with electron microscopy.

Their presence in both diseased and healthy animals makes determination of their significance uncertain but a chronic disease with fistulating subcutaneous wounds and possible secondary joint involvement that was refractory to most antibiotics was reported in cats (Carro *et al.*, 1989) and thought to be caused by a *Mycoplasma* L-form. The source of infection could be a cat bite or application of infected ointment (Keane, 1983). Affected animals had non-specific systemic disease and swollen, crepitant joints from which discharged purulent material. The disease appeared responsive to tetracyclines.

An L-form of *Nocardia asteroides* (Buchanan *et al.*, 1983) was retrieved from a dog with progressive polyarthritis that was unresponsive to steroids and antibiotics. Erythromycin and chloramphenicol have been used in canine infections.

Radiographs may show periarticular swelling, periosteal proliferation and, with time, articular cartilage and subchondral bone destruction. Diagnosis may be speculative, absolute confirmation often being difficult.

Chlamydial arthritis

Although rare, systemic disease associated with pyrexia, lymphadenopathy and arthropathy of several joints in which *Chlamydia* spp. was implicated has been described (Lambrechts *et al.*, 1999).

Mycobacterial arthritis

In the developed world mycobacterial infection has appeared rare in the dog and cat, but in recent years, it is being reported more commonly in the cat (Gunn-Moore *et al.*, 2013) and infective arthritis may occur. Due to the zoonotic potential of the infection (can be transmitted in either direction) and implications of human infection, specifically with *M. bovis*, treatment of affected animals is controversial (Möstl *et al.*, 2015).

Bartonella

Bartonellosis is an emerging zoonotic infectious bacterial disease (Breitschwerdt et al., 2010) caused by the Gram-negative bacterium Bartonella, and may be of increasing clinical importance. Bartonella spp. are transmitted to dogs by fleas, sand flies, lice and ticks. Clinical signs are extremely variable and there is a wide spectrum of disease; infective endocarditis is the most common manifestation, but arthritis also occurs (Diniz et al., 2009). Treatment is usually with doxycycline, azithromycin or a fluoroquinolone though optimum treatment is unknown.

Viral arthritis

Calicivirus: In the cat, infection can occasionally cause acute synovitis, polyarthritis and lameness. While vaccine strains can cause clinical signs (Dawson et al., 1994), field strains and possibly passaged vaccine strains (Davidson, 1993) have a greater propensity to do so.

Polyarthritis typically affects kittens 5–7 days after first vaccination. They are frequently febrile and may show oral and respiratory signs too. Joints are painful to manipulate and synovial fluid shows a variable increase in nucleated cell count, with small mononuclear cells and macrophages predominating.

Feline calicivirus may be isolated from the oropharynx of some affected cats, and rarely from the joint (Levy and Marsh, 1992) but diagnostic investigation may not be required when typical clinical signs and history are present because signs typically resolve after 2–5 days. Short-term treatment with analgesics may be appropriate.

Coronavirus: Synovitis and lameness may accompany the effusive, and sometimes dry, forms of feline infectious peritonitis with yellow, turbid synovial fluid evident on arthrocentesis. In most cases this is likely to be due to immune complex deposition but macrophages can be identified in some coronavirus infected joints.

Feline leukaemia virus and feline syncytial virus: A chronic, progressive polyarthritis not caused by identifiable bacteria or Mycoplasma but aetiologically linked to feline leukaemia virus (FeLV) and feline syncytial virus (FeSV) has been reported by Pederson et al. (1980). Two forms were described, with the first and most common form characterized by osteopenia and periosteal new bone formation and the other exhibiting subchondral marginal erosions and deformity. Post-viral arthropathy is relatively common in humans, perhaps due to immune complex hypersensitivity rather than a direct pathogenic effect of the virus. In the dog, a transient polyarthritis is sometimes seen 5–7 days after vaccination, most commonly associated with multivalent live vaccine. Corticosteroid therapy may be used if lameness is severe and persistent but is usually unnecessary and may interfere with effectiveness of vaccination.

Fungal arthritis

Fungal arthritis is uncommon in the dog and cat and, apart from a case of discospondylitis associated with Aspergillus spp. (Butterworth et al., 1995), has not been reported in the UK. Elsewhere, causative agents have included Coccidioides immitis (Maddy 1958), Cryptococcus neoformans (Kavit, 1958), Blastomyces dermatitidis (Oshin et al., 2009; Woods et al., 2013), Sporothrix shenckii (Goad and Goad, 1986) and Aspergillus fumigatus (Oxenford and Middleton, 1986).

Haematogenous spread following inhalation is thought to be the principal source of infection, though direct contamination or spread from contiguous infected tissues may occur. Clinical and radiographic signs are similar to those of other inflammatory arthritides. Additional signs present depend on which organs are affected and patients should be assessed for signs of systemic disease.

Microscopic examination of joint fluid or synovium will demonstrate inflammatory changes and organisms may be visible. Confirmation of disease is based on fungal culture (in media such as Sabouraud's agar) or serological examination.

Treatment with anti-fungal drugs (± surgical debridement) including amphotericin B, ketoconazole, itraconazole and fluconazole has been variably successful.

Osteoarthritis

Osteoarthritis (also known as degenerative joint disease or osteoarthrosis) is the most common form of arthritis in dogs and cats. It should be thought of as a disease process rather than disease entity because it appears to be a common pathway for the failing joint. Importantly in the dog, it is almost always a secondary phenomenon to an initiating abnormality (e.g. joint laxity or instability, osteochondrosis, trauma).

> Articular cartilage is considered the key tissue in osteoarthritis but it must be remembered that the synovial joint is an organ with cross-talk between the various tissues (cartilage, synovium, bone, ligament, meniscus, synovial fluid, fat)

The relative importance of cross-talk between different joint tissues (e.g. between synovium and cartilage) is still unknown. There is no doubt that a morphological marker of progression of osteoarthritis is the gradual loss of articular cartilage. An understanding of osteoarthritis requires some information on the metabolism of the tissues of the joint.

Pathological processes in osteoarthritis

Because some therapies are designed to influence the metabolism of joint tissues in osteoarthritis, a brief discussion of the underlying pathological processes is relevant background for the practitioner.

Although there is a tendency to think of osteoarthritis as merely a degenerative disease (so-called 'wear and tear'), there are active biological processes within tissues such as cartilage and synovium that gradually lead to the loss of integrity of cartilage and a progression to cartilage erosion and ulceration (Figure 6.18). However, osteoarthritis is a slowly progressive disease and the natural history of the condition typically extends to a number of years. Early in the disease process, there are limited anabolic responses from joint tissues but degradative mechanisms are also activated in osteoarthritis and the tendency is for the balance between synthesis and degradation to gradually swing towards the latter. However, by way of example it takes 3 to 5 years for full-thickness cartilage lesions to appear following cruciate transection in the dog. Of course, the sequence and timeframe of events varies with the joint and the initiating cause. For example, the progression to full-thickness cartilage lesions is generally more rapid in the medial compartment of the elbow with elbow dysplasia.

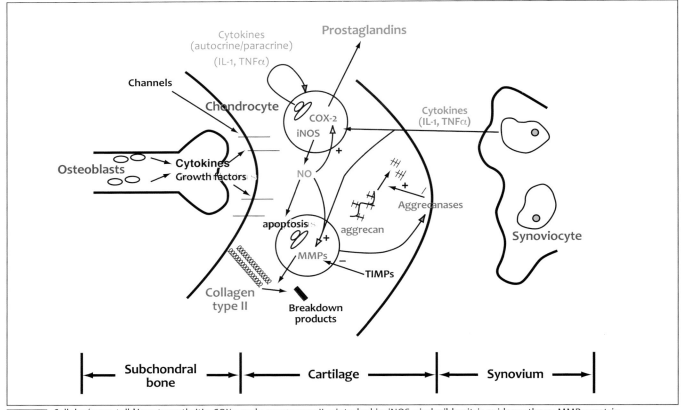

6.18 Cellular 'cross-talk' in osteoarthritis. COX = cyclo-oxygenase; IL = interleukin; iNOS = inducible nitric oxide synthase; MMP = matrix metalloproteinase; NO = nitric oxide; TIMP = tissue inhibitor of metalloproteinase; TNFα = tumour necrosis factor α.

Diagnosis and staging of osteoarthritis

> Osteoarthritis is usually not a diagnosis of sufficient accuracy in canine orthopaedics because the disease is usually the result of some other primary joint abnormality (e.g. instability, laxity, fracture). The clinician should seek to identify why a joint has osteoarthritis

Other chapters in this manual deal with methods to reach such diagnoses and there is often a seamless transition between the primary joint disease and the process of osteoarthritis. Management decisions are more often based on the stage of the disease (Figure 6.19), or perhaps the age of the animal. In cats, it may be difficult to identify a primary joint abnormality (e.g. idiopathic elbow osteoarthritis in older cats).

Obtaining a client history and clinical metrology instruments

General questions to the client with an animal with a musculoskeletal disorder also apply to patients with osteoarthritis. However, following a diagnosis of osteoarthritis, it is important to assess the disease severity because this can guide the clinician as to how best to manage the problem. In recent years there has been progress with validation of client questionnaires (or 'clinical metrology instruments' (CMIs)) for canine osteoarthritis and lameness and these can be of use to clinicians in formalizing and scoring disease severity. In general, management decisions for osteoarthritis should primarily be based on the *functional* effects of the disorder rather than changes on radiographs or other imaging modalities.

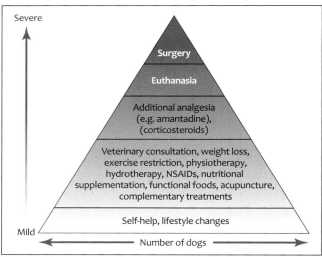

6.19 Staging osteoarthritis can help to guide the clinician with disease management.
(Redrawn after Tobias and Johnston, 2012)

There are several CMIs now published for dogs, including the Liverpool Osteoarthritis in Dogs (LOAD) instrument, the Canine Brief Pain Inventory and the Helsinki Chronic Pain Index. Readers are referred to the individual instruments for information on their use in a clinical setting. In a chronic disorder such as osteoarthritis, CMIs can play a large role in evaluating the impact of the disease on the function and activity of the dog. However, the results should always be combined with the clinician's clinical assessment and other diagnostic tests. The situation for cats is less well developed at the current time although CMIs are emerging.

Clinical signs of osteoarthritis

The clinical signs of osteoarthritis in dogs are similar to many joint-related conditions (Figure 6.20). In cats, behavioural changes are frequently present and should be looked for when taking a history (Figure 6.21).

- Stiffness after inactivity
- Lameness
- Reluctance to exercise
- Reluctance to climb or descend stairs or to jump
- Muscle atrophy
- Reduced range of motion
- Crepitus
- Altered gait (reduced stride length, altered swing phase)
- Altered behaviour (aggression, reduced general activity)

6.20 Clinical signs of osteoarthritis in dogs.

- Reluctant to jump up or down; smaller jumps; less frequent jumps
- Reduced activity
- Lameness
- Reduced fluidity of movement
- Less playing and hunting, more time sleeping
- Less interaction with owner and other cats
- Reduced range of motion
- Crepitus
- Altered gait (reduced stride length, altered swing phase)
- Unkempt appearance

6.21 Clinical signs of osteoarthritis in cats.

Radiographic signs of osteoarthritis

The radiographic signs of osteoarthritis are non-specific. The features that are associated with osteoarthritis are listed in Figure 6.22. All joints with osteoarthritis will show osteophyte formation eventually. However, this can occur at different rates. In dogs with complete cranial cruciate ligament rupture, osteophytes are usually visible radiographically within 3–4 weeks. Conversely, in some dogs with elbow dysplasia, osteophytes may take several months to develop despite significant cartilage loss. In addition, data from the PennHIP® scheme indicates that some breeds produce more osteophytes than others, given the same degree of hip laxity. This highlights the heterogeneity of osteoarthritis between joints and between individuals. The relationship between osteophyte severity and cartilage pathology is poorly defined in dogs and cats but it is likely to change with disease progression. In other words, osteophytes seem to appear early in disease but they may remodel and appear less severe with time, despite the progression of cartilage pathology (Hielm-Bjorkman *et al.*, 2003).

- Osteophytosis
- Enthesophytosis
- Intra-articular mineralization
- Subchondral sclerosis
- Subchondral cysts (geodes)
- Soft tissue enlargement

6.22 Radiographic features of osteoarthritis in dogs and cats.

Intra-articular mineralization in dogs seems to occur only in some individuals. It probably represents deposition of hydroxyapatite crystals within soft tissues such as menisci and ligaments. The significance of this change in dogs is unknown. In cats, mineralization of the medial meniscus is associated with osteoarthritis of the medial compartment of the stifle joint.

Subchondral sclerosis is a change traditionally associated with chronic disease. Care must be taken when using plain radiographs to derive information regarding bone density. CT scanning can provide more accurate information.

> **WARNING**
>
> Although the osteophyte and enthesophyte are used as markers of osteoarthritis, it should be remembered that these occur with other forms of joint disease

Advanced imaging techniques

Arthroscopy can be used to help diagnose and stage osteoarthritis but this is not usually necessary from a purely clinical standpoint. Arthroscopy can be used to grade the depth and extent of cartilage loss in a semi-quantitative way; a modification of the Outerbridge classification system is often used (Figure 6.23).

CT scanning can provide detailed information on the bony changes associated with osteoarthritis, including bone density. However, the direct clinical relevance of such examinations remains unknown at the present time. MRI is now the established gold standard for assessing the loss of cartilage from human joints. There are several methods to acquire and process the MRI data including estimating whole cartilage volumes, thickness mapping and delayed gadolinium enhanced MRI of cartilage (dGEMRIC). In the context of imaging canine cartilage, there are technical issues caused by the thinness of canine cartilage and, as such, the technique is likely to remain a clinical research tool.

Outerbridge score	Outerbridge descriptors (original)	Modified Outerbridge descriptors
0	Normal	Normal
1	Cartilage softening and swelling	Chondromalacia or cartilage softening assessed by probing
2	Partial thickness defect with surface fissures that are <15 mm in diameter or do not reach subchondral bone	Partial thickness fibrillation
3	Fissures >15 mm diameter or reach the subchondral bone	Deep fibrillation
4	Exposed subchondral bone	Full thickness cartilage loss
5	n/a	Subchondral bone eburnation

6.23 The Outerbridge and modified Outerbridge classification scoring systems used to classify the severity of articular cartilage damage.

Synovial fluid analysis

The characteristics of synovial fluid in osteoarthritis can change as the disease progresses (see Chapter 4). Early in disease there may be significant effusion but later on there may be a reduced synovial fluid volume. The viscosity of the fluid is usually near-normal and the colour is clear to light straw coloured. The cell count is usually low (1.0–5.0 x 10^9/l) with only 2–5% neutrophils. Hydroxyapatite crystals may be seen under polarized light microscopy.

Management of osteoarthritis

Identification of the primary cause of osteoarthritis may direct the clinician to surgical treatment of that condition (e.g. cranial cruciate ligament rupture, fragmentation of the medial coronoid process, hip laxity) but because most joint disorders will cause some degree of osteoarthritis, consideration must also be given to the disease process. This chapter will only discuss the medical management of osteoarthritis. In severe or end-stage disease, surgical treatment may be considered (e.g. total joint replacement or arthrodesis) and the reader is referred to the relevant chapters for appropriate discussion of such techniques. Conservative management of osteoarthritis can be sub-divided into the following categories:

- Client education
- Weight control
- Exercise control
- Physiotherapy (including hydrotherapy)
- Medical management
  - Symptom-modifying drugs for osteoarthritis
  - Structure-modifying drugs for osteoarthritis
  - Cell-based therapies
- Nutritional supplementation (nutraceuticals and functional foods)
  - Nutritional supplementation for pain relief
  - Nutritional supplementation for structure modification.

Client education and clinical monitoring

> Education of the client is very important in managing osteoarthritis. An understanding of the disease keeps the client motivated and 'onside'

The client needs to know that the disease can only be managed, rather than cured, and that this may have an impact on the patient's (and the owner's) lifestyle. The use of a variety of educational aids and strategies is extremely useful at the start of the management process. Nurse-led arthritis clinics can also aid this process and reinforce management concepts.

> **PRACTICAL TIP**
>
> The use of clinical metrology instruments (CMIs) which ask the client to score the activity of their pet and the severity of the osteoarthritis can be very helpful in transferring knowledge to the client and assisting their understanding of the disease process. It can also be a useful means to stage the disease and track response to treatment

Weight control

In humans, there is a strong epidemiological link between osteoarthritis and obesity, particularly for the knee. There are fewer data for the dog, but previous studies have shown a link between higher body condition score and progression of osteoarthritis secondary to hip dysplasia. Within the constraints of the current knowledge base, it does seem sensible to recommend avoidance of obesity in dogs and cats with joint disease. Body condition scoring is a useful and accessible way to assess the level of obesity in dogs and cats. Proprietary weight-reduction diets are available and participation in veterinary nurse-led weight control clinics is recommended as a means to encourage compliance of owners in this respect. For a full discussion of weight control strategies, the reader is referred to the *BSAVA Manual of Canine and Feline Rehabilitation, Supportive and Palliative Care: Case Studies in Patient Management*. There are studies indicating that in clinically affected overweight or obese dogs, weight reduction can have a positive benefit on the signs of osteoarthritis. Of course, the reduction in bodyweight is also somewhat dependent on activity levels, and other aspects of disease management (e.g. analgesia) are aimed at increasing activity which will in turn help to manage obesity.

Exercise control

> The aim of exercise control is a balance between avoiding excessive stress on the osteoarthritic joint, and limiting the joint stiffness often noted following prolonged inactivity

The effect of exercise regimens on canine osteoarthritis is relatively poorly understood. The traditional recommendation is that exercise should be controlled (leash) and in moderation, with perhaps an increased frequency, but decreased duration. Exercise on flat, even ground is likely to be less problematic than rough, uneven ground and slightly soft surfaces (grass, firm sand) may be preferred to concrete. However, there are few firm data to guide the clinician in this respect and the majority of advice is based on intuition or extrapolated from reports of human patients. The effects of exercise on canine osteoarthritis have received little attention in the literature to date. One recent study investigated a small group of dogs with osteoarthritis and showed that ground reaction forces were decreased after 1.2 km of lead exercise (Smith *et al.*, 1995). However, another study suggests a beneficial effect of exercise for canine hip osteoarthritis. On a very practical level, some clients who work may have different expectations of their animal during their leisure time (e.g. weekends) compared to when they are busy working. It may be that exercise may vary with the day of the week and due allowance for this might need to be built in to the management protocol (e.g. increasing the dose of analgesics at these times).

Physiotherapy

There is increasing evidence that physiotherapy can help the injured canine joint. Most of this information concerns the postoperative joint and for a more detailed discussion of physiotherapy modalities, the reader is referred to Chapter 17. Certainly in human medicine, physiotherapy and exercise protocols have shown functional and pain-relieving benefits for patients with osteoarthritis (Innes *et al.*, 2004). It seems likely that selected physiotherapy techniques may help the arthritic joint. Swimming and hydrotherapy have become very popular for dogs but, to date, the effects for dogs with osteoarthritis have not been widely documented. Swimming does result in a greater range of motion of joints and there appears to be some benefit of hydrotherapy in human patients with arthritis; however, a systematic review of non-surgical management of canine hip osteoarthritis indicated that further information is required on the role of swimming and hydrotherapy in dogs with osteoarthritis.

Medical management

Medications for osteoarthritis may affect symptoms (clinical signs) and/or modify structure (joint pathology). The Osteoarthritis Research Society International has suggested that the term 'symptom-modifying osteoarthritis drug' (SYMOAD) be used for agents that relieve pain, including both those with a rapid and a slow onset of action. Agents with the potential for structure modification in osteoarthritis (STMOADs) have previously been labelled as 'chondroprotective', 'disease-modifying drugs for osteoarthritis' (DMOADs), 'anatomy-modifying agents', etc., although STMOAD is the current recommended group name (Beraud et al., 2010). The demonstration of structure modification in osteoarthritis requires randomized, controlled clinical trials with appropriate outcome measures. Such measures (e.g. MRI of cartilage) are not yet developed for dogs.

Symptom-modifying osteoarthritis drugs:
Non-steroidal anti-inflammatory drugs:

- Mode of action: NSAIDs act to inhibit cyclooxygenase (COX) and therefore decrease the production of proinflammatory prostaglandins, e.g. PGE2. For some time, cyclooxygenase has been known to exist in two isoforms: the constitutive COX-1 and the inducible COX-2. COX-2 is induced at sites of inflammation and has been an important target for drug development by pharmaceutical companies for some years. Effective inhibition of COX-2 appears to reduce pain and inflammation, and sparing of COX-1 appears to reduce the side effects of NSAID administration (e.g. gastrointestinal irritation, reduced renal blood flow). The currently available NSAIDs for veterinary species vary somewhat in their selectivity for COX-1 and COX-2. Those licensed for long-term use tend to be either non-selective or have a preference for COX-2. This has theoretical advantages in terms of reducing side effects while maintaining efficacy. It is probably better to describe these newer agents as COX-1-sparing drugs because of their rapidly reversible blockade of COX-1.
- Use of NSAIDs in dogs: NSAIDs have been the mainstay for medical management of osteoarthritis for some considerable time. The NSAIDs licensed for use in the

dog in Europe and the USA are listed in Figure 6.24. Because the pain of osteoarthritis is likely to be chronic and persistent, veterinarians need to think about long-term treatment and not merely short-term treatment for an acute flare in pain. In cats, however, this may be a necessity because of limited treatment options. In dogs, there is evidence that longer term, continuous treatment provides improved efficacy. The licence for some drugs facilitates long-term use in osteoarthritis; currently, examples of such drugs include carprofen, deracoxib, etodolac, firocoxib, meloxicam and robenacoxib. In the UK, paracetamol (acetaminophen) is only licensed for up to 5 days in combination with codeine (Pardale V®, Upjohn), but it does not appear to inhibit COX peripherally. Various studies have compared these agents in terms of efficacy but there is likely to be publication bias in the literature and it is difficult to give a firm opinion as to the preferred agents based on efficacy. Clinical trials, including those using objective measures such as force platform evaluation, have indicated that this class of drug is effective in reducing synovial joint pain and lameness.

> The efficacy of individual agents in individual patients appears somewhat variable and it may be necessary to try different agents to find the most effective one for a particular patient. Clinicians should take note of product data sheets when switching between agents and adhere to the required wash-out period between NSAIDs to avoid compounding gastrointestinal tract or other side effects

- Use of NSAIDs in cats: the use of NSAIDs in cats can be problematic because of toxicity issues. Currently only meloxicam, robenacoxib (up to 6 days) and ketoprofen are licensed for cats in the UK (Figure 6.24).
- Side effects of NSAIDs: by virtue of their action on COX-1, NSAIDs may be associated with adverse events. The pharmacology of individual agents influences the frequency and severity of these but the common adverse events are vomiting and diarrhoea due to irritation of the gastrointestinal mucosa. COX-1 is also involved in control of renal blood flow and so

Drug	Formulation	Dogs[a]	Cats[a]
Carprofen	Tablet	2–4 mg/kg q24h	C/I
Cimocoxib	Tablet	2 mg/kg q24h	C/I
Deracoxib[b]	Tablet	1–2 mg/kg q24h[c]	C/I
Etodolac[b]	Tablet	10–15 mg/kg q24h[c]	C/I
Firocoxib	Tablet	5 mg/kg q24h	N/A
Ketoprofen	Tablet	1 mg/kg q24h for up to 5 days	1 mg/kg q24h for up to 5 days
Mavacoxib	Long-acting tablet	2 mg/kg on days 0 and 14, then every 30 days	C/I
Meloxicam	Oral suspension	0.2 mg/kg on day 1, then 0.1 mg/kg q24h	0.1 mg/kg on day 1, then at maintenance dose of 0.05 mg/kg q24h
Pardale V (paracetamol and codeine)	Tablet	Suggested 10 mg/kg paracetamol q8h	C/I
Phenylbutazone	Tablet	2–20 mg/kg q24h for 14 days, then review	C/I
Robenacoxib	Tablet	1–2 mg/kg q24h	1–2.4 mg/kg q24h for up to 6 days
Tolfenamic acid	Tablet	4 mg/kg q24h for up to 3 days. May be repeated every 7 days	N/A (only licensed for febrile syndromes)

6.24 Licensed non-steroidal anti-inflammatory drugs for dogs and cats in Europe and the USA. [a] licensed dose in the UK; [b] not available in Europe; [c] licensed dose in the USA; C/I = contraindicated; experience indicates this drug is not suitable for long-term use in the cat or no information available regarding use in cats; N/A = no current licence for use in cats for osteoarthritis.

care should be taken in any patient with renal impairment. This is also true of cardiovascular impairment where renal perfusion may be decreased. NSAIDs inhibit platelet COX to a variable degree and this should be borne in mind in patients with bleeding disorders or immunosuppressed patients. NSAIDs may be metabolized in the liver; thus, hepatic disease may also be a contraindication to the use of NSAIDs. Furthermore, the displacement of protein-bound agents in animals on concomitant treatment is also sometimes a concern. The gastrointestinal side effects of NSAIDs may be ameliorated with gastroprotectants such as sucralfate (Antepsin), histamine (H2) receptor antagonists such as ranitidine and cimetidine, or proton pump inhibitors such as omeprazole. Prostaglandin E_1 agonists such as misoprostol can be used in severe incidents. The reader is referred to the *BSAVA Manual of Canine and Feline Gastroenterology* for further information.

Corticosteroids: The use of corticosteroids for the treatment of osteoarthritis is controversial. For a local disease such as osteoarthritis, corticosteroids are generally used as intra-articular agents. Suppression of local joint inflammation by corticosteroids is rapid and pronounced, and may be achieved with only minor systemic effects. However, this suppression usually is only temporary. Long-acting preparations such as methylprednisolone acetate, triamcinolone acetonide, and triamcinolone hexacetonide are the preferred intra-articular corticosteroids. A number of potential adverse effects of intra-articular corticosteroids stress the importance of their judicious use. The risk of cartilage damage and progressive joint destruction is a controversial issue. Results of animal studies are ambiguous. Although corticosteroids are potent anti-inflammatory agents, and some evidence suggests that they can protect articular cartilage in experimental canine osteoarthritis and can provide significant alleviation of clinical signs, they also can have deleterious effects on joint tissues with repeated use, caused by the suppression of cartilage matrix synthesis. Despite case reports of severe arthropathy, most studies involving their use in humans suggest that, when used appropriately, the beneficial effects of intra-articular corticosteroids exceed the harmful effects. Nevertheless, it is recommended for human beings that corticosteroid injections into the same joint should be limited, for instance to one injection every 6 weeks and no more than three to four injections in any single year; it would seem prudent to adopt similar guidelines for small animals. Before intra-articular corticosteroid injections are given, the indications and contraindications should always be considered. In particular, infection should be ruled out. Strict aseptic technique is essential to avoid iatrogenic septic arthritis.

Potential structure-modifying agents: Many of the candidate structure-modifying agents actually remain in the nutritional supplementation class and the reader is referred to the discussion of these agents. There are a few licensed drugs that purport structure-modifying properties but, to date, none have satisfied appropriate criteria such as those described by the Osteoarthritis Research Society International.

Polysulphated glycosaminoglycans: Polysulphated glycosaminoglycan (PSGAG) is licensed for the treatment of osteoarthritis in dogs in some countries, including the USA. The exact mode of action of PSGAG *in vivo* is not known. The recommended dose of Adequan® Canine

(Novartis Animal Health, Basel, Switzerland) is 2 mg/lb bodyweight by intramuscular injection only, twice weekly for up to 4 weeks (maximum of eight injections). Two systematic reviews of treatments for canine osteoarthritis concluded that there was a moderate level of comfort in recommending the use of PSGAG for canine osteoarthritis.

Pentosan polysulphate: Pentosan polysulfate (PPS) is a semisynthetic GAG prepared from beech hemicellulose. It is structurally similar to heparin and has anticoagulant properties. Laboratory studies have shown that *in vitro* PPS can retard articular cartilage degradation and stimulate the synthesis of hyaluronan by synovial cells and proteoglycan by chondrocytes. PPS also acts as a fibrinolytic and thrombolytic agent. For a review of the potential effects of this drug the reader is referred elsewhere (Foley *et al.*, 2003). PPS is licensed for osteoarthritis in dogs in several European countries, as well as in Australia, New Zealand, and Canada. It is prepared as the sodium salt for parenteral administration. The calcium salt exhibits higher bioavailability when delivered orally, but this version of the product is not licensed currently for use in canine osteoarthritis. There are three published clinical trials of PPS in dogs. The first trialled the injectable sodium salt of PPS against placebo in dogs with established osteoarthritis and used clinical scores as the primary outcome measure (Crook *et al.*, 2007); results showed positive benefit on clinical signs of osteoarthritis. A second study compared the use of PPS against surgical treatment (fragment removal via arthrotomy) in dogs with elbow dysplasia; the results failed to show a difference between the two treatment regimens (Bouck *et al.*, 1995). The third study was a one-year, placebo-controlled trial that investigated use of the oral calcium salt of PPS in dogs immediately after surgery for cruciate ligament deficiency; the results failed to show any clinical benefit. Thus there is conflict in the literature as to the efficacy of this agent; anecdotally, it may be that the drug is more useful for pain relief in chronic osteoarthritis. Systematic reviews of treatments for canine osteoarthritis have concluded that there was a *moderate* level of comfort in recommending the use of PPS for canine osteoarthritis.

Cell-based and biological therapies: In recent years there has been much interest in cell-based therapies for a variety of disorders, including musculoskeletal problems such as osteoarthritis. Mesenchymal stem cells (MSCs) are multipotent stem cells that can differentiate into a variety of cell types, including chondrocytes and osteoblasts. In the past decade or so, there has been a surge of interest in the use of MSCs to repair damaged connective tissue. This discipline, known as regenerative medicine, aims to develop biological, cell-based therapies to repair or replace injured or eroded tissues such as cartilage. At the current time, techniques offered commercially for osteoarthritis in dogs involve harvesting of autologous adipose tissue and extraction of stromal cells (the 'stromal vascular fraction' (SVF)). The SVF may be injected intra-articularly after extraction or, alternatively, cultured in the laboratory to produce an expanded population of MSCs. The mode of action of such procedures is unclear at the current time and may involve soluble factors released by MSCs or actions of the cells themselves. Early clinical trials, including one placebo-controlled trial, suggest some efficacy in dogs with osteoarthritis of the hip and elbow. However, this is currently an emerging treatment modality and there are many unanswered questions regarding its efficacy, safety and indications.

Platelet-rich plasma (PRP) is an autologous derivative of whole blood that contains high concentrations of growth factors including transforming growth factor-β, insulin-like growth factor, platelet-derived growth factor, basic fibroblast growth factor, and vascular endothelial growth factor, as well as bioactive proteins. Through the effects of the various growth factors, PRP has been shown to have a positive effect on chondrogenesis and mesenchymal stem cell proliferation. PRP has also been shown to increase anti-inflammatory and decrease pro-inflammatory mediators. These combined effects of PRP make it a potential injectable option for management of osteoarthritis. Published data on PRP in dogs are limited but studies in experimental dogs suggest some clinical benefits (Bozynski *et al.*, 2016; Upchurch *et al.*, 2016).

Nutritional supplementation

In recent years, the use of nutritional supplementation to support synovial joint health has become very popular. Nutritional supplementation may be provided in the form of a 'nutraceutical' which is typically a tablet, capsule or liquid which is added to the diet, or as a 'functional food' which is a complete diet enriched with specific nutrients. Regulation of these products is inconsistent in that in some countries, some nutraceuticals are licensed, whereas in many countries, products such as glucosamine, chondroitin sulphate and omega-3 fatty acids are unlicensed with unrestricted availability.

The majority of nutritional supplement products marketed for osteoarthritis in veterinary species are combination products consisting of glucosamine, chondroitin sulphate and fatty acids, often with other ingredients added (e.g. methylsulphonylmethane, turmeric, manganese ascorbate). In addition, the majority of clinical studies have used combination products, although there are a very limited number of peer-reviewed studies in the veterinary literature. One double-blind comparator study involved 71 osteoarthritic dogs and compared the efficacy, tolerance and ease of administration of two routinely prescribed NSAIDs, carprofen and meloxicam, and a combination glucosamine sulphate–chondroitin sulphate (GS–CS) nutraceutical (Moreau *et al.*, 2003). The authors found significantly improved ground reaction forces for the index limbs following NSAID treatment, but not following nutraceutical therapy. It was concluded that both NSAIDs had a beneficial functional effect, while the GS–CS nutraceutical did not. A systematic review of the evidence regarding the efficacy of such nutritional supplements in the management of osteoarthritis in companion animals concluded that the general strength of evidence was weak but the best evidence was for omega-3 fatty acids in dogs.

Immune-mediated arthritis

The term 'immune-mediated arthritis' (IMA) encompasses a group of conditions which are manifest by an aberrant and profound synovial inflammation and which result in joint pain and, potentially, other systemic signs of illness. IMA is also termed immune-mediated polyarthritis (IMPA) because, in the vast majority of patients, multiple joints are affected. Although uncommon, IMAs are frequently undiagnosed or misdiagnosed, and should be considered in ANY dog or cat with persistent lameness, joint pain, joint effusion, lymphadenopathy and/or pyrexia where the underlying cause is not immediately apparent. Any synovial joint can be affected by the disease. Most commonly, the major appendicular joints are affected, although on occasion synovial joints of the axial skeleton can also be affected.

Historically, IMAs have been classified into different types on the basis of the presence or absence of periarticular bone erosion, the involvement of other organ systems and the identification of an underlying aetiopathological event that may have triggered the disease (Figure 6.25). This further classification is important as both the treatment and prognosis can be influenced by the diagnosis.

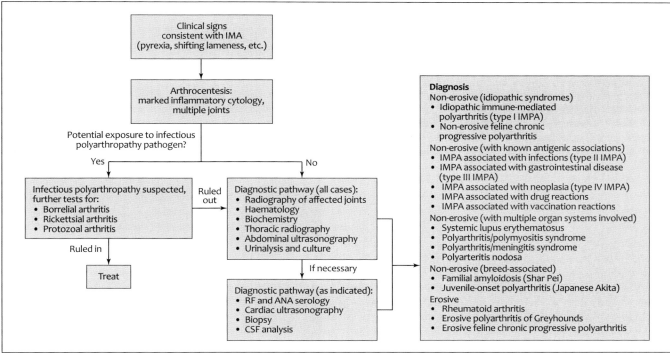

6.25 The diagnostic pathway and classification of immune-mediated arthritides. ANA = antinuclear antibody; CSF = cerebrospinal fluid; IMA = immune-mediated arthritis; IMPA = immune-mediated polyarthritis; RF = rheumatoid factor.

Aetiopathogenesis

Marked synovial inflammation is the predominant feature of IMAs. The aetiology of this inflammation is believed to be an antigenic stimulus in or around the joint, producing antigen–antibody bound complexes, which produce a type III hypersensitivity reaction. The synovial inflammation results in proinflammatory cytokine release and neutrophil chemotaxis into the joint space, which in turn perpetuates the inflammatory reaction.

In some types of immune-mediated arthritides, the inciting antigen may be identified (such as a neoplasm, microbial agent, drug or virus), but in many cases it may not. The chronic nature of the inflammation, which is a feature of many IMAs, may be due to persistence or recurrence of the antigenic stimulus, or a loss of the 'tolerance' of the immune system to normal host antigens.

The major aetiological feature of the autoimmunity which characterizes IMAs in humans is genetic risk, and in particular, the association of major histocompatibility (MHC) alleles with disease. MHC molecules present antigens exclusively to CD4-positive T 'helper' cells, which help to trigger an appropriate immune response, such as the recruitment of phagocytes or the activation of B cells. Similar associations have been made in dogs with IMA and the canine MHC equivalent, the dog leucocyte antigen (DLA) class II alleles (Ollier *et al.*, 2001; Wilbe *et al.*, 2009).

Diagnosis

Immune-mediated polyarthritis should be considered in any patient with single or multiple limb lameness or stiffness, particularly if more generalized signs of systemic illness including lymphadenopathy, pyrexia, inappetence or general malaise are also reported. IMA is the most commonly diagnosed condition causing pyrexia of unknown origin in dogs (Dunn and Dunn, 1998), but a significant proportion of dogs presenting with the condition do not demonstrate pyrexia (Clements *et al.*, 2004). Waxing and waning clinical signs may be reported as the disease can go into a degree of remission or relapse.

Multiple and symmetrical joint involvement is commonly recognized with IMA. Given the frequently cyclical nature of the disease, lameness can affect multiple limbs at different times. Joints will often be effused and painful on manipulation, although this is not always the case. Where the disease is severe and chronic in nature, joint effusion, joint thickening and deformities may be marked.

The first diagnostic investigative step in any patient where IMA is suspected is arthrocentesis of multiple joints. Typically joints selected for arthrocentesis will be those which are painful or effused. Where overt signs of joint disease are not readily identified, the major, more distal joints (elbow, antebrachiocarpal, stifle and talocrural joints) should all be considered for sampling, as these are more likely to be affected. Gross changes in the appearance of the synovial fluid recovered (increased synovial fluid volume, turbid appearance and decreased viscosity) may be recognized, although this is not pathognomonic for the disease. Normal gross synovial fluid appearance does not exclude IMA; therefore, cytological evaluation is mandatory. The characteristic cytological finding in cases with IMA is an increased white cell count that is predominantly polymorphonuclear in nature (see Chapter 4).

The main alternative diagnosis for polyarticular synovial joint inflammation is that caused by an infectious aetiology. These two conditions cannot be differentiated on the appearance of the synovial fluid cytology alone. Most polyarticular infectious agents are vector-borne and, thus, a history of potential exposure to the vector (e.g. a recent history of a tick bite, or travel history to an area where the diseases are known to be endemic) warrants caution. Where an element of doubt exists, the diagnostic tests for borrelial, rickettsial and protozoal infections should be instigated (see Chapter 4). In the UK, the prevalence of these diseases as causes of polyarthritis is very low and further diagnostic investigation can be continued while the results of these tests are pending.

Further diagnostic investigations

Radiography is performed to evaluate for the presence of bone erosions (Figure 6.26). With non-erosive forms of IMA, the radiographic changes will typically be non-specific; namely periarticular soft tissue swelling (indicative of synovitis and synovial effusion) with or without osteophyte deposition (which often develops with prolonged uncontrolled disease). The radiographic features will usually be bilaterally symmetrical. Where erosive changes are not identified (which is the case for the majority of cases), further diagnostic steps should be taken to try and identify an underlying antigenic stimulus which might be causative.

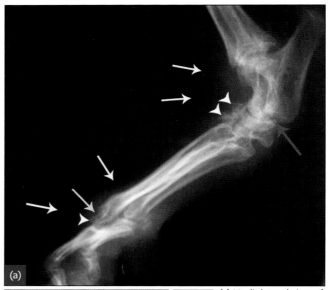

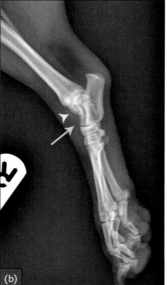

6.26 (a) Mediolateral view of the tarsus and pes of a 1-year-old crossbreed dog with an erosive arthopathy. Note the extensive soft tissue swelling (white arrows), periarticular new bone formation and joint destruction at all joints (arrowheads) with subluxation of the proximal intertarsal joint (red arrow). In particular, note the erosive changes in the distal joints (yellow arrow). (b) Mediolateral view of the tarsus and pes of a 6-year-old Cocker Spaniel with type I IMPA. Note the subtle periarticular soft tissue swelling (yellow arrow) and new bone formation (arrowhead) on the dorsal aspect of the talus.

In all cases the following diagnostic tests are recommended:

- **Haematology:** many cases will show a leucocytosis, but there can be leucopenia, neutrophilia with left shift, anaemia (of chronic disease or immune-mediated aetiology) and/or thrombocytopenia
- **Biochemistry:** urea, creatinine, alkaline phosphatase, alanine transferase and aspartate transferase concentrations may be elevated. Raised creatine kinase may be associated with concurrent myositis. Globulins may be raised as a result of increased antibody production
- **Thoracic radiography and abdominal ultrasonography:** these techniques facilitate the evaluation of the thoracic and abdominal cavities to screen for the presence or absence of an inflammatory or neoplastic focus
- **Urinalysis:** may reveal proteinuria if concurrent glomerulonephropathy or urinary tract infection is present. Urine culture is routinely performed.

In selected cases, the following diagnostic tests may be helpful:

- **Serology for anti-nuclear antibody (ANA):** this may be helpful if there is concurrent immune-mediated disease confirmed in another organ system (in addition to the polyarthritis), to confirm or refute the diagnosis of systemic lupus erythematosus (SLE). It is not routinely performed in other cases, however, as it is neither highly specific nor sensitive for the disease. Rheumatoid factor (RF) is neither specific nor sensitive for the identification of rheumatoid arthritis, and thus is only of value in cases where bony erosions have been identified on radiography
- **Cerebrospinal fluid analysis:** this should only be performed in the presence of spinal pain, to rule in concurrent aseptic meningitis. The author [DC] does not do this routinely, as the diagnosis of concurrent aseptic meningitis does not appear to affect the treatment or prognosis
- **Cardiac ultrasonography:** this should be performed where a cardiac murmur is auscultated and endocarditis needs to be ruled out; blood culture is performed if suspected
- **Biopsy of skin, muscle, liver or the kidney:** this is performed to investigate concurrent immune-mediated disease where there is a high index of suspicion.

Non-erosive immune-mediated arthropathies

Idiopathic immune-mediated polyarthritis (type I IMPA)

The most common IMA is idiopathic (type I) IMPA; it has been reported to account for 50% of cases of IMA (Bennett, 1987b), but in the author's [DC] experience, it accounts for a much higher proportion of IMA cases. No source of antigenic stimulus can be found, although patients often have non-specific changes on diagnostic tests (such as raised liver enzymes). The prognosis with chemotherapeutic immunosuppression is complete cure in 54% of patients, with 18% of cases requiring continuous treatment, 13% of cases developing recurrence and 15% of cases dying or requiring euthanasia as a result of their disease (Clements *et al.*, 2004).

Non-erosive feline chronic progressive polyarthritis

Two forms of feline chronic progressive polyarthritis (FCPP) exist: erosive and non-erosive. Both are characterized by the development of profound periarticular new bone and enthesophyte formation (Figure 6.27) (Pedersen *et al.*, 1980). Affected cats may be seropositive for feline syncytial virus (FeSV) and feline leukaemia virus (FeLV), although a causal relationship has never been demonstrated. The prognosis for both forms of the condition is guarded.

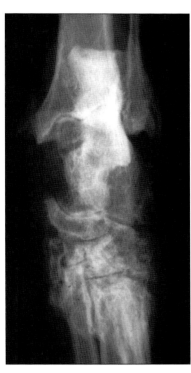

6.27 Dorsoplantar view of the tarsus of a cat with the non-erosive form of FCPP. There is periarticular new bone formation but no evidence of erosion. Symmetrical changes were present in the contralateral limb.

Non-erosive immune-mediated arthropathies with known antigenic associations

Immune-mediated polyarthritis associated with an infection (type II IMPA)

Type II IMPA is associated with an infection remote from the joint, such as a respiratory tract infection or a urinary tract infection (Bennett, 1987b). The hypothesis is that the primary infection is an antigenic source which results in immune complex disease in the joints. Resolution of the primary infection should facilitate resolution of the polyarthritis, although it is important to ascertain the joint disease is not simply an extension of the primary infection. Some cases will require immunosuppression to fully resolve the IMA, even after the primary infection has resolved. In these cases, it can be challenging to differentiate whether the infectious process has truly resolved or not, which will govern whether immunosuppressive treatment is started or not.

Immune-mediated polyarthritis associated with gastrointestinal disease (type III IMPA)

Gastrointestinal disease (most commonly manifest as vomiting or diarrhoea) can trigger IMPA (Bennett, 1987b). Both the intestinal microflora and food particles could act as potential sources of antigens to stimulate immune complex disease. It should be borne in mind that a clear temporal relationship between the development of gastrointestinal disease and the IMPA should be made for the diagnosis of type III IMPA, as gastrointestinal upset is not uncommon in dogs, and spurious associations can easily be made. If the gastrointestinal disease can be addressed successfully, the prognosis is good.

Immune-mediated polyarthritis associated with neoplasia (type IV IMPA)

While any tumour could potentially provide the antigenic source to drive IMPA (Bennett, 1987b), myeloproliferative diseases have been most commonly associated. Therefore, cats with type I IMPA which do not respond to therapy may require bone marrow aspiration and analysis. The prognosis will depend on whether the antigenic stimulus of the tumour can be resolved or not.

Vaccination reactions

Vaccination reactions typically occur 5–7 days after the primary vaccination course, and in most cases the lameness is transient, lasting 1–2 days. The calicivirus component of the vaccine has been associated with the disease in cats (Dawson et al., 1993), and the distemper virus component may be the cause in dogs, although no evidence exists to support this theory. The prognosis is very good for resolution of the disease, although re-vaccination may cause recurrence of the disease. Avoidance of the inciting antigenic component of the vaccine is difficult when a direct causal relationship is not fully understood, but as some measure of the level of protection to the suspected component can be made (through demonstration of a protective antibody titre), then the risks of re-vaccination are balanced with the risks of becoming infected with the wild-type disease.

Drug-induced IMPA

Occasionally, IMPA can be seen as a side effect of drug therapy, for example with sulphonamide administration in Dobermanns. It is hypothesized that the hypersensitivity reaction arises as a result of drug–antibody interactions; as such, other organ systems can also be involved. Withdrawal of the drug is usually sufficient to effect resolution of the condition within a short period of time and the prognosis is excellent providing the same class of drugs is avoided in that patient.

Non-erosive immune-mediated arthropathies with multiple organ systems involved

Systemic lupus erythematosus

SLE is a multi-organ disease, in which affected individuals can concurrently develop one or more autoimmune diseases affecting organ systems in addition to the IMA, such as autoimmune haemolytic anaemia, immune-mediated thrombocytopenia, leucopenia, glomerulonephritis, dermatitis, polymyositis, pleuritis and aseptic meningitis (Fournel et al., 1992). The disease is characterized by the development of autoimmunity (antibodies to nuclear antigen) and immune complex formation, which triggers the disease in the various organ systems.

ANA levels can be measured in dogs and cats; they can be elevated in other disease states so raised levels do not constitute a diagnosis. The accepted criteria for diagnoses are confirmed autoimmune disease of two organ systems and a positive ANA titre or alternatively, confirmed autoimmune disease of three organ systems. The prognosis for SLE is guarded as it often requires aggressive immunosuppression and remission can be difficult to maintain, ultimately leading to euthanasia. Other non-erosive IMAs with additional organ system involvements are characterized by the absence of antinuclear antibodies.

Polyarthritis/polymyositis syndrome

Polyarthritis/polymyositis syndrome is marked by profound stiffness, myalgia and in time, muscle wastage. Spaniel breeds are most commonly affected (Bennett and Kelly, 1987). The prognosis is reported to be poor, with only 30% of dogs making a full recovery.

Polyarthritis/meningitis syndrome

Polyarthritis/meningitis syndrome is typically manifest as pyrexia, stiffness and neck pain; occasionally neurological signs will be present. The prognosis is reported to be good in most cases. Meningitis can be present in a proportion of dogs with type I IMPA where spinal pain is noted on physical examination (Webb et al., 2002).

Polyarteritis nodosa

Polyarteritis nodosa is an inflammatory condition resulting in polyarthritis, but which can also affect the meninges, muscles and kidneys. The condition is characterized by a generalized granulomatous necrotizing vasculitis of the small and medium arteries of the affected tissues; the condition can only be diagnosed with histological evaluation of affected tissues. The prognosis for the condition is reported to be good in dogs.

Non-erosive immune-mediated arthropathies with breed associations

Immune-mediated arthritis in the Chinese Shar Pei

A recurring inflammatory disease of the distal limbs, particularly the hocks, with concurrent episodes of profound pyrexia (40.5–41.5°C) is recognized in the Chinese Shar Pei (May et al., 1992), and is also called 'Shar Pei fever'. Young dogs tend to be affected and episodes may be triggered by stress. The inflammation tends to be periarticular; therefore, synovial fluid analysis may be normal. An association with the development of amyloidosis has been made in some individuals, which may lead to hepatic and/or renal failure. Affected dogs will often respond to immunosuppressive treatment early in life, but the development of concurrent amyloidosis is associated with a high rate of mortality.

Juvenile-onset polyarthritis in the Japanese Akita

Polyarthritis of young Akitas (less than 1 year of age) has been reported (Dougherty et al., 1991), sometimes in association with meningitis. The prognosis for the condition is poor as dogs often respond poorly to immunosuppressive treatment and require euthanasia.

Erosive immune-mediated arthropathies
Rheumatoid arthritis

Rheumatoid arthritis is a severe, debilitating IMA which is rarely encountered in dogs and cats. The disease is characterized by the radiographic appearance of subchondral and periarticular lucencies, which can progress with time to complete destruction of the articular surface, gross joint malformation and luxation or subluxation (see Figure 6.26a). Cases can typically be diagnosed when having two of the following features: a serological positive test for RF, erosive changes on radiographs, and histopathological changes consistent with rheumatoid arthritis. A set of 11 diagnostic criteria, including those listed, have been used to define canine rheumatoid arthritis (Figure 6.28) (Bennett, 1987a), with seven criteria required for the diagnosis, including two of criteria 7, 8 and 10. However the criteria 1–5 and 9 are observed in many dogs with IMAs and are not unique to rheumatoid arthritis, and thus do not provide a particularly useful method for discriminating the disease from other types of IMA.

The author [DC] urges caution in the over-interpretation of serological tests for rheumatoid arthritis. RF is an antibody to the Fc component (the tail region which interacts with cell surface receptors) of IgG or IgM; it is neither specific nor completely sensitive for the disease. One should also note that the erosive changes may not be visible in the early stages of the disease, so repeating diagnostic imaging of the joints is warranted if the disease is suspected. The prognosis for the disease in dogs is poor, although aggressive multimodal immunosuppression may delay the time until euthanasia is required. The prognosis for cats has been reported to be good with a combination treatment of oral methotrexate and leflunomide (Hanna, 2005).

Diagnosis of rheumatoid arthritis requires the presence of seven of the 11 criteria below, including two or three of the changes in **bold**

1. Stiffness after rest persisting for at least 6 weeks
2. Pain or tenderness on motion of at least one joint persisting for 6 weeks
3. Swelling of at least one joint persisting for at least 6 weeks
4. Swelling of at least one other joint within 3 months
5. Symmetrical joint swelling persisting for at least 6 weeks
6. Subcutaneous nodules (rare in dogs)
7. **Erosive changes on joint radiographs**
8. **Positive serological test for rheumatoid factor**
9. Synovial fluid cytology consistent with IMA
10. **Synovial membrane histology typical of rheumatoid arthritis**
11. Subcutaneous nodule histology consistent with rheumatoid arthritis

6.28 Simplified diagnostic criteria for rheumatoid arthritis.

Erosive polyarthritis of Greyhounds

Erosive IMA of young Greyhounds has been reported in both the USA and Australia. Although the articular pathology of these cases is very similar to canine rheumatoid arthritis, there has been a suggestion that the condition actually represents an infective arthropathy, with a *Mycoplasma* sp. implicated (Barton *et al.*, 1985). The prognosis for these cases is extremely poor, as they will not return to a normal athletic performance and often respond poorly to immunosuppressive treatment.

Erosive feline chronic progressive polyarthritis

The erosive form of FCPP is characterized by the development of radiolucencies in addition to the extensive new bone formation which is the predominant feature of the non-erosive form of the disease (Pedersen *et al.*, 1980). It is unclear whether the two forms of the disease are related.

Treatment

The treatment of IMA is determined in each separate case by the diagnosis, but can be simplified as follows:

* If an inciting cause is identified, it should be eliminated (i.e. type II, III and IV IMPA, drug and vaccination reactions)
* Where no inciting cause is identified or its elimination does not resolve the IMA, then immunosuppressive treatment needs to be instigated.

The goals of immunosuppressive therapy are:

* To relieve the clinical signs of the disease
* To suppress the synovial inflammation sufficiently to return the synovial fluid characteristics to normal
* To prevent damage to articular cartilage, ligament or bone
* To facilitate complete remission of the disease, or determine the minimum doses of medication where remission is maintained.

This must be balanced against the fact that all immunosuppressive agents currently available can have significant side effects. The relatively low prevalence of IMAs means that large-scale controlled clinical trials of different therapeutic regimens for the treatment of the disease do not exist for dogs or cats. The lack of standardization of diagnoses or treatment regimens further compounds the problem, which renders meaningful and objective assessment of different treatment regimens impossible.

Regardless of treatment, success is gauged as an improvement (clinical remission) or resolution of clinical signs and the return of synovial fluid parameters to normal (complete remission). Clinical improvements can often be reported when the synovial inflammation has not been addressed (as assessed by synovial fluid analysis); consequently, the decision to change the treatment regimen must be made with the synovial fluid parameters in mind. Recent work has suggested that C-reactive protein can also be used as a measure of clinical response to treatment with prednisolone in cases of IMPA (Foster *et al.*, 2014), although a further study found that it was a poorly sensitive marker for the control of IMPA (Grobman *et al.*, 2017), which concurs with the author's experience [DC]. One should also note that reductions in the synovial fluid abnormalities without their complete normalization do not constitute remission. Once a patient is in remission, synovial fluid analysis is generally not repeated unless clinical signs become evident again (Figure 6.29).

Note: for ALL immunosuppressive treatments, readers should refer to the latest edition of the *BSAVA Small Animal Formulary* to familiarize themselves with the safety practices, adverse reactions, drug interactions, contraindications and suggested doses. In particular, the requirement for monitoring of side effects (for example regular haematological analysis for the evaluation of myelosuppression) should be ascertained for any immunosuppressive agent used.

Prednisolone has been the primary treatment for IMA in dogs and cats. The drug is usually initiated at 2–4 mg/kg daily in a divided dose, for 2 weeks. Providing remission is attained, the dose can generally be reduced over a 6–8-week period, at which point the drug can be stopped.

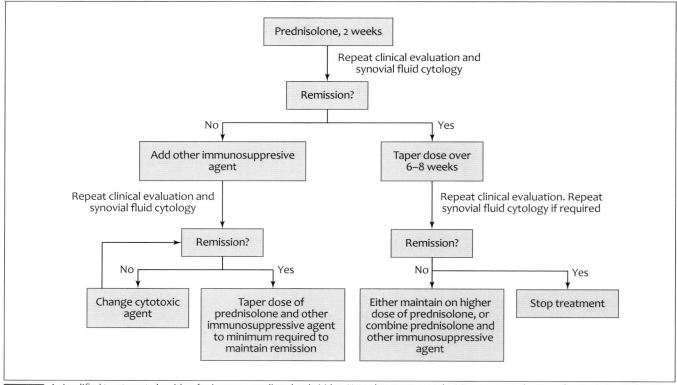

6.29 A simplified treatment algorithm for immune-mediated arthritides. Note that treatment decisions on re-evaluation of patients treated with immunosuppressive agents must also be influenced by the potential side effects of the agents used. The suggestions are guidelines; the duration of treatment and time to taper doses need to be gauged on an individual basis.

If remission is not obtained with prednisolone alone, it can be used in combination with other immunosuppressive drugs (Figure 6.30). Once remission has been achieved, the dose of prednisolone and/or the other immuno-suppressive agent can be tapered to the lowest effective dose. The response to other immunosuppressive thera-peutic agents varies from individual to individual, but often a number of agents may need to be trialled before remis-sion can be achieved. The costs associated with repeated diagnostic evaluation for the side effects of each chemo-therapeutic agent can be significant, and owners of affected dogs should be warned at the outset of treatment that repeated investigations may be required and that remission cannot always be achieved.

One of the mainstays of treating human rheumatoid arthritis when conventional drug treatments fail is the use of so-called biological therapies or immunotherapies. The most popular are antibody-based treatments that bind and sequester TNFα, a key cytokine in the pathogenesis of the disease. The efficacy of such treatments can be high, and they can be combined with conventional chemotherapeutic regimens. To date, the costs of such products and their human specificity has precluded their use in canine IMAs, but canine-specific antibody preparations are becoming available (Gearing et al., 2013), and the availability of one specific for canine TNFα is likely to become available in the near future.

Drug	Loading dose	Suggested tapering strategy	Major side effects
Prednisolone	1–2 mg/kg, orally, twice daily (2–3 mg/kg, twice daily in cats)	Reduce dose by half every 2 weeks, then give every other day when reach 0.5 mg/kg	Suppression of the hypothalamic–pituitary axis; gastrointestinal ulceration
Chlorambucil	2 mg/m², orally, once daily	Give every other day, then reduce dose by half	Myelosuppression; gastrointestinal signs
Azathioprine	2 mg/kg, orally, once daily	Give every other day, then reduce dose by half	DO NOT USE IN CATS; myelosuppression in dogs
Leflunomide	3–4 mg/kg, orally, once daily; 10 mg (total dose) orally once daily in cats in combination with methotrexate	Reduce dose after 6 weeks	Myelosuppression; hepatotoxicity
Levamisole	2–5 mg/kg, orally, every other day	Reduce dosing frequency	Maximum dose 150 mg
Methotrexate	2.5 mg/m², orally, twice weekly	Reduce dose	Myelosuppression; vomiting
Ciclosporin	5 mg/kg, orally, once daily	Generally do not reduce dose	Gastrointestinal signs
Cyclophosphamide	1.5 mg/kg, orally, 4 consecutive days each week; 2.5 mg/kg, orally, once daily in cats	Reduce dose of frequency	Myelosuppression; haemorrhagic cystitis

6.30 Drugs commonly used in the treatment of immune-mediated arthritis. The drugs are listed in the order of preference they are used by the author [DC].

Surgical treatment

With severe forms of IMA (such as rheumatoid arthritis) or IMA which does not respond to immunosuppressive treatment, the chronicity of disease can eventually lead to irreversible joint destruction (see Figure 6.25a). While it is tempting to immediately consider a salvage procedure (such as arthrodesis or joint replacement), extreme caution should be exercised. Consideration must be given to the general health of the patient and the status of other joints. Multiple joint involvement can result in the requirement for multiple surgical procedures or the inability to treat the disease effectively elsewhere in the limb (for example in the metacarpophalangeal, metatarsophalangeal and proximal interphalangeal joints). In severe cases, euthanasia may need to be considered as the most humane option, when no other effective treatment options are available.

References and further reading

Altman R, Brandt K, Hochberg M et al. (1996) Design and conduct of clinical trials in patients with osteoarthritis: Recommendations from a task force of the Osteoarthritis Research Society – Results from a workshop. Osteoarthritis and Cartilage 4, 217–243

Aragon CL, Hofmeister EH and Budsberg SC (2007) Systematic review of clinical trials of treatments for osteoarthritis in dogs. Journal of the American Veterinary Medical Association 230, 514–521

Barton MD, Ireland L, Kirschner JL and Forbes C (1985) Isolation of Mycoplasma spumans from polyarthritis in a Greyhound. Australian Veterinary Journal 62, 206–210

Benito J, Depuy V, Hardie E et al. (2013a) Reliability and discriminatory testing of a client-based metrology instrument, feline musculoskeletal pain index (FMPI) for the evaluation of degenerative joint disease-associated pain in cats. Veterinary Journal 196, 368–373

Benito J, Hansen B, Depuy V et al. (2013b) Feline musculoskeletal pain index: responsiveness and testing of criterion validity. Journal of Veterinary Internal Medicine 27, 474–482

Bennett D (1987a) Immune-based erosive inflammatory joint disease of the dog: canine rheumatoid arthritis. Journal of Small Animal Practice 28, 779–797

Bennett D (1987b) Immune-based non-erosive inflammatory joint disease of the dog. 3. Canine idiopathic polyarthritis. Journal of Small Animal Practice 28, 909–928

Bennett D and Kelly DF (1987) Immune-based non-erosive inflammatory joint disease of the dog. 2. Polyarthritis/polymyositis syndrome. Journal of Small Animal Practice 28, 891–908

Bennett D and Taylor DJ (1988) Bacterial infective arthritis in the dog. Journal of Small Animal Practice 29, 207–230

Beraud R, Moreau M and Lussier B (2010) Effect of exercise on kinetic gait analysis of dogs afflicted by osteoarthritis. Veterinary and Comparative Orthopaedics and Traumatology 23, 87–92

Black LL, Gaynor J, Adams et al. (2008) Effect of intraarticular injection of autologous adipose-derived mesenchymal stem and regenerative cells on clinical signs of chronic osteoarthritis of the elbow joint in dogs. Veterinary Therapeutics 9, 192–200

Black LL, Gaynor J, Gahring D et al. (2007) Effect of adipose-derived mesenchymal stem and regenerative cells on lameness in dogs with chronic osteoarthritis of the coxofemoral joints: a randomized, double-blinded, multicenter, controlled trial. Veterinary Therapeutics 8, 272–284

Bonilla HF, Chenoweth CE, Tully JG et al. (1997) Mycoplasma felis septic arthritis in a patient with hypogammaglobulinemia. Clinical Infectious Diseases 24, 222–225

Bouck GR, Miller CW and Taves CL (1995) A comparison of surgical and medical treatment of fragmented coronoid process and osteochondritis-dissecans of the canine elbow. Veterinary and Comparative Orthopaedics and Traumatology 8, 177–183

Bozynski CC, Stannard JP, Smith P et al. (2016) Acute management of anterior cruciate ligament injuries using novel canine models. Journal of Knee Surgery 29, 594–603

Breitschwerdt EB, Maggi RG, Chomel BB and Lappin MR (2010) Bartonellosis: an emerging infectious disease of zoonotic importance to animals and human beings. Journal of Veterinary Emergency and Critical Care 20, 8–30

Brisson BA, Bersenas A and Etue SM (2004) Ultrasonic diagnosis of septic arthritis secondary to porcupine quill migration in a dog. Journal of the American Veterinary Medical Association 224, 1467–1470

Brown A and Bennett D (1988) Gentamicin-impregnated polymethylmethacrylate beads for the treatment of septic arthritis. Veterinary Record 123, 625–626

Brown DC, Boston RC, Coyne JC and Farrar JT (2008) Ability of the Canine Brief Pain Inventory to detect response to treatment in dogs with osteoarthritis. Journal of the American Veterinary Medical Association 233, 1278–1283

Brown DC, Boston R, Coyne JC and Farrar JT (2009) A novel approach to the use of animals in studies of pain: validation of the Canine Brief Pain Inventory in canine bone cancer. Pain Medicine 10, 133–142

Buchanan AM, Beamen BL and Pederson NC (1983) Nocardia asteroides recovery from a dog with steroid and antibiotic unresponsive idiopathic arthritis. Journal of Clinical Microbiology 18, 702–709

Butterworth SJ, Barr FJ, Pearson GR and Day MJ (1995) Multiple discospondylitis associated with Aspergillus species infection in a dog. Veterinary Record 136, 38–41

Buttin P, Bismuth C, Genevois JP and Carozzo C (2013) Contribution of computed tomography in chronic septic arthritis and osteomyelitis management in a dog. Revue de Médecine Vétérinaire 164, 226–229

Carro T, Pederson NC, Beaman BL and Munn R (1989) Subcutaneous abscesses and arthritis caused by a probable bacterial L-form in cats. Journal of the American Veterinary Medical Association 194, 1583–1588

Clarke SP and Ferguson JF (2012) Bacterial infective arthritis following a penetrating stick injury of the stifle joint in a dog. Journal of Small Animal Practice 53, 483–486

Clements DN, Gear RN, Tattersall J, Carmichael S and Bennett D (2004) Type I immune-mediated polyarthritis in dogs: 39 cases (1997–2002). Journal of the American Veterinary Medical Association 224, 1323–1327

Clements DN, Owen MR, Mosley JR et al. (2005) Retrospective study of bacterial arthritis in 31 dogs. Journal of Small Animal Practice 46, 171–176

Cowell RL, Tyler RD, Clinkenbeard KD and Meinkoth JH (1988) Ehrlichiosis and polyarthritis in three dogs. Journal of the American Veterinary Medical Association 192, 1093–1095

Crook T, McGowan C and Pead M (2007) Effect of passive stretching on the range of motion of osteoarthritic joints in 10 labrador retrievers. Veterinary Record 160, 545–547

Cuervo B, Rubio M, Sopena J et al. (2014) Hip osteoarthritis in dogs: a randomized study using mesenchymal stem cells from adipose tissue and plasma rich in growth factors. International Journal of Molecular Sciences 15, 13437–13460

Davidson A (1993) Vaccination against feline calicivirus. Veterinary Record 132, 418–419

Dawson S, Bennett D, Carter SD et al. (1994) Acute arthritis of cats associated with feline calicivirus infection. Research in Veterinary Science 56, 133–143

Dawson S, McArdle F, Bennett D et al. (1993) Investigation of vaccine reactions and breakdowns after feline calicivirus vaccination. Veterinary Record 132, 346–350

Diniz PPV de P, Wood M, Maggi RG et al. (2009) Co-isolation of Bartonella henselae and Bartonella vinsonii ssp. berkhoffii from blood, joint and subcutaneous seroma fluids from two naturally infected dogs. Veterinary Microbiology 138, 368–372

Dougherty SA, Center SA, Shaw EE and Erb HA (1991) Juvenile-onset polyarthritis syndrome in Akitas. Journal of the American Veterinary Medical Association 198, 849–856

Dunn KJ and Dunn JK (1998) Diagnostic investigations in 101 dogs with pyrexia of unknown origin. Journal of Small Animal Practice 39, 574–580

Dyce J and Olmstead ML (2002) Removal of infected canine cemented total hip prosthesis using a femoral window technique. Veterinary Surgery 31, 552–560

Eps HA, Utley M, Southwood T et al. (2002) A multi-centred randomised controlled trial investigating the effectiveness of hydrotherapy in children with juvenile idiopathic arthritis. Arthritis and Rheumatism 46, S608

Foley A, Halbert J, Hewitt T and Crotty M (2003) Does hydrotherapy improve strength and physical function in patients with osteoarthritis – a randomised controlled trial comparing a gym based and a hydrotherapy based strengthening programme. Annals of the Rheumatic Diseases 62, 1162–1167

Foster JD, Sample S, Kohler R et al. (2014) Serum biomarkers of clinical and cytologic response in dogs with idiopathic immune-mediated polyarthropathy. Journal of Veterinary Internal Medicine 28, 905–911

Fournel C, Chabanne L, Caux C et al. (1992) Canine systemic lupus erythematosus. I: A study of 75 cases. Lupus 1, 133–139

Freire M, Brown J, Robertson ID et al. (2010) Meniscal mineralization in domestic cats. Veterinary Surgery 39, 545–552

Gearing D, Virtue E, Gearing R and Drew A 2013. A fully caninised anti-NGF monoclonal antibody for pain relief in dogs. BMC Veterinary Research 9, 226

German A (2010) Obesity and weight management. In: BSAVA Manual of Canine and Feline Rehabilitation, Supportive and Palliative Care, ed. S Lindley and P Watson, pp. 60–77. BSAVA Publications, Gloucester

Ghosh P (1999) The pathobiology of osteoarthritis and the rationale for the use of pentosan polysulfate for its treatment. Seminars in Arthritis and Rheumatism 28, 211–267

Goad DL and Pecquet Goad ME (1986) Osteoarticular sporotrichosis in a dog. Journal of the American Veterinary Medical Association 189, 1326–1328

Goossens HAT, van den Bogaard AE and Nohlmans MKE (2001) Dogs as sentinels for human Lyme Borreliosis in the Netherlands. Journal of Clinical Microbiology 39, 844–848

Greene LM, Marcellin-Little DJ and Lascelles BDX (2013) Associations among exercise duration, lameness severity, and hip joint range of motion in Labrador Retrievers with hip dysplasia. Journal of the American Veterinary Medical Association 242, 1528–1533

Grobman M, Outi H, Rindt H and Reinero C (2017) Serum Thymidine Kinase 1, Canine-C-Reactive Protein, Haptoglobin, and Vitamin D Concentrations in Dogs with Immune-Mediated Hemolytic Anemia, Thrombocytopenia, and Polyarthropathy. Journal of Veterinary Internal Medicine 31, 1430–1440

Gruen ME, Griffith E, Thomson A, Simpson W and Lascelles BDX (2014) Detection of clinically relevant pain relief in cats with degenerative joint disease associated pain. Journal of Veterinary Internal Medicine 28, 346–350

Gunn-Moore DA, Gaunt C and Shaw DJ (2013) Incidence of mycobacterial infections in cats in Great Britain: estimates from feline tissue samples submitted to diagnostic laboratories. *Transboundary and Emerging Diseases* **60**, 338–344

Hall EJ, Simpson JW and Williams DA (2005) *BSAVA Manual of Canine and Feline Gastroenterology, 2nd edn.* BSAVA Publications, Gloucester

Hanna FY (2005) Disease modifying treatment for feline rheumatoid arthritis. *Veterinary and Comparative Orthopaedics and Traumatology* **18**, 94–99

Hercock C, Pinchbeck G, Giejda A, Clegg PD and Innes JF (2009) Validation of a client-based clinical metrology instrument for the evaluation of canine elbow osteoarthritis. *Journal of Small Animal Practice* **50**, 266–271

Hielm-Bjorkman AK, Kuusela E, Liman A et al. (2003) Evaluation of methods for assessment of pain associated with chronic osteoarthritis in dogs. *Journal of the American Veterinary Medical Association* **222**, 1552–1558

Hillman TJ and Shaw SE (2010) Imported vector transmitted diseases in dogs – part 2. *Irish Veterinary Journal* **63**, 380–383

Hooper PT, Ireland LA and Carter A (1985) *Mycoplasma* polyarthritis in a cat with probable severe immune deficiency. *Australian Veterinary Journal* **62**, 352

Impellizeri JA, Tetrick MA and Muir P (2000) Effect of weight reduction on clinical signs of lameness in dogs with hip osteoarthritis. *Journal of the American Veterinary Medical Association* **216**, 1089–1091

Innes JF, Barr ARS and Sharif M (2000) Efficacy of oral calcium pentosan polysulphate for the treatment of osteoarthritis of the canine stifle joint secondary to cranial cruciate ligament deficiency. *Veterinary Record* **146**, 433–437

Innes JF, Clayton J and Lascelles BDX (2010) Review of the safety and efficacy of long-term NSAID use in the treatment of canine osteoarthritis. *Veterinary Record* **166**, 226–230

Innes JF, Costello M, Barr FJ, Rudorf H and Barr ARS (2004) Radiographic progression of osteoarthritis of the canine stifle joint: A prospective study. *Veterinary Radiology and Ultrasound* **45**, 143–148

Jalava J, Skurnik M, Toivanen A, Toivanen P and Eerola E (2001) Bacterial PCR in the diagnosis of joint infection. *Annals of the Rheumatic Diseases* **60**, 287–289

Kaandorp CJE, Dinant HJ, van de Laar MAFJ et al. (1997) Incidence and sources of native and prosthetic joint infection: a community based prospective survey. *Annals of the Rheumatic Diseases* **56**, 470–475

Kavit AY (1958) Cryptococcic arthritis in a Cocker Spaniel. *Journal of the American Veterinary Medical Association* **133**, 386–388

Kealy RD, Lawler DF, Ballam JM et al. (1997) Five-year longitudinal study on limited food consumption and development of osteoarthritis in coxofemoral joints of dogs. *Journal of the American Veterinary Medical Association* **210**, 222–225

Keane DP (1983) Chronic abscesses in cats associated with organisms resembling *Mycoplasma*. *Canadian Veterinary Journal* **24**, 289–291

Kirkby KA and Lewis DD (2012) Canine hip dysplasia: reviewing the evidence for nonsurgical management. *Veterinary Surgery* **41**, 2–9

Lambrechts N, Picard J and Tustin RC (1999) *Chlamydia*-induced septic arthritis in a dog. *Journal of the South African Veterinary Association* **70**, 40–42

Lawler DF, Larson BT, Ballam JM et al. (2008) Diet restriction and ageing in the dog: major observations over two decades. *British Journal of Nutrition* **99**, 793–805

Levy JK and Marsh A (1992) Isolation of calicivirus from the joint of a kitten with arthritis. *Journal of the American Veterinary Medical Association* **201**, 753–755

Liehmann L, Degasperi B, Spergser J and Niebauer GW (2006) *Mycoplasma felis* arthritis in two cats. *Journal of Small Animal Practice* **47**, 476–479

Lindley S and Watson P (2010) *BSAVA Manual of Canine and Feline Rehabilitation, Supportive and Palliative Care.* BSAVA Publications, Gloucester

Littman MP, Goldstein RE, Labato MA, Lappin MR and Moore GE (2006) ACVIM small animal consensus statement on Lyme disease in dogs: diagnosis, treatment and prevention. *Journal of Veterinary Internal Medicine* **20**, 422–434

Maddy KT (1958) Disseminated coccidioidmycosis of the dog. *Journal of the American Veterinary Association* **137**, 483–489

Marchevsky AM and Read RA (1999) Bacterial septic arthritis in 19 dogs. *Australian Veterinary Journal* **77**, 233–237

Marshall WG, Hazewinkel HAW, Mullen D et al. (2010) The effect of weight loss on lameness in obese dogs with osteoarthritis. *Veterinary Research Communications* **34**, 241–253

Mathews CJ, Weston VC, Jones A, Field M and Coakley G (2010) Bacterial septic arthritis in adults. *Lancet* **375**, 846–855

May C, Carter SD, Barnes A et al. (2008) *Borrelia burgorferi* infection in cats in the UK. *Journal of Small Animal Practice* **35**, 517–520

May C, Hammill J and Bennett D (1992) Chinese shar pei fever syndrome: a preliminary report. *Veterinary Record* **131**, 586–587

McConkey SE, Lopez A, Shaw D and Calder J (2002) Leishmanial polyarthritis in a dog. *Canadian Veterinary Journal* **43**, 607–609

Mlacnik E, Bockstahler BA, Muller M et al. (2006) Effects of caloric restriction and a moderate or intense physiotherapy program for treatment of lameness in overweight dogs with osteoarthritis. *Journal of the American Veterinary Medical Association* **229**, 1756–1760

Moise NS, Crisman JW, Fairbrother JF and Baldwin C (1983) *Mycoplasma gateae* arthritis and tenosynovitis in cats: case report and experimental reproduction of the disease. *American Journal of Veterinary Research* **44**, 16–21

Montgomery RD, Long IR and Milton JL (1989) Comparison of aerobic culturette, synovial membrane biopsy and blood culture medium in detection of canine bacterial arthritis. *Veterinary Surgery* **18**, 300–303

Moreau M et al. (2003) Clinical evaluation of a nutraceutical, carprofen and meloxicam for the treatment of dogs with osteoarthritis. *Veterinary Record* **152(11)**, 323–330

Möstl K, Addie DD, Boucraut-Baralon C et al. (2015) Update of the 2009 and 2013 ABCD guidelines on prevention and management of feline infectious diseases. *Journal of Feline Medicine and Surgery* **17**, 570–582

Muir P, Oldenhoff WE, Hudson AP et al. (2007) Detection of DNA from a range of bacterial species in the knee joints of dogs with inflammatory knee arthritis and associated degenerative anterior cruciate ligament rupture. *Microbial Pathogenesis* **42**, 47–55

Ollier WE, Kennedy LJ, Thomson W et al. (2001) Dog MHC alleles containing the human RA shared epitope confer susceptibility to canine rheumatoid arthritis. *Immunogenetics* **53**, 669–673

Oshin A, Griffon D, Lemberger K, Naughton J and Barger A (2009) Patellar blastomycosis in a dog. *Journal of the American Animal Hospital Association* **45**, 239–244

Owen MR, Moores AP and Coe RJ (2004) Management of MRSA septic arthritis in a dog using gentamicin-impregnated collagen sponge. *Journal of Small Animal Practice* **45**, 609–612

Oxenford CJ and Middleton DJ (1986) Osteomyelitis and arthtits associated with *Aspergillus fumigatus* in a dog. *Australian Veterinary Journal* **63**, 59–60

Pedersen NC, Pool RR and O'Brien T (1980) Feline chronic progressive polyarthritis. *American Journal of Veterinary Research* **41**, 522–535

Queneau P, Francon A and Graber-Duvernay B (2001) Methodological reflections on 20 randomized clinical hydrotherapy trials in rheumatology. *Therapie* **56**, 675–684

Ramsey I (2017) BSAVA *Small Animal Formulary, 9th edn., Part A: Canine and Feline.* BSAVA Publications, Gloucester

Read RA, Cullishill D and Jones MP (1996) Systemic use of pentosan polysulfate in the treatment of osteoarthritis. *Journal of Small Animal Practice* **37**, 108–114

Sanderson RO, Beata C, Flipo RM et al. (2009) Systematic review of the management of canine osteoarthritis. *Veterinary Record* **164**, 418–424

Sbrana S, Marchetti V, Mancianti F, Guidi G and Bennett D (2014) Retrospective study of 14 cases of canine arthritis secondary to *Leishmania* infection. *Journal of Small Animal Practice* **55**, 309–313

Smith GK, Popovitch CA, Gregor TP and Shofer FS (1995) Evaluation of risk factors for degenerative joint disease associated with hip dysplasia in dogs. *Journal of the American Veterinary Medical Association* **206**, 642–647

Spreng D (1993) Leishmanial polyarthritis in two dogs. *Journal of Small Animal Practice* **34**, 559–563

Stener-Victorin E, Kruse-Smidje C and Jung K (2004) Comparison between electro-acupuncture and hydrotherapy, both in combination with patient education and patient education alone, on the symptomatic treatment of osteoarthritis of the hip. *Clinical Journal of Pain* **20**, 179–185

Stenske KA, Bemis DA, Hill K and Krahwinkel DJ (2005) Acute polyarthritis and septicaemia from *Mycoplasma edwardii* after surgical removal of bilateral adrenal tumors in a dog. *Journal of Veterinary Internal Medicine* **19**, 768–771

Stern L, McCarthy R, King R and Hunt K (2007) Imaging diagnosis – discospondylitis and septic arthritis in a dog. *Veterinary Radiology and Ultrasound* **48**, 335–337

Stockham SL, Schmidt DA, Curtis KS et al. (1992) Evaluation of granulocytic ehrlichiosis in dogs of Missouri, including serological status to *Ehrlichia canis*, *Ehrlichia equi* and *Borrelia burgdorferi*. *American Journal of Veterinary Research* **53**, 63–68

Stockham SL, Schmidt DA and Taylor JW (1986) Polyarthritis associated with canine granulocytic ehrlichiosis. *Veterinary Clinical Pathology* **15**, 8

Tobias KM and Johnston SA (2012) *Veterinary Surgery: Small Animal.* Saunders Elsevier, Philadelphia

Upchurch DA, Renberg WC, Roush JK, Milliken GA and Weiss ML (2016) Effects of administration of adipose-derived stromal vascular fraction and platelet-rich plasma to dogs with osteoarthritis of the hip joints. *American Journal of Veterinary Research* **77**, 940–951

Vandeweerd JM, Coisnon C, Clegg P et al. (2012) Systematic review of efficacy of nutraceuticals to alleviate clinical signs of osteoarthritis. *Journal of Veterinary Internal Medicine* **26**, 448–456

Vilar JM, Batista M, Morales M, et al. (2014) Assessment of the effect of intraarticular injection of autologous adipose-derived mesenchymal stem cells in osteoarthritic dogs using a double blinded force platform analysis. *BMC Veterinary Research* **10**, 143

Walton MB, Cowderoy E, Lascelles D and Innes JF (2013) Evaluation of construct and criterion validity for the 'Liverpool Osteoarthritis in Dogs' (LOAD) clinical metrology instrument and comparison to two other instruments. *PLoS One* **8**, e58125

Walton MB, Cowderoy EC, Wustefeld-Janssens B, Lascelles BDX and Innes JF (2014) Mavacoxib and meloxicam for canine osteoarthritis: a randomised clinical comparator trial. *Veterinary Record* **175**, 280

Webb AA, Taylor SM and Muir GD (2002) Steroid-responsive meningitis-arteritis in dogs with noninfectious, nonerosive, idiopathic, immune-mediated polyarthritis. *Journal of Veterinary Internal Medicine* **16**, 269–273

Wilbe M, Jokinen P, Hermanrud C, et al. (2009) MHC class II polymorphism is associated with a canine SLE-related disease complex. *Immunogenetics* **61**, 557–564

Wilson HE, Mugford AR, Humm KR and Kellett-Gregory LM (2013) *Ehrlichia canis* infection in a dog with no history of travel outside the United Kingdom. *Journal of Small Animal Practice* **54**, 425–427

Wolshrijn CF, Meyer HP, Hazewinkel HAW and Wolvekamp WT (1996) Destructive polyarthritis in a dog with leishmaniasis. *Journal of Small Animal Practice* **37**, 601–603

Woods KS, Barry M and Richardson D (2013) Carpal intra-articular blastomycosis in a Labrador Retriever. *Canadian Veterinary Journal* **54**, 167–170

Zeugswetter F, Hittmair KM, Arespacochaga AG, Shibly S and Spergser J (2007) Erosive polyarthritis associated with *Mycoplasma gateae* in a cat. *Journal of Feline Medicine and Surgery* **9**, 226–231

Chapter 7

Diseases and disorders of bone

Gareth Arthurs and Sorrel Langley-Hobbs

Introduction

This chapter will address a variety of metabolic bone diseases and some otherwise poorly categorized bone disorders such as bone cysts and infarcts. These can all cause lameness in dogs and cats. There are many more bone disorders but it is beyond the scope of this chapter to cover them all. Conditions affecting the physes are covered in Chapter 8, neoplastic bone disease in Chapter 11 and conditions specific to certain joints, such as ischaemic necrosis of the femoral head, are covered in the anatomy-specific chapters, such as Chapter 22.

Metabolic bone diseases affect all parts of the skeleton to different degrees. Most conditions are characterized by either an increase in bone formation or by bone loss. They can, therefore, be classified into hyperostotic or osteopenic conditions.

Hyperostotic bone conditions

Panosteitis

Panosteitis is a self-limiting, episodic disease affecting the long bones of puppies and young adult dogs. It is characterized by focal areas of endosteal bone proliferation. Synonyms include juvenile osteomyelitis, eosinophilic panosteitis and enostosis.

Aetiology/pathogenesis

Canine panosteitis is a disease of the adipose bone marrow characterized by degeneration of medullary adipocytes. This is followed by stromal cell proliferation, intramembranous ossification, resorption and remodelling. Medullary vascular congestion and hyperaemia may account for the associated pain.

The precise aetiology of panosteitis has not been elucidated but there are many hypotheses. Bacterial osteomyelitis was originally thought to be the underlying cause, but blood cultures from affected puppies are typically negative and they have normal white blood cell counts; in one necropsy study of 18 affected dogs, no bacteria were isolated (Zeskov, 1960).

Panosteitis has been successfully transmitted from affected to healthy dogs by intramedullary inoculation of bone marrow (Zeskov, 1960), although the radiographic changes were equivocal. No bacteria were isolated from inocula and transmission was achieved with and without filtration to remove most bacteria; this suggests viral rather than bacterial aetiology. Canine distemper virus has been implicated. However, when German Shepherd Dogs and Pointer puppies were reared together, only the German Shepherd Dogs developed panosteitis. Distemper virus, therefore, seems unlikely be the cause, although breed susceptibilities may exist.

A hereditary cause is another possibility as the condition can be seen in whole litters of puppies. The incidence in German Shepherd Dogs might support this suggestion but it does not explain why the condition is also seen sporadically in so many other breeds. Other hypotheses include transient vascular anomalies, allergies, a metabolic phenomenon, hyperoestrogenism, parasite migration or autoimmune reaction following viral infection.

It has also been suggested that the risk of developing panosteitis by 3 to 4 months of age in German Shepherd Dog puppies is increased by a high dietary calcium intake. However, one study investigating puppy nutrition found that some preparations of puppy milk replacers had 17 times the recommended level of vitamin D and three times that of bitch milk, but there was no direct link to panosteitis (Corbee *et al.*, 2012)

Signalment

Panosteitis is typically seen in young, large-breed dogs, 6–18 months of age. Very occasionally middle-aged dogs, usually German Shepherd Dogs, are affected (Bohning *et al.*, 1970). There is a male:female ratio of 4:1 (Bohning *et al.*, 1970). For females, the first episode is usually associated with the first oestrus. The most common breed affected is the German Shepherd Dog but panosteitis has also been reported in the Labrador Retriever, Bassett Hound, Dobermann, Great Dane, Golden Retriever and other large breeds.

History and clinical signs

Lameness is usually acute in onset and severe, often progressing over the first few days to severe and occasionally non-weight-bearing lameness. Bouts of lameness usually last 2 to 3 weeks and the lameness typically has a migratory pattern as the severity of disease shifts from bone to bone. Different bones in the same limb can be affected, which causes prolonged single limb lameness. As the puppy gets older, episodes of lameness usually become less pronounced and the interval between successive episodes increases.

Pain is elicited by deep palpation of the affected area of the bone. A normal dog should be able to tolerate firm bone palpation (pressure that causes blanching of the veterinary surgeon's fingernails) without showing signs of pain. Care should be taken when palpating dogs with panosteitis as they can react unpredictably and aggressively, even with relatively gentle bone palpation.

Dogs with panosteitis can become systemically ill and exhibit pyrexia and tonsillitis; haematology may show elevated white blood counts, but these signs are unusual. Panosteitis may also occur coincidentally to common developmental orthopaedic disorders such as elbow dysplasia, osteochondrosis and hip dysplasia. Attributing clinical significance to such disorders can be challenging as the signs associated with panosteitis can be severe and predominant. In such cases re-examination after resolution of signs of panosteitis is advised.

Diagnostic imaging

Radiographic changes can be subtle and good quality images are required. The radiographic changes and pathological features of panosteitis are summarized in Figure 7.1. Radiographic changes are often seen in the mid-diaphysis close to the nutrient foramen. If changes are not apparent on the initial radiographs then further images should be taken 2 to 3 weeks later if the clinical suspicion remains. It is worthwhile taking radiographs of multiple long bones when suspicious of panosteitis, as radiographic changes (severity or location) do not necessarily correlate with clinical signs or the degree of pain exhibited on clinical examination. The disease usually begins in the thoracic limb with the proximal ulna most commonly affected, followed by the central radius, distal humerus, proximal and central femur and proximal tibia. Metacarpal bones and the pelvis can also be involved. Radiographic examples of panosteitis in the humerus, ulna and femur are illustrated in Figures 7.2, 7.3 and 7.4.

Scintigraphy has been found to be more sensitive than radiography in detecting focal areas of increased blood flow as a result of increased osteoblastic activity. Although scintigraphy localizes these changes, it cannot characterize them, therefore radiography is more sensitive and specific in establishing a definitive diagnosis of panosteitis, albeit at a later stage in the disease process (Turnier and Silverman, 1978).

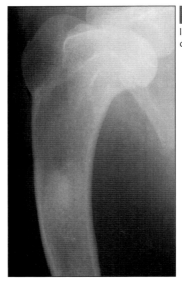

7.2 An early and fairly subtle panosteitis lesion in the proximal humeral diaphysis.

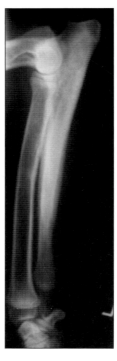

7.3 Severe panosteitis lesion affecting the entire ulna with increased medullary bone opacity, loss of corticomedullary distinction and thickened ulnar cortices.

Day of cycle	Radiographic phases	Pathogenesis
0	Very early – increased radiolucency to medullary bone	Degeneration of medullary adipocytes adjacent to nutrient foramen
10–14	Early – subtle poorly marginated and occasionally granular increased radiodensity evident in medullary canal. Medullary blurring and loss of corticomedullary contrast results	Proliferation of stromal and adventitial cells of bone marrow – intramembranous ossification starts
20–30	Middle – obvious patchy mottled increase in radiodensity, approaching that of cortical bone. Endosteal roughening and an accentuated coarsened trabecular pattern may be visible. Periosteal and endosteal new bone formation usually develops such that cortices may appear thickened and indistinct in affected areas – bone is usually smooth and laminar in appearance	Nidus enlarges, becoming attached to endosteal surface. Fibrous bone trabecular pattern replaced by laminar bone. Periosteal reaction appears secondary to medullary osseous reaction
70–90	Late – medullary canal regains normal appearance and patchy radiodensities disappear as lesions are gradually remodelled	Remodelling and re-establishment of vascularization. Osteolysis begins at area of initial nidus formation

7.1 Radiographic and pathological changes seen with panosteitis.

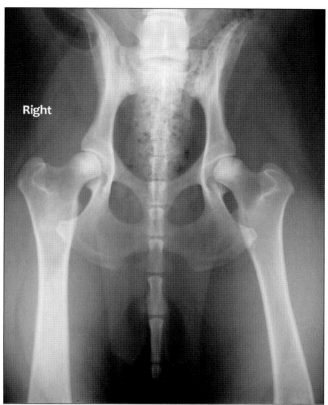

7.4 Panosteitis of the right femur. Note the increased opacity of the mid-femoral diaphysis of the right femur (left of the image), with subtly patchy texture and reduced corticomedullary distinction; compare with the left femur.

Differential diagnoses

Common causes of lameness in immature large-breed dogs include:

- Metaphyseal osteopathy
- Osteomyelitis
- Hip dysplasia
- Elbow dysplasia
- Shoulder osteochondrosis
- Cranial cruciate ligament rupture.

Treatment

Treatment is supportive, with a combination of restriction of activity and administration of non-steroidal anti-inflammatory drugs (NSAIDs) together with oral analgesics such as paracetamol and codeine (Pardale V) or tramadol and parenteral buprenorphine or methadone for the more severe cases. Corticosteroids can be effective but should not be the first line of treatment. The prognosis is good for a complete recovery.

Prognosis

Panosteitis is usually self-limiting with spontaneous recovery after several weeks, although lameness may persist or migrate from limb to limb for longer in some dogs. Relapses are possible, usually occurring about 1 month apart (Bohning et al., 1970). Dogs with panosteitis are generally sound in between bouts of lameness. In contrast, dogs with other developmental orthopaedic diseases, such as osteochondrosis or hip dysplasia, usually have a persistent, low grade, less variable lameness.

Metaphyseal osteopathy

Metaphyseal osteopathy (MO) is a condition seen in immature medium and large-breed dogs. It is characterized by severe lameness, pyrexia, depression and bilaterally symmetrical distal metaphyseal bone changes. Synonyms include hypertrophic osteodystrophy, Möller-Barlow's disease, skeletal scurvy, infantile scurvy, osteodystrophy II and metaphyseal dysplasia.

Aetiology/pathogenesis

The cause of MO is unknown but many hypotheses exist including:

- Vitamin C deficiency – levels have been described as being low in affected dogs but vitamin C levels also vary with exercise, food intake and stress. As dogs suffering from MO are under stress and often anorexic, low vitamin C levels should not be unexpected. The results of vitamin C supplementation have been disappointing
- Dietary over-supplementation – dogs fed on diets with high levels of calcium and/or carbohydrates have developed MO
- Infectious agents – some dogs have a prior history of illness, so the possibility of an infectious cause has been cited. The multifocal perivascular infiltrations of neutrophils seen histologically may be suggestive of osteomyelitis, but this histological presentation is more typical of bacterial rather than viral infection.

Canine distemper virus has been isolated from bone samples from three dogs affected with MO (Mee et al., 1992). However, no convincing evidence has been found linking MO with canine distemper virus in the general population (Munjar et al., 1998). To attempt to fulfil Koch's postulates, blood from distemper affected dogs was transfused into 3-month-old puppies. Clinical signs of acute distemper developed 2 weeks later and the puppies died, but with no signs of MO (Grondalen, 1979).

In Weimaraners, severe clinical signs and classic bone changes have developed following vaccination (Abeles et al., 1999; Harrus et al., 2002). One study investigated an association between MO in Weimaraners and the major histocompatibility complex alleles on the DLA-DQA1 locus of unrelated dogs (Crumlish et al., 2006). Of 12 dogs, all developed clinical signs of MO within 6 weeks of vaccination but no association was found between DQA1 alleles and MO; it was concluded that, while recent vaccination may be a trigger for the disease, there is no specific vaccine responsible for disease expression. It is likely that the development of MO in both Weimaraners and Irish Setters has a multifactorial aetiology related to a compromised immune system, neutrophil dysfunction and canine distemper virus. The response to corticosteroids has been promising, but dogs should be thoroughly evaluated first for bacterial infections.

MO has been reported in three Border Collie puppies in association with polyarthritis, neutropenia and trapped neutrophil syndrome; a good response was achieved following treatment with antibiotics and corticosteroids (Mason et al., 2014).

Signalment

The disease affects young, rapidly growing medium and large-breed dogs. Puppies present between the ages of 2 and 6 months, and males may be slightly predisposed. Many breeds are affected including the Boxer, Weimaraner, Great Dane, Irish Wolfhound, St Bernard and Border Collie. It is rarely seen in smaller breeds.

History and clinical signs

While affected puppies may have been vaccinated up to 6 weeks prior to developing signs of the disease, this may be coincidental. The extent and nature of clinical signs of MO range from mild lameness to a severely affected and collapsed animal. Affected puppies have swollen metaphyseal areas, usually affecting the distal radius and ulna and the distal tibia (Figure 7.5); lesions of the proximal humerus have also been reported (Franklin *et al.*, 2008). Palpation and manipulation should distinguish metaphyseal swelling from joint swelling or effusion. There may be a history of diarrhoea prior to the first appearance of MO; ocular and nasal discharge, tonsillitis and hyperkeratosis of footpads have also been reported. The most severely affected puppies may be presented for the systemic manifestations of the disease, including pyrexia, anorexia, depression and collapse, rather than lameness.

There is a single case report involving a German Shepherd Dog puppy that suffered bilateral distal femoral fractures thought to be secondary to MO; the fractures healed and normal function was restored with conservative management (Arnott *et al.*, 2008).

Laboratory analysis

Laboratory analysis is generally not helpful in making a diagnosis of MO, but may be useful to document normal parameters and exclude differentials such as a consumptive septicaemia. Haematology may show a mildly decreased red blood cell count and haemoglobin concentration, and a slightly increased white blood cell count. Bacteraemia has been reported in one dog; therefore, blood culture has been recommended in severely affected dogs (Schulz *et al.*, 1991). However, such infection may represent a secondary manifestation in an immunocompromised dog rather than the primary cause.

Diagnostic imaging

The definitive diagnosis is made from observing pathognomonic changes on radiographs. Changes are seen in the metaphyses of the long bones, most commonly the distal radius and ulna, and the distal tibia. In more chronic cases, the more proximal metaphyses may be involved. Other less commonly affected bones include the mandible, scapula, ribs and metacarpal bones. Changes are usually bilaterally symmetrical. In one study of 53 cases, 94% had radiographic lesions of hypertrophic osteodystrophy at the time of disease onset (Safra *et al.*, 2013).

The characteristic radiographic changes include a linear area of increased radiopacity in the metaphysis adjacent and parallel to the normal growth plate (Figure 7.6). Adjacent and parallel to the radiopaque zone, there is a radiolucent zone (the Trummerfield zone). The epiphysis and growth plates may appear normal or slightly wide. In the later phases of the disease, periosteal mineralization occurs around and proximal to the metaphysis; this probably reflects mineralization of subperiosteal haematoma. In severe cases, metaphyseal periosteal mineralization may extend to involve the whole diaphysis. At this later stage the metaphyseal radiolucent zone may no longer be visible.

Histology

Histologically the metaphyseal lesions are characterized by the following changes, progressing from the physis to the metaphysis:

- Normal to slightly widened growth plate, caused by increased height of columns of hypertrophied chondrocytes

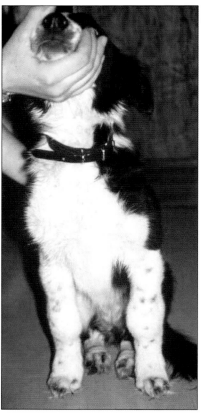

7.5 A 5-month-old Border Collie with metaphyseal osteopathy, showing marked swelling of the metaphyseal areas of the distal and proximal antebrachia.

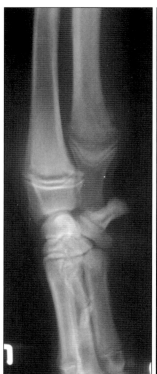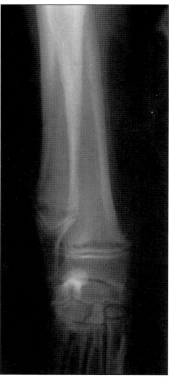

7.6 Radiographs of the left antebrachium of a puppy with metaphyseal osteopathy, showing typical changes to the distal ulnar and radial metaphyses; there are radiopaque and radiolucent zones immediately parallel and adjacent to the physes, and there is a small amount of periosteal mineralization of the caudolateral ulnar metaphysis.

- Narrow zone of increased radiopacity immediately adjacent to the physis caused by trabecular collapse and mineralization of trabecular haemorrhage
- Towards the diaphysis, the spongiosa becomes more disorganized; there is a broad band of cellular infiltration, while trabecular bone becomes necrotic to absent, reflecting the lucent zone seen radiographically
- Secondary trabeculae of woven bone are deposited on the pre-existing trabecular remnants (often necrotic)
- Sub-periosteal haemorrhage, inflammation and fibrosis with periosteal thickening, mineralization and new bone formation.

Differential diagnoses

As with panosteitis, differential diagnoses to consider include all conditions causing lameness in the immature large-breed dog. Osteomyelitis is an important differential diagnosis for MO as the clinical and radiographic signs can appear very similar, although physeal and metaphyseal osteomyelitis is uncommon in dogs.

Treatment

As with panosteitis, treatment for MO is symptomatic and supportive and is aimed primarily at managing the dog's pain using NSAIDs and analgesics (including opioids as necessary) until the metaphyseal pathology resolves. Severely affected animals may require hospitalization and aggressive analgesia. In one study, 55% of Weimaraners treated with NSAIDs did not achieve remission within 7 days of treatment but all dogs treated with corticosteroids achieved remission within 48 hours (Safra et al., 2013). NSAIDs and corticosteroids should not be given together. The extent and intensity of required treatment is dependent on the severity of the presentation but the following should be considered:

- Intravenous fluids – if the patient is anorexic, pyrexic or shows evidence of dehydration
- Antibiotics – if osteomyelitis is a differential diagnosis
- Diet – a balanced commercial diet should be given; anorexic animals may need encouragement to eat. There is no indication to add mineral, vitamin or any other supplements to the diet
- Nursing – painful recumbent animals should be provided with appropriate bedding and turned frequently to avoid pressure sores
- Physiotherapy and hydrotherapy – puppies that are reluctant to move may benefit from gentle range-of-motion exercises and hydrotherapy to reduce joint stiffness and muscle atrophy
- Cold pack application – applied three to four times daily may reduce metaphyseal heat, alleviate pain and encourage movement.

Many dogs recover within a week with no recurrence, but relapses are common. Death has been reported in 25–33% of cases, and occasionally euthanasia may be considered because of the distressing appearance of the puppy. Residual skeletal deformities can occur in more severely affected puppies, e.g. if metaphyseal pathology results in a mismatch in growth rates of the paired radius and ulna bones of the antebrachium. Similarly, lateral patellar luxation has been seen secondary to premature closure of the lateral distal femoral physis; such puppies have been noted to be 'cow-hocked' and have carpal valgus (Lenehan and Fetter, 1985).

Craniomandibular osteopathy

Craniomandibular osteopathy (CMO) is a proliferative bone disease seen in immature dogs. It is neither inflammatory nor neoplastic. It most commonly affects the bones of the skull, specifically the mandibular body, occipital bone, tympanic bullae and temporomandibular joint (TMJ). Bone changes are usually bilaterally symmetrical. Synonyms include mandibular periostitis, temporomandibular osteodystrophy and lion jaw.

Aetiology

The condition is hereditary with an autosomal recessive mode of inheritance in West Highland White Terriers (Padgett and Mostosky, 1986). Given its high prevalence in other breeds, there are probably other hereditary predispositions. There appears to be a lower but unproven risk of CMO after neutering, suggesting a possible hormonal influence (Watson et al., 1995). A viral aetiology has also been proposed, but there is no conclusive evidence to support this (Munjar et al., 1998).

Signalment

The onset of signs is usually between 4 and 10 months of age. There is no reported sex predisposition. The breeds most commonly affected are the West Highland White and Scottish Terriers but other breeds have been reported including the Boston Terrier, Cairn Terrier, Great Dane, Dobermann and Labrador Retriever (Alexander and Kallfelz, 1975). Irish Setters can suffer a similar bony abnormality of the mandible but this is associated with a serious and ultimately fatal disease: canine leucocyte adhesion deficiency (Trowald-Wigh et al., 1995).

A related condition, calvarial hyperostosis syndrome, resembles CMO except that there is progressive and asymmetric involvement of the calvarium; this affects young male Bullmastiff dogs (McConnell et al., 2006). The condition has also been reported in other breeds including an English Springer Spaniel (Mathes et al., 2012) and an 8-month-old Pit Bull Terrier presented with periosteal new bone formation and hyperostosis on the frontal, parietal and mandibular bones bilaterally (Thompson et al., 2011).

Clinical signs

Affected puppies suffer pain, mandibular swelling, inability to open the mouth completely, drooling, weight loss and intermittent pyrexia. Lymphadenopathy and temporal muscle atrophy may also be present.

Variations of the condition have been reported. Antebrachial angular limb deformity associated with gross clinical, radiographic and histological ulnar thickening and concomitant rostral mandibular and calvarial thickening of CMO occurred in a 4-month-old West Highland White Terrier (Pettitt et al., 2012). A 4-month-old male Akita suffered generalized hyperostotic lesions including endosteal thickening of multiple bones including femora, ilium and cranial bones; the latter caused compression of the cerebellum and brain stem and associated neurological deficits; histopathology of multiple bone lesions was consistent with craniomandibular osteopathy (Ratterree et al., 2011).

Diagnostic imaging

Typical changes will be identified on good quality orthogonal radiographs or by computed tomography (CT) examination, which is particularly useful in assessing involvement of the TMJ. Proliferative palisading bone affects the mandible and petrous–tympanic area (Figure 7.7). The disease usually affects both regions but occasionally will just be confined to one (Figure 7.8). The precise size and location of periosteal new bone can be much better appreciated with a CT scan (Figure 7.9). Other bones that may be affected include the occipital, parietal, frontal, tentorium osseum, maxilla and, rarely, appendicular bones. The medullary cavity and cortices of affected bones may be indistinguishable because of the superimposition of new bone. Changes are usually bilateral but can be asymmetrical.

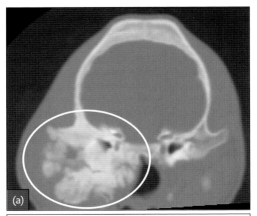

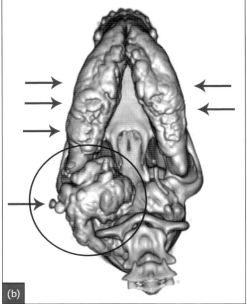

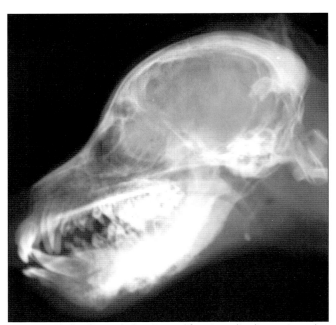

7.7 Skull radiograph showing proliferative palisading periosteal bone affecting the mandible of a dog with craniomandibular osteopathy. There is also smooth laminated bone production over the frontal and parietal bones.

7.9 (a) CT image showing a transverse slice through the skull just caudal to the temporomandibular joint of a dog suffering from severe craniomandibular osteopathy; a large amount of new bone formation is seen (circled) with secondary deviation/deformation of the overlying soft tissues and the oropharynx. (b) Three-dimensional volume rendered image of the skull of the same dog viewed ventrally; severe thickening of the entire ventral mandible (arrowed) is seen in addition to the remodelling in the region of the right temporomandibular joint (circled).
(Courtesy of Gordon Brown)

Laboratory analysis

No significant abnormalities have been found on haematological or biochemical analysis of blood, but there may be mild elevations in serum alkaline phosphatase, phosphate, cholesterol and gammaglobulins. Multiple blood cultures from four West Highland White Terriers were all negative (Riser *et al.*, 1967).

Histology

There is osteoclastic resorption of the lamellar bone followed by replacement with primitive woven bone that expands beyond the normal periosteal boundaries. Normal bone marrow spaces are replaced with a highly vascular fibrous stroma and are invaded by inflammatory cells including neutrophils, lymphocytes and plasma cells. The orientation pattern of bone formation is compatible with alternating periods of bone formation and resorption. Frontal and parietal bones are thickened without disrupting the outer or inner surfaces.

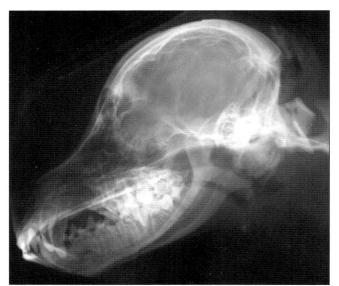

7.8 Skull radiograph of a West Highland White Terrier with craniomandibular osteopathy. Bone production is isolated to the petrous–tympanic area and there is some thickening of the frontal/ parietal bones.

Differential diagnoses

Usually the signalment, history, clinical and radiographic findings are diagnostic. However, differential diagnoses to consider include canine leucocyte adhesion deficiency, osteomyelitis, traumatic periostitis, calvarial hyperostosis syndrome and neoplasia, particularly in atypical breeds or if the bony changes are asymmetric.

Treatment

NSAIDs should be prescribed initially but this may be insufficient to alleviate the clinical signs. Corticosteroids may be more effective in retarding bone pathology. If food prehension and mastication is impaired, liquefied food should be provided and, in very severe cases, oesophagostomy tube feeding should be considered. In rare cases, it is reported that mandibulectomy may be considered to allow oral intake of food if bone deposition prevents or severely limits mouth opening. One attempt to remove excess bone surgically was unsuccessful (Pool and Leighton, 1969).

Prognosis

The prognosis depends on which bones are involved and how severely. New bone production slows by 7–8 months of age, then becomes static and is subsequently gradually resorbed (Alexander and Kallfelz, 1975). However, bone deposition can interfere with TMJ function and movement and therefore can impair eating and even respiration. The poorest prognosis is associated with bone deposition around the TMJ; euthanasia may be considered if the puppy's pain or inability to eat is severe.

Hypervitaminosis A

Hypervitaminosis A is a condition seen in cats exposed to excessive levels of dietary vitamin A, usually as a result of being fed mostly or exclusively liver. It is characterized by extensive confluent exostoses of the cervical and thoracic vertebrae and the appendicular skeleton. The condition is rare in the United Kingdom as the majority of cats are fed commercial diets, but it is seen sporadically, usually in indoor cats fed liver. Historically, the condition was more common in Australia and New Zealand where it was more common for cats to be fed offal.

Pathogenesis

Vitamin A causes increased sensitivity of the periosteum to trauma. Vitamin A renders lysosomal membranes more labile and therefore susceptible to rupture and release of enzymes. The cervical and cranial thoracic region is particularly sensitive because of the grooming activity of cats.

Signalment

Affected cats are presented for treatment typically between 2 and 9 years of age.

History and clinical findings

Signs of hypervitaminosis A include malaise, anorexia, lethargy, irritability, exophthalmos and a scurfy dull coat. The cervical and cranial thoracic spine may be immobile so the cat presents with a very stiff neck that it cannot move, and movement is not possible on manipulation. As a result, the cat cannot groom so the coat is unkempt. If the new bone formation encroaches on the intervertebral foramina and compresses the cervical, thoracic or lumbosacral nerve root outflow tracts, neurological signs such as pain, ataxia, paralysis and urinary incontinence may be seen. Serum vitamin A concentration may also be elevated (Polizopoulou et al., 2005).

Diagnostic imaging

On radiographic examination, confluent exostoses occur on the ventral aspect of the cervical and cranial thoracic spine producing ankylosis (Figure 7.10). Exostoses can also be seen associated with the elbow, shoulder, hip, stifle, ribs and sternebrae.

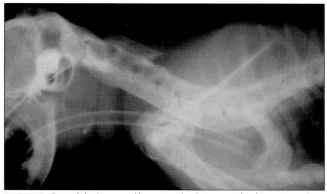

7.10 Spondylosis caused by extensive intervertebral exostoses in a 12-year-old cat with hypervitaminosis A. The first rib and sternum also show new bone deposition.

Histopathology

Subperiosteal proliferation of new woven bone occurs around the apophyseal (facet) joints. Proliferation of cartilage from the margins of articular hyaline cartilage overgrows the joint and replaces synovial membrane. Myeloid marrow becomes resorbed and replaced with fibrous marrow.

Treatment and prognosis

Removal of liver from the diet and restoration of a balanced diet prevents further progression of the lesions and clinical signs can improve markedly within a couple of weeks. Despite restoration of a normal diet and normalization of vitamin A levels, the proliferative new bone that has already formed does not resorb or regress, i.e. range of neck movement does not improve. There is no known effective treatment.

Hypertrophic osteopathy

Hypertrophic osteopathy is most frequently recognized as a paraneoplastic syndrome affecting human and canine cancer patients. It is characterized by swelling and periosteal new bone production affecting primarily the small long bones of the distal limbs, i.e. the metacarpal, metatarsal and phalangeal bones. It occurs secondary to thoracic or abdominal mass lesions, and is most frequently seen secondary to thoracic neoplasia. Synonyms include hypertrophic pulmonary osteopathy, hypertrophic pulmonary osteoarthropathy and Marie's disease.

Primary causes

The most common underlying cause of hypertrophic osteopathy is primary or metastatic pulmonary neoplasia (55 of 60 cases in one report: Brodey, 1971). Other causes in the thorax include pulmonary granulomatous disease, pulmonary abscess, chronic bronchopneumonia, pulmonary tuberculosis, oesophageal granulomas caused by *Spirocerca lupi*, dirofilariasis, rib tumours and bacterial endocarditis. Abdominal causes include liver adenocarcinoma, adrenocortical carcinoma and primary neoplasia of the bladder, with or without pulmonary metastases. Hypertrophic osteopathy has been reported in cats associated with renal adenoma (Johnson and Lenz, 2011), megaoesophagus (Mills, 2010), and in seven cats it was reported with no detectable underlying disease (Huang *et al.*, 2010)

Pathogenesis

There are extensive and detailed published accounts of the proposed pathophysiology of hypertrophic osteopathy in human and veterinary patients. The most commonly accepted explanation is a neurovascular mechanism whereby stimulation of the afferent fibres in the vagal or intercostal nerves by a thoracic mass causes stimulation of efferent fibres to the connective tissue and periosteum of the limbs. This results in an increased vascular supply to the limbs; plethysmographic studies have shown an increase in blood flow of two to three times normal in affected limbs (Holling *et al.*, 1961). The excess blood flow passes through arteriovenous shunts, bypassing the capillary bed. This produces local passive congestion and poor tissue oxygenation, stimulating proliferation of the connective tissues including the periosteum. It has been postulated that the afferent fibres originate in the thorax and join the vagus in the mediastinum; an alternative pathway might be from the parietal pleura and along the intercostal nerves. The extrapulmonary lesions are thought to exert their effects via the vasopharyngeal and vagus nerves. Release of humoral substances produced by neoplastic and inflammatory cells, megakaryocytic/platelet clumping and the production and activity of vascular endothelial growth factor and platelet-derived growth factor may be involved, particularly in cases of hypertrophic osteopathy without thoracic involvement.

Signalment

Hypertrophic osteopathy has been reported most frequently in humans and dogs, but it occurs in a variety of other species including cats. As hypertrophic osteopathy occurs secondary to other disease processes, a wide variety of ages and breeds can be affected but, reflecting the higher incidence of neoplasia, the majority are in middle to old age and Boxers may be over-represented.

Clinical signs

Animals usually present with acute or gradual onset lameness or limb swelling. Ocular discharge, episcleral injection, lameness and lethargy may also occur. Signs attributable to the primary lesion are rare at initial presentation. Affected animals may have palpably to visibly thickened non-oedematous distal limbs. The thickening is warm and pulsatile, and the overlying skin is taut. Anaemia, neutrophilia and elevated serum alkaline phosphatase may be features of baseline haematology and serum biochemistry investigations.

Diagnostic imaging

In very early cases, only appendicular soft tissue swelling is seen. Bony changes consist of palisading proliferative new bone formation affecting the metacarpal and metatarsal bones and the bones of the distal limbs. The first bones to be affected are the abaxial aspects of the second and fifth metacarpal and metatarsal bones (Figure 7.11). Changes are usually bilaterally symmetrical. In advanced cases, the lesions extend proximally to affect the tibia, radius and ulna, humerus and femur, and occasionally the ribs, scapula and vertebrae. Once the radiographic diagnosis is made, the primary mass lesion should be located; the thorax should be imaged by radiography or CT, and the abdomen may be imaged by radiography, ultrasonography or CT.

Treatment and prognosis

Treatment of hypertrophic osteopathy relies on treating the primary disease. The bone lesions may resolve after resection of the primary mass lesion, thoracotomy, vagotomy and/or rib resection (Becker *et al.*, 1999). Lameness gradually improves, the heat and pain diminish within a couple of weeks and all signs of lameness resolve within 3–4 months. Radiographic changes take longer to disappear completely but the periosteal bone gradually becomes smoother and less reactive.

The prognosis for hypertrophic osteopathy depends on the primary disease. It is, however, usually guarded to poor as the underlying disease is most commonly pulmonary neoplasia, a thoracic mass lesion or abdominal mass. Consequently, survival times following diagnosis are usually limited.

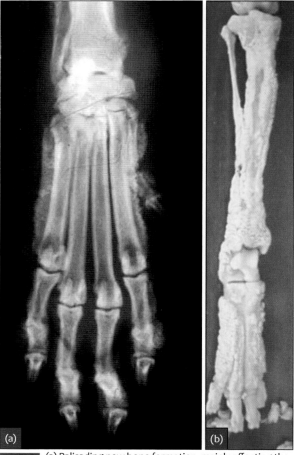

7.11 (a) Palisading new bone formation, mainly affecting the abaxial aspects of metacarpal bones 2 and 5, in a dog with hypertrophic osteopathy. (b) Anatomical specimen of a dog suffering from hypertrophic osteopathy; note the periosteal new bone affecting the pes, tarsus and crus.

Medullary bone infarcts

There are several reports in the literature of multifocal medullary bone infarcts associated with primary bone sarcomas, usually osteosarcomas (Ansari, 1991). Dogs are usually presented with signs attributable to the primary tumour and the infarcts are incidental radiographic findings. Femoral medullary infarction can be seen following total hip replacement; the incidence may be reduced from 20% to 3% with a modification of reaming technique that limits depth (Haney and Peck, 2009). There is a single case report of a male Samoyed that developed osteosarcoma at the site of bone infarction 5 years previously (Marcellin-Little et al., 1999).

Histopathogenesis

Obliteration of intramedullary arteries with collagen leads to the production of poorly differentiated osteoid and necrosis of bone marrow as a result of hypoxia.

Signalment

Infarcts tend to affect smaller breeds, with the Miniature Schnauzer being over-represented in a case series of 13 bone sarcomas associated with multifocal bone infarctions in dogs (Dubielzig et al., 1981).

Clinical findings

Dogs usually present with signs attributable to the primary bone tumour(s). These are more likely to affect the pelvic limb and multiple tumours may be present.

Diagnostic imaging

Infarcts are characterized by irregularly demarcated areas of radiopacity in the medullary cavity (Figure 7.12). Bones distal to the elbow and distal to the distal third of the femur are more likely to be affected.

Osteomyelitis

The term osteomyelitis means inflammation of bone and marrow. This is most commonly caused by a bacterial infection although fungal osteomyelitis should be

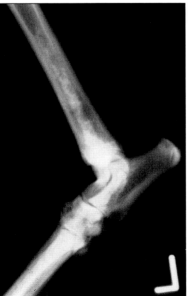

7.12 Infarcts in the distal tibia of an 11-year-old crossbreed dog. The contralateral tibia was affected by a poorly differentiated bone tumour.

considered in immunosuppressed individuals and in animals imported from tropical or semi-tropical environments. There are three main forms of osteomyelitis: acute haematogenous, acute post-traumatic and chronic post-traumatic forms.

Acute haematogenous osteomyelitis

This is a very uncommon form of osteomyelitis in dogs and cats and occurs most commonly in the neonate.

Pathogenesis: Emboli of bacteria from septicaemia lodge in the metaphyseal region of bone. The initial source of infection may be the umbilicus. Disruption to the metaphyseal vasculature causes necrosis, hyperaemia and migration of leucocytes. The tortuous anatomy of blood vessels at the physis combined with greater permeability of the vessels in young dogs may be contributory factors. The infection can spread along the bone, or break into the joint resulting in septic arthritis. If bone destruction is severe, pathological fracture may occur.

Clinical signs: Affected patients may be pyrexic, depressed, lethargic and exhibit focal pain or lameness. Several limbs or a single bone may be affected. The affected metaphyses are swollen and painful, and septic arthritis may follow.

Diagnostic imaging: In the early stages, only soft tissue swelling may be appreciable. Later, irregular areas of bone lysis become apparent within the affected metaphysis. In severe cases, cortical lysis may be evident. Differentiating aggressive osteomyelitis from neoplasia may be impossible based on radiographs alone; bone biopsy may be necessary.

Culture: Fine-needle aspirate or bone biopsy samples from affected bone should be submitted for culture and sensitivity testing, and a smear evaluated for the presence of bacteria. Blood culture may also be helpful to check for septicaemia.

Treatment and prognosis: Antibiotics should be administered immediately after collection of samples for culture. Sensitivity results direct antibiotic selection but until available, a broad-spectrum antibiotic such as co-amoxiclav should be used. High levels of antibiotics should be used for 3 to 4 weeks following the cessation of signs. If the disease is recognized early and treatment instituted quickly, the prognosis should be good. Coexistent joint infections should be treated as a matter of urgency (see Chapter 6). Polyostotic bone involvement can carry a guarded prognosis (Rabillard et al., 2011).

Acute post-traumatic osteomyelitis

Bacteria enter through a traumatic wound such as a bite, gunshot wound, or foreign object such as a nail. More commonly, osteomyelitis occurs as a complication of orthopaedic surgery, e.g. following fracture reduction and internal fixation.

Clinical signs: Signs typical of inflammation are seen, i.e. heat, swelling, pain, redness and loss of function. There may be wound disruption and a draining tract. If these signs occur and there has been a history of recent surgery or wounding then deep surgical site infection should be suspected.

Diagnostic imaging: Radiographs at an early stage may show only soft tissue swelling. Radiographs will also help determine the status of internal fixation devices and fracture/osteotomy stability or healing, if present. Radiographs should be taken every 2–4 weeks to monitor progress and response to treatment. With respect to bone formation and resorption, radiographs lag behind the clinical event by 10–14 days, so clinical presentation is equally important in assessing response to treatment. The use of advanced imaging such as CT or MRI including contrast or a contrast fistulogram may be useful in identifying the nature of the swelling, and whether a foreign body is present.

Treatment: Treatment should be instigated as soon as possible. Depending on the wound, therapy should consist of debridement, lavage and stabilization. Haematoma, fluid and necrotic material should be debrided and samples submitted for culture and sensitivity. Following debridement and lavage, the wound may be primarily closed or a closed-suction drain placed. Appropriate antibiotics (based on culture and sensitivity results) should be given at the high end of the therapeutic dose range for a sufficient period of time, usually for a minimum of 6 weeks. Fracture stability is one of the most important factors to address with fracture-associated osteomyelitis. Adequate stability of the fracture will allow the bone to heal in the face of infection, allowing the osteomyelitis to be effectively treated. External skeletal fixation is often the method of choice to confer stability without placing metal implants directly into an infected area. When necessary, however, internal fixation is appropriate but implants will probably need to be removed after the bone has healed.

Chronic post-traumatic osteomyelitis

Following inadequate treatment of acute post-traumatic osteomyelitis, the condition may become chronic. Chronic osteomyelitis can become apparent weeks, months or even years later, particularly if implants are present and is rarely cured until they are removed.

Clinical signs: Lameness is usually present but may not be severe. There is usually pain, disuse atrophy and tenderness around the affected limb or bone. Discharging sinuses may be present that drain intermittently; i.e. they respond to antibiotic therapy but then recur when antibiotics are discontinued. The patient is generally well systemically.

Diagnostic imaging: Radiographs may show few abnormalities. Soft tissue swelling associated with a draining sinus may be seen. The most frequent radiographic appearance of chronic osteomyelitis is a lytic region of bone at the bone–implant interface with a sclerotic margin of bone immediately adjacent. On digital radiographs, apparent radiolucency at the bone–implant interface must be carefully differentiated from Überschwinger artefact (see Chapter 3). If periosteal reaction is present it may be irregular if sub-acute, or regular, smooth and well organized if chronic. Periosteal new bone may be local or extend along the length of the diaphysis; this should be differentiated from healing callus, which is local specifically to the region directly over the fracture. Sequestra are dead, nonvascularized pieces of bone which appear radiographically as opaque pieces of bone with very sharp margins and no connection to the adjacent bone. Sequestra can be surrounded by a radiolucent zone and a sclerotic bony margin – the involucrum (Figure 7.13). Sequestra are uncommon in small animals.

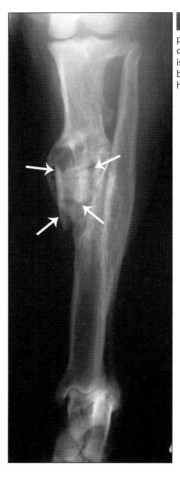

7.13 Radiograph of the tibia of a mature dog presenting with a history of discharging sinuses. A sequestrum is present (arrowed) surrounded by an involucrum. There is massive hypertrophy of the fibula.

Treatment: The underlying cause should be established and addressed. If a fracture is present, the fracture needs to be stabilized to resolve the infection and facilitate fracture healing (see the *BSAVA Manual of Canine and Feline Fracture Repair and Management*). If the fracture has healed completely then implants should be removed if osteomyelitis is recurrent. Principles of treatment are outlined in Figure 7.14.

1. Identification of underlying cause: often motion at the fracture site or sequestra.
2. Assessment of the likelihood of successful treatment; amputation is considered if there is loss of joint funtion, neurological defects or severe muscle or soft tissue loss.
3. Addressing underlying cause:
   - Removal of loose or broken implants
   - Debridement of sequestra and avascular tissue
   - Restoration of stability (external skeletal fixator/plate and screw fixation/interlocking nail); ultimately the stability achieved is more important than the choice of implant.
4. Placement of a bone graft or graft substitute.
5. Closure of incision and placement of either a:
   - Closed-suction drain
   - Ingress/egress system
   or initial primary closure.
6. Submission of samples for culture and sensitivity prior to starting on antibiotics.
7. Treatment with broad-spectrum bactericidal antibiotics whilst awaiting sensitivity results.
8. Treatment for 4–6 weeks after cessation of clinical signs with appropriate antibiotics.
9. If implants are still present, these may need removal once fracture has healed and if infection persists.

7.14 Principles of treatment of post-traumatic osteomyelitis.

Fungal osteomyelitis

Fungal osteomyelitis is very rare in temperate climates and more common in hot, wet regions. Young animals and immunosuppressed patients seem to be more at risk. The disease is frequently part of a systemic fungal infection such as systemic aspergillosis, for which the German Shepherd Dog is over-represented (Schulz *et al.*, 2008). Clinical signs are often non-specific and may include general malaise, anorexia, weight loss, respiratory signs, ocular signs or diarrhoea. Abnormalities may be detectable on haematological and biochemical blood analysis. It is advisable to image the thorax by radiography or CT, as the route of infection is often by inhalation of spores and respiratory tract signs are common (Figure 7.15). Pulmonary granulomas seen in association with bone lesions may be mistaken for lung metastases; the bone lesions themselves can be misdiagnosed as being neoplastic unless thoroughly investigated. When osteomyelitis is present, animals may present with lameness and obvious limb swelling or palpable bony nodules. Spinal pain and neurological signs may be associated with fungal discospondylitis or vertebral osteomyelitis. A summary of the fungal osteomyelitides is given in Figure 7.16. The prognosis is guarded and dependent on the severity and extent of the infection and on the underlying cause of immunosuppression; long-term survival is uncommon.

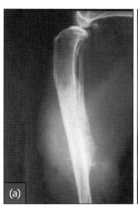
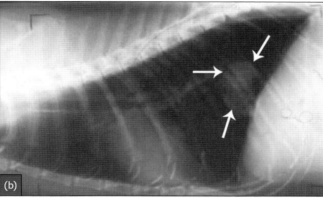

7.15 (a) Proliferative osteomyelitic skeletal lesion in a cat with *Cryptococcus neoformans* infection. (b) A pulmonary granulomatous lesion was also present in the caudal lung lobes (arrowed).

Species	Distribution	Route of infection	Common clinical signs	Radiographic signs	Diagnostic tests	Treatment options
Coccidioides immitis	South-western USA and South America	Inhalation of spores	Dry non-productive cough, pyrexia	Areas of increased bone density, periosteal elevation and joint involvement	Cytology, culture, serology	Ketoconazole or itraconazole
Blastomyces dermatitidis	USA and Canada	Inhalation of yeast	Respiratory signs, lymphadenopathy, skin papules, ocular signs	Bone destruction or production, often multiple appendicular lesions	Direct microscopic examination of pus	Itraconazole or amphotericin B
Histoplasma capsulatum	Temperate and subtropical areas of the world	Inhalation or ingestion of macroconidia	Variable – multisystemic disease	Mixed bone production and destruction; joints may be involved	Cytology, histopathology, culture	Itraconazole or amphotericin B
Actinomycetes: *Actinomyces bovis* – commensal	Worldwide	Invades penetrating wound	Jaw and scapular enlargement. Thick mucoid tenacious greenish yellow non-odorous pus with sulphur granules	Bone destruction without formation – early, reaction pronounced	Direct microscopic examinaton of pus	Iodine solution and systemic antibiotics
Nocardia – soil saprophyte	Worldwide	Inhalation, ingestion or direct inoculation into tissue	Mass with numerous sinuses, pyothorax (respiratory signs)	Chronic suppurative osteomyelitis – vertebral, nasal, hock	Culture, direct Gram stain of pus	Penicillin and streptomycin or sulfadiazine for 6–12 weeks. Surgical excision of masses
Cryptococcus neoformans (see Figure 7.15)	Worldwide – avian habitats, especially USA and Australia	Inhalation, bird droppings	Sinusitis, nasopharyngeal and pulmonary granulomas. Neural and ocular involvement	Skeletal lesions seen in diaphyses (25% of cases have musculoskeletal involvement)	Cytology, histopathology, culture, serology	Amphotericin B or flucytosine

7.16 Summary of the characteristics of selected fungal osteomyelitides. (continues) ▶

Species	Distribution	Route of infection	Common clinical signs	Radiographic signs	Diagnostic tests	Treatment options
Aspergillus fumigatus	Wordlwide	Inhalation	Nasal: nasal discharge, epistaxis, nasal pain	Loss of nasal turbinates with radiolucency and opacity	Radiology, cytology, histopathology, serology	Topical clotrimazole or enilconazole
			Disseminated: vertebral pain, paraparesis/lameness	Focal bone lucencies and soft tissue mineralization	Urinalysis, serology	Itraconazole

7.16 (continued) Summary of the characteristics of selected fungal osteomyelitides.

Osteopenic bone conditions

Nutritional secondary hyperparathyroidism

Nutritional secondary hyperparathyroidism (NSH) is usually associated with an absolute deficiency of dietary calcium, which is most commonly caused by a boneless, all meat diet. NSH can also be caused by an inability to absorb dietary calcium, or excessive dietary phosphate. Synonyms include osteitis fibrosa, juvenile osteoporosis and paper bone.

Balanced commercial diets are in widespread use and therefore diseases of dietary deficiency, such as NSH, are rare. Despite this, occasionally pet owners and breeders may unwittingly feed an imbalanced diet through ignorance.

Pathogenesis

When serum calcium levels drop, parathyroid hormone (PTH) synthesis and secretion is stimulated (Figure 7.17). Released PTH increases bone calcium resorption, and renal calcium resorption, phosphorus excretion and synthesis of active vitamin D (calcitriol). Calcitriol stimulates intestinal absorption of calcium and phosphorus through increased synthesis of intestinal calcium-binding protein.

Hyperphosphataemia does not stimulate the parathyroid gland directly, but does so indirectly by lowering blood calcium levels.

Signalment

NSH is primarily a disease of growing animals because of the increased calcium demand required for bone growth. Adult animals still develop osteoporosis but more slowly. Dogs and cats can be affected; NSH should be considered as a differential diagnosis particularly in growing dogs or cats with spontaneous fractures or seizures.

Clinical signs

Clinical signs include bone pain, lameness, reluctance to move and play, and difficulty chewing food. Affected animals may exhibit a plantigrade/palmigrade stance (Figure 7.18) and carpal valgus. Affected kittens may present with lordosis caused by spinal fractures; other neurological signs include ataxia, paraparesis, paraplegia and seizures. Acute deterioration may occur after pathological fractures. Tooth eruption and development can also be abnormal.

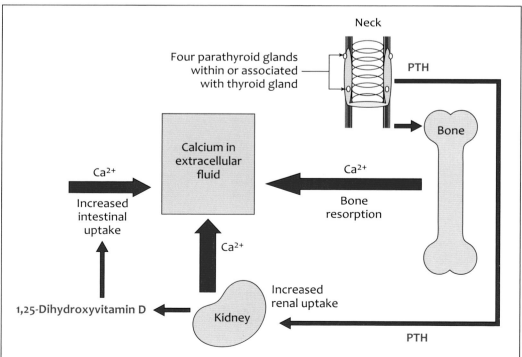

7.17 Schematic diagram of calcium homeostasis.
Ca^{2+} = calcium ions;
PTH = parathyroid hormone.

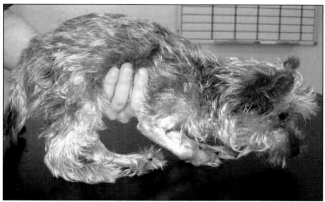

7.18 Nutritional secondary hyperparathyroidism in a 6-month-old Yorkshire Terrier. The dog had recent bilateral radial and ulnar fractures, healed femoral, humeral and pelvic fractures, a fused cervical spine and a plantigrade stance.

Laboratory investigations

Abnormalities detectable on laboratory analysis of blood and urine from dogs and cats suffering from NSH are listed in Figure 7.19.

Parameter	Finding in NSH
Calcium	Normal or low
Parathyroid hormone (PTH)	Elevated
Phosphorus	Usually elevated but can be low
Alkaline phosphatase	Increased
25-hydroxyvitamin D$_3$ (25(OH)D$_3$)	Low/normal
1,25-dihydroxyvitamin D$_3$ (1,25(OH)$_2$D$_3$, calcitriol)	Normal/elevated
Urine	Decreased urinary calcium

7.19 Abnormalities detectable on laboratory analysis of blood and urine from dogs and cats with nutritional secondary hyperparathyroidism (NSH).

Diagnostic imaging

There is extensive osteopenia of the diaphyses of the long bones and vertebrae, and the thinned cortical bone develops a similar radiopacity to medullary bone; the bones appear 'ghost-like' (Figure 7.20). A double cortical line may also be seen (Lamb, 1990) that reflects intracortical resorption of bone. The epiphyses are normal but there may be an area of increased metaphyseal opacity that probably represents an area of preferential mineralization. If bone demineralization is severe enough, pathological fractures occur. Any bone can fracture, with compression fractures of metaphyseal bone of the vertebrae, pelvis, scapula and proximal humerus and folding type fractures of the long bone diaphyses often seen. Diffuse bone resorption of the skull can also occur (see renal secondary hyperparathyroidism below). Bone mineralization must decrease by at least 50% before it is detectable radiographically; therefore the radiographic changes observed with NSH reflect demineralization to levels lower than 50% normal.

Histology

Resorption of bone proceeds at a faster rate than repair by fibrous connective tissue proliferation. This results in decreased bone volume and is called hypostotic fibrous osteodystrophy.

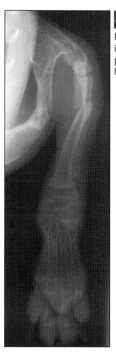

7.20 'Ghost-like' bones of a dog with nutritional secondary hyperparathyroidism. The density of the bone is similar to that of the soft tissue density of the pads. There are radial and ulnar fractures and a healed mid-diaphyseal humeral fracture.

Treatment

The diet should be corrected. This is best achieved by feeding an appropriate commercial diet; supplements should not be necessary, but parenteral calcium should be administered if seizures occur. Cage rest is advisable to allow fractures to heal while bone mineralization progresses. Internal fixation should be used cautiously as implants do not hold well in the very weak osteopenic bone; the use of intramedullary pins, locking plates and elastic osteosynthesis may be advantageous.

Prognosis

The prognosis is good for uncomplicated cases. Improvement in demeanour should be seen within a week of initiating a balanced diet. The prognosis may be guarded if neurological signs are present secondary to vertebral fractures. Healed pelvic fracture malunions can lead to constipation and megacolon.

Renal secondary hyperparathyroidism

Renal secondary hyperparathyroidism is a complication of chronic renal failure. The mandible and maxilla appear to be particularly affected.

Pathogenesis

When renal disease is at an advanced stage, phosphorus retention occurs, resulting in hyperphosphataemia. As a result of the law of mass action (i.e. the product of calcium and phosphate must remain stable), this causes relative hypocalcaemia, resulting in release of PTH and secondary hyperparathyroidism. Subsequently, excessive bone resorption occurs with the cancellous bone of the skull particularly affected; in particular the resorption of alveolar bone can result in loose teeth.

Chronic renal disease also leads to reduced production of vitamin D and therefore impaired intestinal absorption of calcium, causing problems of impaired mineralization of osteoid with features of rickets/osteomalacia. Mandibular bone becomes softened and pliable (fibrous osteo-dystrophy) and proliferation of connective tissue occurs. The abnormalities of mineral metabolism cause extra-osseous calcification with deposition of mineral in peri-articular, visceral and vascular tissues.

Clinical signs

Predominantly, clinical signs relate to renal disease and include polyuria, polydipsia, vomiting and depression. Signs relating to osteopenia and osteomalacia include loose teeth, a pliable mandible, and inability to close the jaw properly resulting in drooling of saliva and protrusion of the tongue. Mandibular fractures can occur unexpect-edly following minimal trauma such as dental extractions or dog fights. Signs can be more severe in puppies with congenital renal disease; in particular swelling of the jaw and disruption of tooth eruption can occur. Renal second-ary hyperparathyroidism should be considered as a differ-ential diagnosis in any patient presenting with mandibular fractures but minimal trauma.

Laboratory investigations

Blood biochemistry findings include elevations in phos-phate, urea, creatinine and alkaline phosphatase. Calcium is normal to low, although paradoxically may be elevated in 5 to 10% of cases. PTH levels are elevated, often to a level above that seen with primary hyperparathyroidism.

Diagnostic imaging

Generalized osteopenia of the skull and soft tissue min-eralization is evident on radiographs. Teeth may appear as if they are 'floating' in the osteopenic skull (Figure 7.21). Parathyroid glands may appear evenly enlarged on ultrasonography.

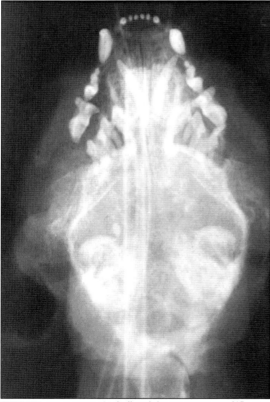

7.21 An osteopenic skull and the appearance of 'floating teeth' in a cat with renal secondary hyperparathyroidism.

Histology

Much of the bone has generalized fibrous osteodystrophy. In adults, the volume of bone is usually normal (isostotic fibrous osteodystrophy); in immature dogs hyperostotic lesions can be seen, often as facial swellings.

Treatment and prognosis

The aim is to address renal disease with a reduction in dietary phosphate intake, oral phosphate binders, and erythropoietin injections if anaemia exists. If fractures are present, traditional methods of fracture stabilization may not be effective as implants are unlikely to hold well in such osteopenic bone, but use of locking implants may be advantageous. Salvage options, such as hemimandibulec-tomy can be considered. Ultimately the prognosis is deter-mined by the progress of renal failure.

Primary hyperparathyroidism

Primary hyperparathyroidism occurs when excess PTH is produced by functional tumours of the parathyroid glands. These are generally adenomas, but adenocarcinomas and glandular hyperplasias also occur. The excess PTH causes increased calcium resorption from bone and renal tubules, increased absorption from the intestines, and increased phosphate excretion by the kidneys. There is accelerated bone resorption and bone is replaced by fibrous tissue. The cancellous bone of the skull is particularly affected.

Clinical signs

These are often attributable to the systemic effects of hypercalcaemia rather than bone demineralization. Signs include polyuria, polydipsia, anorexia, vomiting, consti-pation, muscle weakness and listlessness. Occasionally animals may present with fractures of long bones or verte-brae. Other bony changes include facial hyperostosis due to the deposition of excess woven bone.

Laboratory investigations

Laboratory findings include elevations in serum calcium, alkaline phosphatase and PTH, and low or normal phos-phate levels. Serum calcium exists as free calcium, protein-bound calcium and complexed calcium; free calcium (fCa^{2+}) is biologically active and it is this that should be measured when assessing pathology; fCa^{2+} can help to differentiate primary and secondary hyperparathyroidism.

Diagnostic imaging

Radiographic features of primary hyperparathyroidism include subperiosteal cortical resorption, loss of lamina dura dentes (bone adjacent to the periodontal ligaments), soft tissue mineralization, bone cysts and a generalized decrease in bone opacity. In advanced cases fractures may be present, particularly in cancellous bone. Nephro-calcinosis and urolithiasis may be detected on radiography, ultrasonography or CT of the urinary tract.

Ultrasonography of the parathyroid glands may show enlargement of one or more glands. All four glands should be assessed; if there is no obvious enlargement, the anterior mediastinal area near the base of the heart should be assessed for ectopic tissue.

Treatment

The aim of therapy is to eliminate the source of PTH production and surgical excision of the abnormal para-thyroid tissue is the treatment of choice. The negative effects of hypercalcaemia should be addressed preoperatively. Diuresis and the use of bisphosphonates can decrease the hypercalcaemia, while surgical excision of the abnormal tissue should result in a rapid resolution of hypercalcaemia. As PTH has a half-life of approximately 20 minutes, serological assessment can be a quick and useful indicator of the success of therapy. The patient must be monitored for postoperative hypocalcaemia which typically develops in 1 to 6 days. If calcium levels remain elevated for a week or more after surgery, the presence of a second adenoma or metastases should be suspected. Parathyroidectomy surgery was successful in 45 of 48 dogs in one study (Rasor et al., 2007).

Rickets

Rickets is an extremely rare bone disease in dogs and cats that typically affects puppies and kittens. It is characterized by a failure in mineralization of newly formed osteoid (enchondral mineralization) and caused by insufficient availability of calcium and/or phosphorus.

Pathogenesis

Systemic levels of calcium and phosphorus, and therefore bone mineralization, are regulated in part by the steroid hormone, calcitriol, which is one of the vitamin D family of steroid molecules. Vitamin D has multiple effects on bone. Its metabolic pathway is illustrated in Figure 7.22. Canine

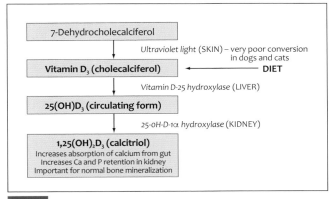

7.22 The metabolic pathway of vitamin D.

and feline skin contains much less 7-dehydrocholesterol than other mammals. The dermal production of vitamin D_3 is very inefficient in dogs and absent in cats; as a result, dogs and cats are dependent on dietary vitamin D.

Rickets can be caused by a dietary deficiency of cholecalciferol (hypovitaminosis D), a hereditary defect in vitamin D metabolism, failure of vitamin D to bind at the vitamin D receptor (vitamin D-independent rickets), or defective renal tubular resorption of phosphate.

The different types of rickets are summarized in Figure 7.23. In normal animals, a diet deficient in either calcium and/or phosphorus and a lack of vitamin D are necessary to produce the disease (Malik et al., 1997).

Vitamin D deficiency causes production of cartilage matrix that is highly stable and difficult to mineralize and resorb. In the young animal, this results in cartilage cells that fail to degenerate and capillaries from the metaphysis that are unable to penetrate the physeal cartilage. Epiphyseal lines become thickened and irregular. In adults, osteomalacia occurs because vitamin D is needed for osteoclasts and osteocytes to respond to PTH and allow bone resorption.

Clinical signs

Affected animals are usually young, severely stunted, bowlegged and plantigrade. Metaphyseal areas and costochondral junctions (the so-called 'rachitic rosary') are prominent. Signs may be attributable to the systemic effects of hypocalcaemia rather than the effects on bone; i.e. muscle weakness, tremors or seizures may be the predominant features (Schreiner and Nagode, 2003).

Diagnostic imaging

Puppies and kittens with rickets show characteristic cup-shaped and widened physes on radiography due to the accumulation of cartilage at the epiphyses (Figure 7.24). In adults, the bones appear osteopenic and folding fractures may be present.

Treatment and prognosis

The treatment of rickets depends on the subtype of the disease. If due to dietary deficiency of minerals or cholecalciferol, then providing a balanced diet should suffice,

Type of rickets	Laboratory analysis	Treatment	Reference
Nutritional: vitamin D deficiency. Diet deficient in vitamin D, calcium and/or phosphate	Low 1,25(OH)$_2$D$_3$ Hypophosphataemia and/or hypocalcaemia Secondary hyperparathyroidism	Balanced diet, exposure to sunlight	Malik et al., 1997
Hereditary: X-linked hypophosphataemic rickets. Defect in renal tubular resorption of phosphate	Hypophosphataemia High urinary fractional clearance of phosphorus Normocalcaemia Normal 25(OH)D$_3$ Normal to low 1,25(OH)$_2$D$_3$ Secondary hyperparathyroidism	Phosphate salts	Henik et al., 1999
Hereditary: Vitamin D-dependent rickets type I: defect in calcitriol production	Very low 1,25(OH)$_2$D$_3$ Hypocalcaemia Secondary hyperparathyroidism	Calcitriol supplementation	Johnson et al., 1988
Hereditary: Vitamin D-dependent rickets type II: impaired responsiveness of target organs to calcitriol because of defects in vitamin D receptors	Normal 25(OH)D$_3$ Elevated 1,25(OH)$_2$D$_3$ Hypocalcaemia Secondary hyperparathyroidism	Oral calcium supplementation Additional calcitriol	Schreiner and Nagode, 2003
Transient: non-type I, non-type II vitamin D metabolism rickets	Reduced total ALKP Increased PTH Very low 25(OH)D$_3$ and 1,25(OH)$_2$D$_3$	Calcitriol supplementation	Phillips et al., 2011

7.23 The different forms of rickets recognized in dogs and cats.

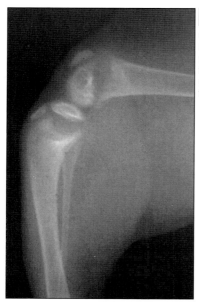

7.24 Epiphyseal widening, or cup-shaped growth plates, in a kitten with congenital rickets (vitamin D-dependent type II) caused by a deficiency or lack of binding to vitamin D receptors.

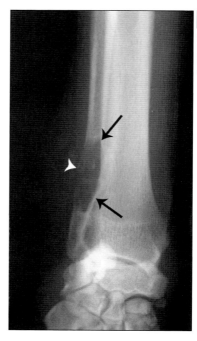

7.25 A bone cyst (arrowed) in the distal ulna of a 3-year-old Boxer. The dog presented lame after fracture of the cyst wall (arrowhead).

but there may be permanent growth plate damage (Malik *et al.*, 1997). The prognosis for the hereditary forms is more guarded for a complete resolution of signs and return to normality.

Bone cysts

Bone cysts in dogs are rare and the nomenclature is confusing but three types of bone cyst are recognized: simple bone cysts (which may be uni- or multicameral), aneurysmal bone cysts, and subchondral cysts. The cause of bone cysts is unknown but potential causes include physeal trauma causing ischaemic necrosis, haemorrhage and congenital or acquired vascular malformations. Subchondral cysts are very rare and occur either secondary to osteochondrosis and failure of enchondral ossification, or osteoarthritis and herniation of synovial fluid into the subchondral bone through hyaline cartilage fissures (Basher *et al.*, 1988); subchondral bone cysts are not covered further.

Fibrous dysplasia is a similar but probably distinct condition from simple bone cysts, although the distinction is poorly defined. The term 'fibrous dysplasia' emphasizes the one feature that all these conditions have in common, namely the replacement of bone by fibrous tissue that may contain areas of cystic degeneration.

Simple bone cysts

Simple bone cysts may be monostotic or polyostotic, i.e. in single or multiple bone locations. Uncommon in dogs and cats, they are found in in the long bone metaphyses and adjacent diaphyses of young, large-breed dogs (Figure 7.25); the epiphysis and physis are not affected. Males are affected twice as frequently as females.

Histopathogenesis: Lesions are lytic and expansile and usually contain serous to serosanguinous fluid. A single cyst cavity may be present (unicameral) or it may be divided into several cavities (multicameral) by septa of variably dense fibrous connective tissue, or woven to lamellar bone. The histopathological diagnosis of bone cyst must be carefully interpreted against clinical and radiographic presentation and progression of disease; the only purely cystic lesion is seen at the ends of the

large cylindrical bones of the extremities of the growing skeleton. Other cyst-like lesions should be designated as areas of liquefaction necrosis rather than cysts because they are merely areas of degeneration in proliferative processes. Biopsy of cystic cavitation within a tumour lesion could lead to misdiagnosis.

Signalment: Polyostotic cystic bone lesions have been reported in families of Dobermanns (Figure 7.26) and Old English Sheepdogs, and a genetic aetiology has been suggested. Monostotic lesions have been reported in Great Danes, Weimaraners, Irish Wolfhounds, German Shepherd Dogs and other large breeds.

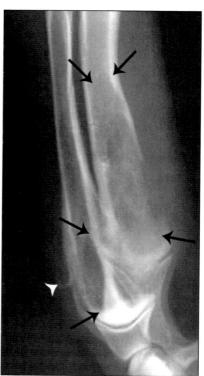

7.26 Polyostotic multicameral bone cysts (fibrous dysplasia) (arrowed) affecting the distal radius and ulna in a Dobermann. A pathological fracture is present (arrowhead).

Clinical signs: Many bone cysts do not produce clinical signs and may be an incidental diagnosis. If the cyst reaches sufficient size then pain, swelling and stiffness of the adjacent joint may be noted. Very large cysts may cause bone fracture.

Diagnostic imaging: A bone cyst appears as an expansile radiolucent area of the metaphysis and adjacent diaphysis, and does not affect the physis or epiphysis. The expanding cyst may cause cortical thinning.

Treatment: Drainage, curettage and packing with cancellous bone graft is the accepted method of treatment, if necessary. Fractures can be challenging to repair given the metaphyseal location and thin cortices (Dueland and Van Enkevort, 1995) but would involve drainage, curettage, packing with bone graft and fracture stabilization. Elbow arthrodesis was performed in a 10-month-old Yorkshire Terrier that suffered pathological humeral lateral condyle fracture secondary to a polyostotic bone cyst (Choate and Arnold, 2011).

Aneurysmal bone cysts

Aneurysmal bone cysts are benign, rapidly expansile and destructive bone lesions filled with free-flowing blood or serosanguinous fluid. The name aneurysmal derives from the cyst's gross resemblance to aortic aneurysms seen in humans. Aneurysmal bone cysts are common in humans but rare in dogs and cats.

Pathogenesis: The cause of aneurysmal bone cysts is unknown but in humans trauma and a benign bone tumour have been suggested as initiating events. These could lead to disrupted vascular blood flow (venous obstruction) and subsequent arteriovenous shunting. Venous obstruction or arteriovenous fistula formation results in haemorrhage, lysis and subperiosteal expansion, resulting in a rapidly expanding lesion that damages mesenchymal bone and causes endosteal bone resorption with expansile eccentric periosteal proliferation. However, no evidence for this aetiology has been present in canine or feline cases. Benign and malignant neoplasia, fibrous dysplasia, unicameral bone cysts and trauma have also been proposed as inciting factors for aneurysmal cyst formation. Malignant transformation to chondrosarcoma has been reported (Barnhart, 2002).

Signalment: Aneurysmal bone cysts are rare. Of the reported cases in dogs and cats, affected bones include the scapula, humerus, ulna, pelvis, tibia, rib, sacral and coccygeal vertebrae. Dogs are aged 6 months to 13 years, with most being older, and cats between 1 and 14 years, with most being young. Small bone cysts are more commonly reported in the appendicular skeleton, particularly the tibia. In cats they mainly affect the axial skeleton. In dogs the gender ratio is approximately even while in cats, a 5:1 female to male ratio is reported.

Clinical signs: Swelling over the cysts with pain and tenderness are reported clinical findings. Some animals present with signs attributable to an obstructive lesion and others present when the cyst acutely fractures.

Diagnostic imaging: The cysts are usually thin-walled, non-reactive expansile bone lesions. When affecting the appendicular skeleton, they are often eccentric in the metaphysis. They can have a characteristic soap-bubble appearance within the bone. Radiography, ultrasonography and MRI can be used to make the diagnosis (Benamou et al., 2012).

Histopathology: The cyst consists of a thin bony shell divided by bony and fibrous septa that contains serosanguinous fluid and fibrovascular tissue with a honeycomb-like structure of very large vascular channels. The septa are lined with fibroblasts and multinucleated giant cells. Lytic areas of bone contain extensive zones of haemorrhage and dilated coalescent spaces filled with blood, but blood clots are rare. Differential diagnoses include telangiectatic osteosarcoma, haemangiosarcoma and giant cell tumours.

Treatment: Therapy depends on location. As lesions can develop secondary to malignancy, multiple representative biopsy specimens from various areas are mandatory. There is a lack of information in the veterinary literature regarding treatment protocols and these are therefore adapted from those reported for humans. Treatment of axial lesions is by curettage, bone grafting, local excision and irradiation. Treatment of appendicular lesions is similar but in addition *en bloc* resection with reconstruction or amputation may be considered. Super-selective embolization using cyanoacrylate can provide definitive therapy in humans.

Fibrous dysplasia

Fibrous dysplasia is a rare condition in which the medullary cavity of bones is replaced by fibrous tissue. This results in intramedullary expansion of the lesion and secondary cortical thinning, as for bone cysts. The cause is unknown but appears not to be hereditary. It affects young animals and is probably a developmental defect. It may be monostotic or polyostotic and typically affects the skull, mandible and long bones. If clinically significant, the condition can cause bone swelling and pain, irregular bone growth and deformity; there is also increased risk of fracture.

References and further reading

Abeles V, Harrus S, Angles JM et al. (1999) Hypertrophic osteodystrophy in six Weimeraner puppies associated with clinical signs. *Veterinary Record* **145**, 130–134

Alexander JW and Kallfelz FA (1975) A case of craniomandibular osteopathy in a Labrador Retriever. *Veterinary Medicine: Small Animal Clinician* **70**, 560–563

Ansari MM (1991) Bone infarcts associated with malignant sarcomas. *Compendium on Continuing Education for the Practicing Veterinarian* **13**, 367–370

Arnott JL, Pilbey AW and Bennett D (2008) Pathological fractures secondary to metaphyseal osteopathy in a dog. *Veterinary Comparative Orthopaedics and Traumatology* **21**, 177–180

Barnhart MD (2002) Malignant transformation of an aneurysmal bone cyst in a dog. *Veterinary Surgery* **31**, 519–524

Barrett RB, Schall WD and Lewis RE (1968) Clinical and radiographic features of eosinophilic panosteitis. *Journal of the American Animal Hospital Association* **4**, 94–104

Basher AWP, Doige CE and Presnell KR (1988) Subchondral bone cysts in a dog with osteochondrosis. *Journal of the American Animal Hospital Association* **24**, 321–326

Becker TJ, Perry RL and Watson GL (1999) Regression of hypertrophic osteopathy in a cat after surgical excision of an adrenocortical carcinoma. *Journal of the American Animal Hospital Association* **35**, 499–505

Benamou J, Lussier B, Alexander K, Gains MJ and Savard C (2012) Use of magnetic resonance imaging and histopathologic findings for diagnosis of an aneurysmal bone cyst in the scapula of a cat. *Journal of the American Veterinary Medicine Association* **240**, 69–74

Biller DS, Johnson GC, Birchard SJ and Fingland RB (1987) Aneurysmal bone cyst in a rib of a cat. *Journal of the American Veterinary Medical Association* **190**, 1193–1195

Bohning RH, Suter PF, Hohn RB and Marshall J (1970) Clinical and radiologic survey of canine panosteitis. *Journal of the American Veterinary Medical Association* **156**, 870–883

Bowles MH and Freeman K (1987) Aneurysmal bone cyst in the ischia and pubes of a dog: a case report and literature review. *Journal of the American Animal Hospital Association* **23**, 423–427

Brodey R (1971) Hypertrophic osteoarthropathy in the dog. A clinicopathological study of 60 cases. *Journal of the American Veterinary Medical Association* **159**, 1242–1256

Capen CC (1985) Calcium-regulating hormones and metabolic bone disease. In: *Textbook of Small Animal Orthopaedics*, ed. CD Newton and DM Nunamaker, pp. 690–693. JB Lippincott, Philadelphia

Choate CJ and Arnold GA (2011) Elbow arthrodesis following a pathological fracture in a dog with bilateral humeral bone cysts. *Veterinary and Comparative Orthopaedics and Traumatology* **24**, 398–401

Corbee RJ, Tryfonidou MA, Beckers IP and Hazewinkel HA (2012) Composition and use of puppy milk replacers in German shepherd puppies in the Netherlands. *Journal of Animal Physiolology and Animal Nutrition (Berl)* **96**, 395–402

Crumlish PT, Sweeney T, Jones B and Angles JM (2006) Hypertrophic osteodystrophy in the Weimeraner dog: Lack of association between DQA1 alleles and the canine MHC and hypertrophic osteodystrophy. *The Veterinary Journal* **171**, 308–313

Dittmer KE and Thompson KG (2011) Vitamin D metabolism and rickets in domestic animals: a review. *Veterinary Pathology* **48**, 389–407

Dubielzig RR (1985) Medullary bone infarction in dogs. In: *Textbook of Small Animal Orthopaedics*, ed. CD Newton and DM Nunamaker, pp. 615–619. JB Lippincott, Philadelphia

Dubielzig RR, Biery DN and Brodey RS (1981) Bone sarcomas associated with mulitfocal bone infarction in dogs. *Journal of the American Veterinary Medicine Association* **179**, 64–68

Dueland RT and Van Enkevort B (1995) Lateral tibial head buttress plate: use in a pathological femoral fracture secondary to a bone cyst in a dog. *Veterinary and Comparative Orthopaedics and Traumatology* **8**, 196–199

Duval JM, Chambers JN and Newell SM (1995) Surgical treatment of an aneurysmal bone cyst in a dog. *Veterinary and Comparative Orthopaedics and Traumatology* **8**, 213–217

Franklin MA, Rochat MC and Broaddus KD (2008) Hypertrophic osteodystrophy of the proximal humerus in two dogs. *Journal of the American Animal Hospital Association* **44**, 342–346

Gemmill TJ and Clements DN (2016) *BSAVA Manual of Canine and Feline Fracture Repair and Management, 2nd edn.* BSAVA, Gloucester

Goldschmidt MH and Biery DN (1985) Bone cysts in the dog. In: *Textbook of Small Animal Orthopaedics*, ed. CD Newton and DM Nunamaker, pp. 611–613. JB Lippincott, Philadelphia

Grondalen J (1976) Metaphyseal osteopathy (hypertrophic osteodystrophy) in growing dogs. A clinical study. *Journal of Small Animal Practice* **17**, 721–735

Grondalen J (1979) Letter to the editor re: metaphyseal osteopathy. *Journal of Small Animal Practice* **20**, 124

Haney DR and Peck JN (2009) Influence of canal preparation depth on the incidence of femoral medullary infarction with Zurich Cementless Canine Total Hip arthroplasty. *Veterinary Surgery* **38**, 673–676

Harrus S, Waner T, Aizenberg I et al. (2002) Development of hypertrophic osteodystrophy and antibody response in a litter of vaccinated Weimeraner puppies. *Journal of Small Animal Practice* **43**, 27–31

Henik RA, Forrest LJ and Friedman AL (1999) Rickets caused by excessive renal phosphate loss and apparent abnormal vitamin D metabolism in a cat. *Journal of the American Veterinary Medical Association* **215**, 1644–1649

Holling H, Brodey R and Boland C (1961) Pulmonary hypertrophic osteoarthropathy. *Lancet* **2**, 1269–1274

Huang CH, Jeng CR and Yeh LS (2010) Feline hypertrophic osteopathy: a collection of seven cases in Taiwan. *Journal of the American Animal Hospital Association* **46**, 346–352

Johnson KA, Church DB, Barton RJ and Wood AKW (1988) Vitamin-D dependent rickets in a Saint Bernard dog. *Journal of Small Animal Practice* **29**, 657–666

Johnson RL and Lenz SD (2011) Hypertrophic osteopathy associated with a renal adenoma in a cat. *Journal of Veterinary Diagnostic Investigation* **23**, 171–175

Kidder AC and Chew D (2009) Treatment options for hyperphosphataemia in feline CKD: what's out there? *Journal of Feline Medicine and Surgery* **11**, 913–924

Krook L and Whalen JP (2010) Nutritional secondary hyperparathyroidism in the animal kingdom: report of two cases. *Clinical Imaging* **34**, 458–461

Lamb CR (1990) The double cortical line: a sign of osteopenia. *Journal of Small Animal Practice* **31**, 189–192

Lenehan TM and Fetter AW (1985a) Hypertrophic osteodystrophy. In: *Textbook of Small Animal Orthopaedics*, ed. CD Newton and DM Nunamaker, pp. 597–602. JB Lippincott, Philadelphia

Lenehan TM and Fetter AW (1985b) Metaphyseal osteopathy. In: *Textbook of Small Animal Orthopaedics*, ed. CD Newton and DM Nunamaker, pp. 603–607. JB Lippincott, Philadelphia

Lenehan TM, Van Sickle DC and Biery DN (1985) Canine panosteitis. In: *Textbook of Small Animal Orthopaedics*, ed. CD Newton and DM Nunamaker, pp. 591–596. JB Lippincott, Philadelphia

Liu S, Dorfman HD and Patnaik AK (1974) Primary and secondary bone tumours in the cat. *Journal of Small Animal Practice* **15**, 141–156

Liu S and Thacher C (1991) Case report 673. *Skeletal Radiology* **20**, 311–334

Malik R, Laing C and Alan GS (1997) Rickets in a litter of racing greyhounds. *Journal of Small Animal Practice* **38**, 109–114

Marcellin-Little DJ, DeYoung DJ, Thrall DR and Merrill CL (1999) Osteosarcoma at the site of bone infarction associated with total hip arthroplasty in a dog. *Veterinary Surgery* **28**, 54–60

Mason SL, Jepson R, Maltman M and Batchelor DJ (2014) Presentation and management of trapped neutrophil syndrome (TNS) in UK border collies. *Journal of Small Animal Practice* **55**, 57–60

Mathes RL, Homes SP, Coleman KD, Radlinksy MA and Moore PA (2012) Calvarial hyperostosis presenting as unilateral exophthalmos in a female English springer spaniel. *Veterinary Ophthalmology* **14**, 263–270

McConnell JF, Hayes A, Platt SR and Smith KC (2006) Calvarial hyperostosis in two bullmastiffs. *Veterinary Radiology and Ultrasound* **47**, 72–77

Mee A, Bennett D and May C (1992) Canine distemper virus in bone. *Veterinary Record* **131**, 496

Mills J (2010) Hypertrophic osteopathy and megaoesophagus in a cat. *Veterinary and Comparative Orthopaedics and Traumatology* **23**, 218–222

Muir P, Dubielzig RR and Johnson KA (1996) Panosteitis. *Compendium on Continuing Education for the Practicing Veterinarian* **18**, 29–33

Muir P, Dubielzig RR, Johnson KA and Shelton GD (1996) Hypertrophic osteodystrophy and calvarial hyperostosis. *Compendium on Continuing Education for the Practicing Veterinarian* **18**, 143–151

Munjar TA, Austin CC and Breur GJ (1998) Comparison of risk factors for hypertrophic osteodystrophy, craniomandibular osteopathy and canine distemper virus infection. *Veterinary and Comparative Orthopaedics and Traumatology* **11**, 37–43

Nunamaker DM (1985) Osteomyelitis. In: *Textbook of Small Animal Orthopaedics*, ed. CD Newton and DM Nunamaker, pp. 499–510. JB Lippincott, Philadelphia

Padgett GA and Mostosky UV (1986) Animal model: the mode of inheritance of craniomandibular osteopathy in West Highland white terriers. *American Journal of Medical Genetics* **25**, 9–13

Pernell RT, Dunstan RW and DeCamp CE (1992) Aneurysmal bone cyst in a six-month-old dog. *Journal of the American Veterinary Medical Association* **201**, 1897–1899

Pettitt R, Fox R, Comerford EJ and Newitt A (2012) Bilateral angular carpal deformity in a dog with craniomandibular osteopathy. *Veterinary and Comparative Orthopaedics and Traumatology* **25**, 149–154

Phillips AM, Fawcett AC, Allan GS et al. (2011) Vitamin D-dependent non-type 1, non-type 2 rickets in a 3-month-old Cornish Rex kitten. *Journal of Feline Medicine and Surgery* **13**, 526–531

Polizopoulou ZS, Kazakos G, Patsikas MN and Roubies N (2005) Hypervitaminosis A in a cat: a case report and review of the literature. *Journal of Feline Medicine and Surgery* **7**, 263–368

Pool RR and Leighton RL (1969) Craniomandibular osteopathy in a dog. *Journal of the American Veterinary Medical Association* **154**, 657–660

Rabillard M, Souchu L, Niebauer GW and Gauthier O (2011) Haematogenous osteomyelitis: clinical presentation and outcome in three dogs. *Veterinary and Comparative Orthopaedics and Traumatology* **24**, 146–150

Rasor L, Pollard R and Feldman EC (2007) Retrospective evaluation of three treatment methods for primary hyperparathyroidism in dogs. *Journal of the American Animal Hospital Association* **43**, 70–77

Ratterree WO, Glassman MM, Driskell EA and Havig ME (2011) Craniomandibular osteopathy with a unique neurological manifestation in a young Akita. *Journal of the American Animal Hospital Association* **47**, 7–12

Renegar WR, Thornburg LP, Burk RL and Stoll SG (1979) Aneurysmal bone cyst in the dog. A case report. *Journal of the American Animal Hospital Association* **15**, 191–195

Riser WH and Newton CD (1985) Craniomandibular osteopathy. In: *Textbook of Small Animal Orthopaedics*, ed. CD Newton and DM Nunamaker, pp. 621–626. JB Lippincott, Philadelphia

Riser WH, Parkes LJ and Shirer JF (1967) Canine craniomandibular osteopathy. *Journal of the American Veterinary Radiological Society* **8**, 23–29

Safra N, Johnson EG, Lit L et al. (2013) Clinical manifestations, response to treatment, and clinical outcome for Weimaraners with hypertrophic osteodystrophy: 53 cases (2009–2011). *Journal of the American Veterinary Medical Association* **242**, 1260–1266

Sakalas SA, Gillick MS, Kerr ME and Boston SE (2010) Diagnosing the aetiology of hypercalcaemia in the dog: a case of primary hyperparathyroidism. *Veterinary Pathology* **47**, 579–581

Savary KCM, Price GS, Vaden SL (2000) Hypercalcaemia in cats: a retrospective study of 71 cases (1991–1997). *Journal of Veterinary Internal Medicine* **14**, 184–189

Schreiner CA and Nagode LA (2003) Vitamin D-dependent rickets type 2 in a four-month-old cat. *Journal of the American Veterinary Medical Association* **3**, 337–339

Schulz RM, Johnson EG, Wisner ER et al. (2008) Clinicopathological and diagnostic imaging characteristics of systemic aspergillosis in 30 dogs. *Journal of Veterinary Medicine* **22**, 851–859

Schulz KS, Payne JT and Aronson E (1991) *Escherichia coli* bacteraemia associated with hypertrophic osteodystrophy in a dog. *Journal of the American Veterinary Medical Association* **199**, 1170–1173

Seawright AA, English PB and Gartner RJW (1970) Hypervitaminosis A of the cat. *Advances in Veterinary Science and Comparative Medicine* **14**, 1–27

Shiroma JT, Weisbrode SE, Biller DS and Olmstead ML (1993) Pathological fracture of an aneurysmal bone cyst in the lumbar vertebra of a dog. *Journal of the American Animal Hospital Association* **29**, 434–437

Tabaoda J (2000) Systemic mycoses. In: *Textbook of Veterinary Internal Medicine: Diseases of the Dog and Cat, 5th edn*, ed. SJ Ettinger and EC Feldman, pp. 453–476. WB Saunders, Philadelphia

Thompson DJ, Rogers W, Owen MC and Thompson KG (2011) Idiopathic canine juvenile cranial hyperostosis in a Pit Bull Terrier. *New Zealand Veterinary Journal* **59**, 201–205

Tomsa K, Glaus T, Hauser B *et al.* (1999) Nutritional secondary hyperparathyroidism in six cats. *Journal of Small Animal Practice* **40**, 533–539

Trostel CT, Pool RR and McLaughlin RM (2003) Canine lameness caused by developmental orthopaedic diseases: panosteitis, Legg-Calve-Perthes disease and hypertrophic osteodystrophy. *Compendium on Continuing Education for the Practicing Veterinarian* **25**, 282–294

Trowald-Wigh G, Ekman S, Hannsson K *et al.* (1995) Clinical, radiological and pathological features of 12 Irish Setters with canine leucocyte adhesion deficiency. *Journal of Small Animal Practice* **41**, 211–217

Turnier JC and Silverman S (1978) A case study of canine panosteitis: comparison of radiographic and radioisotope studies. *American Journal of Veterinary Research* **39**, 1550–1552

Vanbrugghe B, Blond L, Carioto L, Carmel EN and Nadeau M (2011) Clinical and computed tomography features of secondary renal hyperparathyroidism. *Canadian Veterinary Journal* **52**, 177–180

Van Sickle D (1975) Canine panosteitis. In: *Selected Orthopaedic Problems in the Growing Dog*, pp. 20–28. Monograph, American Animal Hospital Association, South Bend

Walker MA, Duncan JR, Shaw JW and Chapman MD (1975) Aneurysmal bone cyst in a cat. *Journal of the American Veterinary Medical Association* **167**, 933–935

Watson ADJ, Adams WM and Thomas CB (1995) Craniomandibular osteopathy in dogs. *Compendium on Continuing Education* **17**, 911–922

Withers SS, Johnson EG, Culp WT *et al.* (2015) Paraneoplastic hyperthrophic osteopathy in 30 dogs. *Veterinary Comparative Oncology* **13**, 157–165

Zeskov B (1960) A contribution to 'eosinophilic panosteitis' in dogs. *Zentralblatt für Veterinarmedizin* **7**, 671–680

Chapter 8

Disturbances of growth and bone development

Gareth Arthurs and Sorrel Langley-Hobbs

Introduction

A range of conditions in dogs and cats can affect bone growth and development. Problems affecting the growth plates (physes) are caused by abnormalities of cartilage formation (chondrogenesis), cartilage transformation, or bone formation (ossification). Underlying causes may be hormonal (including excess or lack of growth hormone, thyroid hormones and steroid hormones), congenital, nutritional, metabolic or traumatic.

Dogs experience a rapid growth spurt between approximately 4 and 5 months of age. The rate of growth then slows considerably from about 6 months and is 95% complete by 7 months (in Greyhounds). The physes of larger breed dogs remain open and growing for longer than those of smaller breeds. The timing of individual physeal closure is variable and dependent on many factors, including species, breed (size) and the individual bone under consideration. The stimulus for closure is an alteration in secretion of a variety of hormones. This results in an arrest in cartilage proliferation, allowing multiple bony bridges to traverse the physis. Conditions that affect the growth plate usually cause premature closure or retarded growth, resulting in reduced length of the affected bone and a resultant disparity in the relative lengths of paired bones. An increase in length or delay in physeal closure is much less common but has been reported in association with neutering (May *et al.*, 1991) and with fractures (Denny, 1989; Lefebvre *et al.*, 2008).

Angular limb deformities as a result of physeal injuries

The cartilaginous physis in the skeleton of the growing animal is relatively weak, being only 20–50% as strong as adjacent mineralized bone or ligaments. Therefore trauma in immature animals is more likely to result in physeal fracture than diaphyseal fracture, tendon/ligament injury or joint luxation. The management and diagnosis of physeal fractures is covered in the *BSAVA Manual of Canine and Feline Fracture Repair and Management*.

Premature growth plate arrest occurs if there is injury to the germinal cells or blood supply. This chapter will consider the secondary effects of premature and abnormal physeal closure, the consequences of which are dependent on a wide variety of factors, including age and the specific bone affected; a summary of pertinent considerations is presented in Figure 8.1.

- **Age of the animal at time of injury:** How much potential is there for further growth? (95% of growth is complete by 7 months of age in Greyhounds)
- **Which bone is affected?** Complete closure of a growth plate in a single bone, such as the femur, is less likely to be a problem than closure of a growth plate of a paired bone such as the radius, ulna, tibia or fibula
- **Is the closure complete or partial?** Complete closure may cause shortening, which may be compensated for by alteration in joint angles. Partial closure is likely to cause angulation of the affected bone as the unaffected part of the growth plate continues to grow
- **Is there joint subluxation?** This is likely to be the cause of lameness and is the most important aspect to address. Is there secondary osteoarthritis?
- **Shortening (leg length discrepancy):** Generally, shortening is not a problem if it is less than 20% of the total length of the mature bone
- **Rotational deformity:** Often a significant problem
- **Angular deformity:** May be less serious than rotational deformity. Mediolateral deviation is more of a problem than craniocaudal deviation

 8.1 Factors to consider when assessing the effect of premature physeal closure.

Investigation

When an animal is presented with an angular limb deformity, relevant history should include: when the problem was first noticed; whether the patient has suffered any previous trauma; its diet (both previous and current); and whether any siblings are affected. A general physical and full orthopaedic examination as well as gait assessment should be performed. The affected and contralateral limbs should be assessed for lameness, limb alignment in the sagittal, dorsal and transverse planes, limb length including limb length discrepancy, joint pain and range of movement.

Further investigation usually involves imaging the limbs under sedation or general anaesthesia; radiography and/or computed tomography (CT) may be performed. Radiographic examination is readily available and usually cheaper than advanced imaging, but may be more time-consuming. Multiple radiographic views of both affected and contralateral limbs are essential for a complete assessment of the deformities. However, radiography only gives a two-dimensional (2D) image and representation of what can be a complex three-dimensional (3D) deformity. For this reason, CT is superior as 2D and 3D reconstructions of the limb in any plane and orientation can be visualized and assessed. For complex deformities, data from the CT scan can be used to produce a model of the deformity by 3D laser printing. This allows precise understanding of the deformity, and corrective surgery can be rehearsed on the model. It is important to follow basic principles when imaging a patient with angular deformity secondary to physeal disturbance (Figure 8.2).

Measurements can be made from radiographs or CT images to define and quantify the deformities present. When using radiographs, frontal plane alignment (varus/valgus) is measured from a craniocaudal image, and sagittal plane alignment (procurvatum/recurvatum) from a mediolateral image. Rotational deformity is very difficult to quantify from radiographs, but is more readily measured from a CT scan. Alignment may be quantified by comparing the alignment of the joints proximal and distal to the deformity, for example the alignment of the elbow and carpal joints for an antebrachial deformity. A more intricate methodology of assessment termed centre of rotation of angulation (CORA) has been derived from human surgery (Fox *et al.*, 2006). More precise comparison of joint angulation and longitudinal bone axis allows the exact location and degree of deformity to be defined. A bone may have one (uniapical), two (biapical) or more than two (multiapical) points of deformity or CORAs (Figure 8.3). Once the CORA is defined, the correct location for osteotomy is also defined (see below).

- Both the affected and unaffected contralateral limb are imaged
- The whole bone is imaged, including the joints above and below the affected bone, and as much of the affected limb as possible is included on the films in order to assess deviation
- The leg is positioned so the most proximal joint is 'normal' or straight. The distal joints can be then be assessed for rotational deformity by comparison with the limb. For example, when taking craniocaudal views of the antebrachium, the elbow is positioned so it is in a true craniocaudal position and then rotation can be assessed or estimated from the carpal rotation
- If there is concern or suspicion of joint subluxation, specific films are taken centred on affected joints
- Adjacent bones in the limbs are imaged to enable measurement for compensatory overgrowth; if present this should be taken into account when estimating the limb length discrepancy

8.2 Basic principles of diagnostic imaging for angular limb deformity.

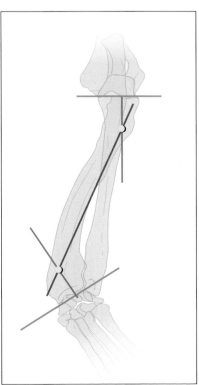

8.3 Example of CORA calculation for frontal plane antebrachial angular limb deformity; two centres of rotation angulation deformities are identified and illustrated.

Management of deformities as a result of premature physeal closure

A number of principles apply when correcting a deformity that has occurred after premature physeal closure; these are often referred to as Paley's principles of deformity correction. The main aim is restoration of normal bone geometry by correction of angular, rotational and length deformities. Restoration of alignment in the frontal (medial–lateral) plane and rotational deformities are most important. Restoration of limb length and alignment in the sagittal (cranial–caudal) plane are ideal but less important to achieve because dogs and cats can usually cope well with minor length discrepancy and deformity in this plane. Restoration of joint congruity is also very important, but it is often difficult or impossible to achieve 'normal' joint congruity and consequently the development of a degree of degenerative joint disease/osteoarthritis is often inevitable.

Angular limb deformities are usually corrected by cutting the bone, improving or correcting alignment and then maintaining the limb segment in the new position with implants while the bone heals. If there is a growth discrepancy between two bones, e.g. the radius and ulna, and there is remaining growth potential, it may be adequate to simply cut the slower growing bone and thereby neutralize its retarding effect on the other bone (e.g. an ulnar osteotomy to alleviate retarding radial growth, see later). Angular limb deformities in horses and humans caused by abnormal physeal growth can be corrected by a temporary transphyseal bridging device such as a staple or screws and wire. This technique retards growth of one half of the physis while the other half continues to grow at a normal rate; hence the bone gradually straightens and the angular deformity reduces. This is rarely possible to perform satisfactorily in puppies and kittens because physeal growth is so rapid and quickly complete that the angular limb deformity is often recognized too late to take advantage of any remaining physeal growth.

An osteotomy is a cut in the bone, compared with an ostectomy which is removal of a piece of bone. Both techniques can be used successfully for correction of angular limb deformity. Typically the bone is cut and the angular limb deformity corrected and then immobilized using internal or external fixation devices. For definitive (rather than dynamic) osteotomy procedures, temporary K-wires may be placed parallel to the joints and in the plane of the proximal and distal segments of bone. The K-wires are then used during correction as guides to ensure alignment; if the K-wires are aligned parallel and in the correct plane, then the proximal and distal joints become parallel, thus achieving one of the most important principles of angular limb deformity correction. The temporary K-wires may be used as 'full pins' in a simple two-pin, type II external skeletal fixator frame to confer temporary stability on the realigned limb segment following correction. This can facilitate the application of definitive plate and screw fixation. Once the segments are secured the K-wire frame is removed. Alternatively, if an external skeletal fixator (ESF) is to be used as the definitive fixation then the proximal and distal full pins placed initially will remain as part of the frame and therefore centrally threaded pins are used and not simple K-wires. When the limb segments are realigned following osteotomy, the remaining pins in the frame are inserted.

The range of available osteotomy/ostectomy techniques includes:

BSAVA Manual of Canine and Feline Musculoskeletal Disorders: A Practical Guide to Lameness and Joint Disease

- Transverse osteotomy. A transverse bone cut is made. It is used for correction of rotational, angular or combinations of deformities but is most useful for rotational and opening wedge osteotomies (Figure 8.4a)
- Opening wedge. A transverse osteotomy is performed and the bone wedged open. No bone is removed, bone length is maintained and even lengthened slightly. Angular limb deformity and rotation can be corrected simultaneously. Muscle tension can limit the amount of opening possible (Figure 8.4b)
- Cuneiform (closing wedge) ostectomy. A pre-calculated segment of bone is removed from the point of maximal deformity (Figure 8.4c). This is simpler to reduce than the opening wedge and gives better stability postoperatively as the bone can be apposed so there is bone–implant load sharing. However, bone length is lost unless the technique is combined with distraction osteogenesis, in which case the advantages of postoperative bone apposition are lost
- Oblique osteotomy. An oblique cut is made parallel to the distal articular surface. The proximal part is 'wedged' and apposed with the medullary canal of the distal fragment. This increases length slightly and can be used to correct rotation and valgus or varus deformity. It is most frequently used in corrective surgery for radius curvus (Figure 8.4d)
- Segmental (partial) ostectomy. Part of a bone is removed, usually after two parallel cuts. This allows bone shortening, or prevents or delays bone healing (Figure 8.4e)
- Dome osteotomy. A curved osteotomy is made using a curved oscillating blade such as a tibial plateau levelling osteotomy (TPLO) saw blade. The axis of rotation of the blade is aligned with the point of maximal deformity (Figure 8.4f). The main advantage of this technique is that the point of deformity correction is located as close to the point of deformity as possible, while preserving as much bone as possible for implant placement and stabilization
- Distraction osteogenesis with angular deformity correction. Following careful preoperative assessment and planning from bone images, a circular ESF (cESF) frame including hinges and motors is applied to the abnormal bone and an osteotomy is made as close as possible to the point of maximal deformity. Rotational deformity is corrected immediately; then sagittal and frontal plane deformities and limb lengthening are gradually corrected during the postoperative period as the cESF is gradually and progressively adjusted several times daily. This is a complex and challenging procedure to learn and master; the results can be excellent but the procedure is unforgiving of errors. Dynamic limb lengthening can also be achieved using a linear ESF, but dynamic correction of angular deformity needs a circular ESF.

Corrective surgery should be performed early to avoid or minimize irreversible pathological changes in adjacent joints. However, it is an elective procedure, not an emergency, and planning is essential. The whole limb and the entire patient must be examined thoroughly. Non-traumatic premature physeal closure or retarded growth may be bilateral. Orthogonal radiographs (craniocaudal and mediolateral planes) should be taken that include the joint above and below the affected limb segment. Tracings of the bones from the radiographs on to paper with virtual rehearsal surgeries and reconstructions can help to plan the definitive osteotomy and correction. However, rotational

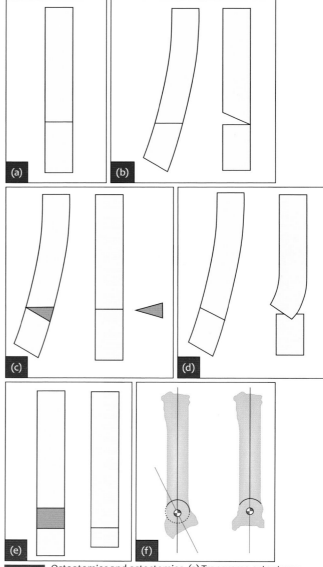

8.4 Osteotomies and ostectomies. (a) Transverse osteotomy. (b) Opening wedge osteotomy. (c) Closing wedge after cuneiform osteotomy. (d) Oblique osteotomy. (e) Segmental osteotomy. (f) Dome osteotomy.

abnormalities are hard to appreciate from radiographs, and soft tissue tension may limit the ability to fully correct alignment of the bone intraoperatively.

Deciding which is the optimal surgical technique to perform will depend on the degree of deformity, the age of the dog, surgeon experience and availability of implant systems. The timing of physeal closure is variable but important as it gives an indication of the approximate remaining growth potential in skeletally immature dogs (Figure 8.5).

Correction of angular limb deformity can be very challenging. A single plane deformity is relatively straightforward; the level of complexity is similar to a moderate fracture repair. However, most deformities are multiplanar which is much more challenging; broad general orthopaedic experience and attendance at an appropriate training course is recommended.

For angular deformity correction, the osteotomy should be made as close to the point of maximal deformity as possible, while preserving as much bone as possible in the proximal and distal bone segments for implant placement

Breed type	Skeletally immature: 2–3 months' growth potential remains	Skeletally mature: growth plates not necessarily completely closed but little potential for further growth remaining
Giant breed	<7–8 months	>8 months
Large breed	<5–6 months	>7 months
Small breed	<3 months	>4 months

8.5 Indication of remaining physeal growth potential in puppies. (Data from Piermattei and Flo, 1997)

and stabilization. The further away the osteotomy is positioned on the bone from the point of maximum deformity, the less straight the final shape of the bone will be regardless of the type of osteotomy (Figure 8.6). This may be acceptable so long as the joints above and below the bone segment are parallel and the resultant longitudinal translation is not excessive. Intraoperatively, final limb alignment and joint function is always checked visually using joint manipulation, particularly flexion and extension, and ensuring that all the long bones and the pes are parallel. It is very important to be able to assess this intraoperatively, i.e. the entire limb should be draped into the surgical field.

The nature of the surgical approach depends on the intended osteotomy as determined by presurgical planning and the type of stabilization/fixation intended. If the bone is to be stabilized with an ESF or minimally invasive plate application, a very limited approach may be made to the bone. If standard internal fixation is planned, the approach to the bone will need to be more extensive. Either way, the periosteum is incised longitudinally and elevated using a periosteal elevator. The bone is then cut as planned using an oscillating saw, Gigli wire or osteotome and mallet. An osteotome and mallet is not ideal as the brittle nature of bone makes it liable to fissure or crack; pre-drilling small holes and then linking them with the osteotome is safer. Bone grafts can be used at the osteotomy site in mature animals, and stabilization needs to be appropriate for the fracture gap created (see *BSAVA Manual of Canine and Feline Fracture Repair and Management*). Radiographs should be taken until full healing is documented; usually every 2 to 6 weeks depending on the age of the animal.

Radius and ulna

In the dog, the distal radial and ulnar physes are, either individually or together, the most commonly affected physes as they are in a location where they are susceptible to damage and the unique conical shape of the distal ulnar physis predisposes it to premature closure. Both bones have to develop in synchrony and their distal growth plates contribute significantly to overall length. The distal radial physis accounts for 60% of radial growth and while the distal ulnar physis accounts for 85% of ulnar growth, its contribution to the potential development of incongruity at

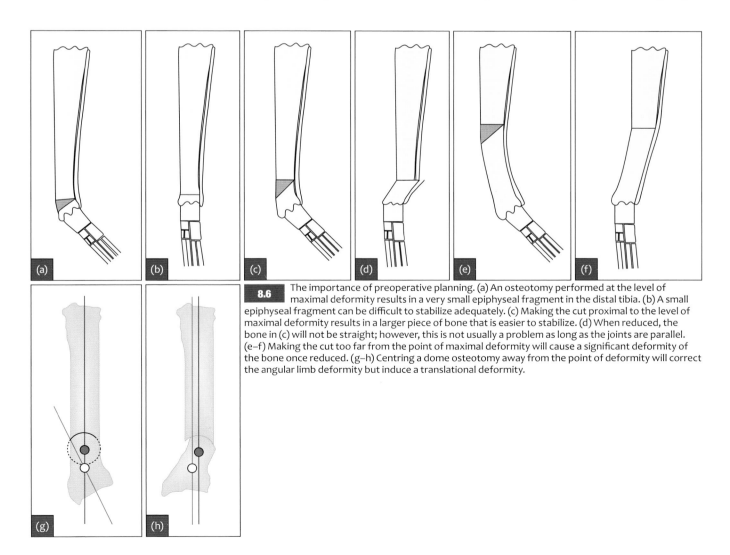

8.6 The importance of preoperative planning. (a) An osteotomy performed at the level of maximal deformity results in a very small epiphyseal fragment in the distal tibia. (b) A small epiphyseal fragment can be difficult to stabilize adequately. (c) Making the cut proximal to the level of maximal deformity results in a larger piece of bone that is easier to stabilize. (d) When reduced, the bone in (c) will not be straight; however, this is not usually a problem as long as the joints are parallel. (e–f) Making the cut too far from the point of maximal deformity will cause a significant deformity of the bone once reduced. (g–h) Centring a dome osteotomy away from the point of deformity will correct the angular limb deformity but induce a translational deformity.

the elbow joint is even more significant as the proximal physis contributes minimally to overall length of the bone.

If a generalized physeal disorder is suspected such as metaphyseal osteopathy or rickets, the distal radial and ulnar physes are often affected. As they are biologically very active, it is very important to evaluate them for evidence of abnormalities.

Distal ulnar physis: premature closure/retarded growth

This is the commonest cause of canine thoracic limb growth deformity. Although often termed premature closure of the distal ulnar physis, it may be more accurately described as retarded growth of the distal ulnar physis. It is often bilateral and is most frequently seen in chondrodystrophic breeds such as Spaniels, Bassett Hounds, Terriers and occasionally some large-breed dogs. Dogs are usually presented because of visible antebrachial deformity and lameness as a result of elbow incongruity or subluxation. There is usually no known history of trauma and the cause is unknown, but can include unseen trauma, retained cartilaginous cores of the distal ulna (Johnson 1981), metaphyseal osteopathy (Figure 8.7), or a form of dwarfism seen in dogs such as the Skye Terrier (Lau, 1977). It is not reported in cats.

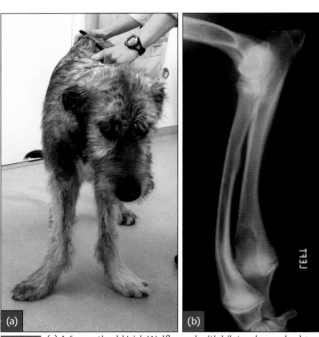

(a) (b)

8.7 (a) A 6-month-old Irish Wolfhound with bilateral carpal valgus secondary to metaphyseal osteopathy. (b) Mediolateral radiograph of the antebrachium of a 7-month-old Irish Wolfhound with radius curvus and a retained cartilaginous core in the distal ulna.

Imaging: The entire antebrachium should be radiographed to include the elbow and carpus, and images acquired of both thoracic limbs. If elbow subluxation is suspected, elbow-centred images should also be taken. CT is more informative, particularly with respect to elbow congruity and pathology.

Radiographic changes and clinical signs relate to retarded ulnar growth resulting in a short ulna which acts as a limiting factor or 'bowstring' on the radius (Carrig *et al.*, 1975). This causes the growing radius to bow around the ulna with resultant radius curvus and associated deformities (Figure 8.8). Some or all of these changes may be present in an individual case. Large-breed

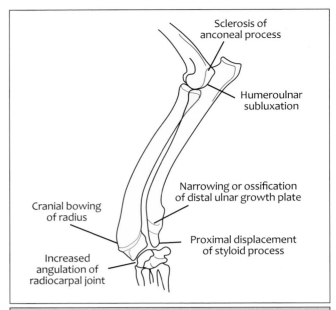

Sclerosis of anconeal process

Humeroulnar subluxation

Narrowing or ossification of distal ulnar growth plate

Cranial bowing of radius

Proximal displacement of styloid process

Increased angulation of radiocarpal joint

- Bowing:
  - Cranial and medial bowing of the radius
- Carpal valgus:
  - Lateral angulation of the foot
- Supination:
  - Radius rotates externally around a short ulna leading to external rotation of the paw
- Elbow:
  - Subluxation of the humeroulnar and radioulnar joints
  - Possible ununited anconeal process
- Carpus:
  - Caudolateral subluxation of antebrachiocarpal joint

8.8 Changes associated with retarded growth of the distal ulnar growth plate (radius curvus).

longer-limbed dogs such as the Irish Wolfhound and Great Dane may be more prone to angular limb deformity, and shorter-limbed breeds such as the Jack Russell Terrier and Bassett Hound are more prone to elbow subluxation (Figure 8.9).

Most physes are flat and discoid but the distal ulnar physis is not; it is conical or V-shaped. The conical shape means the distal ulnar physis has approximately 50% more surface area than a normal flat physis; this may be how the distal ulnar physis contributes so much to ulnar longitudinal growth (85%). However, the conical physis as a result of its anatomical geometry is at higher risk of permanent damage from external trauma. Laterally applied forces that would result in a shear force across other physes, are readily converted to compressive forces resulting in damage (Salter–Harris type V injury) to the germinal layer and predisposing it to premature closure.

Treatment: The choice of treatment option depends on the type and degree of deformity and disability, the presence of joint subluxation, and the age of the animal, in particular with respect to potential for further growth (Figure 8.10).

- **Skeletally immature animals:** early surgery is indicated to minimize further deformity, muscle shortening or contracture, and degenerative joint changes. For mild carpal valgus in a dog with potential for further growth, an ulnar ostectomy/osteotomy (see Operative Technique 8.1) may be sufficient, but this may only be effective in young dogs (median age 5 months) with less than 25 degrees of carpal valgus, or

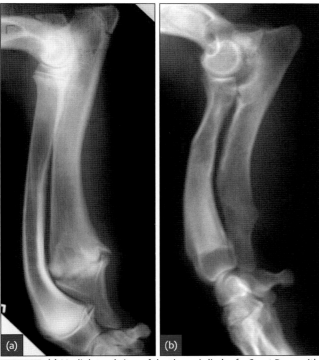

8.9 (a) Mediolateral view of the thoracic limb of a Great Dane with carpal valgus, showing premature closure of the distal ulnar growth plate and radius curvus but no elbow joint subluxation. (b) Mediolateral view of the thoracic limb of a Bassett Hound with carpal valgus, showing premature closure of the distal ulnar growth plate, radius curvus and humeroulnar subluxation. The dog also had panosteitis.

be considered; this should allow the triceps to 'pull' the proximal ulna proximally and improve elbow congruency (see Operative Technique 19.8). However, the surgeon should recognize the associated risk of this procedure is destabilization of the elbow joint because of radioulnar and radiohumeral instability.

- **Skeletally mature animals:** corrective radial and ulnar osteotomies are necessary (see Operative Technique 8.2).

Although the commonest cause of carpal valgus is premature closure of the distal ulnar growth plate, partial closure of the caudolateral aspect of the distal radial growth plate can result in carpal valgus. Careful radiographic evaluation of the distal radial physis and distal ulnar physis is essential, as premature closure of both growth plates can occur concurrently.

Retained cartilaginous cores

Retained cartilaginous cores can affect the distal ulna and are a reflection of the very active growth that occurs at around 5 months of age. They are usually of little clinical significance but they may cause slower growth or premature physeal closure. In such cases, the cores may be irregular with ill-defined borders as compared to cartilage cores in normal dogs that have smooth well defined borders (Fox, 1984). The core is composed of columns of hypertrophic cartilage cells that fail to develop normally. The matrix septa in the hypertrophic zone fail to calcify, and vascularization is impeded. The aetiology is unknown but as the condition is seen in giant breeds, genetics and/or nutrition may play a role in its development and it has also been classified as a form of metaphyseal osteochondrosis. Decreasing the plane of nutrition to slow growth is recommended in the 3- to 4-month-old puppy. In the older skeletally immature puppy, a segmental ulnar ostectomy (see Operative Technique 8.1) may be helpful. Radial and ulnar corrective osteotomies may be indicated in a mature dog with functional problems due to deformity (see Operative Technique 8.2).

for older animals (median age 6.5 months) when valgus is less than 13 degrees (Shields and Gambardella, 1989). If carpal valgus exceeds 25 degrees in an immature dog, segmental ulnar ostectomy combined with corrective osteotomy of the radius is advisable (see Operative Technique 8.2). If elbow (humeroulnar) subluxation is marked, a proximal ulnar osteotomy can

Deformity	Growth plate affected	Age and severity	Corrective surgery	Comments
Carpal valgus	Distal ulnar	Skeletally immature; <25 degrees	Segmental ulnar ostectomy distally	Moderate humeroulnar subluxation of the elbow will correct following distal ostectomy but more severe disease requires proximal ulnar osteotomy
	Distal ulnar	Skeletally immature; >25 degrees	Segmental ulnar ostectomy and wedge ostectomy of radius	
	Distal ulnar	Skeletally mature; >13 degrees	Segmental ulnar ostectomy and wedge ostectomy of radius	
	Radial – caudolateral aspect	Skeletally mature	Segmental ulnar ostectomy and wedge ostectomy of radius	
	Retained cartilaginous cores	Skeletally immature	Try a decreased plane of nutrition initially	
	Retained cartilaginous cores	Skeletally mature	Segmental ulnar ostectomy and wedge ostectomy of radius	
Humeroulnar subluxation	Distal ulnar	Skeletally mature	Dynamic proximal ulnar osteotomy	
Humeroradial subluxation	Distal or proximal radial	Skeletally immature	Segmental ulnar ostectomy OR proximal radial osteotomy and dynamic fixation	Distraction osteogenesis to increase limb length using an Ilizarov or ring fixator may be necessary
Distal tibial valgus/varus	Distal tibial	Skeletally mature	Opening or closing wedge ostectomy of distal tibia and external skeletal fixator (ESF) application	

8.10 Procedures for surgical correction of an angular deformity.

Premature closure of the distal radial physis

Closure of the distal radial growth plate is much less common than closure of the distal ulnar growth plate. When it occurs, closure may be symmetrical or asymmetrical. Symmetrical physeal closure results in a short radius but the limb is usually straight (Figure 8.11); varus deformity of the manus rarely results from continued ulnar growth. Conversely, asymmetrical distal radial physeal closure may result in valgus or varus deformity, depending on which part of the radial physis is affected. Premature closure of the caudolateral part of the distal radial growth plate is most common and results in carpal valgus, mimicking premature closure of the distal ulnar growth plate distally, but the radius is short (Figure 8.12).

Lameness is often attributable to proximal luxation of the humeroradial joint (Olson *et al.*, 1979). As the ulna continues to grow with respect to a more slowly growing (proximal) radius, the net effect is that the proximal radius drifts distally causing increased joint space between the radial head and humeral condyle. Subsequently, the humeral condyle drifts distally and humeroulnar incongruity occurs, i.e. an increased distance between the anconeal process and the humeral condyle. Increased pressure on the medial coronoid process through the distal humeral condyle may cause medial coronoid process fragmentation (Macpherson *et al.*, 1992). Distally, there may be relative overgrowth of the styloid process of the ulna and increased width of the antebrachiocarpal joint space (Vandewater and Olmstead, 1983). The presenting complaint is usually lameness associated with elbow incongruity, pain or degenerative joint disease. If partial closure is present then the complaint may be one of angular limb deformity. Affected animals should be assessed particularly for limb length, angular and rotational deformity and joint pain.

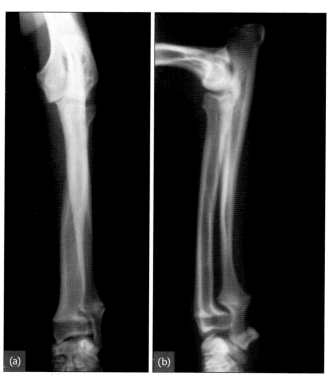

8.11 (a) Craniocaudal and (b) mediolateral views of a 9-month-old Cavalier King Charles Spaniel with premature closure of the distal radial growth plate. The radius has lost its normal cranial bowing, there is a marked humeroradial subluxation and secondary humeroulnar subluxation. There is no significant angular deformity.

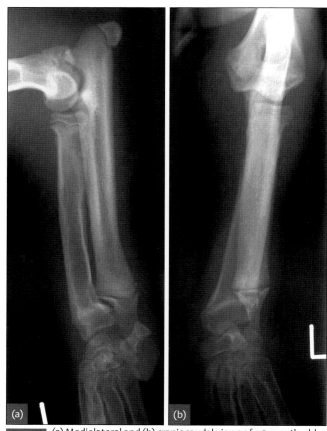

8.12 (a) Mediolateral and (b) craniocaudal views of a 5-month-old crossbreed dog with partial closure of the caudolateral aspect of the distal radial growth plate, combined with an abnormal appearance of the distal ulnar growth plate probably associated with delayed growth. There is humeroradial and humeroulnar subluxation. The radius has lost its normal cranial bow and has a straight appearance. There is a carpal valgoid deformity induced by the partial growth plate closure.

Imaging: The features associated with premature closure of the distal radial physis are illustrated in Figure 8.13; radiography or CT may be used to make a diagnosis, but CT is more sensitive to concurrent pathology such as fragmented medial coronoid process.

Treatment: Elbow incongruity can be addressed by a number of surgical techniques including lengthening the radius or shortening the ulna. Fragmentation of the medial coronoid process can occur, and the elbow joint should be inspected for this (see Chapter 19).

Radial lengthening is arguably the best option as it maintains limb length, but it can be a challenging and complex procedure, and perfect radiohumeral and elbow congruity may not be achievable because of pre-existing conformational deformity of the radial head. Mid or proximal radial osteotomy is performed that is then followed by gradual proximal distraction of the proximal segment either using pins and elastic bands from radial head to humeral condyle, or by use of a circular or linear ESF to achieve distraction osteogenesis (see Operative Techniques 8.3 and 19.10). Alternatively, definitive lengthening can be achieved at the time of osteotomy using internal fixation to stabilize the radius in the distracted position; this has the disadvantage that perfect lengthening may not be achieved or may become inadequate if further ulnar growth and humeroradial incongruence develop. The two big challenges with radial lengthening are achieving perfect position of the radial head, and whether normal

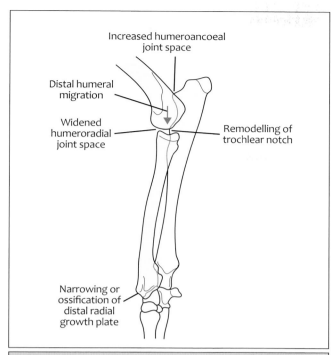

- Elbow joint:
  - Increase in width of the humeroradial joint
  - Abnormal development of the trochlear notch
  - Fragmentation of the medial coronoid process of ulna
- Secondary humeroulnar subluxation
- Short radius or short antebrachium
- Straight radius: loss of normal cranial bow
- Reduction of cortical thickness and bone diameter
- Antebrachiocarpal joint: subluxation and secondary osteoarthritis

8.13 Imaging changes seen with premature closure of the distal radial physis.

elbow congruity is ever possible to achieve because the radial head may be dysplastic due to chronic non-articulation with the humerus; such dysplasia is unlikely to be corrected by establishing humeroradial contact.

Alternatively the ulna may be shortened with an ulnar ostectomy. A distal ulnar ostectomy (see Operative Technique 8.1) is safer as the risk of proximal elbow instability is abolished, but bearing in mind these risks, a proximal ulnar ostectomy (see Operative Technique 19.8) may facilitate better relative ulnar migration and resultant elbow congruity, but with higher risk of ulnar instability and elbow subluxation. Postoperative stabilization is generally not required but the risk of ulnar instability can be reduced by performing a bi-oblique ulnar osteotomy, or by stabilizing the ulna using an intramedullary pin or a plate. Regardless of location, segmental ulnar ostectomy should remove a section of bone equal to or slightly greater in length than the measured humeroradial gap.

If significant distal antebrachial deformity is present, angular limb correction of the distal antebrachium may be necessary (see Operative Technique 8.2). In the most severe cases if carpal function is judged to be beyond recovery, pancarpal arthrodesis might be considered (see Operative Technique 20.1).

Premature closure of the distal radial and ulnar physes

Partial or complete premature closure of both the distal radial and ulnar physes can occur in the same limb. Both the radius and ulna will be short which is often the major

concern, particularly in a very young puppy. Humeroulnar subluxation may be present due to continued growth of the proximal radial physis. Although the proximal ulnar physis is unaffected, it is only responsible for growth of the ulna/olecranon proximal to the elbow. Radial and ulnar osteotomies are used to correct angular and rotational deformities as previously described (see Operative Technique 8.2). If the limb length deficiency is significant, distraction osteogenesis should also be considered.

Synostosis

Synostosis is fusion of two bones that are not normally fused. The most common example of this is synostosis between the radius and ulna that occurs following antebrachial fracture repair, often when only the radius is stabilized without ulnar stabilization. In the immature dog, normal antebrachial development and growth occurs as the radius and ulna grow simultaneously but independently, and are able to 'slide' past each another. Synostosis of the radius and ulna in the growing puppy would be rare but could result in humeroulnar subluxation due to continued growth in the proximal radial growth plate (Figure 8.14) (Alexander *et al.*, 1978). Humeroulnar subluxation can be treated by ulnar osteotomy (see Operative Techniques 8.1 and 19.8). Overgrowth of the styloid process may also occur at the carpus, but this would be unlikely to cause a clinical problem.

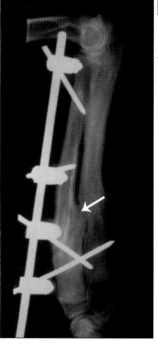

8.14 Synostosis (arrowed) between the radius and ulna in a 6-month-old Pointer after a mid-diaphyseal fracture was stabilized with external skeletal fixation. Continued growth of the proximal radial growth plate in this immature dog could result in humeroulnar subluxation.

Premature closure of the distal femoral and/or proximal tibial physes

Genu valgum ('knock-knees') is an uncommon condition that is diagnosed in large breeds such as the Great Dane, St Bernard and Mastiff at 4–6 months of age (Newton, 1985b). It is frequently a bilateral problem and clinical signs include:

- Genu valgum with medial bowing at the stifle joint as a result of relative overgrowth of the medial condylar regions of the distal femur or proximal tibia

- Lateral patellar luxation; lameness can be severe
- Progressive femoral bowing which may cause coxa valga and femoral neck anteversion leading to hip subluxation
- External rotation of the distal tibia and paw.

This growth deformity probably occurs during the rapid long bone growth phase and has been associated with retained cartilaginous cores (Newton, 1985b). There is overgrowth of the medial femoral condyle and medial tibia compared to the lateral aspects that are relatively hypoplastic. Other deformities may also be present in the thoracic limbs such as carpal valgus secondary to distal ulnar physeal closure. Affected puppies need comprehensive assessment prior to contemplating surgical intervention.

Genu varum ('bow legs') is most often associated with medial patellar luxation in small- and large-breed dogs. Affected dogs have mild lateral bowing of the distal femur (distal femoral varus) and a compensatory opposite bend (proximal tibial valgus) with a resultant S-shape of the tibia. Medial patellar luxation is usually the cause of lameness and can be addressed surgically; simultaneous corrective osteotomy to correct femoral varus is occasionally performed but the selection criteria for this have not been clearly defined (see Chapter 23).

Premature closure, fracture or growth deformity of the caudal proximal tibial physis

This can result in an increased tibial plateau angle (TPA) that could cause altered stifle mechanics and possibly predispose to rupture of the cranial cruciate ligament. However, the aetiology of cranial cruciate ligament disease is complex, and absolute correlation with TPA has not been established. High TPA can occur secondary to fracture of the tibial plateau with caudal displacement relative to the metaphysis (Pratt, 2001). High TPA has also been recognized in large- and small-breed dogs (e.g. West Highland White Terrier) with no history of trauma. When high TPA is clinically significant (usually only if cranial cruciate ligament disease is present) or another proximal tibial conformation anomaly is present, corrective osteotomy may be undertaken, i.e. a cranial closing wedge ostectomy or TPLO that is usually achieved using a curvilinear proximal tibial metaphyseal osteotomy (see Chapter 23).

Premature closure of the tibial tuberosity physis

This can result in 'distal tuberosity drift': the proximal tibial plateau continues to grow but if the tibial tuberosity apophysis is prematurely and abnormally fused to the tibial diaphysis it becomes progressively more distal in position relative to the stifle. This is usually asymptomatic but has the potential to cause problems in athletic breeds such as Greyhounds due the abnormally distal insertion point of the patellar ligament.

Premature closure of the distal tibial or fibular physis

Tarsal varus (pes varus) is most frequently seen in the Dachshund (Johnson et al., 1989) (Figure 8.15). A hereditary cause is suspected as the condition is often bilateral with no

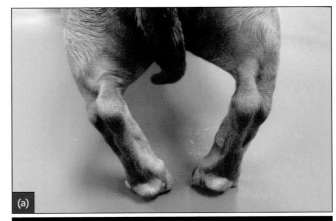

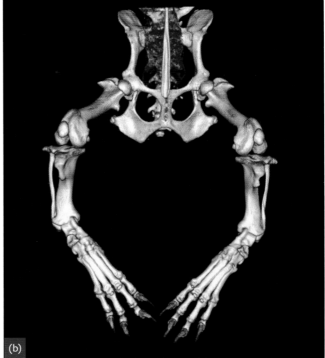

8.15 (a) An adult Dachshund with marked bilateral pes varus and (b) a 3D volume rendered image from the same dog illustrating the severity of the deformity.
(Courtesy of Gordon Brown)

history of trauma. Clinical signs first appear at 5–6 months of age and surgical correction is recommended; tibial medial opening wedge osteotomy and stabilization with external skeletal fixation or locking plate fixation have been described (Johnson et al., 1989; Petazzoni et al., 2012).

Tarsal valgus has been reported in Shetland Sheepdogs and an Anatolian Sheepdog (Figure 8.16). It is thought to arise from premature closure of the distal fibular growth plate. If longitudinal tibial growth is constrained laterally by a static fibula, the result is lateral deviation of the distal tibia (Vaughan, 1987; Jevens and DeCamp, 1993). A number of tibial osteotomy/ostectomy and realignment techniques may be considered (see Figure 8.4 and Operative Technique 8.4) combined with possible fibular osteotomy. If limb length discrepancy is minimal, medial closing wedge ostectomy is most straightforward and the repair is stable because of immediate bone–implant load sharing (Altunatmaz et al., 2007; Burton and Owen, 2007).

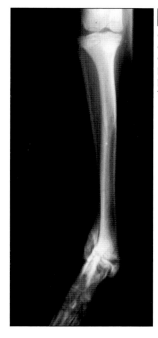

8.16 Radiograph of a Shetland Sheepdog with a valgoid deformity of the tibia. The deformity developed subsequent to premature closure of the distal fibular growth plate, either alone or combined with partial closure of the lateral aspect of the distal tibial growth plate.

Genu recurvatum

Genu recurvatum means a stifle with a deformity that results in apparent hyperextension, i.e. the joint is 'bent backwards in the wrong direction' (Figure 8.17). It is seen in puppies and kittens as a rare congenital abnormality. Affected animals present with a hyperextended pelvic limb. It is possible to partially flex the stifle in the early stages, which differentiates it from quadriceps contracture, but the flexor muscles or hamstrings seem to be too weak and inadequate to maintain the stifle in a normal slightly flexed position. As the animal ages, the stifle becomes fixed in extension. Radiographically, the distal femur and proximal tibia develop abnormally and the stifle is abnormally extended. Treatment can be attempted in early cases, for example using transarticular ESFs to maintain stifle flexion, but the prognosis is guarded; stifle arthrodesis or amputation can be considered as salvage options.

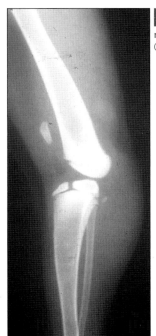

8.17 Lateral radiograph of the stifle of a kitten with genu recurvatum.
(Courtesy of Matthew Pead)

Bone dysplasias – genetic bone disorders

Many genetically determined disorders that occur in dogs and cats, including those of the osseous skeleton, have been positively selected by breeders and some may be considered 'normal' for the breed. Most diseases that are recognized in dogs and cats have a similar if not identical disease that affects humans. A 1997 system of classification for constitutional (intrinsic) disorders of bone in humans is of limited application in dogs and cats because although much of what we know about bone dysplasias is extrapolated from the equivalent disease in man, the pathology, signs and significance cannot necessarily be translated directly between species.

Osteochondrodysplasias

Osteochondrodysplasias are a group of inherited disorders of cartilage and bone development and all are associated with varying degrees and types of dwarfism. In dogs and cats, most conditions are identified during development rather than at birth. Details of specific conditions, breeds affected and other details are given in Figure 8.18.

Chondrodysplasia

Chondrodysplasia means abnormal growth of cartilage which results in disproportionate dwarfism. Chondrodysplastic dwarfs have been developed by selective breeding; examples include the Dachshund and Basset Hound. These disproportionate dwarfs have short bent legs but dolichocephalic or mesocephalic heads (normal to elongated skulls). This form of dwarfism, with reduced limb length relative to the trunk, is also known as rhizomelic or micromelic disproportionate dwarfism. Radiographic features considered normal for the breed but abnormal in other breeds include:

- Short, thick long bones
- Short vertebrae
- Wide physes with delayed closure
- Accentuated shape of bones with prominent tuberosities and flared epiphyses.

Lameness can occur secondary to joint pathology resulting from conformational abnormalities, e.g. humero-ulnar subluxation, shoulder dysplasia, ununited anconeal process, hip dysplasia, tarsal varus or patellar luxation.

Osteochondrodysplasia

This is a disorder of bone and cartilage development that causes dwarfism. Chondrodystrophic puppies are occasionally recognized in breeds that are not overtly chondrodystrophic but may have mild chondrodystrophic traits, including the Labrador Retriever, Alaskan Malamute, Norwegian Elkhound, Great Pyrenees, Miniature Poodle, Newfoundland, German Shepherd Dog, St Bernard, Clumber Spaniel and Scottish Deerhound (Breur *et al.*, 1989; Bingel and Sande, 1994). Osteochondrodysplastic dwarfs have short bowed thoracic limbs with carpal valgus, cubital varus and external rotation of the paws (Figure 8.19). Radiographic features include humeroulnar subluxation and caudolateral subluxation of the radial head. The distal ulnar metaphysis is wide and ragged with an obliquely running depression and radiolucent insertion

Disorder	Synonyms	Breeds affected	Radiographic changes	Other	Genetics
Chondrodysplasia punctate	Multiple epiphyseal dysplasia	Beagle, Miniature Poodle	Short limbs, enlarged joints, stippled epiphyses. May be dysplastic hips	Present from birth or develops in late puppyhood	Autosomal recessive (Beagle)
Achondroplasia		Shih Tzu, Pekingese, Pug	Limb shortening, flared metaphyses, depressed nasal bridge, short maxilla, small foramen magnum, wedge/hemivertebrae	Soft tissue airway problems, medial patellar luxation, elbow luxation	Autosomal dominant
Hypochondroplasia		Dachshund, Welsh Corgi, Scottish Terrier, Irish Setter	Limb shortening	Disc disease, elbow dysplasia	Autosomal dominant
Metaphyseal chondrodysplasia		Small breeds	Medial patellar luxation, hypoplasia of medial femoral condyle		
		Dachshund	Tarsal varus due to distal medial tibial dysplasia		
		Giant breeds	Retained cartilaginous cores	Carpal valgus, osteochondrosis	
Osteochondrodysplastic dwarfism	Artho-ophthalmopathy, dyschondrosteosis	Labrador Retriever, Samoyed	Short radius and ulna: mesomelic dwarfism	Cataract, detached retina	Autosomal recessive
	Alaskan Malamute chondrodysplasia	Alaskan Malamute, Norwegian Elkhound	Short radius and ulna: mesomelic dwarfism	Anaemia (Alaskan Malamute)	Autosomal recessive (Alaskan Malamute)
Pseudochondroplasia		Miniature Poodle	Enlarged joints, stippling and patchy densities of epiphyses in young animals; in older animals bones are short and deformed	Stiff joints	
Enchondrodystrophy		English Pointer	Flared metaphyses, wide growth plates	Cystic degeneration of articular cartilage	Autosomal recessive

8.18 Osteochondrodysplasias: abnormalities of cartilage and/or bone growth and development.

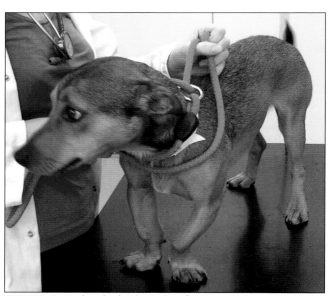

8.19 Osteochondrodysplastic dwarfism in a crossbreed dog. The dog has marked curvature of the antebrachium with cubital varus, carpal valgus and external rotation of the foot. The pelvic limbs are relatively straight.

groove seen cranially. The condition is not usually recognized until puppies are 4 to 5 months old and males may be predisposed. Heritability may be due to a single autosomal recessive gene with complete penetration but with variable phenotypic expression (Fletch *et al*., 1973; Bingel and Sande, 1994). Surgery can be attempted to correct the elbow incongruity and straighten the limbs.

Concurrent abnormalities have been recognized in specific breeds including macrocytic anaemia in Alaskan Malamutes (Fletch *et al*., 1973), retinal abnormalities and cataracts in the Samoyed (Meyers *et al*., 1983), glycosuria in Norwegian Elkhounds and ocular anomalies in Labrador Retrievers (Carrig *et al*., 1977). In the Labrador, oculo-skeletal dysplasia is characterized by the presence of cataracts, retinal dysplasia, folds or detachments in dogs with shorter than normal thoracic limbs and an abnormal morphological appearance of the radius and ulna (osteo-chondrodysplastic dwarfism). The syndrome is caused by one abnormal gene with recessive effects on the skeleton and incompletely dominant effects on the eye. Carrier dogs (i.e. heterozygotes) have a clinically normal skeleton and mild ocular deformities, whereas homozygotes have skeletal abnormalities and severe ocular abnormalities. A DNA test is available commercially to indicate either normal, carrier or affected.

Achondroplasia

In humans, achondroplasia is an autosomal dominant condition that causes dwarfism with specific characteristics such as failure of the skull fontanelle to fuse, and missing collar bones. Failure of cartilaginous growth results in proportionate short-limbed dwarfs. In dogs, it is also an autosomal dominant condition perpetuated by selective breeding in the Bulldog, Shi Tzu, Lhaso Apso and Pekingese. Features include short limbs, flared metaphyses, brachycephalic skulls, a depressed nasal bridge and short maxilla. Numerous defects are seen including mandibular prognathism (lower jaw overshot), stenotic nares, overlong soft palate, hemivertebrae and cardiac defects. Lameness can occur secondary to congenital elbow luxation and patellar luxation (Jezyk, 1985). Histologically there is evidence of retarded endochondral ossification.

Enchondrodystrophy in the English Pointer

This is an inherited dwarfism thought to be homozygous recessive in nature (Whitbread, 1983). Signs of growth plate deformity appear before weaning; the pups have a stiff, stilted gait and experience difficulty in turning. They may exhibit a 'bunny-hopping' motion when moving at speed. The affected animals remain considerably smaller than their normal litter mates.

Radiographically, there is widening of the growth plates (similar to rickets) with flaring of the metaphyses and periosteal bone production around the physes. The distal ulnar, radial and tibial physes are worst affected but vertebral bodies are also affected. Late changes include limb deviation and elbow or hip deformity with secondary osteoarthritic changes.

Scottish Fold osteodystrophy

This affects the Scottish Fold breed of cats and the defining feature is a cartilage defect causing the folded ears. The breed originated in Scotland by breeding naturally occurring, spontaneously mutated farm cats with folded ears to British and American Shorthair cats. The breed is rare because it is not recognized by a number of feline breed standards and governing bodies, due to health concerns including deafness, ear infections and persistent ear mite infestations. Autosomal dominant individuals also suffer severe osteochondrodysplasia including malformed bones and joints and severe crippling degenerative joint disease. The pathogenesis is related to disordered endochondral ossification in the epiphyses. Most affected individuals have a short, thick, inflexible tail that precedes other problems. The presence or absence of the deformed tail is not a reliable indicator of more severe problems and is unreliable as a breeding selection indicator (Mathews *et al*., 1995).

Canine osteochondromas

Canine osteochondromas are characterized by ossified protuberances arising from the metaphyseal cortical surfaces of long bones, ribs and vertebrae. They can occur singly or as multiple lesions; multiple lesions may be referred to as hereditary multiple exostoses and there may be a familial tendency. Dogs are first affected from 4 to 6 months of age. The osseous nodules are trophic and cease growth at maturity. They are asymptomatic unless the bone enlargement encroaches on neurovascular, tendinous or ligamentous structures (Figure 8.20). Synovial osteochondromatosis is a separate condition characterized by chondrometaplasia of the synovial membrane and the formation of benign osteochondral nodules. Malignant transformation of one synovial osteochondroma lesion to chondrosarcoma has been documented (Aeffner *et al*., 2012).

It is suspected that osteochondromas develop from chondrocytes displaced from the growth plate, which undergo osseous differentiation in a juxtacortical position. Signs vary from usually asymptomatic incidental findings to discomfort and lameness, or rarely paralysis, depending on the location. On palpation they are firm swellings. Radiographically, lesions appear as pedunculated sessile

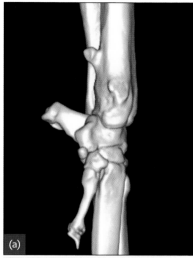

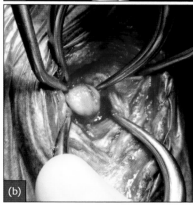

8.20 (a) CT 3D volume rendered image showing a caudally directed osteochondroma of the distal radius in a 1-year-old Deerhound with lameness due to impingement of the flexor tendons. (b) An intraoperative image showing removal of the lesion in the same dog.
(Courtesy of Gordon Brown)

masses with a smooth or irregular outline arising from cortical surfaces. Histopathology shows a layer of cartilage overlying trabecular bone. Prognosis is usually reasonable but may be guarded for patients with multiple or compressive vertebral lesions.

Feline osteochondromas

Feline osteochondromas are rare, sessile bony masses that are either single or multiple. They account for 20% of feline primary bone tumours seen in feline leukaemia virus (FeLV) positive cats and can transform into osteosarcomas or chondrosarcomas. Cats are usually 2 to 6 years old and Siamese cats may be over-represented for multiple lesions. The prognosis is guarded when cats are positive for FeLV; lesions can recur after excision, necessitating euthanasia.

Solitary osteochondromas have also been reported in the Burmese cat and the elbow is a site of predilection (Figure 8.21). For solitary lesions, the prognosis is better and surgical excision can be successful, but metaplastic change with late neoplastic transformation can occur. Complete treatment is not possible because of the underlying FeLV positive status (Rosa and Kirberger, 2012)

Multiple enchondromatosis

This is a rare polyostotic disease with chondroma-like proliferations in the metaphyseal and diaphyseal region of cartilaginous bones. It has been reported in Toy Poodles (Krauser *et al*., 1989) and a Bull Terrier (Watson *et al*., 1991). Dogs present with pathological fractures or lameness between 4 months of age and adulthood; multiple bones can be affected. The Poodles were also chondrodysplastic.

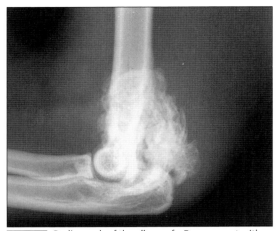

8.21 Radiograph of the elbow of a Burmese cat with an osteochondroma. The cat was sound for 6 months after local excision; however, the lesion recurred and a sarcoma developed. Amputation was curative.

Radiological characteristics included rounded or oval eccentrically situated metaphyseal areas of increased radiolucency. The areas were usually sharply defined, extended into the diaphysis or epiphysis and were only found in bones that develop by endochondral ossification. The lesions are thought to develop as a result of internal remodelling disorders from the remains of the epiphyseal physis, or due to aberrant formation of cartilage instead of bone in the ossification zone. In humans, the equivalent condition is called Ollier disease; enchondromas are benign cartilaginous tumours that develop in the metaphysis and typically affect the short bones of the hands and feet. Malignant transformation occurs in 15–25% of cases and is characterized by increased pain. Solitary lesions are treated by curettage and bone grafting.

Abnormalities of density of cortical diaphyseal structure and/or metaphyseal modelling

Osteogenesis imperfecta

This is an inherited bone disease also called brittle bone disease, or Lobstein syndrome in humans. It is a congenital bone disorder caused by genetic defects usually affecting the *COL1A1* and *COL1A2* genes that encode the procollagen molecules of type I collagen. Type I collagen constitutes more than 85% of the organic matrix of bone and provides the framework for mineralization. In osteogenesis imperfecta, qualitative and quantitative abnormalities of its formation occur, leading to defective connective tissue formation and, consequently, excessive bone fragility. In humans, there are eight types whose genetic and physical attributes are well characterized; signs vary from mild to lethal in the perinatal period. In puppies and kittens, the disease mimics nutritional secondary hyperparathyroidism. Osteogenesis imperfecta should be suspected in young animals fed on a normal diet and presenting with multiple fractures but no signs or history of trauma. Clinical signs are usually seen between 10 and 18 weeks of age. Affected animals are susceptible to pathological fractures and often have deformed limbs secondary to multiple historic fracture malunions or folding fractures. Radiography may show poor mineralization (but not always), osteopenia or thinning cortices and pathological fractures (Figure 8.22). The teeth may have a translucent

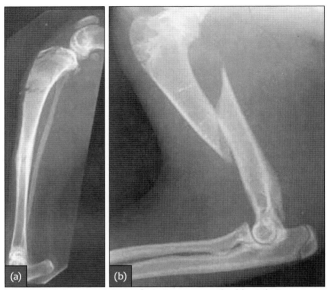

8.22 Osteogenesis imperfecta in an 11-month-old cat that presented with a tibial fracture. Radiographs showed (a) the presence of healed fractures in the same bone (and in the opposite tibia). (b) The cat suffered spontaneous bilateral humeral fractures while being caged during hospitalization. Bone density in this cat was not grossly reduced radiographically.

appearance and tooth fractures are reported (known as dentinogenesis imperfecta in humans; dentine also contains type I collagen). Blue sclerae may be seen. Skin abnormalities are rarely reported but the skin may be thin.

Histologically, cortical bone quantity is reduced and the bone is woven with increased porosity. In one series of three dogs, analysis of type I collagen from cultured skin fibroblasts was used to confirm the diagnosis of osteogenesis imperfecta (Campbell *et al.*, 1997); in a kitten, a presumed diagnosis was made (Evason *et al.*, 2007). There is no effective treatment but bisphosphonates have been used in humans to retard osteoclast activity and thus limit bone resorption; this increases bone mineral density and decreases fracture frequency.

Osteopetrosis

This is an extremely rare congenital and familial developmental abnormality of skeletal growth. Synonyms include osteosclerosis fragilis, chalk bones, marble bones and Albers-Schönberg disease. The disease manifests as an abnormality of bone turnover relating to abnormal osteoclast function and therefore reduced bone resorption. The exact mechanism of osteoclast dysfunction is unknown but in humans an osteoclast deficiency of carbonic anhydrase is recognized. The bone becomes abnormally dense because it is being formed normally but not resorbed properly. Clinical signs either relate to pathological fracture due to the brittle nature of the bone, or obliteration of normal marrow that can result in aplastic anaemia. The condition may also be detected as an incidental finding (Figure 8.23). There is a paucity of reports in the dog. Riser and Fankhauser (1970) reported the post-mortem results of three Dachshund puppies and there is a single case report in an Australian Shepherd Dog (Lees and Sautter, 1979), which presented at 1 year of age with anaemia. There may be decreased activity of lysosomal and oxidative enzymes, or an absolute decrease in osteoclasts.

Osteopetrosis has been described rarely in cats, characterized by endosteal lamellar bone formation and anaemia (Kramers *et al.*, 1988). There is also a distinct

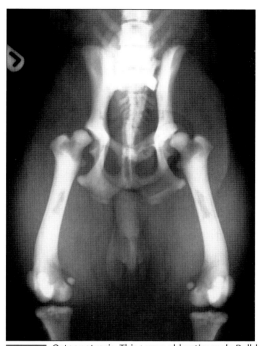

8.23 Osteopetrosis. This 1-year-old entire male Bulldog presented because of lameness secondary to hip dysplasia.
(Courtesy of George Papadopoulos)

condition of medullary osteosclerosis as a result of trabecular bone formation within the medullary cavity that can occur in association with FeLV infection. Recently a generalized idiopathic hyperostosis was described in an 11-year-old adult cat (Fawcett *et al.*, 2014).

Dysostoses

Dysostosis is a broad term encompassing a group of congenital bone disorders that are characterized by abnormal development of whole bones or parts of bones. In humans, dysostoses are divided into three groups but this is not particularly helpful in dogs and cats. However, it can be helpful to divide dysostoses depending on whether the appendicular skeleton (dysmelia) or axial skeleton is affected. The cause of dysostoses may be hereditary (spontaneous mutations) or as a result of exposure to teratogens usually in the first trimester of gestation.

Axial dysostoses may affect the craniofacial bones, the vertebral column or the thoracic skeleton (ribs and sternum). Dysostoses with cranial and facial involvement are common in certain dog breeds. Mandibular hypoplasia (undershot lower jaw or brachygnathism) is seen in mesocephalic and dolichocephalic breeds such as Cocker Spaniels, Poodles, Greyhounds and Whippets. This abnormality can cause dental occlusion problems. Vertebral dysostoses are also common and include hemivertebrae and fused or block vertebrae (Figure 8.24). Such abnormalities are often incidental findings, although they can occasionally cause spinal cord compression.

Appendicular dysostoses are often more striking and occur sporadically in dogs and cats.

Embryological limb development commences with a projection of mesoderm covered by ectoderm that has an inductive ectodermal ridge. Subsequently the individual bones form from a cartilage anlage. Three mesodermal rays, the ulnar, radial and central rays, contribute to pectoral limb formation. Disturbances of one or more of these rays result in abnormal formation of the soft tissues and corresponding bones.

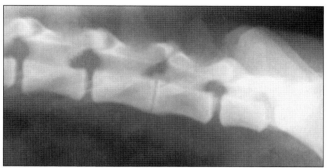

8.24 Partial fusion of the fifth and sixth lumbar vertebrae. Block vertebrae are examples of axial dysostoses and are often incidental findings.

Amelia

Amelia is the absence of one or more limbs caused by failure of limb bud formation or growth. A small number of dogs and cats have been reported with amelia and they all had concurrent life-threatening conditions (Towle, 2004).

Hemimelia

Hemimelia is the absence of one or more bones either whole or in part. Different subtypes of hemimelia are recognized with different patterns of deficits: e.g. terminal hemimelia (bones at the end of the limb are missing), longitudinal hemimelia (bones along the axis of the limb are missing; often a complete long bone, e.g. radius or tibia), and transverse hemimelia (bones are absent across the width of the limb). Radial agenesis is one of the commonest hemimelic defects (Winterbotham *et al.*, 1985); agenesis of the tibia has also been reported (Jezyk, 1985). In cases of radial hemimelia, the affected limb or limbs are shortened with a varus and flexion deformity of the carpus and elbow; such limbs cannot function as the ulna cannot support the animal's weight.

Phocomelia

This condition is characterized by the absence of a limb segment. The radius and ulna may be absent with the paw attached to the trunk like a seal flipper. The proximal aspect of the femur was absent in a Dalmatian in one report. In humans, it is a rare genetic disease and historically caused by thalidomide.

Segmental hemiatrophy

Segmental hemiatrophy has been reported in a dog (Hardie *et al.*, 1985). One limb was significantly smaller and shorter than the other. Limb hypoplasia may be a more accurate descriptive term than atrophy which suggests the limb was once normal size (Johnson and Watson, 2000). The cause may be uneven blood supply. In humans, an enlargement or increase in length is more commonly termed hemihypertrophy. Treatment of all these conditions is very challenging but bespoke surgery to improve limb conformation and function is possible; intraosseous transcutaneous amputation prostheses may have a role in terminal hemimelia.

Ectrodactyly

This is also called split-hand, cleft hand or lobster claw and is a congenital thoracic limb abnormality whereby the digital cleft extends proximally beyond the metacarpophalangeal joints (Barrand, 2004). The split results from failure of fusion of the embryonic precursors of the bones of the thoracic limb. There is separation of the medial and lateral aspects of the limb between any of the metacarpal bones and this can extend proximally between the radius and ulna. There may also be absence or hypoplasia of carpal and metacarpal bones (Figure 8.25). The condition occurs sporadically in dogs but may be inherited in cats as an autosomal dominant defect with variable expression. Treatment depends on the severity of the deformity, which may just be cosmetic. Reconstructive surgery is possible for more severely affected animals.

If the deformity continues proximally, elbow luxation or subluxation may be present (Montgomery and Tomlinson, 1985). The elbow joint should be carefully examined and radiographed in dogs affected with proximal ectrodactyly.

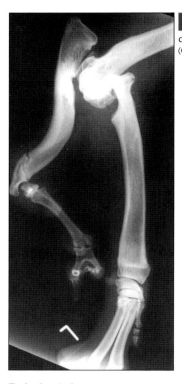

8.25 Ectrodactyly in a dog with associated elbow deformity and luxation.
(Courtesy of John Innes)

Polydactyly

Polydactyly is the presence of one or more extra digits and is seen most commonly in cats (Jezyk, 1985). In cats and dogs, it is thought to be an autosomal dominant trait with variable expression, except for pre-axial pelvic limb polydactyly in St Bernards and Collies that is presumed to be autosomal recessive. A similar inheritance pattern appears to apply to the occurrence of multiple dewclaws in the dog, such as in the Pyrenean Mountain Dog. In some giant breeds there may also be anomalous tarsal bones; some have a large curved bone that seems to be an extension of the central tarsal bone on the medial aspect of the proximal row of tarsal bones. These tarsal anomalies are often bilateral and incidental findings. The condition is typically of no clinical importance but the supernumerary digits may be amputated.

Syndactyly

The congenital lack of differentiation between two or more digits, i.e. persistent bone or soft tissue union, is known as syndactyly. Cases may be unilateral or bilateral. Simple syndactyly is a lack of cutaneous separation between the digits; this causes lameness because the skin is stretched during weight-bearing; it can be treated surgically by simply separating the digits (Richardson *et al.*, 1994). Complex syndactyly is when the bones are fused; typically this does not cause lameness.

Adactyly

Adactyly is a congenital defect whereby one or more digits are missing. It is an example of terminal transverse hemimelia. A cat has been reported with bilateral hindlimb adactyly; both tarsi terminated abnormally early with no digits present; despite this, the cat coped well with the deformity and no treatment was undertaken (Barrand and Cornillie, 2008).

Chromosomal aberrations: lysosomal storage diseases

Mucopolysaccharidosis

Mucopolysaccharidosis (MPS) comprises a group of metabolic disorders caused by abnormalities of the lysosomal enzymes that break down glycosaminoglycan molecules (also known as GAGs or mucopolysaccharides). GAGs are an important cell constituent found throughout body tissues including bone, cartilage, tendon, cornea, skin, connective tissue and synovial fluid. There are 11 enzymes necessary to break down GAGs; if insufficient breakdown occurs, GAGs build up in the cells causing progressive damage.

In humans, seven distinct types of mucopolysaccharidosis are recognized and there are further subtypes. The disease manifests as the level of GAGs increases in the cells, so not necessarily at birth. Symptoms include impaired mental function, hearing loss, coarse facial features, short stature, thickened skin, excessive hair growth and enlarged abdominal organs. The disease is rare in dogs and cats and reports of cases in the literature span back to the 1980s; types I, II, VI and VII have been reported in the cat, and I, II, IIIA, IV and VI in the dog. Signs vary depending on the subtype but include skeletal deformities such as dwarfism, and bony proliferation of joints and spine including vertebral fusion, multifocal neurological defects, and facial deformities including small ears, wide-spaced eyes, thickened eyelids and tear staining secondary to blocked nasolacrimal ducts.

Diagnosis is made from clinical signs, characteristic radiographic findings (Figure 8.26), urine examination (excess GAGs are excreted in the urine with different GAGs

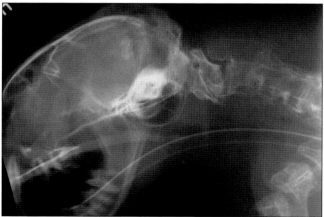

8.26 Cervical spine, skull and shoulder of a cat with mucopolysaccharidosis. There is vertebral fusion, with widened intervertebral disc spaces and abnormally shaped vertebral bodies. The shoulder joint shows irregular bone proliferation on the humeral head.

associated with different MPS types), cytological examination of peripheral leucocytes (coarse granular material in neutrophils that stain metachromatically to toluene blue), enzyme assays of cells or body fluid to test enzyme deficiency, or genetic testing.

There is no effective treatment beyond supportive care, although enzyme replacement therapy or neonatal gene therapy may play a role in the future.

Mucopolysaccharidosis I: This is a deficiency of α-L-iduronidase and has been recognized in the Plott Hound, Rottweiler and Boston Terrier and in cats. Inheritance is thought to be autosomal recessive. Features include a short and depressed nose, prominent forehead, corneal opacity, crouching of the forelimbs, wide asymmetrical and fused cervical vertebrae, and a concave sternum. Cardiac abnormalities including mitral and aortic valve abnormalities are seen in older cats (Sleeper *et al.*, 2008). Affected cats can survive comfortably for several years, and treatment with recombinant enzyme replacement therapy has been reported.

Mucopolysaccharidosis II: This is a deficiency of iduronate-2-sulfatase and has only been confirmed in one 7-month-old female Domestic Shorthaired cat (Hubler *et al.*, 1996), and one 5-year-old Labrador Retriever (Wilkerson *et al.*, 1998). Characteristics include abnormal facial features, corneal dystrophy, thickened skin, retarded growth, de-formed spinal column and joints, incoordination and pelvic limb paresis.

Mucopolysaccharidosis IIIA: This is a deficiency of *N*-sulfoglucosamine sulfohydrolase that causes a primarily neurodegenerative disorder that has been recognized in two Wire-haired Dachshunds and Huntaway dogs (Jolly *et al.*, 2007). Cerebellar signs may be seen from 18 months of age.

Mucopolysaccharidosis VI: This is a deficiency of arylsulfatase B and is recognized in Siamese cats and crosses, the Miniature Poodle, Pinscher and Schnauzer, the Chesapeake Bay Retriever and the Welsh Corgi. Features may not be recognized until adulthood and can include broadening of the maxilla, corneal clouding, pectus excavatum, diffuse neurological abnormalities, a crouching gait with abduction of the stifles, pain and crepitus in several joints and chronic diarrhoea.

Mucopolysaccharidosis VII: This is a deficiency of β-glucuronidase and has been reported in a family of mixed breed dogs (Jezyk, 1985), a cat (Gitzelmann *et al.*, 1994), and is recognized in the Brazilian Terrier and German Shepherd Dog, in which a genetic test is available. Features include a large head with a shortened maxilla, glossoptosis, peg-shaped and widely spaced teeth, corneal clouding, pelvic limb paresis, dorsoventrally compressed rib cage, short, curved limbs, and lax, swollen and crepitant joints.

Mannosidosis

Alpha-mannosidosis is a rare autosomal recessive genetic lysosomal storage disease. Intralysosomal accumulation of mannose-rich oligosaccharide occurs secondary to deficient activity of acidic D-mannosidase. The diagnosis is made by measuring enzymatic activity of α-D-mannosidase in leucocytes. The condition has been recognized in a litter of Persians and a Domestic Shorthaired cat (Blakemore, 1986) but not in the dog. Characteristics

included dwarfism, limb deformity, ataxia and an intention tremor. Radiographs showed osteolytic lesions in the vertebrae and generalized osteopenia. Corneas were clear but suture line cataracts were present.

Mucolipidosis

Mucolipidosis is a group of autosomal recessive metabolic disorders. In humans, four forms are recognized. It has been recognized in a 7-month-old female cat with abnormal facial features and gait, that was found to have a deficiency of *N*-acetylglucosamine-1-phosphotransferase (Hubler *et al.*, 1996). Inclusion bodies in lysosomes contained oligosaccharides, mucopolysaccharides and lipids. A urine test was negative for glycosaminoglycans.

Bone abnormalities due to disturbances of extraskeletal systems
Congenital hypothyroidism

Congenital hypothyroidism is a rare disease of dogs and cats that has been recognized in the Boxer, Scottish Deerhound, Giant Schnauzer, Abyssinian cat and Japanese cats (Mooney and Anderson, 1993; Bojanic *et al.*, 2011). It is caused by anomalies of the thyroid or pituitary glands.

Clinical signs can be variable. Skeletal development is affected, resulting in disproportionate dwarfism with a large head and short limbs and spine. Mental development is also abnormal and lethargy and apathy are seen. There is muscle weakness, the hair coat is thin and juvenile and there may be myxoedematous facial features. Kyphosis may be present and radiography may show lack of epiphyseal ossification, metaphyseal flaring, delayed physeal closure, ragged epiphyses, shortened facial bones and open suture lines in the skull.

Definitive diagnosis is by thyroid stimulation tests; the basal serum thyroxine level is low and it fails to increase following administration of thyroid stimulating hormone (TSH). In one dog, repeated administration of TSH resulted in reactivation of the thyroid gland, suggesting a central rather than primary problem (Mooney and Anderson, 1993). If hormone replacement therapy is started early and particularly before permanent abnormalities have developed, the prognosis can be favourable.

Congenital growth hormone deficiency (pituitary dwarfism)

Pituitary dwarfism (proportionate) is a rare congenital autosomal recessive condition recognized in German Shepherd Dogs (Allan *et al.*, 1978), the Karelian Bear Dog, Weimaraner, Spitz and Toy Pinscher; a single case has been reported in a cat. Lack of growth hormone production occurs following cystic or abnormal development of the pituitary gland. Other hormones may be deficient, including thyroxine, androgens and antidiuretic hormone.

Affected animals are usually recognized by 2–3 months of age. The appendicular skeleton shows retarded growth; the physes remain open longer but are inactive. Epiphyses may show disordered ossification suggestive of hypothyroidism. The os penis has delayed mineralization from the normal 4–5 months to 15 months (Figure 8.27). Animals are usually proportionate dwarfs (Figure 8.27). Affected dogs retain deciduous dentition, often have an undershot mandible, shrill puppy bark, puppy hair coat and a 'rat tail'. As they mature they develop hyperpigmentation and bilateral symmetrical alopecia. Other abnormalities include behavioural

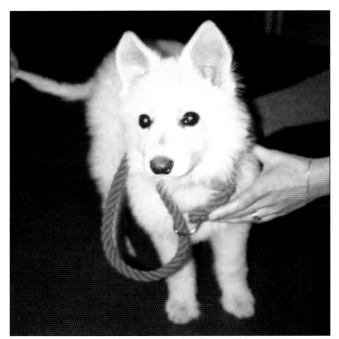

8.27 A 6-month-old German Shepherd Dog with pituitary dwarfism. The dog is a proportionate dwarf with a retained puppy coat and 'rat tail'.

and cardiac disorders, cryptorchidism and megaoesophagus. The diagnosis is made by measuring plasma growth hormone, including stimulation testing, or by genetic testing in the dog. Advanced imaging may show pituitary cysts. The disease can be treated by administering porcine growth hormone, which is identical to canine growth hormone; however, the dog needs to be monitored carefully for side effects. Without treatment the prognosis is poor, but treatment with thyroxine and growth hormone can give a good prognosis.

References and further reading

Aeffner F, Weeren R, Morrison S, Grundmann INM and Weisbrode SE (2012) Synovial osteochondromatosis with malignant transformation to chondrosarcoma in a dog. *Veterinary Pathology* **49**, 1036–1039

Alexander JW, Walker TL, Roberts RE and Dueland R (1978) Malformation of canine forelimb due to synostosis between the radius and ulna. *Journal of the American Veterinary Medical Association* **173**, 1328–1330

Allan GS, Huxtable CR, Howlett CR *et al.* (1978) Pituitary dwarfism in German shepherd dogs. *Journal of Small Animal Practice* **19**, 711–727

Altunatmaz K, Ozsoy S and Guzel O (2007) Bilateral pes valgus in an Anatolian Sheepdog. *Veterinary and Comparative Orthopaedics and Traumatology* **20**, 241–244

Barrand KR (2004) Ectrodactyly in a West Highland white terrier. *Journal of Small Animal Practice* **45**, 315–318

Barrand KR and Cornillie PKLN (2008) Bilateral hindlimb adactyly in an adult cat. *Journal of Small Animal Practice* **49**, 252–253

Bingel SA and Sande RD (1982) Chondrodysplasia in the Norwegian elkhound. *American Journal of Veterinary Pathology* **107**, 219–229

Bingel SA and Sande RD (1994) Chondrodysplasia in five Great Pyrenees. *Journal of the American Veterinary Medical Association* **205**, 845–848

Blakemore WF (1986) A case of mannosidosis in the cat: clinical and histopathological findings. *Journal of Small Animal Practice* **27**, 447–455

Bojanic K, Acke E and Jones BR (2011) Congenital hypothyroidism of dogs and cats: a review. *New Zealand Veterinary Journal* **59**, 115–122

Breur GJ, Zerbe CA, Slocombe RF, Padgett GA and Braden TD (1989) Clinical, radiographic and pathologic and genetic features of osteochondrodysplasia in Scottish Deerhounds. *Journal of the American Veterinary Medical Association* **195**, 606–612

Burton NJ and Owen MR (2007) Limb alignment of pes valgus in a giant breed dog by plate-rod fixation. *Veterinary and Comparative Orthopaedics and Traumatology* **20**, 236–240

Campbell BG, Wootton JAM, Krook L, DeMarco J and Minor RR (1997) Clinical signs and diagnosis of osteogenesis imperfecta in three dogs. *Journal of the American Veterinary Medical Association* **21**, 183–187

Carrig CB, MacMillan A, Brundage S, Pool RR and Morgan JP (1977) Retinal dysplasia associated with skeletal abnormalities in Labrador retrievers. *Journal of the American Veterinary Medical Association* **170**, 49–57

Carrig CB, Morgan JP and Pool RR (1975) Effects of asynchronous growth of the radius and ulna on the canine elbow joint following experimental retardation of longitudinal growth of the ulna. *Journal of the American Animal Hospital Association* **11**, 560–567

Carrig CB, Sponenburg DP, Schmidt GM and Tvedten HW (1988) Inheritance of associated ocular and skeletal dysplasia in Labrador retrievers. *Journal of the American Veterinary Medical Association* **193**, 1269–1272

Chastain CB, McNeel SV, Graham CL and Pezzanite SC (1983) Congenital hypothyroidism in a dog due to an iodide organification defect. *American Journal of Veterinary Research* **44**, 1257–1265

Cohn LA and Meuten DJ (1990) Bone fragility in a kitten: an osteogenesis imperfecta-like syndrome. *Journal of the American Veterinary Medical Association* **197**, 98–100

Cowell KR, Jezyk PF, Haskins ME and Patterson DF (1976) Mucopolysaccharidosis in a cat. *Journal of the American Veterinary Medical Association* **169**, 334–339

Denny H (1989) Femoral overgrowth to compensate for tibial shortening in the dog. *Veterinary and Comparative Orthopaedics and Traumatology* **1**, 47–48

Evason MD, Taylor SM and Bebchuk TN (2007) Suspect osteogenesis imperfecta in a male kitten. *Canadian Veterinary Journal* **48**, 297–298

Fawcett A, Malik R, Howlett RC *et al.* (2014) Polyostotic hyperostosis in a domestic shorthair cat. *Journal of Feline Medicine and Surgery* **16**, 432–440

Fetter AW, Siemering GH and Riser WH (1985) Osteoporosis and osteopetrosis. In: *Textbook of Small Animal Orthopaedics*, ed. CD Newton and DM Nunamaker, pp. 627–631. Lippincott, Philadelphia

Fletch SM, Smart ME, Pennock PW and Subden RE (1973) Clinical and pathologic features of chondrodysplasia (dwarfism) in the Alaskan Malamute. *Journal of the American Veterinary Medical Association* **162**, 357–361

Fox SM (1984) Premature closure of distal radial and ulnar physes in the dog: Part 1 pathogenesis and diagnosis. *Compendium of Continuing Education for the Practicing Veterinarian* **6**, 128–144

Fox DB, Tomlinson JL, Cook JL and Breshears LM (2006) Principles of Uniapical and Biapical Radial Deformity Correction Using Dome Osteotomies and the Center of Rotation of Angulation Methodology in Dogs. *Veterinary Surgery* **35**, 67–77

Franczuszki D, Chalman JA, Butler HC, DeBowes RM and Leipold H (1987) Postoperative effects of experimental shortening in the immature dog. *Journal of the American Animal Hospital Association* **23**, 429–437

Gemmil T and Clements D (2016) *BSAVA Manual of Canine and Feline Fracture Repair and Management, 2nd edn.* BSAVA Publications, Gloucester

Gitzelmann R, Bosshard NU, Superti-Furga A *et al.* (1994) Feline mucopolysaccharidosis VII due to α-glucuronidase deficiency. *Pathology* **31**, 435–443

Hansen JS (1968) Historical evidence of an unusual deformity in dogs ('short-spine dog'). *Journal of Small Animal Practice* **9**, 103–107

Hanssen I, Falck G, Grammeltvedt AT, Haug E and Isaksen CV (1998) Hypochondroplastic dwarfism in the Irish Setter. *Journal of Small Animal Practice* **39**, 10–14

Hardie EM, Chambers JM and Mahaffey MB (1985) Segmental hemiatrophy in a dog. *Journal of the American Veterinary Medical Association* **186**, 1315–1317

Hubler M, Haskins ME, Arnold S *et al.* (1996) Mucolipidosis type II in a domestic shorthaired cat. *Journal of Small Animal Practice* **37**, 435–441

Jevens DJ and DeCamp CE (1993) Bilateral distal fibular growth abnormalities in a dog. *Journal of the American Veterinary Medical Association* **202**, 421–422

Jezyk PF (1985) Constitutional disorders of the skeleton in dogs and cats. In: *Textbook of Small Animal Orthopaedics*, ed. CD Newton and DN Nunamaker, pp. 637–654. Lippincott, Philadelphia

Johnson KA (1981) Retardation of endochondral ossification at the distal ulnar growth plate in dogs. *Australian Veterinary Journal* **57**, 474–478

Johnson SG, Hulse DA, Vangundy TE and Green RW (1989) Corrective osteotomy for pes varus in the dachshund. *Veterinary Surgery* **18**, 373–379

Johnson KA and Watson ADJ (2000) Skeletal diseases. In: *Textbook of Veterinary Internal Medicine – Diseases of the Dog and Cat, 5th edn*, ed. SJ Ettinger, pp. 1887–1916. WB Saunders, Philadelphia

Jolly RD, Hopwood JJ, Marshall NR *et al.* (2012) Mucopolysaccharidosis type VI in a Miniature Poodle-type dog caused by a deletion in the arysulphatase B gene. *New Zealand Veterinary Journal* **60**, 183–188

Jolly RD, Johnstone AC, Norman EJ, Hopwood JJ and Walkley SU (2007) Pathology of mucopolysaccharidosis IIIA in Huntaway dogs. *Veterinary Pathology* **44**, 569–578

Kene ROC, Lee R and Bennett D (1982) The radiological features of congenital elbow luxation/subluxation in the dog. *Journal of Small Animal Practice* **23**, 621–630

Kramers P, Fluckiger MA, Rahn BA, Cordey J (1988) Osteopetrosis in cats. *Journal of Small Animal Practice* **29**, 153–164

Krauser K, Matis U, Schwartz-Porsche D and Putzer-Brenig AV (1989) Multiple enchondromatosis in the dog. Clinical findings. *Veterinary and Comparative Orthopaedics and Traumatology* **4**, 144–151

Langweiler M, Haskins ME and Jezyk PF (1978) Mucopolysaccharidosis in a litter of cats. *Journal of the American Animal Hospital Association* **14**, 748–751

Lau RE (1977) Inherited premature closure of the distal ulna physis. *Journal of the American Animal Hospital Association* **13**, 609–612

Lees GE and Sautter HJH (1979) Anaemia and osteopetrosis in a dog. *Journal of the American Veterinary Medical Association* **175**, 820–824

Lefebvre JGNG, Robertson TRA, Baines SJ, Jeffrey ND and Langley-Hobbs SJ (2008) Assessment of humeral length in dogs after repair of Salter–Harris Type IV fracture of the lateral part of the humeral condyle. *Veterinary Surgery* **37**, 545–551

Lindley S and Watson P (2010) *BSAVA Manual of Canine and Feline Rehabilitation, Supportive and Palliative Care.* BSAVA Publications, Gloucester

Lodge D (1966) Two cases of epiphyseal dysplasia. *Veterinary Record* **79**, 136–138

Macpherson GC, Lewis DD, Johnson KA, Allen GS and Yovich JC (1992) Fragmented coronoid process associated with premature distal radial physeal closure in four dogs. *Veterinary and Comparative Orthopaedics and Traumatology* **5**, 93–99

Mathews KG, Koblik PD, Knoeckel MJ, Pool RR and Fyfe JL (1995) Resolution of lameness associated with Scottish fold osteodystrophy following bilateral ostectomies and pantarsal arthrodeses: a case report. *Journal of the American Animal Hospital Association* **31**, 280–288

May C, Bennett D and Downham DY (1991) Delayed physeal closure associated with castration in cats. *Journal of Small Animal Practice* **32**, 326–328

Meyers VN, Jezyk PF, Aguirre GD and Patterson DF (1983) Short-limbed dwarfism and ocular defects in the Samoyed dog. *Journal of the American Veterinary Medical Association* **183**, 975–979

Montgomery M and Tomlinson JL (1985) Two cases of ectrodactyly and congenital elbow luxation in the dog. *Journal of the American Animal Hospital Association* **21**, 781–785

Mooney CT and Anderson TJ (1993) Congenital hypothyroidism in a boxer dog. *Journal of Small Animal Practice* **34**, 31–35

Newton CD (1985a) Radial and ulna osteotomy. In: *Textbook of Small Animal Orthopaedics*, ed. CD Newton and DM Nunamaker, pp. 533–544. JB Lippincott, Philadelphia

Newton CD (1985b) Genu valgum. In: *Textbook of Small Animal Orthopaedics*, ed. CD Newton and DM Nunamaker, pp. 633–636. JB Lippincott, Philadelphia

Olson NC, Carrig CB and Brinker WO (1979) Asynchronous growth of the canine radius and ulna: effects of retardation of longitudinal growth of the radius. *American Journal of Veterinary Research* **40**, 351–355

Petazzoni M, Nicetto T, Vezzoni A, Piras A and Palmer R (2012) Treatment of pes varus using locking plate fixation in seven Dachshund dogs. *Veterinary and Comparative Orthopaedics and Traumatology* **25**, 231–282

Piermattei DL and Flo G (1997) Correction of abnormal bone growth and healing. In: *Brinker, Piermattei and Flo's Handbook of Small Animal Orthopaedics and Fracture Repair, 3rd edn*, pp. 686–714. WB Saunders, Philadelphia

Pratt JN (2001) Avulsion of the tibial tuberosity with separation of the proximal tibial physis in seven dogs. *Veterinary Record* **149**, 352–356

Rasmussen PG (1971) Multiple epiphyseal dysplasia in a litter of beagle puppies. *Journal of Small Animal Practice* **12**, 91–97

Richardson EF, Wey PD and Hoffman LA (1994) Surgical management of syndactyly in a dog. *Journal of the American Veterinary Medical Association* **205**, 1149–1151

Riser WH and Fankhauser R (1970) Osteopetrosis in the dog. A report of three cases. *Journal of the American Veterinary Radiology Society* **11**, 29–34

Riser WH, Haskins ME, Jezyk PF and Patteson DF (1980) Pseudo-achondroplastic dysplasia in Miniature Poodles: clinical, radiologic, and pathologic features. *Journal of the American Veterinary Medical Association* **176**, 335–341

Rosa C and Kirbeger RM (2012) Extraskeletal osteochondroma on a cat's elbow. *Journal of the South African Veterinary Association* **83**, 104

Sande RD and Bingel SA (1982) Animal models of dwarfism. *Veterinary Clinics of North America: Small Animal Practice* **13**, 71–89

Shields LH and Gambardella PC (1989) Premature closure of the ulnar physis in the dog: a retrospective clinical study. *Journal of the American Animal Hospital Association* **25**, 573–581

Sleeper MM, Kusiak CM, Shofer FS et al. (2008) Clinical characterization of cardiovascular abnormalities associated with feline mucopolysaccharidosis I and VI. *Journal of Inherited Metabolic Disease* **31**, 424–431

Towle HAM and Bruer GJ (2004) Dysostoses of the canine and feline appendicular skeleton. *Journal of the American Veterinary Medicine Association* **225**, 1685–1692

Vandewater AL and Olmstead ML (1983) Premature closure of the distal radial physis in the dog – a review of 11 cases. *Veterinary Surgery* **12**, 7–12

Van Vechten BJ and Vasseur PB (1993) Complications of mid-diaphyseal radial ostectomy performed for treatment of premature closure of the distal radial physis in two dogs. *Journal of the American Veterinary Medical Association* **202**, 97–100

Vaughan LC (1987) Disorders of the tarsus in the dog II. *British Veterinary Journal* **143**, 498–505

Watson AFJ, Miller AC, Allan GC, Davis PE and Howlett PE (1991) Osteochondrodysplasia in bull terrier littermates. *Journal of Small Animal Practice* **32**, 312–317

Whitbread TJ (1983) An inherited endochondrodystrophy in the English Pointer dog. *Journal of Small Animal Practice* **24**, 399–411

Wilkerson MJ, Lewis DC, Marks SL and Prieur DJ (1998) Clinical and morphologic features of mucopolysaccharidosis type II in a dog: naturally occurring model of Hunters syndrome. *Veterinary Pathology* **35**, 230–233

Winterbotham EJ, Johnson KA and Francis DJ (1985) Radial agenesis in a cat. *Journal of Small Animal Practice* **26**, 393–398

OPERATIVE TECHNIQUE 8.1

Distal ulnar osteotomy/segmental ostectomy

POSITIONING

Lateral recumbency with affected limb uppermost.

ASSISTANT

Useful.

EQUIPMENT EXTRAS

Hohmann or Gelpi retractors (two); oscillating saw, or Gigli saw, or mallet and osteotome.

SURGICAL APPROACH

A skin incision is made over the lateral aspect of the ulna, extending from the distal third of the antebrachium to the ulnar styloid process (Figure 8.28).

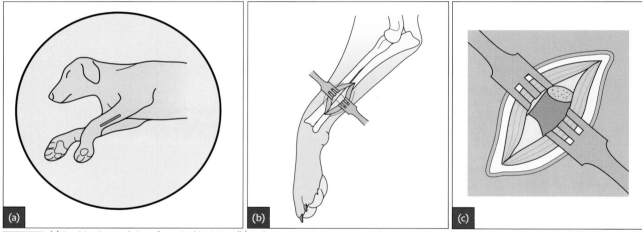

8.28 (a) Positioning and site of surgical incision. (b) Hohmann retractors are used to retract muscles prior to cutting the ulna. (c) When performing a segmental ulnar ostectomy, the length of ulna resected should be approximately 1.5 times the diameter of the bone.

SURGICAL TECHNIQUE

The ulna is approached by blunt dissection between the ulnaris lateralis (caudally) and the lateral digital extensor (cranially) muscles. A longitudinal incision is made through the periosteum which is then elevated; length should be approximately equal to twice the diameter of the bone. Hohmann or Gelpi retractors are used cranially and caudally to protect and elevate the soft tissues. Hohmann retractors should help prevent inadvertent cutting of the radius but Gelpi retractors will not. The ulna is then cut using a Gigli wire, oscillating saw, or mallet and osteotome. The length of the excised ulnar segment should be approximately 1.5 times the diameter of the bone (Figure 8.29). The periosteum should be removed to reduce the chance of premature fusion of the segmental ulnar ostectomy; bleeding may occur when dissecting the periosteum.

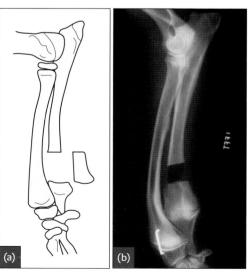

8.29 (a) Illustration of segmental distal ulnar ostectomy and (b) radiograph of procedure performed to address short ulna syndrome with elbow incongruence. (b, courtesy of Dr. Catharina Arthurs)

→ OPERATIVE TECHNIQUE 8.1 CONTINUED

Closure

Soft tissues should be apposed to minimize the dead space. Skin closure is routine.

A firm padded support bandage may be applied for 7–10 days postoperatively.

WARNING

With Gigli wire there should be no risk of cutting or 'nicking' the radius but this is a potential risk with the oscillating saw or mallet and osteotome: great care should be taken to avoid such injury

IMPORTANT NOTE:

Performing distal ulna osteotomy/ostectomy removes the risk of proximal ulnar and elbow instability that is a serious complication that can occur secondary to proximal ulnar osteotomy/ostectomy (PUO). However, it may be less effective than proximal ulnar osteotomy in managing significant elbow incongruity and where this is an issue, PUO using guidelines and heeding warnings in Operative Technique 19.8 should be considered

OPERATIVE TECHNIQUE 8.2

Radial and ulnar corrective osteotomies

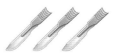

INDICATIONS

This technique is indicated for carpal valgus in a mature animal, or for an immature animal with valgus of more than 25 degrees.

PLANNING

Orthogonal radiographs are taken of the antebrachium, including the elbow and carpus. Planes and angles of deformity and surgical planning can be calculated in a number of ways, including using computer software. A simple method is to trace the radiographs and calculate the angle of maximal deformity by simple trigonometry; two techniques are illustrated in Figures 8.30 and 8.31. The level of osteotomy is adjusted if necessary to ensure an adequate size of the distal fragment for adequate stabilization. The proposed wedge ostectomy is drawn on the diagram. Correct alignment is checked by 'cutting out' the wedge and trial 'reconstruction' of the bone using the paper tracings. Implant placement can be preplanned on the diagram by measuring bone dimensions and using implant (plate) outline acetates.

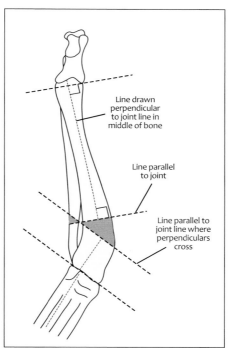

8.30 The lining technique for calculating the point of maximal deformity and the size of the cuneiform (wedge) ostectomy.

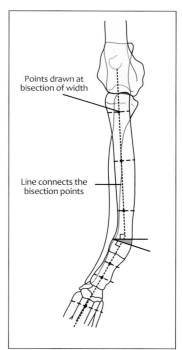

8.31 The bisection technique for calculating the point of maximal deformity and the size of the cuneiform (wedge) ostectomy.

→ OPERATIVE TECHNIQUE 8.2 CONTINUED

POSITIONING

Dorsal recumbency with limb suspended, or lateral recumbency with access to the medial and lateral aspects of limb.

ASSISTANT

Useful.

EQUIPMENT EXTRAS

Oscillating saw (or mallet and osteotome or Gigli wire); periosteal elevator; Hohmann retractors; Gelpi retractors; drill and drill bits; internal fixation or external fixation kit (linear or circle).

SURGICAL APPROACH AND TECHNIQUE

It is very helpful to place a pin (either a temporary K-wire or a definitive positive profile centrally threaded ESF pin) medial to lateral across the proximal radius parallel to the elbow joint, and a second pin or K-wire medial to lateral across the distal radius parallel to the carpal joint. Hypodermic needles can be used to identify the joints and avoid intra-articular pin placement. These K-wires or ESF pins are then used to ensure correct alignment of the limb after the osteotomies have been performed i.e. once the pins are aligned to be parallel, the elbow and carpal joints should be parallel.

Ulnar ostectomy

A limited skin incision is made over the lateral aspect of the distal ulna, extending from the distal third of the antebrachium to the ulnar styloid process. The ulna is approached by blunt dissection between the ulnaris lateralis and lateral digital extensor muscles. A longitudinal incision is made through the periosteum and an area, of length approximately equal to twice the diameter of the bone, is elevated cranially and caudally. Hohmann retractors are used cranially and caudally to protect and elevate the soft tissues, to prevent the inadvertent cutting of the radius. The bone is cut using a Gigli wire, oscillating saw, or mallet and osteotome at approximately the same level as the proposed radial osteotomy. If required, to avoid premature fusion of the ulnar ostectomy site, the periosteum should be removed.

WARNING

With Gigli wire there should be no risk of cutting or 'nicking' the radius but this is a potential risk with the oscillating saw or mallet and osteotome: great care should be taken to avoid such injury

Radial osteotomy

It may be possible for both osteotomies to be performed through a craniolateral skin incision, depending on the size of the dog, but usually, a separate skin incision is made craniomedially at the level of the proposed radial cut. A wedge ostectomy of the radius is performed, according to the preoperative calculations. Ideally, the distal cut should be parallel to the distal articular surface. The craniocaudal direction of the cut is also angled to correct cranial bowing, with more bone being removed from the cranial aspect of the limb than the caudal aspect.

Osteotomy stabilization

Regardless of the intended method of definitive fixation, temporary alignment and fixation of the radius using the pre-placed K-wire or ESF pins, followed by placement of a simple 2 bar type II ESF construct is a useful intraoperative technique, as definitive stabilization is then straightforward. Alternatively cross K-wires may be used temporarily. The radial osteotomy can be stabilized with an ESF (Figure 8.32) or using internal fixation, e.g. a cranial and/or medial plate (Figure 8.33). Ulnar fixation may also be considered to augment construct stability if necessary. The principles of internal and external fixation should be closely followed for implant placement (see *BSAVA Manual of Canine and Feline Fracture Repair and Management*). Prior to definitive stabilization, alignment in all planes should be carefully checked by visual assessment and evaluation of flexion and extension of the limb. The paw should be in line with the humerus when viewed from the cranial aspect (Figure 8.34), and the carpal pad should be in line with the olecranon when viewed from the caudal aspect. When the elbow and carpus are flexed there should not be rotation or deviation of the paw medially or laterally. It is often difficult to fully correct the cranial bowing of the radius, due to tension in the flexor muscles.

➜ **OPERATIVE TECHNIQUE 8.2 CONTINUED**

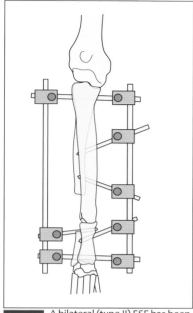

8.32 A bilateral (type II) ESF has been used to stabilize the antebrachium after a corrective closing wedge ostectomy.

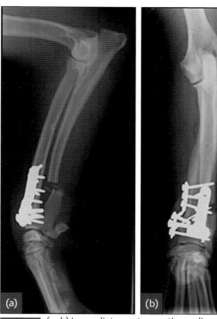

8.33 (a–b) Immediate postoperative radiographs following corrective radial and ulnar ostectomies showing cranial and medial radial plates, with a K-wire used for intraoperative stabilization.

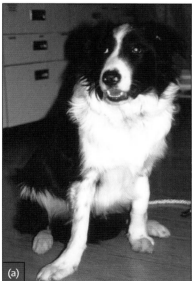

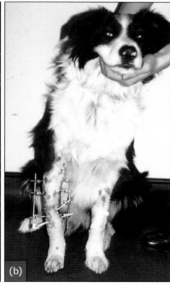

8.34 (a) Border Collie with carpal valgus subsequent to a distal radial fracture and a Salter–Harris type V closure of the distal ulnar growth plate. (b) A bilateral ESF has been applied after a closing wedge ostectomy to correct the carpal valgus. The ostectomy was performed more proximally than the true point of maximal deformity, to give a large enough distal piece of the bone to stabilize. This has resulted in a slight bow to the antebrachium; however, the foot and humerus are in line and the elbow and carpal joints are parallel, so the antebrachial deformity should not cause a problem.

Closure

Bone grafting is generally not necessary but if an ostectomy has been performed, the resected bone can be morselized and placed at the surgical site as an autograft. Routine skin closure is carried out after flushing with sterile saline.

POSTOPERATIVE CARE

A bandage can be placed for a few days to prevent postoperative swelling, and control bleeding associated with ESF pins, if placed. The radius is radiographed every 2 to 4 weeks to evaluate healing. If an ESF has been placed, it is removed once bone healing is sufficiently mature and strong; if internal fixation has been used, removal is not necessary.

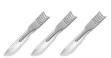

OPERATIVE TECHNIQUE 8.3

Dynamic lengthening of the radius using an external skeletal fixator

PLANNING

Orthogonal radiographs of both antebrachia and additional images centred on the elbow joint are taken. The radial length deficit is calculated by comparative measurement of the radius, ulna and the humeroradial and humeroulnar joints from mediolateral and craniocaudal radiographs of left and right limbs. The need for angular and/or rotational correction is assessed from careful examination of the dog and the radiographs.

POSITIONING

Dorsal recumbency with limb pulled caudally.

ASSISTANT

Useful.

EQUIPMENT EXTRAS

Oscillating saw (or mallet and osteotome or Gigli wire); Hohmann or Gelpi retractors; periosteal elevator; battery drill and drill bits; linear or circular ESF frames with distractors/motors.

SURGICAL APPROACH AND TECHNIQUE

The ESF is applied to the most proximal and distal aspects of the radius. A small medial skin incision is made centred over the mid to proximal third of the radius and dissection is performed on to the radius between the extensor muscles. The periosteum is incised and elevated. Two Hohmann retractors, or Gelpi retractors, are placed orthogonally to reflect and protect the soft tissues (Figure 8.35). The radius is cut at the predetermined location using an oscillating saw, osteotome and mallet, or Gigli wire. Application of the ESF is then completed (see *BSAVA Manual of Canine and Feline Fracture Repair and Management* for principles of application). Radial lengthening may be achieved using a type II modified ESF (Figure 8.36) or a circular fixator (Figure 8.37).

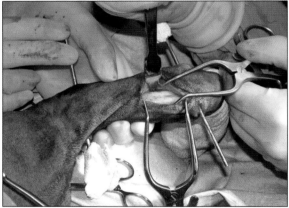

8.35 An intraoperative view of the radius being exposed prior to osteotomy.

> **PRACTICAL TIP**
>
> If an osteotome and mallet are used, small holes should be drilled along the osteotomy line first – this is to reduce the risk of the osteotome shattering the radius or propagating a fissure

Closure

The periosteum and fascia over the osteotomy site are sutured using a slowly absorbable synthetic suture material, such as polydioxanone. Subcutaneous tissue and skin are closed in a routine fashion.

POSTOPERATIVE CARE

Depending on patient age and ESF construct type, a latent period of 1–2 days elapses after the osteotomy before distraction is started. Distraction of 0.5 mm twice daily then starts for an average-sized dog. The limb is radiographed regularly (usually every 1 to 2 weeks) to assess the humeroradial joint space, radial osteotomy gap and bone regeneration. Once elbow subluxation is reduced and no further antebrachial growth is anticipated, the distraction stops and the ESF is left in place until radial osteotomy bone regeneration consolidates enough to allow fixator removal. This usually takes another 2 to 4 weeks.

→ **OPERATIVE TECHNIQUE 8.3 CONTINUED**

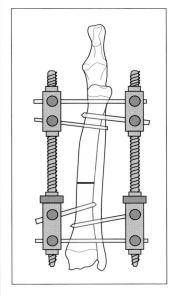
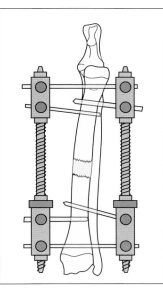

8.36 Diagrams showing a type IIB ESF applied to the radius to achieve radial lengthening. Note the distraction of the proximal radial segment, lengthening of the radial osteotomy gap, and proximal translation of the radial head to a more normal position relative to the ulnar trochlea.

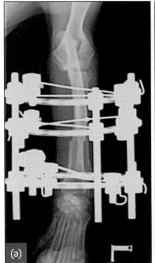
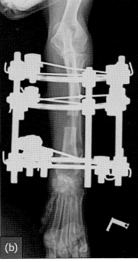
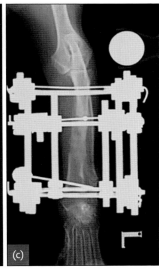

(a) (b) (c)

8.37 Correction of short radius with a mid-radial osteotomy and dynamic lengthening using a circular ESF. (a) Immediately postoperatively: note the radial osteotomy, radiohumeral and humeroulnar incongruence, and circular ESF in place. (b) Three weeks postoperatively: note the distracted radial gap with early mineralization and improved radiohumeral congruency. (c) Seven weeks postoperatively: note the improved radiohumeral congruency and mature bridging of the radial osteotomy; the circular ESF was removed at this point.

A second osteotomy may be needed in immature dogs if healing occurs before complete correction of the short radius. Alternatively, both the radius and ulna can be cut. Lengthening can then be continued until the length of the affected limb approaches that of the unaffected side, including continued growth. If the ulna continues to grow after radial healing, recurrence of short radius and elbow luxation is a risk; removal of the distal ulnar growth plate or segmental distal ulnar ostectomy may prevent this.

IMPORTANT NOTE:

It can be very challenging or even impossible to achieve normal radiohumeral and elbow congruency, because radial head dysplasia secondary to chronic abnormal humeroradial contact pressures may preclude normal radiohumeral articulation. If so, progression of elbow degenerative joint disease is inevitable

---

OPERATIVE TECHNIQUE 8.4

Tibial osteotomy for tarsal varus or valgus

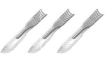

PLANNING

Orthogonal images of the affected and normal tibia are taken, including the hock and stifle. The point of deformity and amount of deformity is calculated preoperatively. This can be done by tracing the outline of the tibia, identifying the axes of the stifle and hock and the longitudinal axes of the proximal and distal tibial diaphysis (Figures 8.38 and 8.39). The corrective osteotomy/ostectomy is carefully calculated; its position depends on the intended nature of postoperative stabilization (external skeletal fixation or internal fixation) as there needs to be enough room in the distal tibial segment for implant placement.

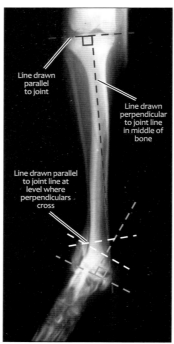

Line drawn parallel to joint

Line drawn perpendicular to joint line in middle of bone

Line drawn parallel to joint line at level where perpendiculars cross

8.38 Application of the lining method for determining the point of maximal deformity and size of wedge required in order to straighten the tibia.

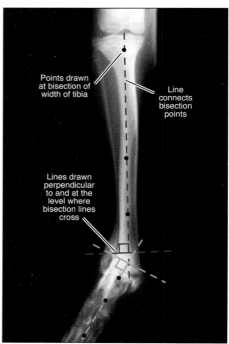

Points drawn at bisection of width of tibia

Line connects bisection points

Lines drawn perpendicular to and at the level where bisection lines cross

8.39 Application of the bisection technique for determining the point of maximal deformity and size of wedge required in order to straighten the tibia. Dots indicate the midpoint of the tibia and tarsus, and the dotted line connects these bisection points to define the long axis of the tibia and tarsus respectively.

POSITIONING

Dorsal recumbency.

ASSISTANT

Useful.

EQUIPMENT EXTRAS

Periosteal elevator; oscillating saw; two Hohmann retractors; internal or external skeletal fixation equipment.

SURGICAL APPROACH AND TECHNIQUE

It can be helpful to place a pin (either a temporary K-wire or a definitive positive profile centrally threaded ESF pin) medial to lateral across the proximal tibia parallel to the stifle joint, and a second pin or K-wire medial to lateral across the distal tibia parallel to the tarsal joint. Hypodermic needles can be used to identify the joints. These K-wires or ESF pins are used to ensure correct alignment of the limb after the osteotomies have been performed: if the pins are aligned parallel to each other, the stifle and tarsus joints should be parallel.

A small skin incision is made over the medial aspect of the tibia over the point of the deformity. If a closing wedge ostectomy is to be performed, a predetermined wedge of bone is removed using an oscillating saw. If an opening wedge ostectomy is intended, a single osteotomy is made in the tibia and if possible the medial cortex/periosteum is preserved. The soft tissues are protected with Hohmann or Gelpi retractors. The distal tibia is oriented to be parallel with the proximal tibia by aligning the pre-placed K-wires or ESF pins; angulation and rotation are corrected simultaneously. Alignment is reassessed and confirmed then the tibia is stabilized definitively by application of internal or external fixation. Figure 8.40 shows application of an ESF with closing wedge ostectomy, and Figure 8.41 shows opening wedge osteotomy for tibial varus in Dachshunds.

→

→ OPERATIVE TECHNIQUE 8.4 CONTINUED

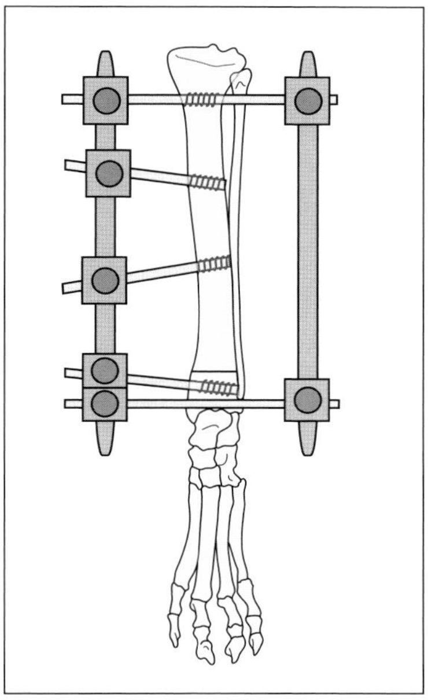

8.40 A bilateral ESF has been applied with three half pins medially after closing wedge ostectomy for tarsal valgus correction.

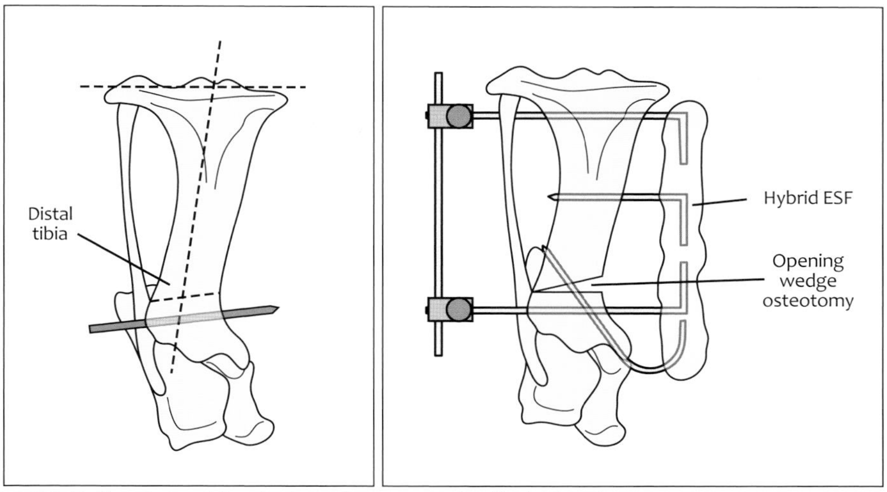

8.41 Opening wedge osteotomy for pes varus in a Dachschund. (Modified from Johnson *et al.*, 1989, with permission)

Closure

The skin incision is closed routinely.

POSTOPERATIVE CARE

A bandage can be placed for a few days to prevent postoperative swelling and control bleeding associated with ESF pins if placed. The tibia is radiographed every 2 to 4 weeks to evaluate healing. If an ESF has been placed, it is removed once bone healing is sufficiently mature and strong; if internal fixation has been used, removal is not necessary.

Chapter 9

Muscle, tendon and ligament injuries

Angus Anderson

Anatomy and physiology of muscle, tendon and ligament

Muscle

Skeletal muscle constitutes the single largest tissue mass in the body and equates to 40–50% of bodyweight. The basic structural element of muscle is the muscle fibre, which is a syncytium of many cells fused together with multiple nuclei surrounded by a connective tissue layer called endomysium. Individual muscle fibres are organized in groups by a connective tissue layer called perimysium that binds them together to ensure integrated movement. This connective tissue also provides a scaffold for regenerating muscle fibres following injury (Figure 9.1). Skeletal muscle is innervated by neuronal axons that terminate at the motor endplate. The neuron and all the muscle fibres that it contacts are referred to as a motor unit. The number of muscle fibres per motor unit varies enormously. Where fine control is required (e.g. extraocular muscles), the number of muscle fibres per unit may be small, whereas in large muscles, such as the triceps, the number may be very large. Skeletal muscles are attached to bone or cartilage by cord-like tendons or flat aponeuroses. Some muscles attach directly to the periosteum with no demonstrable tendon or aponeuroses and these are referred to as fleshy attachments (e.g. the origin of the middle gluteal muscle on the ilium).

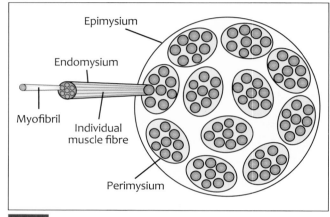

9.1 Schematic drawing of the structure of normal muscle.

Tendon and ligament

Tendon is a composite material consisting of predominantly type I collagen (~85% of dry weight), which is organized in a highly structured way, along with elastin and proteoglycans, resulting in a tissue with one of the highest tensile strengths in the body. Individual collagen fibrils embedded in a matrix of proteoglycans associate to produce fibres. There is a relative paucity of cells, the majority of which are fibroblasts arranged in parallel rows between collagen fibres (Figure 9.2). Tendons that bend sharply,

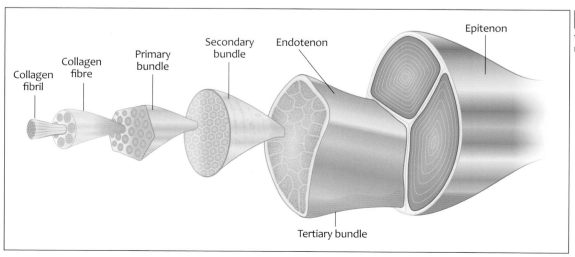

9.2 Schematic drawing of the structure of a normal tendon.

such as the flexor tendons of the digits, are enclosed by a sheath that helps to direct their path and allows the tendon to move smoothly. A mesotenon originating on the side of the bend opposite the friction surface joins the epitenon covering the tendon. Sliding of the tendon is facilitated by the presence of synovial fluid that also provides the tendon with nutrition by diffusion. In regions where tendons wrap around an articular surface, large compressive stresses are generated and in these areas tendon can take on a cartilage-like appearance (Woo *et al.*, 1994). Tendons not enclosed in a sheath move in a straight line and are surrounded by a loose areolar connective tissue called the paratenon. Sheathed tendons have a poor blood supply compared with non-sheathed tendons, and this has a profound influence on the healing response following injury.

Ligaments are similar structurally to tendons and consist of predominantly type I collagen longitudinally arranged in fibrils that combine to form fibres. They unite two or more bones and prevent excess distortion of the joint (varus or valgus angulation and rotation). Most ligaments are extra-articular but some are intra-articular (e.g. cruciate ligaments, teres ligament).

Tendons and ligaments attach to bone through a fibrous or fibrocartilaginous transition zone known as the enthesis.

Muscle injury, healing and treatment

Muscle injury can result from direct trauma, such as laceration or blunt trauma, and indirect trauma, such as strain, ischaemia or neurological dysfunction. The phases of muscle injury are the destruction and inflammatory phase (1–3 days), repair phase (3–4 weeks) and remodelling phase (3–6 months). When injury occurs, myofibres rupture and a haematoma forms. Inflammatory cells (neutrophils) appear first, followed by monocytes that transform into macrophages. These remove necrotic myofibres and, together with fibroblasts, produce a range of cytokines and growth factors that activate myogenic precursor cells (satellite cells). The repair phase involves regeneration of myofibres and the formation of a connective tissue scar. Motor nerves that are left intact can regenerate and form new neuromuscular junctions but sensory nerves cannot regenerate their specialized sensory receptors (Fitch *et al.*, 1997a). Excessive scar tissue formation can interfere with the muscle regenerative processes and contributes to incomplete functional recovery during the remodelling phase. During the remodelling phase, myofibres mature and scar tissue organizes and contracts.

A rare form of muscle injury occurs in compartment syndrome; this is defined as a sustained elevation of tissue pressure in an osteofascial compartment that reduces capillary perfusion below a level required for tissue viability (Basinger *et al.*, 1987). The consequence is ischaemic muscle and nerve injury that may be irreversible. It has been reported following trauma, surgery and neoplasia (Basinger *et al.*, 1987; Radke *et al.*, 2006).

Muscle injuries can be classified as contusions, strains and lacerations (Figure 9.3). The clinical signs of muscle injury vary depending on the severity and chronicity of injury, and the function of the affected muscle.

Muscle contracture

Muscle contracture or fibrotic myopathy is a permanent irreversible state of muscle shortening not caused by active contraction (Vaughan, 1979). The condition is the

Injury	Comments
Contusion	Non-penetrating blunt injury causes an initial inflammatory response and haematoma Over time, scar tissue forms and variable amounts of muscle regeneration may be seen Severe blunt injury may result in the formation of bone within muscle (myositis ossificans)
Strain	Injuries to the muscle–tendon unit are often referred to as strains and usually involve the muscle–tendon junction They result from overstretching, overuse or due to active contraction simultaneous with forced passive extension of the muscle unit They can be classified as: • Grade I: oedema or haemorrhage with little or no structural damage • Grade II: partial rupture (up to 50%) • Grade III: complete rupture. Assessing the severity of injury may not be possible on clinical examination and may require ultrasonography, MRI or surgical exploration (Mueller-Wohlfahrt *et al.*, 2013) They are more common in athletic dogs, such as Greyhounds, and muscles that cross more than one joint (e.g. biceps and gastrocnemius muscle may be more prone to injury)
Laceration	This usually results from direct trauma by sharp objects or may be an iatrogenic surgical injury

9.3 Classification of muscle injuries. MRI = magnetic resonance imaging.

result of the replacement of muscle by fibrous connective tissue that occurs secondary to degenerative change induced by trauma or damage to the nerve or blood supply (Taylor and Tangner, 2007). However, it may also be congenital or result from other disease processes, such as infection or immune-mediated disease, and can be a component of fracture disease. The underlying cause in some instances may be unclear (e.g. semitendinosus or gracilis contracture in German Shepherd Dogs).

Treatment of muscle injuries

Treatment of muscle injury depends on whether the injury is acute or chronic, its severity and on the likely effect of any loss of function on limb use. This may be of particular significance in racing dogs where small tears may result in loss of performance. Mild to moderate contusions and strains are initially treated with rest, cryotherapy (using an ice pack) and compression. Rest or immobilization prevents further retraction of ruptured muscle fibre ends, reduces the size of any haematoma and, consequently, the size of the connective tissue scar. Early cryotherapy and compression (first 24–72 hours) reduces inflammation and haematoma formation (Jarvinen *et al.*, 2013). If the initial response to treatment is good, controlled activity can be started after about a week and then gradually increased. Pain relief can be provided by non-steroidal anti-inflammatory drugs.

Severe contusions, severe strains and lacerations require surgery. If surgery is performed, it should be done without delay. Because muscles have an inherently poor ability to hold sutures, these should be placed through the muscle sheath using a horizontal mattress pattern (Figure 9.4a). A tension-relieving suture pattern such as near–far, far–near can be useful where retraction of the muscle edges makes apposition difficult (Figure 9.4b). Monofilament non-absorbable or slowly absorbable suture material (polydioxanone or polyglyconate) should be used. The latter should retain its tensile strength for long enough to allow healing.

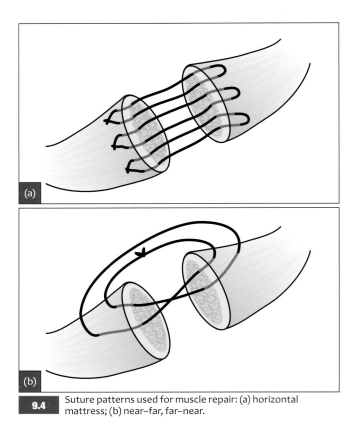

9.4 Suture patterns used for muscle repair: (a) horizontal mattress; (b) near–far, far–near.

The requirement to immobilize the joint or joints that are flexed or extended by the repaired muscle following surgery will depend on the location of the muscle and the severity of the injury. Joints can be immobilized in a position that reduces or eliminates tension across the site of repair using non-weight-bearing slings, splinted dressings, transarticular external skeletal fixators (TESFs) or other implants, such as a calcaneotibial screw to immobilize the tarsal joint. The length of time the joint is immobilized will depend on the severity of the trauma, but is typically 3–6 weeks, and immobilization methods that allow regular physiotherapy during this period are advantageous. Prolonged immobilization can lead to reduced tensile strength, excessive scar tissue contraction and impaired function, and should be avoided. Following removal of any immobilization device, there should be a very gradual return to normal activity.

Physical therapies and modalities, such as therapeutic ultrasonography, may be of considerable value during the rehabilitation period. Full functional recovery may not occur following surgery but partial recovery is usually possible. Muscles that have suffered significant injury are usually more prone to recurrence of injury.

Tendon and ligament injury and treatment

Tendon injury and healing

Tendon injury can result from direct trauma such as laceration or contusion and from indirect trauma as a result of acute or chronic tensile overload. Indirect injury is often multifactorial since most tendons can withstand tensile forces greater than can be exerted by muscles or sustained by bone. For this reason, avulsion fractures and ruptures at the musculotendinous junction are more common than mid-substance tears. The presence of other pathological processes, such as inflammation, may also influence the tendency for tendons to become injured. Tendon injuries frequently occur with injury to adjacent soft tissues and consequently their healing does not take place in isolation. This often results in the formation of adhesions that can limit movement of the tendon. For intrasynovial tendons (e.g. regions of the digital flexor tendons) restoration of gliding function is less critical in veterinary species compared to humans (for example, following hand surgery), and restoration of adequate tensile strength is more important.

The healing process in tendons is generally slow but varies depending upon whether the tendon is surrounded by paratenon (loose areolar connective tissue) or a tendon sheath. There are a number of overlapping phases in the healing process: an initial haemorrhagic and inflammatory phase (several days); a proliferative phase (about 6 weeks); a remodelling phase (about 6 to 10 weeks) and a maturation phase (up to a year).

Healing responses in intrasynovial tendons are much more limited, as the tendon sheath effectively acts as a barrier to vascular ingrowth and healing. The severed ends of the tendon will distract within the sheath, creating a gap. Following surgical repair of intrasynovial tendons, healing occurs predominantly through the ingrowth of connective tissue from the sheath and the cellular response from the endotenon (Woo *et al.*, 1994).

Ligament injury and healing

Injuries to ligaments can occur by direct or indirect trauma. Most ligament injuries are caused by indirect trauma and are referred to as sprains. Injuries to ligaments are usually acute but in some instances, such as trauma to the cranial cruciate ligament, injury may be chronic and multifactorial. Because of their location they may also be damaged by inflammation in joints, or disease processes adjacent to the joint. Ligament injury may involve avulsion of the origin or insertion, or damage to the main body of the ligament. These can be classified as:

- Grade I: damage to a small number of collagen fibres producing mild local inflammation and pain over the affected ligament
- Grade II: incomplete rupture producing a more severe inflammatory response
- Grade III: complete rupture of the ligament with joint instability.

Grade I and II injuries, in the absence of joint instability, do not normally require surgery, although there are some exceptions, such as some partial cranial cruciate ligament injuries. Grade III avulsion injuries and lacerations require surgery to restore joint stability.

There are many similarities in the responses to trauma and healing of ligaments and tendons. Ligaments typically heal very slowly and ligament repair may be poor, particularly for intra-articular ligaments, e.g. cruciate ligaments.

General principles of tendon repair

Certain general principles must be adhered to in order to optimize the healing process. The goals of surgery and postoperative therapy for tendon injury are to restore functional length, allow healing without stretching and avoid development of adhesions that might limit motion of the tendon. There should be a minimal delay in the timing of the repair unless there is an open injury with severe contamination. When contamination is present, the area should be debrided and lavaged and, if there is adequate healthy soft tissue with an adequate blood supply, primary tenorrhaphy can be performed. If contamination is severe, repair can be delayed, but the limb should be immobilized to reduce the likelihood of the tendon ends distracting.

Suture material

The choice of suture material is, to some extent, determined by the preference of the surgeon but it should have the following qualities:

* Easy to pass through tissue (swaged-on needle)
* Non-irritant
* Good knot security
* Adequate tensile strength that is maintained during the healing process.

The materials that fulfill these properties most effectively are monofilament nylon and polypropylene (non-absorbable); in some situations, where loading on the tendon during healing is not great and blood supply is good, polydioxanone (absorbable) can be used. The loss of tensile strength with polydioxanone (42% by 28 days) is less than with other absorbable materials that are not suitable for tendon repair (Smeak, 1997).

The size of suture is determined by the size of the tendon. There is often a tendency to select a suture with a large diameter but this may distort tissues and may not tie or loop properly. The tensile strength of the repair is initially determined by the holding power of the suture in the tendon and not by the strength of the suture material.

The main challenge to tendon repair is to maintain apposition of tendon ends (or tendon to bone in the case of avulsion injuries) while minimizing tension across the repair for a prolonged period that allows functional healing. Gaps in tendons greater than 3 mm have been shown to result in reduced rates of healing, increased risk of breakdown during healing and lower ultimate strength 6 weeks following repair, compared to repairs with no gap or gaps less than 3 mm (Gelberman *et al.*, 1999; Strickland, 2005). Failure to adequately protect a repair will result in breakdown or suboptimal function in the long term. Ideally, tension is gradually applied following tendon repair and is increased at a time and rate dictated by the strength of the repair, which gradually increases over time. In practice, this can be very difficult to achieve in veterinary patients.

Synthetic implants, such as polypropylene mesh, have been used to augment tendon repairs but there are concerns regarding their ability to resist gap formation (Swiderski *et al.*, 2005; Gall *et al.*, 2009). A synthetic degradable polyurethane mesh has been used successfully to augment repair of a chronic triceps avulsion in a dog (Ambrosius *et al.*, 2015).

Suture pattern

A number of suture patterns have been described for tendon repair. No one suture technique is satisfactory in all cases. The three commonest suture patterns for use in round tendons are shown in Figure 9.5. The locking loop (modified Kessler) is superior to the Bunnell–Mayer because it is less constrictive to the intrinsic blood supply and provides greater tensile strength to the repair (Berg

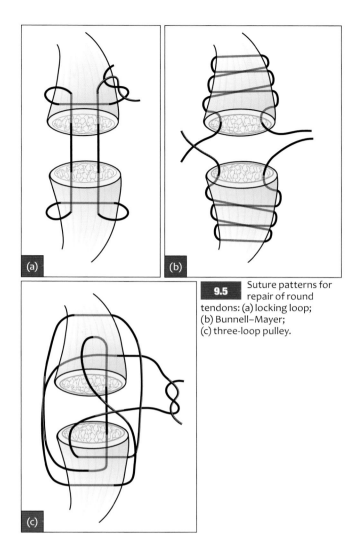

9.5 Suture patterns for repair of round tendons: (a) locking loop; (b) Bunnell–Mayer; (c) three-loop pulley.

and Egger, 1986). The three-loop pulley suture provides greater tensile strength and resistance to gap formation than the locking loop patterns (Berg and Egger, 1986; Moores *et al.*, 2004a) and they can both be modified to attach tendon to bone (Moores *et al.*, 2004b). Gap formation can result in slower healing and increased risk of re-rupture (Gelberman *et al.*, 1999). Short, flat or aponeurotic tendons are most easily repaired with interrupted horizontal mattress sutures or a baseball suture (Figure 9.6).

Whatever suture pattern is chosen, for the first 3 weeks the strength of the anastomosis relies entirely on the suture. A strong anastomosis may allow early mobilization, which may help to maximize final tensile strength.

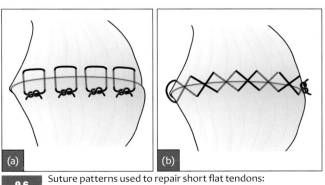

9.6 Suture patterns used to repair short flat tendons: (a) horizontal mattress; (b) baseball.

By 6 weeks after surgery tensile strength is approximately 50% of normal and by 1 year this rises to about 80% (Woo *et al.*, 1994).

Tendons need to be reattached to their bony origin or insertion following avulsion injury. The locking loop and three-loop pulley sutures can be modified to reattach tendon to bone using bone tunnels (Figure 9.7). Following repair, the joint crossed by the tendon will require immobilization that prevents or minimizes tension across the repair for a period of time, typically 6 weeks. This can be achieved by application of a splinted dressing or semi-rigid orthotic device, TESF or other implants, for example a calcaneo-tibial screw following common calcaneal tendon repair.

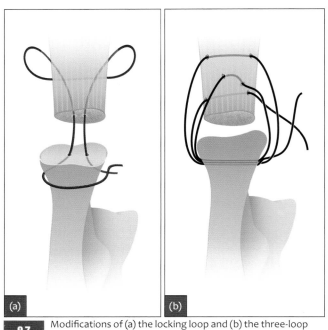

9.7 Modifications of (a) the locking loop and (b) the three-loop pulley suture patterns to reattach tendon to bone.

General principles of ligament repair

The major goals of ligament repair are to restore joint stability and a normal range of joint movement. Many of the principles outlined above for tendons apply to ligaments. Ligaments are usually considerably smaller than tendons and direct suture repair can prove difficult or impossible. The weakest area of a suture repair is the soft tissue–suture interface. When a ligament is repaired or reattached to bone, the main challenge is protection of this repair until there is functional healing or periarticular fibrosis that stabilizes the joint. In most cases, the repair will be augmented or the ligament replaced by a prosthetic ligament and the joint will be immobilized for a period of time. The choice of suture material and suture pattern to repair a torn ligament is the same as for a damaged tendon.

When a ligament has avulsed from bone it can be reattached using staples, or it may be sutured and the ligament–suture construct attached using bone tunnels, screw–washer combinations or suture anchors (Figure 9.8). Depending on location, bone tunnels can be technically difficult and surgically invasive. Bone screws and washers can be bulky and interfere with soft tissues or adjacent joint surfaces. Suture anchors have the advantages of minimal local soft tissue irritation, security of suture fixation and often require only a minimally invasive approach. They can be categorized as transcortical or subcortical (Figure 9.9).

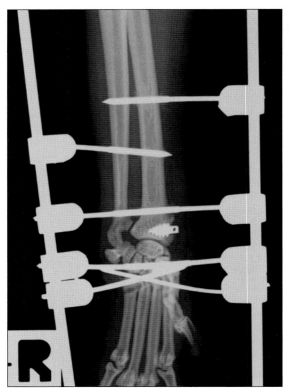

9.8 Dorsopalmar view of a feline carpus following repair of the radial collateral ligament using a suture anchor in the radius; the carpus is immobilized with a transarticular external skeletal fixator (TESF).

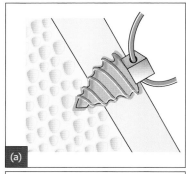

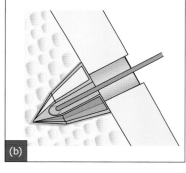

9.9 Suture anchors: (a) transcortical bone anchor; (b) subcortical anchor.

Transcortical anchors engage the cortical bone at their point of insertion whereas subcortical anchors are placed beneath the cortex and resist pull-out by changing their shape following insertion. Eyelet design and orientation have an impact on suture abrasion, and excess friction can increase the risk of suture failure (Giles *et al.*, 2008; Aktay and Kowaleski, 2011).

Subcortical anchors (e.g. BoneBiter™) have the advantage of causing less interference to overlying soft tissues and can be placed very close to joint margins, but are more expensive, have decreased load to failure compared with transcortical anchors (Robb *et al.*, 2005) and are technically more difficult to insert than transcortical anchors.

Frequently, a ligament cannot be repaired because of excessive tissue disruption and under these circumstances it will be replaced by a prosthesis (Figure 9.10) or, under certain circumstances, no attempt is made to replace the ligament and the joint is immobilized using a splinted dressing or TESF (see below).

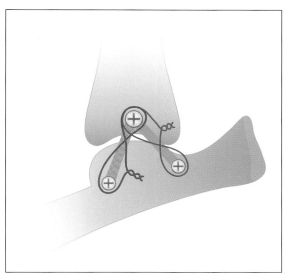

9.10 Prosthetic replacement of the long and short components of the collateral ligament of the tarsal joint. Suture anchors or screws should be inserted to mimic the origin and insertion points of the ligament as closely as possible.

Joint immobilization following surgery

Following ligament repair, the joint will require immobilization for a period of time (typically 4–6 weeks). This can be achieved by application of a cast, semi-rigid orthotic device or TESF (see Figure 9.8). The joint is normally immobilized at a normal standing angle.

Following straight patellar ligament repair, a loop of nylon leader line can be placed from the tibial tuberosity to just proximal to the patella to limit stifle flexion and hence tension on the repair; however, application of a TESF is a more secure and effective method of stifle immobilization (Das *et al.*, 2014).

Splinted dressings can be used to immobilize joints distal to the elbow and stifle. They can also be used to severely restrict movement of the elbow and stifle joints but their application can be more problematic due to anatomical constraints. Complications following splint application are common and can sometimes be significant (Meeson *et al.*, 2011). Advantages of a TESF include rigidity of immobilization and facilitation of wound management, but complications of use, including osteomyelitis and pin loosening, can be significant.

Ligament prostheses

Although there has been a substantial body of work published on suture materials used to stabilize cruciate-deficient stifle joints (see Chapter 23), far less research has been undertaken on ligament prostheses used to stabilize other joints. For collateral ligament repair, non-absorbable suture is generally chosen (stainless steel wire, braided polyester, heavy gauge nylon, e.g. leader line, FiberWire®). The ligament prosthesis is anchored to the bone using one of the methods described above. Suture size will depend on the size of the animal and anticipated loading following surgery. Polypropylene mesh has been used as a prosthetic ligament to replace the medial collateral ligament in stifle joints and was found to have some advantages over a braided polyester prosthesis (Robello *et al.*, 1992). Fascia lata has been used successfully to replace the patellar ligament in dogs (Aron *et al.*, 1997; Gemmill and Carmichael, 2003).

Alternatives to ligament repair and prostheses

Surgery to repair or replace a ligament is not always necessary to achieve the goal of restoring joint stability. In many instances, joint immobilization for a period of time (typically 4–6 weeks) will restore stability by allowing development of scar tissue, e.g. tarsus immobilization with a TESF for tarsal collateral ligament injury in cats (Kulendra *et al.*, 2011) and shearing injuries of this joint in dogs and cats (Figure 9.11). Prolonged joint immobilization may result in irreversible deterioration in the articular cartilage and other joint tissues leading to poor function and should be avoided.

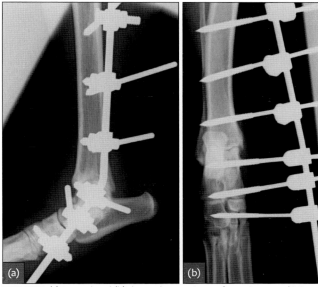

9.11 (a) Lateral and (b) dorsoplantar views of a canine tarsal joint immobilized with a transarticular external skeletal fixator (TESF) following a shear injury. The joint has been immobilized at a normal standing angle.

Specific muscle and tendon injuries of the thoracic and pelvic limbs

These are summarized in Figures 9.12 and 9.13.

Injury to the common calcaneal tendon

The common calcaneal tendon (CCT), also known as the Achilles tendon, is composed of the gastrocnemius tendon, the common tendon of the biceps femoris, gracilis and semitendinosus muscles and the superficial digital flexor tendon (SDFT). The largest component is the tendon of the gastrocnemius muscle, which is the most powerful

Disorder	Signalment, clinical signs and imaging	Treatment and prognosis
Rupture of the serratus ventralis (Bloomberg, 1993)	Dorsal displacement of the scapula when weight-bearing More common in cats	Suture dorsal border of scapula to torn soft tissues; holes drilled in scapula facilitate suture placement Cage rest 3–4 weeks or Velpeau sling 10–14 days Prognosis very good
Avulsion of long head of triceps from scapula (Eaton-Wells, 1998)	Mainly racing Greyhounds Partial avulsion of muscle origin causing local swelling and pain	Conservative Good prognosis
Infraspinatus bursal ossification (McKee *et al.*, 2007) (Figure 9.14)	Calcification of soft tissues between acromion and greater tubercle of humerus on radiographs Other changes in/around shoulder may be detected on MRI/arthroscopy	Conservative; intra-articular methylprednisolone Surgical excision of mineralized bodies if conservative treatment fails
Supraspinatus tendinopathy (Flo and Middleton, 1990; Muir and Johnson, 1994; Kriegleder, 1995; Danova and Muir, 2003; Lafuente *et al.*, 2009) (Figure 9.15)	Some may have mineralization adjacent to greater tubercle of humerus on radiographs MRI changes May be present with other shoulder abnormalities	Conservative; intra-articular methylprednisolone Surgical excision of areas of mineralization Prognosis following resection reported to be good
Avulsion or partial tears of the subscapularis insertion (Murphy *et al.*, 2008)	Acute or chronic shoulder lameness Identified on MRI scanning or shoulder arthroscopy	Conservative unless associated with shoulder instability
Avulsion or rupture of tendon of origin of biceps brachii	Acute lameness Elbow can be fully extended and shoulder fully flexed on examination.	Reattachment of tendon has high failure rate Conservative management usually successful and most dogs will go sound
Avulsion of insertion of biceps brachii and brachialis (Schaaf *et al.*, 2009)	Rare injury of racing Greyhounds Elbow hyperextension and forelimb circumduction	Reattach avulsed tendon(s) using suture anchors Good prognosis
Rupture/avulsion of triceps insertion (Davies and Clayton Jones, 1982; Clarke *et al.*, 2007; Garcia-Fernandez *et al.*, 2014; Ambrosius *et al.*, 2015)	Reported in dogs and cats May be spontaneous rupture or secondary to corticosteroid injection into tendon Pain and swelling at triceps insertion proximal to olecranon and inability to maintain elbow extension on weight-bearing Radiographs may show soft tissue mineralization or avulsed bony fragments	Reattach tendon to olecranon and maintain elbow in extension with splint or transarticular external skeletal fixator for 3–4 weeks Synthetic mesh graft can be used to augment repair Prognosis excellent
Avulsion of origin or insertion of extensor carpi radialis (Anderson *et al.*, 1993; Eaton-Wells, 1998) (Figure 9.16)	Common in Greyhound puppies Also seen in pet dogs Avulsion injury results in pain and swelling and radiographs may show periosteal new bone on humerus Avulsion of insertion seen in racing Greyhounds	Conservative for origin and insertion avulsions Prognosis very good
Flexor carpi ulnaris insertion strain (Roe, 1998)	Pain and swelling proximal to accessory carpal bone where muscle inserts Seen in racing Greyhounds and pet dogs Severe strain/laceration can result in mild to moderate carpal hyperextension	Mild strain managed conservatively Mild to moderate carpal hyperextension managed by surgical repair

9.12 Thoracic limb muscle and tendon injuries.

Disorder	Signalment, clinical signs and imaging	Treatment and prognosis
Injury to tensor fasciae latae muscle (Eaton-Wells, 1998)	Racing Greyhounds Pain on hip extension Swelling and pain over muscle and deficit in muscle may be palpable	Complete or partial avulsions managed with laser therapy or surgery Surgery involves reattaching muscle to fascia Prognosis good
Injury to iliopsoas muscle (Breur and Blevins, 1997; Cabon and Bolinger, 2013)	Pain on hip extension with internal rotation, palpation of muscle insertion on lesser trochanter or of muscle on cranioventral aspect of ilium Contracture of muscle can cause restricted hip extension and femoral neuropathy Radiography may show avulsion injuries/dystrophic calcification on lesser trochanter; the latter does not imply active disease Ultrasonography and MRI scanning show characteristic changes	Acute injury managed conservatively. Chronic injury and contracture may require tenotomy on lesser trochanter Prognosis good
Gracilis injury (Eaton-Wells, 1992, 1998) (Figure 9.17)	Common injury in racing Greyhounds, involving muscular origin and/or tendinous insertion Partial (usually caudal margin) or complete avulsion Avulsion of origin causes ventral displacement of muscle; avulsion of insertion causes dorsal displacement of muscle Subcutaneous haemorrhage along inner thigh in acute injury	Surgical repair if full return to racing desired Avulsions of origin: horizontal incision over origin and sutured with near–far, far–near sutures (pre-placed) of PDS from muscle to subpubic tendon Avulsion of insertion: longitudinal incision with sutures as above to its fascial attachment on tibia Confine to kennel for 1 week; increase exercise over following 6 weeks; return to racing 10–12 weeks

9.13 Pelvic limb muscle and tendon injuries. DDFT = deep digital flexor tendon; PDS = polydioxanone; SDFT = superficial digital flexor tendon. (continues) ▶

Disorder	Signalment, clinical signs and imaging	Treatment and prognosis
Avulsion of origin of lateral or medial head of gastrocnemius (Muir and Dueland, 1994; Prior, 1994; Robinson, 1999) (Figure 9.18)	Uncommon injury causing hyperflexion of hock and semi-plantigrade posture Radiographs show distal displacement of fabella (NB in some breeds, e.g. West Highland White Terrier, the medial fabella can appear more distally located compared to other breeds as a normal feature)	Surgical reattachment of tendon: suture passed around fabella and attached to caudal femur with suture anchor or through bone tunnel Maintain hock extension for 6 weeks to reduce tension on repair Therapeutic ultrasonography also reported to be successful Excellent prognosis
Avulsion of origin of long digital extensor (Pond, 1973; Fitch *et al.*, 1997b)	Rare injury Mainly young, large-breed dogs Radiographs may show avulsed bone fragment or mineralization adjacent to extensor fossa of femur MRI can confirm diagnosis	Reattach avulsed bony fragment with screw In chronic injury attach tendon to proximal tibia Prognosis good
Avulsion of popliteus muscle (Eaton-Wells and Plummer, 1978; Tanno *et al.*, 1996) (Figure 9.19)	Very rare injury; reported in more juvenile dogs than adults Radiographs show distal displacement of popliteal sesamoid and avulsed bony fragment adjacent to lateral aspect of lateral femoral condyle	Reattach avulsed bony origin with screw if large enough; if not, suture tendon to adjacent soft tissues Excellent prognosis
Injury to superficial and deep digital flexor tendons (Figure 9.20)	Usually lacerations to palmar or plantar aspects of pes or avulsion of tendon from insertion Injury to SDFT causes 'flat' toe and is of little clinical significance Avulsion of DDFT from flexor process of third phalanx causes 'knocked-up' toe and is of little clinical significance	Lacerations can be sutured Digits must be kept in flexion; splint (carpus in flexion and hock in extension) to minimize tension on repair for 6 weeks These injuries are not easy to manage postoperatively and prognosis is guarded for return of normal digit posture

9.13 (continued) Pelvic limb muscle and tendon injuries. DDFT = deep digital flexor tendon; PDS = polydioxenone; SDFT = superficial digital flexor tendon.

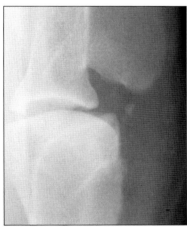

9.14 Craniocaudal view of the shoulder joint showing infraspinatus bursal ossification.

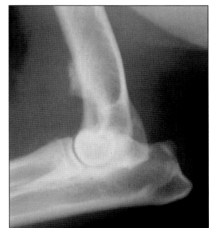

9.16 Radiograph of humerus showing calcification of the origin of the extensor carpi radialis muscle.

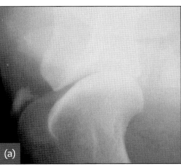
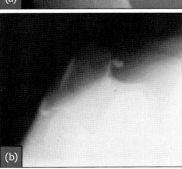

9.15 Mineralization of the supraspinatus muscle. (a) Lateral view of the shoulder joint. (b) Skyline view of the intertubercular groove.

(a)

(b)

9.17 Greyhound with avulsion of the gracilis origin.
(Courtesy of R Eaton-Wells)

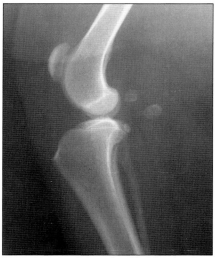

9.18 Lateral view of a stifle joint showing avulsion of the origin of the lateral head of the gastrocnemius muscle.

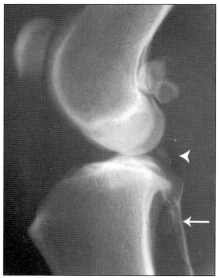

9.19 Lateral view of a stifle joint showing avulsion of the popliteus muscle. The popliteal sesamoid bone is displaced distally (arrowed) and a small avulsion fragment is visible more proximally (arrowhead).
(Courtesy of S Langley-Hobbs)

extensor of the tarsus (Figure 9.21). CCT injuries have been most commonly reported in medium to larger breeds of dog, with Dobermanns, Labrador Retrievers and over-weight neutered bitches over-represented (Corr *et al.*, 2010), and have been classified into three main categories (Meutstege, 1993):

- Tendinosis/tendinitis – can cause swelling of the CCT without any change in joint posture
- Incomplete ruptures – most commonly involve the insertion of the gastrocnemius on the calcaneus and typically result in a semiplantigrade stance with digit hyperflexion if the SDFT is intact (Figure 9.22). This is most frequently seen in middle-aged Dobermanns
- Complete rupture – results in a plantigrade stance and the tarsal joint can be hyperflexed with the stifle held in extension (Figure 9.23).

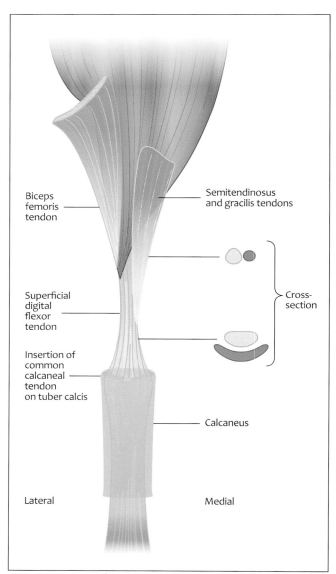

Biceps femoris tendon

Semitendinosus and gracilis tendons

Cross-section

Superficial digital flexor tendon

Insertion of common calcaneal tendon on tuber calcis

Calcaneus

Lateral

Medial

9.21 Anatomy of the common calcaneal tendon. The tendons of the biceps femoris, semitendinosus and gracilis muscles unite with that of the gastrocnemius (shown on cross-section in pale red) and the resulting combined tendon is intimately associated with the superficial digital flexor tendons (shown on cross-section in pale grey) to form the common calcaneal tendon. The combined biceps femoris, semitendinosus, gracilis and gastrocnemius tendon inserts on to the tuber calcis of the calcaneus. The superficial digital flexor tendon courses distally over the tuber calcis and is loosely attached to it by a medial and lateral retinaculum.

9.20 Injury to the superficial digital flexor tendons resulting in 'flat' digits also known as 'dropped toe' (see Chapter 21).

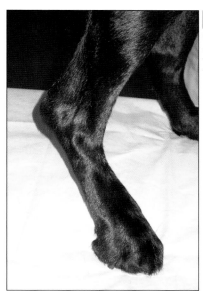

9.22 Avulsion of the gastrocnemius insertion. There is swelling of the soft tissues proximal to the tuber calcis and the toes are held flexed.

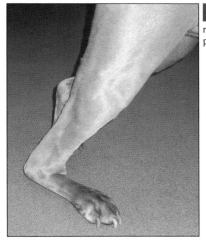

9.23 Common calcaneal tendon rupture resulting in a plantigrade stance.

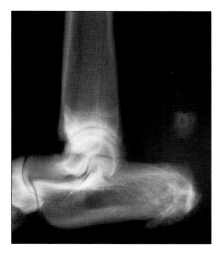

9.24 Lateral view of a tarsal joint showing enthesophytes on the tuber calcis and mineralization in the soft tissues proximal to the tuber calcis.

Although the CCT can be severed by direct trauma, most injuries are the result of internally generated forces. These most commonly involve the insertion of the gastrocnemius tendon on the calcaneus due to degeneration of the tendon at this location, but the cause of this chronic degeneration is not clear (Corr *et al.*, 2010).

Palpation may reveal soft tissue swelling, pain, or a defect in the continuity of the CCT, if complete rupture is present. Radiographs of the tarsus and tibia may show soft tissue swelling at the site of injury, calcification of the soft tissues proximal to the calcaneus and enthesophytes on the calcaneus (Figure 9.24). Ultrasonography or MRI may allow differentiation of partial and complete tears of the tendon and confirm the location of injury (Kramer *et al.*, 2001).

Treatment

Tendinosis/tendinitis: In these cases, there is no evidence of tarsal hyperflexion when the dog is weight-bearing or on physical examination, but the CCT will be thickened. A conservative approach of restricting activity for 6–8 weeks may be successful in some cases. The alternative is to immobilize the tarsus in extension with a splint, TESF or calcaneotibial screw for 6 weeks. Risk of recurrence of lameness and further deterioration in tendon function is possible.

Incomplete ruptures: These most commonly involve avulsion of the gastrocnemius insertion on the calcaneus. Treatment consists of reattaching the end of the gastrocnemius tendon to the calcaneus (through bone tunnels) with one or more modified locking loop sutures or a modified three-loop pulley suture (Moores *et al.*, 2004b). The tarsus should be immobilized after surgery.

Complete ruptures/lacerations: Areas of degenerate or necrotic tendon should be excised and the individual components of the CCT (gastrocnemius and SDFT) should be sutured and the tarsus immobilized.

Options for tarsal immobilization: The tarsal joint can be immobilized in a number of different ways. The tarsus can be maintained in extension with a half cast applied to the dorsal aspect of the limb, a TESF or a calcaneotibial positional screw (usually supplemented with a cranial half cast) (Figure 9.25). Following TESF or screw removal, a semi-flexible dressing can be applied for 2 weeks. Semi-rigid orthotic devices have been used and have the advantage that physiotherapy is facilitated and the angle of immobilization of the tarsus can be varied (Case *et al.*, 2013). The method of immobilization does not appear to affect outcome, but all options can give rise to complications (Nielsen and Pluhar, 2006).

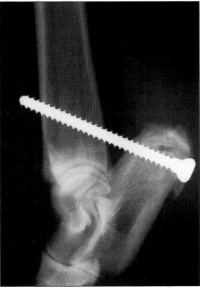

9.25 Stabilization of a tarsal joint with a calcaneotibial screw.

Following removal of external support, exercise should be restricted for 4–6 weeks. Prognosis is generally good but some dogs may be left with a semiplantigrade stance after surgery and athletic dogs may not return to full function (Nielsen and Pluhar, 2006; Corr *et al.*, 2010).

Management of chronic CCT injuries: Chronic injuries of the CCT and those with extensive areas of tendon degeneration or loss represent a significant challenge. Various techniques have been described that utilize autogenous tissue to reconstruct defects. These involve transferring the tendons of the peroneus brevis and peroneus longus muscles and passing them through bone tunnels in the calcaneus, and these can be augmented with strips of fascia lata (Sivacolundhu *et al.*, 2001). Primary repairs of the tendon can also be augmented with a semitendinosus muscle flap (Baltzer and Rist, 2009). Synthetic implants, such as polypropylene mesh, have been used but there are concerns regarding their ability to resist gap formation (Swiderski *et al.*, 2005; Gall *et al.*, 2009). Recently a polyethylene implant has been used with success to treat chronic gastrocnemius tendon ruptures in dogs (Morton *et al.*, 2015). In long-standing injuries, or where primary treatment has failed, pantarsal arthrodesis can be performed to salvage limb function.

Muscle contracture

Contracture of the supra/infraspinatus

Contracture of the infraspinatus, and less commonly the supraspinatus muscle, is an uncommon cause of lameness that has been reported mainly in working dogs (Vaughan, 1979; Bennett, 1986). Usually, medium to larger breeds of dog are affected and, although the lameness is usually unilateral, bilateral lameness has been reported. Typically, lameness is acute in onset at exercise and over a period of several weeks a characteristic gait abnormality develops. At rest the affected limb is held with the elbow joint adducted and the foot and carpus abducted (Figure 9.26). Shoulder flexion is reduced but non-painful and during flexion of the limb, the foot and carpus swing outwards instead of in a straight line. The supra- and infraspinatus are usually atrophied on examination. During locomotion the lower limb is circumducted in a characteristic fashion.

Radiographs of the shoulder joint do not show any specific abnormalities but ultrasonography has been used to identify changes to the affected muscles (Siems *et al.*, 1998). Treatment is by tenotomy of the affected tendon and breaking down adhesions between the tendon and joint capsule. Prognosis is excellent.

Quadriceps contracture

Quadriceps contracture is a condition characterized by a stifle fixed in extension with no, or a very reduced, ability to flex (Figure 9.27). It is less common than it used to be due to improved surgical techniques and a better understanding of its prevention. It is most commonly a sequel to fractures of the distal femur in young dogs. Most cases result from prolonged immobilization of the affected limb where the stifle has been maintained in extension, coupled with inadequate fracture stabilization (Taylor and Tangner, 2007). Muscle trauma appears to have little role in the aetiology. Immobilization of the stifle with concurrent muscle trauma was not found to cause stifle joint stiffness in young dogs (Shires *et al.*, 1982). The condition can also occur as a congenital disorder (Stead *et al.*, 1977) or as a complication of *Toxoplasma* or *Neospora* infection.

The clinical signs of quadriceps contracture include moderate to severe lameness with the stifle fixed in extension. Limited stifle extension may be present in early cases but this may progress to full extension and an inability to flex this joint, or even stifle hyperextension in the young dog (genu recurvatum). The hip joint will not fully extend and the tarsus will not flex, resulting in a very stiff gait with circumduction of the limb. The quadriceps muscle may appear atrophied but not painful. In young dogs the condition can result in secondary hip subluxation with associated degenerative changes. The growth and development of the distal femur and proximal tibia may be affected.

In cases secondary to femoral fracture, the initiating factor is the formation of fibrous adhesions between the quadriceps muscle and the femur. Severe restriction of stifle movement causes progressive degenerative changes in the articular and periarticular tissues that can result in a fibrous ankylosis. Many of these changes to articular tissues, and the generalized muscle atrophy that develops in the limb, reach a stage where they become irreversible.

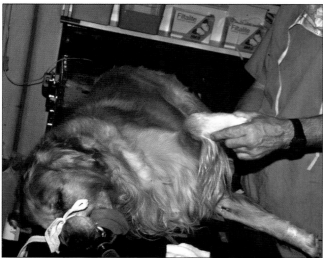

9.26 Infraspinatus contracture in a Golden Retriever showing lateral deviation of the carpus when the limb is flexed.

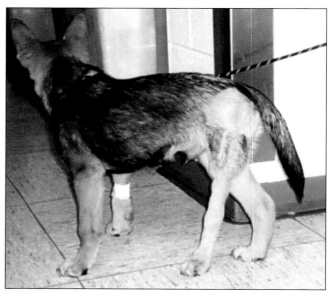

9.27 Quadriceps contracture in a German Shepherd Dog. (Courtesy of S Langley-Hobbs)

Toxoplasma and *Neospora* infections can cause a myositis–polyradiculoneuritis in young dogs (generally under 6 months of age) that causes a progressive ascending paralysis of the hindlimbs. Hindlimb muscle atrophy and contractures result in rigid hyperextension of the stifle and tarsus. Diagnosis is made on histological examination of muscle biopsies. These may show non-suppurative inflammation and tachyzoites within muscle cells. Although some dogs may have high antibody titres to the infecting organism, others may have low titres. If treated early with clindamycin and potentiated sulphonamides, the disease may resolve. However, animals with rigid hyperextension of the hindlimbs do not respond to treatment (Reichel *et al.*, 2007)

Prevention of this condition is far preferable to treatment because the results of treatment are often poor. The key to prevention is rigid fracture stabilization that encourages early limb use. When the condition is recognized early, intervention will improve prognosis.

The goal of surgical treatment is to allow adequate stifle flexion to enable limb function. Surgery involves breaking down the fibrous adhesions between the distal femur and quadriceps. Various materials (e.g. autogenous fat) have been placed between the femur and quadriceps muscle in an effort to prevent recurrence of adhesion. If, following this procedure, the stifle cannot be adequately flexed, a Z-plasty of the quadriceps can be performed to lengthen the muscle (Bloomberg, 1993).

Following surgery, the challenge is preventing the disorder from recurring by maintaining stifle movement. This can be achieved by application of a TESF to maintain stifle flexion and aggressive physiotherapy, which may require heavy sedation and prolonged pain relief. A dynamic stifle flexion apparatus has been described where external fixator pins are placed in the proximal femur and distal tibia and connected by rubber bands (de Haan *et al.*, 1995; Liptak and Simpson, 2000). Alternatively, loops of monofilament nylon can be connected from the ischium to the calcaneus (Moores and Sutton, 2009). These procedures allow stifle movement and physiotherapy but prevent the joint from fully extending.

Stifle arthrodesis may be performed if the above surgery fails, but where there is concurrent significant limb shortening and other abnormalities, such as hip subluxation, amputation is recommended.

Gracilis or semitendinosus contracture (fibrotic myopathy)

Contracture (also referred to as fibrotic myopathy) of the gracilis or, less commonly, the semitendinosus muscles results in a very characteristic gait abnormality that has been reported most frequently in middle-aged German Shepherd Dogs (Vaughan, 1979; Lewis *et al.*, 1997). Lameness in affected dogs may be acute or gradual in onset and may be uni- or bilateral. Affected muscles are palpable as distinct firm bands extending from their origin to the caudomedial aspect of the stifle. Weight-bearing in affected limbs is normal and dogs will exercise normally. Gait abnormality is most obvious when dogs are trotting. When the limb is raised, the tarsus will hyperflex and be rotated rapidly outwards while the foot is turned inwards.

Although lameness can be resolved immediately by surgery (tenotomy, tendinectomy or myectomy), contracture and lameness typically recur within 3–5 months. All forms of adjunctive medical treatment have been reported to be ineffective. Owners should be informed that the lameness is mechanical and not a result of discomfort, and that surgery will not be of benefit.

Sartorius contracture

This condition has been reported in two German Shepherd Dogs with chronic hindlimb lameness characterized by internal rotation of the limb during stifle extension (Lobetti and Hill, 1994; Spadari *et al.*, 2008). The abnormal sartorius muscle may be palpable on the craniomedial aspect of the thigh as a taut, painful band. Tenectomy may resolve lameness in the short term but recurrence of lameness has been reported (Spadari *et al.*, 2008).

References and further reading

Aktay SA and Kowaleski MP (2011) Analysis of suture anchor eyelet position on suture failure load. *Veterinary Surgery* **40**, 418–422

Ambrosius L, Arnoldy C, Waller KR *et al.* (2015) Reconstruction of chronic triceps avulsion using synthetic mesh graft in a dog. *Veterinary Comparative Orthopaedics and Traumatology* **28**, 220–224

Anderson A, Stead AC and Coughlan AR (1993) Unusual muscle and tendon disorders of the forelimb in the dog. *Journal of Small Animal Practice* **34**, 313–318

Aron DN, Selcer BA and Smith JD (1997) Autogenous tensor fascia lata graft replacement of the patellar ligament in a dog. *Veterinary and Comparative Orthopaedics and Traumatology* **10**, 141–145

Baltzer WI and Rist P (2009) Achilles tendon repair in dogs using the semitendinosus muscle: Surgical technique and short-term outcome in five dogs. *Veterinary Surgery* **38**, 770–779

Basinger RR, Aron DN, Crowe DT *et al.* (1987) Osteofascial compartment syndrome in the dog. *Veterinary Surgery* **18**, 427–434

Beale BS, Hulse DA, Schulz KS and Whitney WO (2003) Arthroscopically assisted surgery of the shoulder joint. In: *Small Animal Arthroscopy*, ed. BS Beale, pp. 23–49. WB Saunders, Philadelphia

Bennett RA (1986) Contracture of the infraspinatus muscle in dogs: a review of 12 cases. *Journal of the American Animal Hospital Association* **22**, 481–487

Berg RJ and Egger EL (1986) *In vitro* comparison of the three-loop pulley and locking loop suture patterns for repair of canine weight-bearing tendons. *Veterinary Surgery* **15**, 107–110

Bloomberg M (1993) Muscles and tendons. In: *Textbook of Small Animal Surgery, 2nd edn*, ed. D Slatter, pp. 1996–2020. WB Saunders, Philadelphia

Breur GJ and Blevins WE (1997) Traumatic injury of the iliopsoas muscle in three dogs. *Journal of the American Veterinary Medical Association* **210**, 1631–1634

Cabon Q and Bollinger C (2013) Iliopsoas muscle injury in dogs. *Compendium on Continuing Education for the Practicing Veterinarian* **35**, E1–E6

Case JB, Palmer R, Valdes-Martinez A *et al.* (2013) Gastrocnemius tendon strain in a dog treated with autologous mesenchymal stem cells and a custom orthosis. *Veterinary Surgery* **42**, 355–360

Clarke SP, Jermyn K and Carmichael S (2007) Avulsion of the triceps tendon of insertion in a cat. *Veterinary and Comparative Orthopaedics and Traumatology* **20**, 245–247

Corr SA, Draffan D, Kulendra E *et al.* (2010) Retrospective study of Achilles mechanism disruption in 45 dogs. *Veterinary Record* **167**, 407–411

Danova NA and Muir P (2003) Extracorporeal shock wave therapy for supraspinatus calcifying tendinopathy in two dogs. *Veterinary Record* **152**, 208–209

Das S, Thorne R, Lorenz ND *et al.* (2014) Patellar ligament rupture in the dog: repair methods and patient outcomes in 43 cases. *Veterinary Record* **175**, 370

Davies JV and Clayton Jones DG (1982) Triceps tendon rupture in the dog following corticosteroid injection. *Journal of Small Animal Practice* **23**, 779–787

de Haan JJ, Goring RL, Renberg C *et al.* (1995) Modified transarticular external skeletal fixation for support of Achilles tenorrhaphy in four dogs. *Veterinary and Comparative Orthopaedics and Traumatology* **8**, 32–35

Eaton-Wells RD (1992) Surgical repair of acute gracilis muscle rupture in the racing Greyhound. *Veterinary and Comparative Orthopaedics and Traumatology* **5**, 18–21

Eaton-Wells RD (1998) Muscle injuries in the racing Greyhound. In: *Canine Sports Medicine and Surgery*, ed. MS Bloomberg, JF Dee and RA Taylor, pp. 84–91. WB Saunders, Philadelphia

Eaton-Wells RD and Plummer GV (1978) Avulsion of the popliteal muscle in an Afghan Hound. *Journal of Small Animal Practice* **19**, 743–747

Fitch RB, Montgomery RD and Jaffe MH (1997a) Muscle injuries in dogs. *Compendium on Continuing Education for the Practicing Veterinarian* **19**, 947–957

Fitch RB, Wilson E, Hatchcock JT *et al.* (1997b) Radiographic, computed tomographic and magnetic resonance imaging evaluation of a chronic long digital extensor tendon avulsion in a dog. *Veterinary Radiology and Ultrasound* **38**, 177–181

Flo GL and Middleton D (1990) Mineralization of the supraspinatus tendon in dogs. *Journal of the American Veterinary Medical Association* **197**, 95–97

Gall TT, Santoni BG, Egger EL *et al.* (2009) In vitro biomechanical comparison of polypropylene mesh, modified three-loop pulley suture pattern and a combination for repair of distal canine Achilles tendon injuries. *Veterinary Surgery* **38**, 845–851

Garcia-Fernandez P, Quero Martin P, Mayenco A *et al.* (2014) Surgical management and follow-up of triceps tendon avulsion after repeated local infiltration of corticosteroids: 2 cases. *Veterinary and Comparative Orthopaedics and Traumatology* **27**, 405–410

Gelberman RH, Boyer MI and Brodt ME (1999) The effect of gap formation at the repair site on the strength and excursion of intrasynovial tendons. *Journal of Bone and Joint Surgery (American Volume)* **81**, 975–982

Gemmill TJ and Carmichael S (2003) Complete patellar ligament replacement using fascia lata autograft in a dog. *Journal of Small Animal Practice* **44**, 456–459

Giles JT, Coker D, Rochat MC *et al.* (2008) Biomechanical analysis of suture anchors and suture materials in the canine femur. *Veterinary Surgery* **37**, 12–21

Jarvinen TAH, Jarvinen M and Kalimo H (2013) Regeneration of injured skeletal muscle after injury. *Journal of Muscles, Ligaments and Tendons* **3**, 337–345

Kramer M, Gerwing M, Michele U *et al.* (2001) Ultrasonographic examination of injuries to the Achilles tendon in dogs and cats. *Journal of Small Animal Practice* **42**, 531–535

Kriegleder H (1995) Mineralization of the supraspinatus tendon: clinical observations in seven dogs. *Veterinary and Comparative Orthopaedics and Traumatology* **8**, 91–97

Kulendra E, Grierson J, Okushima S *et al.* (2011) Evaluation of the transarticular skeletal fixator for the treatment of tarsocrural instability in 32 cats. *Veterinary and Comparative Orthopaedics and Traumatology* **24**, 320–325

LaFuente M, Fransson BA, Lincoln JD *et al.* (2009) Surgical treatment of mineralized and nonmineralized supraspinatus tendinopathy in twenty four dogs. *Veterinary Surgery* **38**, 380–387

Lewis DD, Shelton GD, Piras A *et al.* (1997) Gracilis or semitendinosus myopathy in 18 dogs. *Journal of the American Animal Hospital Association* **33**, 177–188

Liptak JM and Simpson DJ (2000) Successful management of quadriceps contracture in a cat using a dynamic flexion apparatus. *Veterinary and Comparative Orthopaedics and Traumatology* **13**, 44–48

Lobetti RG and Hill TP (1994) Sartorius muscle contracture in a dog. *Journal of the South African Veterinary Association* **65**, 28–30

McKee WM, Macias C, May C and Scurrell EJ (2007) Ossification of the infraspinatus tendon-bursa in 13 dogs. *Veterinary Record* **161**, 846–852

Meeson RL, Davidson C and Arthurs GI (2011) Soft tissue injuries associated with cast application for distal limb orthopaedic injuries. *Veterinary and Comparative Orthopaedics and Traumatology* **24**, 126–131

Meutstege FJ (1993) Classification of canine Achilles tendon lesions. *Veterinary and Comparative Orthopaedics and Traumatology* **6**, 53–59

Moores AP, Comerford EJ, Tarlton JF *et al.* (2004b) Biomechanical and clinical evaluation of a modified 3-loop pulley suture pattern for reattachment of canine tendons to bone. *Veterinary Surgery* **33**, 391–397

Moores AP, Owen MR and Tarlton JF (2004a) The three-loop pulley suture versus two locking loop sutures for the repair of canine Achilles tendons. *Veterinary Surgery* **33**, 131–137

Moores AP and Sutton A (2009) Management of quadriceps contracture in a dog using a static flexion apparatus and physiotherapy. *Journal of Small Animal Practice* **50**, 251–254

Morton MA, Thomson DG, Rayward RM *et al.* (2015) Repair of chronic rupture of the insertion of the gastrocnemius tendon in the dog using a polyethylene terephthalate implant. Early clinical experience and outcome. *Veterinary and Comparative Orthopaedics and Traumatology* **28**, 282–287

Mueller-Wohlfahrt HW, Haensel L, Mithoefer K *et al.* (2013) Terminology and classification of muscle injuries in sport: The Munich consensus statement. *British Journal of Sports Medicine* **47**, 342–350

Muir P and Dueland RT (1994) Avulsion of the origin of the medial head of the gastrocnemius in a dog. *Veterinary Record* **135**, 359–360

Muir P and Johnson KA (1994) Supraspinatus and biceps brachii tendinopathy in dogs. *Journal of Small Animal Practice* **35**, 239–243

Murphy SE, Ballegeer EA, Forrest LJ and Schaefer SL (2008) Magnetic resonance imaging findings in dogs with confirmed shoulder pathology. *Veterinary Surgery* **37(7)**, 631–638

Nielsen C and Pluhar GE (2006) Outcome following surgical repair of achilles tendon rupture and comparison between postoperative tibiotarsal immobilization methods in dogs: 28 cases (1997–2004). *Veterinary and Comparative Orthopaedics and Traumatology* **19**, 246–249

Pond MJ (1973) Avulsion of the extensor digitorum longus muscle in the dog: a report of four cases. *Journal of Small Animal Practice* **14**, 785–796

Prior JE (1994) Avulsion of the lateral head of the gastrocnemius muscle in a working dog. *Veterinary Record* **134**, 382–383

Radke H, Spreng D, Sigrist N *et al.* (2006) Acute compartment syndrome complicating an intramuscular haemangiosarcoma in a dog. *Journal of Small Animal Practice* **47**, 281–284

Reichel MP, Ellis JT and Dubey JP (2007) Neosporosis and hammondiosis in dogs. *Journal of Small Animal Practice* **48**, 308–312

Robb JL, Cook JL and Carson W (2005) *In vitro* evaluation of screws and suture anchors in metaphyseal bone of the canine tibia. *Veterinary Surgery* **34**, 499–508

Robello GT, Aron DN, Foutz TL *et al.* (1992) Replacement of the medial collateral ligament with polypropylene mesh or a polyester suture in dogs. *Veterinary Surgery* **21**, 467–474

Robinson A (1999) Atraumatic bilateral avulsion of the origins of the gastrocnemius muscle. *Journal of Small Animal Practice* **40**, 498–500

Roe S (1998) Injuries and diseases of tendons. In: *Canine Sports Medicine and Surgery*, ed. MS Bloomberg, JF Dee and RA Taylor, pp. 92–99. WB Saunders, Philadelphia

Schaaf OR, Eaton-Wells R and Mitchell RAS (2009) Biceps brachii and brachialis tendon of insertion injuries in eleven racing Greyhounds. *Veterinary Surgery* **38**, 825–833

Shires PK, Braund KG and Milton JL (1982) Effect of localized trauma and temporary splinting in immature skeletal muscle and mobility of the femorotibial joint in the dog. *American Journal of Veterinary Research* **43**, 454–460

Siems JJ, Breur GJ, Blevins WE *et al.* (1998) Use of two dimensional ultrasonography for diagnosing contracture and strain of the infraspinatus muscle in a dog. *Journal of the American Veterinary Medical Association* **212**, 77–80

Sivacolundhu RK, Marchevsky AM, Read RA *et al.* (2001) Achilles mechanism reconstruction in four dogs. *Veterinary and Comparative Orthopaedics and Traumatology* **14**, 25–31

Smeak DD (1997) Selection and use of currently available suture materials and needles. In: *Current Techniques in Small Animal Surgery, 4th edn*, ed. MJ Bojrab, pp. 19–26. Williams and Wilkins, Baltimore

Spadari A, Spinella G, Morini M, Romagnoli N and Valentini S (2008) Sartorius muscle contracture in a German shepherd dog. *Veterinary Surgery* **37**, 149–152

Stead AC, Camburn MA and Gunn HM (1977) Congenital hindlimb rigidity in a dog. *Journal of Small Animal Practice* **18**, 39–46

Strickland JW (2005) The scientific basis for advances in flexor tendon surgery. *Journal of Hand Therapy* **18**, 94–110

Swiderski J, Fitch RB, Staatz A and Lowery J (2005) Sonographic assisted diagnosis and treatment of bilateral gastrocnemius tendon rupture in a Labrador retriever repaired with fascia lata and polypropylene mesh. *Veterinary and Comparative Orthopaedics and Traumatology* **18**, 258–263

Tanno F, Weber U, Lang J *et al.* (1996) Avulsion of the popliteus muscle in a malinois dog. *Journal of Small Animal Practice* **37**, 448–451

Taylor J and Tangner CH (2007) Acquired muscle contractures in the dog and cat. A review of the literature and case report. *Veterinary and Comparative Orthopaedics and Traumatology* **20**, 79–85

Vaughan LC (1979) Muscle and tendon injuries in dogs. *Journal of Small Animal Practice* **20**, 711–736

Woo SL-Y, An K-N, Arnoczky SP *et al.* (1994) Anatomy, biology and biomechanics of tendon, ligament and meniscus. In: *Orthopaedic Basic Science*, ed. SS Simon, pp. 45–88. American Academy of Orthopaedic Surgeons, Philadelphia

Chapter 10

Diseases of muscle and the neuromuscular junction

G. Diane Shelton

Introduction

Diseases affecting muscle and the neuromuscular junction are commonly overlooked when evaluating a dog with lameness. Orthopaedic disorders occur more frequently than neuromuscular diseases, but when a diagnosis cannot be reached following thorough orthopaedic evaluation, disorders of muscle and the neuromuscular junction should be considered. Joint diseases such as polyarthritis can appear very similar clinically to polymyositis or myasthenia gravis. This chapter focuses on the most commonly encountered neuromuscular disorders with particular emphasis on those that can present as lameness.

Clinical signs

The clinical signs of muscle or neuromuscular junction disease include:

- Stiff, short-strided gait
- Lameness or limb contractures
- Crouched stance with limbs kept centred under the trunk to support weight
- Normal to decreased muscle tone and reflexes
- Muscle atrophy in chronic myopathies
- Weakness of pharyngeal, laryngeal and oesophageal musculature, resulting in dysphagia, dysphonia and regurgitation
- Pyrexia may be present in inflammatory myopathies (IMs) or associated with megaoesophagus and aspiration pneumonia.

Diagnostic procedures

The diagnostic procedures critical for evaluation of neuromuscular disease include:

- A thorough physical and neurological examination. The clinical phenotype (presentation) should be accurately characterized
- Gait evaluation (including video recordings)
- Routine laboratory analysis of blood, including creatine kinase (CK), electrolytes, lactate, pyruvate, myoglobin and cardiac troponin I (Shelton, 2010a)
- Special testing, including thyroid evaluation and measurement of serum acetylcholine receptor antibodies (see the *BSAVA Manual of Canine and Feline Clinical Pathology*)

- Electromyography (EMG) and measurement of sensory and motor nerve conduction velocities
- Muscle biopsy – this is the single most important diagnostic test for the evaluation of muscle diseases (Dickinson and LeCouteur, 2002).

Muscle biopsy collection

An open surgical approach is made to the muscle and biopsy samples are collected by sharp dissection using a No. 11 scalpel blade.

Two samples (approximately 0.5 x 0.5 x 1.0 cm) should be collected:

- Sample 1 should be wrapped in a saline-dampened (not dripping) gauze sponge and kept chilled
- Sample 2 should be immersed in 10% neutral buffered formalin.

The samples should be handled with care to prevent artefacts.

Both samples should be shipped under refrigeration to a laboratory with expertise in testing for muscle disease.

Myopathies

Myopathies may be classified as either inflammatory or non-inflammatory (Figure 10.1).

- IMs include generalized diseases, such as infectious myositis, immune-mediated polymyositis, dermatomyositis and inclusion body myositis, as well as focal IMs, such as extraocular myositis and masticatory muscle myositis (MMM).
- Non-inflammatory myopathies include muscular dystrophies, congenital myopathies associated with structural defects of myofibres, steroid myopathy, endocrine myopathies associated with hypothyroidism and hyperadrenocorticism (Cushing's syndrome), metabolic myopathies associated with disorders of energy production including glycogen, lipid and mitochondrial metabolism, and myotonic myopathies.

Inflammatory myopathies

- Infectious:
  - Bacteria – clostridia, staphylococci, streptococci
  - Protozoa – *Toxoplasma, Neospora, Leishmania*
  - Parasites – *Trichinella, Ancyclostoma, Sarcocystis*
- Immune-mediated:
  - Masticatory myositis
  - Polymyositis
  - Dermatomyositis
  - Extraocular myositis
  - Inclusion body myositis

Non-inflammatory myopathies

- Acquired:
  - Fibrotic/ossifying/contractures
  - Ischaemic
  - Neoplastic
  - Toxic
  - Endocrine:
    - Hypoadrenocorticism
    - Hypothyroidism
    - Hyperthyroidism
    - Hyperadrenocorticism
- Inherited:
  - Myotonia
  - Muscular dystrophies
    - X-linked, dystrophin deficient
    - Others, dystrophin positive
    - Merosin (laminin α2) deficiency
    - Sarcoglycan deficiency
    - Collagen VI deficiency
  - Breed-associated myopathies
  - Centronuclear myopathy in Labrador Retriever, Great Dane, Border Collie
  - X-linked myotubular myopathy in Labrador Retriever, Rottweiler, Manchester Terrier
  - Nemaline rod myopathy in American Bulldog
  - Metabolic
    - Glycogen storage
    - Mitochondrial
    - Lipid storage
    - Malignant hyperthermia

10.1 Classification of canine myopathies.

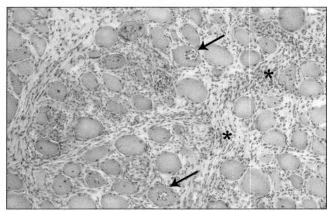

10.2 Fresh-frozen biopsy sample from the vastus lateralis muscle of a dog with chronic inflammatory myopathy. Note the fibrosis and diffuse mononuclear cell infiltration with a perimysial and endomysial distribution (∗), as well as the invasion of non-necrotic fibres by cellular infiltrates (arrowed). (Haematoxylin and eosin stain; original magnification X100)

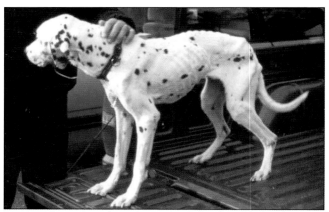

10.3 Severe loss of muscle mass in a Dalmatian with chronic inflammatory myopathy.

Inflammatory myopathies
Generalized inflammatory myopathies

IMs are a result of infiltration of inflammatory cells into striated muscle (Figure 10.2). Reviews of canine IMs have been published (Evans *et al.*, 2004; Shelton 2010b). The prognosis is favourable if they are diagnosed early in the course of the disease and treated appropriately. If there is a delay in reaching a diagnosis or if therapy is inappropriate, severe loss of muscle mass (Figure 10.3) and irreversible fibrosis may result in limb deformities or contractures.

Clinical signs highly suggestive of generalized IMs include:

- Stiff-stilted gait or an unexplained lameness in the absence of detectable orthopaedic abnormalities
- Persistent, mild to moderately (10–20 times normal values) elevated serum CK activity. *Persistently elevated serum CK concentrations must not be ignored*
- Progressive muscle atrophy
- Muscle pain may not be a prominent clinical sign (Evans *et al.*, 2004) although the presence of inflammation in muscle biopsy samples suggests that this should be the case
- Dysphagia, dysphonia and regurgitation may be present if cellular infiltrates invade muscles of the pharynx, larynx or oesophagus.

The single most important diagnostic procedure is muscle biopsy (Dickinson and LeCouteur, 2002). As cellular infiltrates may have a patchy multifocal distribution, biopsy samples should be taken from at least two different muscles. Muscle biopsy is relatively innocuous and well tolerated. For suspected myopathies, biopsy samples should be taken by an open biopsy procedure, from large proximal limb muscles such as the triceps brachii in the thoracic limb and the vastus lateralis or biceps femoris muscles in the pelvic limb. Following a histological diagnosis of inflammatory myopathy, further investigations and therapies can be undertaken (Figure 10.4).

Masticatory muscle myositis

MMM is a focal autoimmune inflammatory myopathy that commonly affects dogs and rarely affects cats. Clinical signs are limited to the muscles of mastication with sparing of limb muscles and other muscle groups.

- It may present in the acute stage with swelling of the masticatory muscles, restricted jaw mobility (trismus) and jaw pain. Inability to open the jaw under anaesthesia is a classic clinical sign.
- A chronic form of MMM can present with slowly progressive atrophy of the masticatory muscles with or without jaw pain or restricted jaw mobility.

- Serum antibody titres against infections (e.g. *Toxoplasma gondii*, *Neospora caninum* and tick-related disorders) are assessed. An infectious aetiology for IMs may be more common than previously thought (Evans *et al.*, 2004).
- Screening thoracic and abdominal radiographs are taken for evidence of oesophageal dilatation, aspiration pneumonia and neoplasia.
- Thoracic and abdominal computed tomography (CT), or thoracic CT and abdominal ultrasonography, may be used as an alternative to routine radiography or during follow-up examinations.
- Specific therapy is administered for an infectious agent or neoplasia, if identified.
- If there is no evidence of an infectious agent or neoplasia, immunosuppressive therapy with prednisolone at a dose of 2 mg/kg orally q12h should be initiated. Serum CK activity is monitored until within the normal range. When clinical signs are controlled, oral prednisolone is gradually decreased to the lowest alternate day dosage that will keep the dog free of clinical signs. Long-term therapy may be required. Other immunosuppressants may be used for steroid-sparing (see Figures 6.29 and 6.30)
- Analgesia must be considered and adjusted to meet the needs of the individual patient. Options for analgesia include buprenorphine, paracetamol, tramadol, methadone, morphine and fentanyl. For further information, see Chapter 17 and the *BSAVA Manual of Canine and Feline Anaesthesia and Analgesia*.
- If aspiration pneumonia is present, appropriate systemic bactericidal antibiotics are given for 24 hours before the onset of corticosteroid therapy.

10.4 Further investigations and possible therapeutic options for inflammatory myopathies.

- Diagnosis of MMM is by biopsy of a masticatory muscle and demonstration of serum antibodies against masticatory muscle type 2M fibres (Shelton, 2010b; test available through the Comparative Neuromuscular Laboratory, University of California San Diego, http://vetneuromuscular.ucsd.edu).
- Immunosuppressive therapy is required as described for polymyositis until jaw pain is no longer apparent and jaw mobility improves (Figure 10.4).
- Relapses are common so low-dose alternate day prednisolone therapy may be required long-term.

Non-inflammatory myopathies
Muscular dystrophies

Muscular dystrophies are a heterogeneous group of over 30 inherited degenerative mostly non-inflammatory disorders, characterized by progressive muscle weakness and wasting (Shelton and Engvall, 2005). A dystrophic myopathy should be considered in any young dog or cat (male or female, mixed breed or purebred) with persistent muscle weakness, muscle atrophy or hypertrophy, gait abnormality, or contractures beginning in the first few months of life. For most disorders that have been identified, neither a cure nor a specific therapy is yet available. It is important to obtain a correct diagnosis because most dystrophic myopathies occur in purebred animals and knowledge of inheritance patterns is of utmost importance to animal breeders.

Clinical signs of muscular dystrophy and appropriate diagnostics include:

- Weakness and muscle atrophy or hypertrophy beginning in the first few months of life (Figure 10.5)
- Dysphagia, regurgitation and dyspnoea as a result of hypertrophy of the lingual, pharyngeal and oesophageal musculature, and the diaphragm
- Cardiomyopathy may result in heart failure
- Dramatically and persistently elevated serum CK activity (10–100 times normal values)

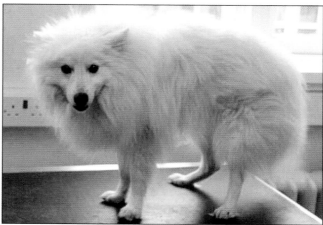

10.5 Young Japanese Spitz diagnosed with muscular dystrophy associated with a truncated form of dystrophin. Note the hunched posture with pelvic limbs tucked under the body.
(Courtesy of Professor Boyd Jones)

- Muscle biopsy is critical for confirmation of the diagnosis and shows a typical dystrophic phenotype which includes myofibre degeneration, regeneration and fibrosis (Figure 10.6). Calcific deposits are found in tissues (Figures 10.6 and 10.7)
- Immunohistochemical evaluation of the expression of relevant muscle proteins including dystrophin, dystrophin associated proteins, laminins and other proteins (Figure 10.8) may determine the type of muscular dystrophy and direct specific mutational analyses. This is a cost-effective and sensitive method, which can be performed directly on fresh-frozen muscle biopsy specimens.

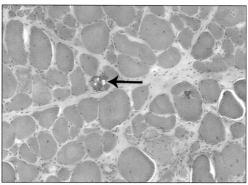

10.6 Fresh-frozen biopsy specimen from the biceps femoris muscle of a 10-month-old Domestic Shorthaired cat with clinical signs of muscle weakness and hypertrophy from an early age. There is variation in myofibre size, endomysial fibrosis and degenerating fibres; a calcific deposit is arrowed. (Haematoxylin and eosin stain; original magnification X100)

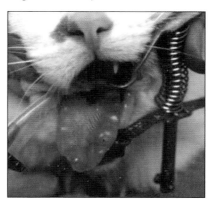

10.7 Numerous calcific deposits were found on the tongue of a young Domestic Shorthaired cat with muscular dystrophy associated with dystrophin deficiency.
(Courtesy of Dr Randy Longshore)

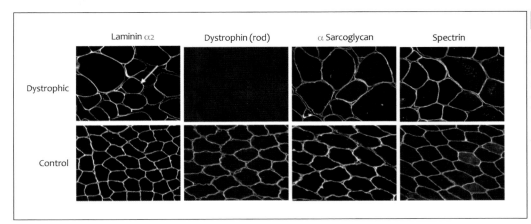

10.8 Examples of immunofluorescence staining performed on muscle biopsy cryosections for the diagnosis of various forms of muscular dystrophy. Sarcolemmal staining for dystrophin (rod) was absent, confirming a dystrophin deficient muscular dystrophy. Staining of the basal lamina for laminin α2 and of the sarcolemma for sarcoglycan and spectrin were similar to the control muscle sample. The arrow in the upper left image shows the positively stained basal lamina.

The most common form of muscular dystrophy in humans is Duchenne muscular dystrophy, caused by a deficiency of the muscle protein dystrophin. A major reason why Duchenne muscular dystrophy is the most common is the extremely large size of the dystrophin gene, making it the target of more frequent mutations than a smaller gene. Dystrophin deficiency is also the most common form of muscular dystrophy in dogs and cats. Muscular dystrophies have also been identified associated with deficiency of merosin (laminin α2) in dogs and cats, and associated with deficiency of sarcoglycans in dogs. Recently, a form of congenital muscular dystrophy has been identified caused by a confirmed mutation in collagen VI.

Dystrophin deficiency in dogs and cats:

- This form of muscular dystrophy is X-linked, typically affects males and has been described in several breeds of dogs, occasionally in mixed breed dogs and females, and in cats.
- Specific mutations in dystrophin have been identified in the Golden Retriever (Sharp *et al.*, 1991), Labrador Retriever (Smith *et al.*, 2007), Cavalier King Charles Spaniel (Walmsley *et al.*, 2010), Akita (Atencia *et al.*, 2013), German Shorthaired Pointer (Schatzberg *et al.*, 1999), Welsh Corgi (Smith *et al.*, 2011) and Rottweiler (Winand *et al.*, 1994). Unpublished mutations have been identified for the Tibetan Terrier and Cocker Spaniel (Kornegay *et al.*, 2012). A hypertrophic form of muscular dystrophy associated with dystrophin deficiency has been described in Domestic Shorthaired cats and mutations identified (Winand *et al.*, 1994; Gambino *et al.*, 2014).

Merosin (laminin α2) deficiency in dogs and cats:

- This form of muscular dystrophy has been described in a young Brittany Springer Spaniel mixed breed dog (Shelton *et al.*, 2001), in Flame Point Siamese and Domestic Shorthaired cats (O'Brien *et al.*, 2001), and in a Maine Coon cat (Poncelet *et al.*, 2003) (Figure 10.9). No specific mutations have yet been described.
- Serum CK activities are moderately elevated (10–20 times normal values).
- The dystrophic phenotype is confirmed in muscle biopsy specimens and the exact classification determined by immunohistochemical staining showing an absence of laminin α2.
- Similar to dystrophin deficiency, no treatments are currently available and the prognosis is poor.

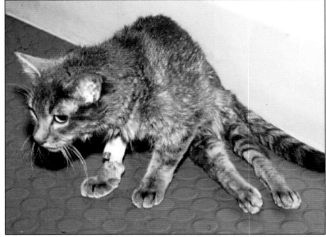

10.9 Muscle contracture resulted in pelvic limb stiffness and rigidity in a young cat with congenital muscular dystrophy, resulting from a deficiency of laminin α2 (merosin).
(Courtesy of Dr Dennis O'Brien)

Sarcoglycan deficiency in dogs:

- The sarcoglycan (SG) complex spans the sarcolemmal membrane, bridging dystrophin and the dystroglycan complexes in muscle. Mutations in the SG complex result in limb girdle muscular dystrophies in humans.
- Deficiency of the SG complex has recently been identified in both male and female Boston Terriers (Deitz *et al.*, 2008), Cocker Spaniels and Chihuahuas (Schatzberg and Shelton, 2004), as well as in a female Dobermann (Munday *et al.*, 2014).
- Presenting clinical signs are similar to those of dystrophin-deficient muscular dystrophy.
- Serum CK concentrations are dramatically elevated (100 times normal values).
- The diagnosis is confirmed by evaluation of muscle biopsy specimens and demonstration of reduced or absent SG complex in immunohistochemical staining.

Congenital muscular dystrophy associated with collagen VI deficiency:

- An 11-month old female spayed Labrador Retriever was presented for progressive gait abnormality and multiple joint deformities of approximately 6 months' duration (Figure 10.10).
- Serum CK activity was mildly increased.

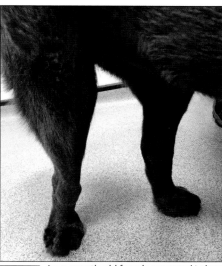

10.10 An 11-month-old female neutered Labrador Retriever with multiple joint deformities, resulting from deficiency of collagen VI. Note the hyperextended stifle and tarsus.
(Courtesy of Dr Katia Marioni-Henry)

- Histopathology and immunofluorescence staining identified an abnormality of collagen VI (Marioni-Henry *et al.*, 2014). A mutation has just been identified in the collagen VI gene (unpublished).
- This case should alert clinicians to the possibility of a congenital myopathy in young dogs with joint deformities.

Endocrine disorders

Weakness, stiffness, myalgia and lameness occur relatively commonly in endocrine disorders, particularly in geriatric animals (Platt, 2002). In some affected dogs and cats, muscle involvement may be an incidental finding or may be subclinical. In other cases, muscle weakness or stiffness may be the first clinical sign of an underlying endocrine disorder and may lead to a diagnosis. It is important to remember that the most common clinical presentations of endocrine disorders, such as the overweight, heat-seeking dog in hypothyroidism, do not have to be present. The most common endocrine disorders that can result in myopathic clinical signs are summarized in Figure 10.11.

Endocrinopathy	Clinical signs	Results of investigations	Treatment and prognosis	Comments
Glucocorticoid excess: Exogenous corticosteroid therapy (steroid myopathy) Endogenous hyperadrenocorticism (Cushing's syndrome)	Steroid myopathy: weakness and muscle atrophy may be profound. Hyperadrenocorticism: muscle atrophy and weakness Progressive limb stiffness can involve all limbs and may be initial clinical sign. Severe pelvic limb rigidity and clinical myotonia may occur in a subset of dogs with chronic hyperadrenocorticism (Figure 10.12)	Type 2 fibre atrophy is a consistent finding in muscle biopsy specimens from dogs with steroid myopathy or spontaneous hyperadrenocorticism	Steroid myopathy: dose reduction if the underlying condition is controlled Exercise may partially prevent weakness Hyperadrenocorticism: muscle weakness and atrophy improve with therapy for hyperadrenocorticism. Clinical myotonia may not resolve	Muscle atrophy resulting from exogenous corticosteroid therapy should be reversible once treatment is discontinued
Hypothyroidism	Classic clinical signs (including lethargy, weight gain, seborrhoea and alopecia) may or may not be obvious Weakness, stiffness and myalgia may be the initial presenting clinical signs. Myopathy and neuropathy may occur in dogs with hypothyroidism	Serum creatine kinase concentration may be mildly elevated if muscle necrosis is present	Prognosis for recovery of muscle strength in hypothyroid myopathy is excellent once a euthyroid state is restored	Response of neuropathy to thyroid replacement may not be as favourable as for myopathy and may take several months
Hyperthyroidism in cats	Generalized weakness, neck ventroflexion, tremors, fatigue, gait disturbances, decreased ability to jump and breathlessness after exertion	Serum creatine kinase activity may be markedly elevated with a normal muscle biopsy. Hypokalaemia may be a complicating factor	Prognosis is good for resolution of muscle weakness following treatment to achieve a euthyroid state	Reversible myasthenia gravis and acetylcholine receptor (AChR) antibodies may occur in cats treated with methimazole. AChR antibody titres return to the normal range following discontinuation of therapy
Hypoadrenocorticism (Addison's disease)	Muscle weakness occurs frequently. Weakness may be generalized or selectively involve the pharyngeal or oesophageal musculature	Hyperkalaemia and hyponatraemia. Minimal or no response to stimulation with adrenocorticotropic hormone (ACTH). Creatine kinase activity may be elevated.	Correction of the electrolyte imbalance and glucocorticoid deficiency usually results in resolution of clinical weakness	Reversible megaoesophagus may occur with hypoadrenocorticism. All cases with acquired megaoesophagus should be tested for glucocorticoid deficiency
Hyperinsulinism secondary to pancreatic islet cell tumours (insulinoma)	Weakness and collapse due to profound hypoglycaemia. Central nervous system signs may predominate. In rare cases, insulinoma causes peripheral neuropathy (see BSAVA *Manual of Canine and Feline Neurology*)	Hypoglycaemia	In general, prognosis for complete remission and recovery from an accompanying peripheral neuropathy, even with surgical intervention, is poor	Pancreatic islet cell carcinoma is a relatively common neoplasm in middle-aged to older dogs

10.11 Common endocrine disorders that can result in myopathic clinical signs.

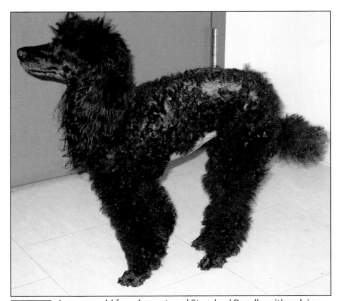

10.12 A 10-year-old female neutered Standard Poodle with pelvic limb spasticity associated with hyperadrenocorticism. Electrophysiology was consistent with a myotonia associated with this endocrine disorder.
(Courtesy of Dr Joan Coates)

Metabolic disorders

Metabolic myopathies make up a diverse group of disorders caused by biochemical defects of the skeletal muscle energy-generating systems (Platt, 2002). These disorders can result in poor exercise tolerance, myalgia, atrophy, cramping, and myoglobinuria. The biochemical defects primarily affect ATP production. Relatively few of these disorders have been characterized in veterinary medicine. In the dog, the presence of predominantly oxidative muscle fibre types, in the absence of classical type 2B fibres (purely glycolytic), may make clinical presentations associated with aberrant glycogen metabolism difficult to recognize. Clinical signs may be referable to abnormalities in other body systems that can overshadow muscle-associated weakness. A good example of this is phosphofructokinase deficiency in English Springer Spaniels, in which the primary clinical signs are associated with haemolytic anaemia. Elevated CK activities and glycogen deposits in muscle biopsy specimens from affected dogs support a concurrent myopathy. The following defects of glycogen metabolism have been confirmed:

- Glycogenosis Type II in Lapland dogs
- Glycogenosis Type III in German Shepherd Dogs and Akitas
- Glycogenosis Type IV in Norwegian Forest cats
- Glycogenosis Type VII (phosphofructokinase deficiency) in English Springer Spaniels and American Cocker Spaniels.

The highly oxidative nature of canine muscle may predispose dogs to disorders of oxidative metabolism, including mitochondrial myopathies and disorders of fatty acid oxidation or of carnitine metabolism. Although confirming a diagnosis of a defect in oxidative metabolism may be difficult, evaluation of plasma lactic and pyruvic acid concentrations (Platt and Garosi, 2004) and muscle biopsy specimens should be helpful diagnostic procedures. To date, the following disorders have been confirmed or suspected in dogs:

- Pyruvate dehydrogenase phosphatase 1 (PDP1) deficiency
- Mitochondrial myopathy
- Lipid storage myopathy.

PDP1 deficiency has been confirmed in Clumber and Sussex Spaniels and the mutation identified in the *PDP1* gene (Cameron *et al.*, 2007). Clinical presentation is one of exercise intolerance. A presumptive diagnosis can be made by demonstration of marked elevations in plasma lactate and pyruvate concentrations with a lactate:pyruvate ratio <10. Confirmation of PDP1 deficiency is made by genetic testing (testing for *PDP1* mutation in Clumber and Sussex Spaniels is offered through Canine Genetic Diseases Network, www.caninegeneticdiseases. net). Although no specific therapy is available, dietary modifications, including feeding a high-fat, low-carbohydrate diet and the addition of thiamine, may be of some benefit (Abramson *et al.*, 2004).

Mitochondrial myopathy associated with altered cytochrome C oxidase activity and reduced mitochondrial mRNA was documented in Old English Sheepdog littermates with exercise intolerance (Vijayasarathy *et al.*, 1994). A young German Shepherd Dog was also described with an absence of cytochrome C oxidase activity and morphologically atypical mitochondria demonstrated by electron microscopy (Paciello *et al.*, 2003).

Lipid storage myopathy has been described in dogs (Shelton *et al.*, 1998) but the precise biochemical defect(s) have not been characterized. The clinical presentation is variable and includes muscle atrophy, weakness and, in some cases, dramatic myalgia. Lactic acidaemia is found in most dogs with lipid storage myopathy. Diagnosis is confirmed by identification of numerous, large lipid droplets within muscle fibres. Therapy includes supplementation of L-carnitine (50 mg/kg twice daily), coenzyme Q_{10} (100 mg daily), and B vitamins.

Myotonic disorders

Myotonia is a myogenic condition defined as prolonged contraction or delayed relaxation of a muscle after voluntary movement or after mechanical or electrical stimulation. Myotonia is characterized by muscle stiffness without cramping (action myotonia), muscle dimpling after being struck by a reflex hammer (percussion myotonia), and characteristic EMG changes (myotonic discharges). Diseases resulting in myotonia may be associated with diminished sarcolemmal chloride conductance, altered sodium channel inactivation, from unknown mechanisms associated with myotonic dystrophy and with various metabolic conditions and intoxications. Vite (2002) provides an in-depth review of myotonia and disorders of muscle cell membrane excitability.

Myotonia congenita: This condition has been reported in dogs and cats.

- Chow Chows affected with myotonia congenita present with evident muscle stiffness soon after pups become ambulatory. The clinical signs of muscle stiffness diminish with exercise.
- In the Miniature Schnauzer, myotonia congenita is inherited as an autosomal recessive trait (Figure 10.13). The mutation has been identified and has been shown to be a result of a missense mutation in both alleles of the gene encoding the skeletal muscle voltage-dependent chloride channel *CLC1* (Bhalerao *et al.*,

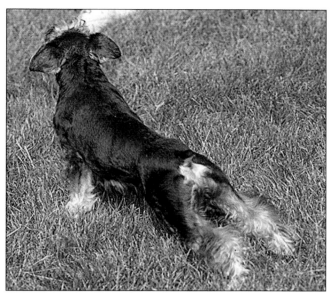

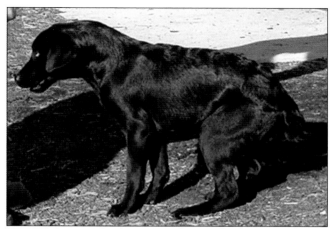

10.14 A young Labrador Retriever diagnosed with centronuclear myopathy. Note that its neck muscles are too weak to lift its head.
(Courtesy of Dr Joan Coates and Dr Dennis O'Brien)

10.13 Muscle stiffness observed in a young Miniature Schnauzer with myotonia congenita. This condition is inherited as an autosomal recessive trait in this breed and is associated with a mutation in the *CLC1* gene.

2002). A DNA-based test capable of detecting the mutant allele in affected and carrier Miniature Schnauzer dogs has been developed and is available at the Josephine Deubler Genetic Testing Laboratory of the University of Pennsylvania (http://research.vet.upenn.edu/AvailableTests/tabid/8242/Default.aspx).
- Myotonia congenita has been described in domestic cats, and a mutation in the skeletal muscle voltage-dependent chloride channel *CLCN-1* was recently identified (Daniel *et al.*, 2014).

Treatment for myotonia congenita is directed at decreasing repetitive activity in muscle by using antagonists to voltage-gated sodium channels. These drugs include procainamide, quinidine, phenytoin and mexiletine. Certain drugs have been reported to worsen myotonia congenita and should be avoided. These include dantrolene, beta-blocking adrenergic agents, fenoterol, diuretics, monocarboxylic aromatic acids, cholesterol-lowering drugs, depolarizing muscle relaxants and anaesthetics acting on the sarcolemma or endplate, including decamethonium, succinylcholine neostigmine and physostigmine. Bromide may also be contraindicated (Vite, 2002).

Miscellaneous breed-associated non-inflammatory myopathies

There are scattered reports of breed-associated non-dystrophic myopathies affecting young dogs in the literature (Shelton and Engvall, 2005). The clinical presentation of muscle weakness and atrophy in a particular breed with age of onset less than one year, combined with typical pathological changes on muscle biopsy specimens, should make a diagnosis of this category of myopathies relatively straightforward.

Centronuclear myopathy in Labrador Retrievers: Centronuclear myopathy (CNM) was previously known as hereditary myopathy of Labrador Retrievers, autosomal recessive muscular dystrophy, type 2 fibre deficiency and colloquially as 'floppy labrador' disease (Figure 10.14). The mutation in the *PTPLA* gene has been identified (Maurer

et al., 2012). A genetic test is available for identification of CNM in Labradors and for carrier detection (www.labradorcnm.com).

X-linked myotubular myopathy: X-linked myotubular myopathy (XLMTM) is associated with a mutation in the myotubularin (*MTM1*) gene and has been identified in Labrador Retrievers (Beggs *et al.*, 2010) and Rottweiler dogs (Shelton *et al.*, 2015). The clinical presentation of this myopathy is very similar to that of CNM; however, onset may be younger at 3–6 months of age and only males are affected.

Both CNM and XLMTM in Labrador Retrievers can readily be distinguished from dystrophin-deficient muscular dystrophy, which also occurs in this breed, by differences in serum CK activity and immunohistochemical staining. Serum CK activity is markedly elevated in dystrophin deficiency and only mildly elevated in CNM and XLMTM. Histopathological examination of muscle and immunohistochemical staining of muscle cryosections for dystrophin reveal normal dystrophin staining in CNM and XLMTM and absence of dystrophin in muscular dystrophy. Genetic testing is also available for CNM and XLMTM.

Centronuclear myopathy in Great Danes: A centronuclear myopathy associated with a mutation in the *BIN1* gene has recently been confirmed in young Great Dane dogs (Bohm *et al.*, 2013). This myopathy was previously known as a 'central-core' myopathy and 'inherited myopathy of the Great Dane' and has distinct histological features. The clinical presentation of muscle weakness and atrophy in this breed with age of onset <1 year, combined with typical pathological changes on muscle biopsy specimens, should make this diagnosis relatively straightforward.

Musladin-Lueke Syndrome: This condition, associated with thick inelastic skin and joint contractures particularly affecting the distal joints (Figure 10.15), has been described in Beagles with a mutation in the *ADAMTSL2* gene (Bader *et al.*, 2010). *ADAMTSL2* interacts with transforming growth factor betaI (TGF-β) and fibrillin 1 in the extracellular matrix. Stiffness persists even under anaesthesia. Affected Beagles appear to be walking on the digits of all four limbs. This gait abnormality may occur in other breeds and should warrant the consideration of a muscle extracellular matrix defect.

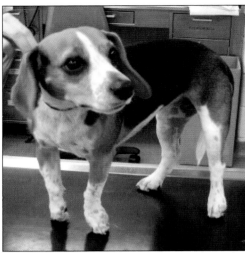

10.15 A young Beagle with Musladin-Lueke syndrome. The puppy appears to be walking on the digits of all four limbs.
(Courtesy of Dr Rebecca Packer)

Disorders of neuromuscular transmission

Myasthenia gravis

Myasthenia gravis is caused by an autoimmune attack against nicotinic acetylcholine receptors, which results in depletion of post-synaptic receptors. Myasthenia gravis is the most completely characterized autoimmune disease affecting the neuromuscular system, and probably the most completely characterized autoimmune disease in general. For a general review of this topic, see Shelton (2002). In the author's opinion, acquired myasthenia gravis is the most common neuromuscular disease that can be diagnosed and treated in dogs. Clinicians should become familiar with the spectrum of clinical signs, as dogs with myasthenia gravis may be misdiagnosed with disc disease and acute abdominal crisis, and undergo anaesthesia and surgical procedures that could potentially exacerbate the myasthenic condition. Although less common in cats, myasthenia gravis should also be considered in any cat that is presented with a recent onset of muscular weakness.

Clinical forms of acquired myasthenia gravis include:

- Focal myasthenia gravis, including oesophageal dilatation and pharyngeal weakness without clinically detectable limb muscle weakness. This is seen in 43% of cases (Shelton et al., 1997). Laryngeal paralysis alone, in the absence of oesophageal or pharyngeal weakness, has not been identified in myasthenia gravis
- Generalized weakness, present in 57% of cases with or without oesophageal or pharyngeal dysfunction (Shelton et al., 1997). The absence of a megaoesophagus cannot eliminate the diagnosis of acquired myasthenia gravis: these dogs are sometimes misdiagnosed with disc disease
- Acute fulminating generalized myasthenia gravis can occur in a small number of cases and these require intensive care, including ventilatory support.

Similar clinical forms occur in cats. Cranial mediastinal masses are more common in cats (52%; Hague et al., 2015) than in dogs (3%).

Diagnosis of acquired myasthenia gravis includes:

- Immunoprecipitation radioimmunoassay to document circulating acetylcholine receptor antibodies continues to be the gold standard for the diagnosis of acquired myasthenia gravis in both dogs and cats. This serum test is sensitive, specific, and documents an autoimmune response. The acetylcholine receptor antibody test is offered through the Comparative Neuromuscular Laboratory, University of California San Diego (http://vetneuromuscular.ucsd.edu)
- The edrophonium chloride challenge test should also be performed as a dramatic response would give a presumptive diagnosis of myasthenia gravis. Edrophonium chloride is a short-acting anticholinesterase drug that prolongs the action of acetylcholine at the neuromuscular junction. Therapy can be initiated based on a dramatic positive improvement in muscle strength. Other myopathies and neuropathies can result in subjective improvement in muscle strength (false-positive) and also false-negative results. A negative test should not rule out a diagnosis of myasthenia gravis. The confirmatory serum test should be performed in all cases of suspected myasthenia gravis
- A decreased amplitude of the compound muscle action potential in response to repetitive nerve stimulation can also provide a presumptive diagnosis of myasthenia gravis; however, there is a lack of sensitivity and specificity, in addition to the requirement for general anaesthesia in a potentially critical patient
- Single-fibre EMG is a sensitive method for detecting delayed or failed neuromuscular transmission, and a methodology has been established for the dog. Specificity is lacking, with positive findings in other disorders of the nerve, muscle and neuromuscular junction. This procedure is also technically difficult and not performed routinely even in specialist neurology practices.

An early and accurate diagnosis of acquired myasthenia gravis, followed by appropriate therapy, is the most important factor in obtaining a good clinical outcome. Megaoesophagus is present in 90% of myasthenic dogs, thus longer term altered feeding procedures (elevation of food and water or placement of a gastrostomy tube) are critical for nutritional support, hydration and drug delivery. Anticholinesterase drugs are the cornerstone of therapy. Available drugs include pyridostigmine (1–3 mg/kg orally q8–12h) and neostigmine (2 mg/kg/day orally in divided doses to effect). Pyridostigmine has fewer cholinergic side effects (salivation, gastrointestinal disturbances) than neostigmine. If an optimal response to therapy is not obtained with supportive care and anticholinesterase drugs alone, low-dose prednisolone therapy is suggested. Immunosuppressive dosages of prednisolone should be avoided early in the course of treatment as increased weakness often occurs, requiring hospitalization and sometimes intensive medical care with respiratory support (Shelton, 2002). Data on the effectiveness of other immunosuppressive agents, such as mycophenolate, ciclosporin and azathioprine, are limited.

In the absence of immunosuppression, determination of acetylcholine receptor antibody titres is a good indicator of disease status and helps to determine duration of therapy, i.e. re-testing and continuing treatment while acetylcholine receptor antibody titres are positive. In dogs, in the absence of immunosuppression, there is an excellent correlation between resolution of clinical signs, including megaoesophagus and return of acetylcholine receptor antibody titres to the normal range (Shelton and Lindstrom, 2001). Spontaneous remissions frequently occur in canine myasthenia gravis (Shelton et al., 2000), but preliminary studies suggest this is not the case in cats (Shelton, unpublished).

Miscellaneous disorders of neuromuscular transmission

Other disorders of neuromuscular transmission encountered in practice include tick paralysis and botulism, organophosphate (OP) intoxication in the cat and drug-induced neuromuscular blockade (Shelton, 2002). These disorders should result in a fairly rapid onset of lower motor neuron tetraparesis and would probably not be a consideration for the lame dog or cat.

References and further reading

Abramson CJ, Platt SR and Shelton GD (2004) Pyruvate dehydrogenase deficiency in a Sussex Spaniel. Journal of Small Animal Practice 45,162–165

Atencia S, Mooney CT, Shiel R, Jones BR and Nolan CM (2013) Muscular dystrophy in the Japanese Spitz: description of the mutation and carrier detection using polymerase chain reaction. Journal of Veterinary Internal Medicine 27, 675

Bader HL, Ruhe AL, Wang LW et al. (2010) An ADAMTSL2 founder mutation causes Musladin-Lueke syndrome, a heritable disorder of Beagle dogs, featuring stiff skin and joint contractures. PLoS One 5, e12817

Beggs AH, Bohm J and Snead E (2010) MTM1 mutation associated with X-linked myotubular myopathy in Labrador Retrievers. Proceedings National Academy of Science USA 107, 14697–14702

Bhalerao DP, Rajpurohit Y, Vite CH and Giger U (2002) Detection of a genetic mutation for myotonia congenita among Miniature Schnauzers and identification of a common carrier ancestor. American Journal of Veterinary Research 63, 1443–1447

Bohm J, Vasli N, Maurer M et al. (2013) Altered splicing of the BIN1 muscle-specific exon in humans and dogs with highly progressive centronuclear myopathy. PLoS Genetics 9, e1003430

Cameron JM, Maj MC, Levandovskiy V et al. (2007) Identification of a canine model of pyruvate dehydrogenase phosphatase 1 deficiency. Molecular Genetics and Metabolism 90, 15–23

Daniel RJ, Cortes A, Gandolfi B et al. (2014) Feline myotonia congenita: clinical, electrophysiologic and histopathologic characteristics with a novel mutation in CLCN-1. Journal of Veterinary Internal Medicine 28, 1016

Deitz K, Morrison JA, Kline K et al. (2008) Sarcoglycan-deficient muscular dystrophy in a Boston Terrier. Journal of Veterinary Internal Medicine 22, 476–480

Dickinson PJ and LeCouteur RA (2002) Muscle and nerve biopsy. Veterinary Clinics of North America: Small Animal Practice 32, 63–102

Duke-Novakovski T, de Vries M and Seymour C (2016) BSAVA Manual of Canine and Feline Anaesthesia and Analgesia, 3rd edn. BSAVA Publications, Gloucester

Evans J, Levesque D and Shelton GD (2004) Canine inflammatory myopathies: a clinicopathologic review of 200 cases. Journal of Veterinary Internal Medicine 18, 679–691

Gambino AN, Mouser PJ, Shelton GD and Winand NJ (2014) Emergent presentation of a cat with dystrophin-deficient muscular dystrophy. Journal of the American Animal Hospital Association 50, 130–135

Hague DW, Humphries HD, Mitchell MA and Shelton GD (2015) Risk factors and outcomes in cats with acquired myasthenia gravis (2001–2012). Journal of Veterinary Internal Medicine 29, 1307–1312

Jones BR, Brennan S, Mooney CT et al. (2004) Muscular dystrophy with truncated dystrophin in a family of Japanese Spitz dogs. Journal of the Neurological Sciences 217, 143–149

Kornegay JN, Bogan JR and Bogan DJ (2012) Canine models of Duchenne muscular dystrophy and their use in therapeutic strategies. Mammalian Genome 23, 85–108

Marioni-Henry K, Haworth P, Scott H et al. (2014) Sarcolemmal specific collagen VI deficient myopathy in a Labrador Retriever. Journal of Veterinary Internal Medicine 28, 243–249

Maurer M, Mary J, Guillaud L et al. (2012) Centronuclear myopathy in Labrador Retrievers: a recent founder mutation in the PTPLA gene has rapidly disseminated worldwide. PLoS One 7, e46408

Munday JS, Shelton GD, Willox S and Kingsbury DD (2014) Muscular dystrophy due to a sarcoglycan deficiency in a female Dobermann dog. Journal of Small Animal Practice 56, 414–416

O'Brien DP, Johnson GC, Liu LA et al. (2001) Laminin α2 (merosin)-deficient muscular dystrophy and demyelinating neuropathy in two cats. Journal of the Neurological Sciences 189, 37–43

Paciello O, Maiolino P, Fatone G and Papparella S (2003) Mitochondrial myopathy in a German Shepherd dog. Veterinary Pathology 40, 507–511

Platt SR (2002) Neuromuscular complications in endocrine and metabolic disorders. Veterinary Clinics of North America: Small Animal Practice 32, 125–146

Platt SR and Garosi LS (2004) Myopathic weakness and collapse. Veterinary Clinics of North America: Small Animal Practice 34, 1281–1306

Platt SR and Olby N (2013) BSAVA Manual of Canine and Feline Neurology, 4th edn. BSAVA Publications, Gloucester

Poncelet L, Resibois A, Engvall E and Shelton GD (2003) Laminin α2 deficiency-associated muscular dystrophy in a Maine coon cat. Journal of Small Animal Practice 44, 550–552

Schatzberg SJ, Olby NJ, Breen M et al. (1999) Molecular analysis of a spontaneous dystrophin 'knockout' dog. Neuromuscular Disorders 9, 289–295

Schatzberg SJ and Shelton GD (2004) Newly identified neuromuscular disorders. Veterinary Clinics of North America: Small Animal Practice 34, 1497–1524

Sharp NJH, Kornegay JN, Van Camp SD et al. (1991) An error in dystrophin mRNA processing in Golden Retriever muscular dystrophy, an animal homologue of Duchenne muscular dystrophy. Genomics 13, 115–121

Shelton GD (2002) Myasthenia gravis and disorders of neuromuscular transmission. Veterinary Clinics of North America: Small Animal Practice 32, 189–206

Shelton GD (2010b) From dog to man: the broad spectrum of inflammatory myopathies. Neuromuscular Disorders 17, 663–670

Shelton GD (2010a) Routine and specialized laboratory testing for the diagnosis of neuromuscular diseases in dogs and cats. Veterinary Clinical Pathology 39, 278–295

Shelton GD and Engvall E (2005) Canine and feline models of human inherited muscle diseases. Neuromuscular Disorders 15, 127–138

Shelton GD, Ho M and Kass PA (2000) Risk factors for acquired myasthenia gravis in cats: 105 cases (1986–1998). Journal of the American Veterinary Medical Association 216, 55–57

Shelton GD and Lindstrom (2001) Spontaneous remission in canine myasthenia gravis: implications for assessing human MG therapies. Neurology 57, 2139–2141

Shelton GD, Liu LA and Guo LT (2001) Muscular dystrophy in female dogs. Journal of Veterinary Internal Medicine 15, 240–244

Shelton GD, Nyhan WL, Kass PH et al. (1998) Analysis of organic acids, amino acids, and carnitine in dogs with lipid storage myopathy. Muscle Nerve 21, 1202–1205

Shelton GD, Rider BE, Child G et al. (2015) X-linked myotubular myopathy in Rottweiler dogs is caused by a missense mutation in exon 11 of the MTM1 gene. Skeletal Muscle 5, 1

Shelton GD, Schule A and Kass PA (1997) Risk factors for acquired myasthenia gravis in dogs: 1,154 cases (1991–1995) Journal of the American Veterinary Medical Association 211, 1428–1431

Smith BF, Kornegay JN, Duan D (2007) Independent canine models of Duchenne muscular dystrophy due to intronic insertions of repetitive dDNA. Molecular Therapeutics 15(Suppl 1), S51

Smith BF, Yue Y, Woods PR et al. (2011) An intronic LINE-1 element insertion in the dystrophin gene aborts dystrophin expression and results in Duchenne-like muscular dystrophy in the Corgi breed. Laboratory Investigation 91, 216–231

Vijayasarathy C, Giger U, Prociuk U et al. (1994) Canine mitochondrial myopathy associated with reduced mitochondrial mRNA and altered cytochrome C oxidase activities in fibroblasts and skeletal muscle. Comparative Biochemistry and Physiology – Part A: Molecular and Integrative Physiology 109, 887–894

Villiers E and Ristic J (2016) BSAVA Manual of Canine and Feline Clinical Pathology, 3rd edn. BSAVA Publications, Gloucester

Vite CH (2002) Myotonia and disorders of altered muscle cell membrane excitability. Veterinary Clinics of North America: Small Animal Practice 32, 169–187

Walmsley GL, Arechavala-Gomeza V, Fernandez-Fuente M et al. (2010) A Duchenne muscular dystrophy gene hot spot mutation in dystrophin deficient Cavalier King Charles spaniels is amenable to exon 51 skipping. PLoS One 5, e8647

Winand NJ, Edwards M, Pradham D et al. (1994) Deletion of the dystrophin muscle promotor in feline muscular dystrophy. Neuromuscular Disorders 4, 433–445

Winand N, Pradham D and Cooper B (1994) Molecular characterization of severe Duchenne-type muscular dystrophy in a family of Rottweiler dogs. Proceedings of Molecular Mechanisms of Neuromuscular Disease. Muscular Dystrophy Association, Tucson, AZ, USA

Chapter 11

Tumours of the musculoskeletal system

Nicholas J. Bacon

> 'In the world of surgical oncology: Biology is King; selection is Queen, and the technical details of surgical procedures are the Princes and Princesses of the realm. Occasionally the Prince and Princess try to usurp the throne; they almost always fail to overcome the powerful forces of the King and Queen.'
>
> Cady, Memorial Sloan Kettering, 1997

Cancer, perhaps more than any other ailment, is an individualized disease. If tumours are viewed and treated the same in every patient without an appreciation of the underlying natural history, biology, response to treatment and prognostic factors, the optimal outcome for owner and animal is rarely achieved.

All tumours in the body fall into one of three broad categories based on cell type:

- Epithelial – of glandular origin, e.g. adenomas, carcinomas
- Round cell – e.g. lymphoma, mast cell tumour, plasma cell neoplasia, histiocytic neoplasia, melanoma
- Mesenchymal – of connective tissue origin, e.g. sarcomas.

Tumours of the musculoskeletal system are therefore predominantly sarcomas that originate from bone, cartilage, joint capsule, nerve, blood vessels and connective tissue. They are usually malignant; benign mesenchymal tumours are sadly rare.

Mesenchymal tumours typically spread haematogenously. Therefore, most metastases are found in large vascular beds such as the lungs (primarily), the liver or spleen; staging tests should be focused accordingly. Lymphatic metastases are significantly less common than epithelial or round cell tumours; lymph nodes should be aspirated on the rare occasion they are enlarged or firm, but nodal disease is uncommon. There are notable exceptions to this rule, the most common being synovial cell sarcoma where nodal metastasis can be present in up to 40% of cases.

Due to the absence of glandular tissue in the musculoskeletal system, if an epithelial tumour is diagnosed (e.g. a carcinoma in bone), it must by definition be a secondary tumour. Round cell tumours in the musculoskeletal system (e.g. plasma cell, mast cell tumour, lymphoma) may be primary or secondary due to the ubiquitous nature of the cell types involved.

Pain is a consistent finding in tumours affecting the skeleton, whether they be appendicular (long bone) or axial (flat bone) in location. In contrast, tumours of soft tissues are usually painless initially and present either because of a visible mass, or from consequences of its physical presence, for example pain from compartment syndrome, compression of a nerve, limb oedema due to lymphatic or venous obstruction, or subcutaneous or muscular haemorrhage.

Most sarcomas, as a result of their behaviour, present two distinct challenges for the clinician:

- A locally invasive primary mass with microscopic extension of tumour 'fingers' along fascial planes and into surrounding tissues
- Possible micro- or macroscopic metastases, either in circulation or settled in remote sites.

Addressing only one of these problems and ignoring the other may undermine the whole treatment plan for the patient. Decision-making for an individual tumour and patient depends on factors such as:

- Tumour type (histogenesis)
- How aggressive the tumour is histologically (the grade, see Figure 11.1)
- Whether or not the tumour has metastasized (see Figure 3.5 in the *BSAVA Manual of Canine and Feline Oncology, 3rd edn*)
- Known prognostic factors for that tumour type
- Anticipated biological behaviour of the tumour type, based on published literature
- Patient factors, e.g. co-morbidities, anatomical location
- Owner factors, e.g. previous experiences with cancer (often another pet, human family member, friend), finances, availability of various treatment modalities (e.g. radiotherapy)
- The goal of treatment; whether diagnostic, palliation, control or cure.

Stage	Grade	Site
1A	Low-grade	Intraosseus/paraosseus
1B	Low-grade	Soft tissue extension
2A	High-grade	Intraosseus/paraosseus
2B	High-grade	Soft tissue extension
3	Any grade	Regional or distant metastasis

11.1 Enneking's classification of musculoskeletal sarcomas, applicable to osteosarcoma in dogs.

Tumour grading

The histological grading of most mesenchymal tumours (where it has been defined) relies on a scale of increasing biological aggressiveness (grade 1, 2, 3). Grading of canine osteosarcomas is modified from the human system and is based (Kirpensteijn *et al.*, 2002) on:

- Degree of nuclear pleomorphism
- Number of mitoses
- Matrix production
- Tumour cell density
- Degree of tumour necrosis.

Applying these published criteria to appendicular osteosarcoma, 4% were identified as grade 1, 21% were grade 2 and 75% were grade 3. A recent reclassification aimed to assess only nuclear pleomorphism, mitotic index and degree of necrosis to give a histological score (1–10) that was then converted into a grade (1, 2 or 3 (Loukopoulos and Robinson, 2007). This latter system was applied to 140 primary canine appendicular and axial osteosarcomas which revealed 28% were grade 1 (low grade), 37% were grade 2 and 35% were grade 3 (high grade). Appendicular osteosarcomas, had a significantly higher mitotic index than axial ones. In all cases grade 3 tumours are associated with a higher rate of metastasis (see Figure 11.1).

Chondrosarcoma grading is also adapted from a previous human scale and is based on:

- Matrix production
- Architecture
- Degree of pleomorphism
- Cellularity
- Necrosis
- Mitosis.

Broadly, tumours can be graded as 24% grade 1, 52% grade 2 and 24% grade 3. The reported rates of pulmonary metastasis are grade 1, 0%, grade 2, 31% and grade 3, 50% (Farese *et al.*, 2009).

Tumour staging

The staging of canine osteosarcoma is modified from Enneking's landmark human paper describing the staging of musculoskeletal sarcomas in man (Enneking *et al.*, 1980). This incorporates grade, local behaviour, and presence/absence of metastasis.

This system is practical for the majority of canine appendicular osteosarcomas in practice, which are typically stage 2B at presentation, before they progress to Stage 3.

For further information on tumour grading and staging, and their relevance to treatment options and prognosis, the reader is referred to the *BSAVA Manual of Canine and Feline Oncology*.

Primary tumours of bone

Canine osteosarcoma

Aetiology

Osteosarcoma is the most common primary bone tumour in dogs, accounting for over 85% of bone tumours; 70% of osteosarcomas affect the long bones and the remainder are axial or extraskeletal. Osteosarcoma is primarily seen in large- to giant-breed dogs, in middle to older age, although it is sporadically seen in younger dogs, smaller breeds and cats. It is a highly heritable disease with some large- and giant-breed dogs at more than ten times increased risk, notably the Greyhound (25% breed mortality due to osteosarcoma; Lord *et al.*, 2007), Irish Wolfhound and Rottweiler. In another study, Rottweilers that were neutered before 1 year of age had a three to four times greater risk of developing osteosarcoma than intact dogs (Cooley *et al.*, 2002). Most tumours originate in the medullary canal and the tumour expands, invades and ultimately destroys the cortex.

Clinical signs

Appendicular osteosarcomas: A variable degree of limping and/or soft tissue swelling is seen; often marked swelling is seen with tumours of the distal radius or tibia where there is little overlying soft tissue. The area of affected bone may be warm to the touch. Bone pain is a consistent feature, either at the walk or on point pressure, and because the tumour is composed of rapidly dividing osteoblasts producing tumour matrix and osteoid, an expanding soft tissue mass is often seen once the cortex is breached (Figure 11.2). Peracute onset or sudden deterioration of lameness can indicate a pathological fracture; these are just as likely to occur during low impact daily routine (rising, sitting, walking) as they are with extreme exercise (Figure 11.3).

Axial osteosarcomas: Axial osteosarcoma is predominantly a large-breed dog disease, with tumours of the ribs, scapula, pelvis and flat bones of the skull seen. Whether the tumour is growing inwardly or outwardly dictates whether or not a mass is visible or palpable.

- **Rib tumours** often present with a visible chest wall mass, but there are times when the mass is predominantly or solely intrathoracic and the animal presents for exercise intolerance due to compression of the great vessels, heart or lungs (Figure 11.4).
- **Scapular tumours** are more likely to cause lameness than any other axial location but the shoulder musculature is often effective at hiding the tumour and so delays diagnosis of a mass for many months if the dog is fully weight-bearing.
- **Pelvic osteosarcomas** present in different ways including lameness, difficulty rising, swelling, obstipation or urinary signs from the mass obstructing the pelvic canal, or fracture (Figure 11.5).

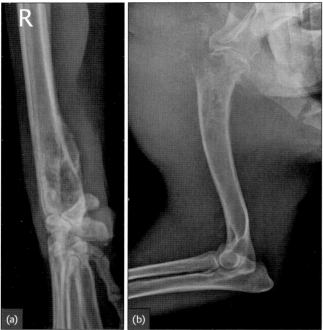

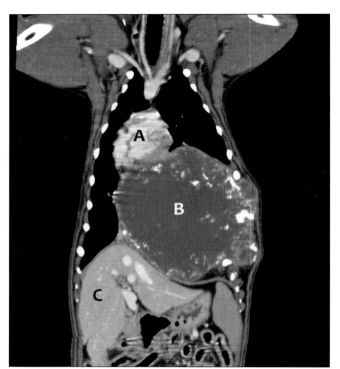

11.2 (a) A primary bone tumour of the distal radial metaphysis. Medullary lysis, sclerosis, cortical thinning, periosteal lifting (forming Codman's triangle) and soft tissue swelling are all apparent. This was confirmed as an osteosarcoma. (b) A permeative lytic pattern of destruction is seen in the proximal humerus with areas of spiculated mineralization extending into the soft tissues. This has hallmarks of being a very aggressive osteosarcoma.

11.4 Dorsal plane CT image showing an osteosarcoma originating in the seventh rib, with minimal external change, but causing significant clinical signs due to compression of thoracic structures. This mass was successfully removed allowing function to return to normal. A = displaced heart; B = rib mass; C = liver.

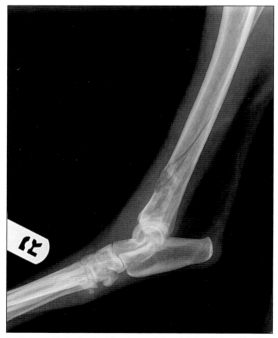

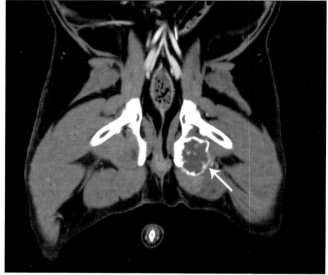

11.3 Pathological fracture of the right tibia in a Greyhound secondary to osteosarcoma. A lytic defect can be seen in the cranial cortex from which the fracture lines are originating.

11.5 Osteosarcoma of the ischium (arrowed) causing the dog to present with pelvic limb lameness. In this case, a hemipelvectomy was performed including an osteotomy at the mid ilial body, and pubic osteotomies cranial and caudal to mid obturator foramen.

- **Skull osteosarcoma** is more commonly seen in the maxilla and mandible, and less often on the calvarium. Halitosis and oral bleeding are often present, in addition to a mass within the mouth. If the tumour has eroded the mucosa, it may appear as a soft pink fleshy mass; otherwise submucosal firm bony swelling is seen. Tooth loosening may occur.

Diagnosis

Radiographs: Plain radiographs (two orthogonal views) of the affected area are indicated to identify areas of bone loss and/or proliferation. Osteosarcoma typically arises in the metaphyses of the long bones, with approximately two-thirds affecting the thoracic limb. It is probably no coincidence that 60% of the dog's weight is carried by the thoracic limbs, prompting theories that osteosarcoma results from chronic weight-bearing microfractures within the metaphyses. The distal radius is the most common location, followed by the proximal humerus. The distribution in the pelvic limb is more or less equal between the proximal and distal ends of the femur and tibia. Primary bone tumours have a variety of radiographic presentations but typically have a characteristic irregularly structured and expansile appearance, are not well marginated and rarely cross joint spaces; many have a marked soft tissue component.

Accurately identifying the extent of disease in the skull, scapula, ribs, pelvis and vertebrae can be very difficult with radiographs alone and computed tomography (CT) is often undertaken to help in surgical planning (Figure 11.6).

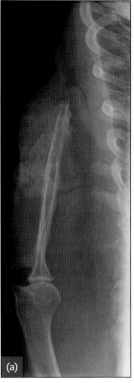
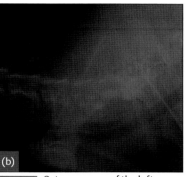

11.6 Osteosarcoma of the left scapula. (a) The cranial–caudal view is the more useful as (b) the lateral view has many superimposed structures, such as the opposite scapula and the cervical/thoracic spine, making determination of the tumour margins difficult. CT will better define the extent of disease and help plan the required osteotomy to remove the proximal scapula if a limb-sparing surgery is intended.

Biopsy: Definitive diagnosis is confirmed by biopsy. Techniques commonly used are an open biopsy, a Jamshidi™ needle core biopsy or a fine-needle aspiration. The main advantages and disadvantages of these are summarized in Figure 11.7.

Open wedge biopsies take both soft tissue and underlying bone in the affected area for maximal chance of a definitive diagnosis, but this comes at a cost to the patient and owner. Jamshidi™ needles are directed into the centre of the tumour (as determined by the most abnormal area on radiographs) and used to retrieve three to four core samples. There is still a sacrifice in terms of possible fracture risk and local tumour dissemination. Fine-needle aspiration is the bone biopsy technique of choice for this author and can be used for aspirating either the soft tissue component or the medullary canal of the affected bone. The latter is easier with ultrasound guidance to pass the needle through any cortical defects into the medullary canal. Unusually for a mesenchymal tumour, osteosarcomas exfoliate well, almost like a round cell tumour, and a diagnosis of 'sarcoma' can often be made cytologically. These slides can also be stained for alkaline phosphatase, whereby negative staining rules out osteosarcoma and positive staining is highly suggestive of osteosarcoma (Britt *et al.*, 2007).

For smaller, deeper, and more osteoblastic masses where fine-needle aspiration may not yield sufficient cells, image-guided Jamshidi™ tissue biopsy, using radiography, fluoroscopy or CT, is occasionally required. This author reserves open biopsy for cases where a diagnosis is absolutely required (usually by the owner) ahead of definitive treatment and the biopsy would not compromise the final procedure (e.g chest wall resection, amputation, hemipelvectomy).

Other diagnostics: A complete blood count, serum biochemistry and urinalysis (including specific gravity) are part of the investigation to rule out the presence of coexisting morbidities that might impact surgical and chemotherapy treatment options or decisions, as well as identifying any possible bone pathology related abnormalities, e.g. hypergammaglobulinaemia (myeloma), hypercalcaemia (myeloma, lymphoma), pancytopaenias (lymphoma), alkaline phosphatase (prognostic marker, osteosarcoma).

	Open biopsy (wedge)	**Jamshidi™ needle core biopsy**	**Fine-needle aspiration**
Advantages	• Large volume of tissue – most reliable • Tissue available for immunohistochemistry • Impression smears might allow for provisional interpretation 'in-house'	• Tissue cores (three or four) retrieved for histological diagnosis • Tissue available for immunohistochemistry • Impression smears might allow for provisional interpretation 'in-house'	• Lowest risk of post-biopsy fracture • Least expensive • Sedation and local anaesthesia • Aspirates of soft tissue extension may be sufficient • Can be provisionally interpreted 'in-house' • Minimal impact on surgical or radiation limb-sparing options or outcomes
Disadvantages	• General anaesthesia required • Open surgical procedure – most expensive • Greatest postoperative pain • Greatest risk of post-biopsy fracture • Greatest local dissemination of tumour cells • May negatively impact options or outcome of surgical or radiation limb-spare due to tumour-contaminated biopsy tract and tumour-bearing local haemorrhage	• General anaesthesia required • Cost of Jamshidi™ needle • Relative risk of post-biopsy fracture • Creates tumour-contaminated biopsy tract • May negatively impact options or outcome of surgical or radiation limb-spare due to tumour-contaminated biopsy tract, especially if needle crosses into soft tissues deep to far cortex	• Ultrasound guidance often useful to help guide needle into cortical defect • No tissue for histological diagnosis • If cortices are intact, it is difficult/impossible to obtain sample from medullary canal

11.7 The relative advantages and disadvantages of different bone biopsy techniques.

Staging:

Thoracic radiographs: Three views of the lungs are required (left and right lateral, and a dorsoventral inflated view taken under anaesthesia); only 10% of dogs will have detectable pulmonary metastases at the time of presentation; however, smaller gross metastases or micrometastatic disease is present in over 95% of cases. The detection limit of radiography for a soft tissue nodule is approximately 7 mm in diameter or greater. CT imaging of the lungs enables identification of smaller soft tissue metastases than radiography does, down to 2–3 mm in diameter. In one study which compared thoracic radiographs and thoracic CT in dogs with appendicular osteosarcoma, pulmonary nodules were found in 5% of dogs by radiography but in 28% of the same dogs by CT (Eberle *et al.*, 2010).

Abdominal ultrasonography: This can be considered, although the incidence of abdominal parenchymal metastasis for appendicular osteosarcoma at presentation is rare (<5%) – it tends to be an end-of-life event with the patient being presented cachexic and emaciated. Abdominal ultrasonography is often omitted at presentation if other diagnostics, especially the blood work, are not suggestive of hepatic/renal disease, or other possible abdominal pathology, e.g. lymphoma, primary epithelial tumour, does not need to be ruled out.

Technetium bone scan: A scan should be performed if available as 8% of patients will have a second bony lesion at the time of presentation in another limb, rib, vertebra, or the skull (see Figure 11.8a).

Skeletal survey radiographs: These are of most benefit as a tool to investigate additional sites of bone pain identified during the course of a thorough orthopaedic examination, or to follow up unexplained 'hot-spots' on technetium bone scans. As a non-specific screening tool they are rather insensitive and are unlikely to find a true secondary bone lesion in the absence of other associated clinical findings.

Lymph node aspiration: If the draining lymph node is enlarged or firm, it should be aspirated but the metastatic rate of osteosarcoma to lymph nodes is reportedly only 4% at the time of diagnosis/amputation.

Occasionally a dog will present with osteosarcoma in two long bones simultaneously, often in two separate metaphyses. It may be difficult to know whether this represents metastatic spread to bone (i.e. Stage 3 disease, worse prognosis) or synchronous primaries (i.e. two primary bone tumours at the same time; Figure 11.8).

Treatment and prognosis

Appendicular osteosarcoma: Appendicular osteosarcoma is fundamentally a terminal disease. Therefore all attempts at treatment should be focused on pain control and improving survival. A number of poor prognostic factors have been described; the most reliable are in bold type:

- **Alkaline phosphatase above the reference range**, and failure to return to normal within 40 days post amputation
- **Lesion in the proximal humerus**
- **Detectable metastases (lung, skeleton, lymph node)**
- **Grade 3 is worse than grades 1 and 2**
- **Appendicular worse than oral osteosarcoma**

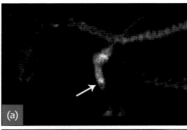

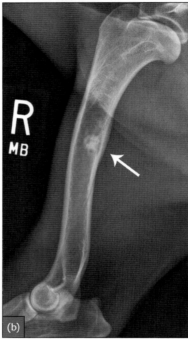

11.8 (a) A technetium bone scan in a Greyhound with a distal femoral osteosarcoma which showed unexpected uptake in the right humeral diaphysis (arrowed). (b) A radiograph confirmed the presence of a bone lesion at this site, subsequently confirmed to be osseous metastasis (arrowed).

- Bodyweight over 40 kg
- Telangiectatic (vascular) subtype.

Assuming the dog or cat has no evidence of macroscopic metastasis, all treatment options outlined below could be considered. In those dogs with macro-metastases, the same options exist, but the relative benefit and risks of the interventions must be carefully weighed against the current clinical condition of the patient, the expectations of the owner, and the experience of the veterinary surgeon in managing patients with advanced and terminal cancer.

Supportive analgesia: It is recommended to start with a single drug and then serially add in more to synergistically address bone pain, which can at times be severe. Pain medications are combined with soft bedding and less intense exercise if the dog is lame:

- Non-steroidal anti-inflammatory drugs
- Paracetamol (in UK only licensed for dogs in combination with codeine as Pardale V™):
  10 mg/kg orally q12h
- Tramadol: 2–5 mg/kg orally q8h
  For bone pain, doses as high as 10 mg/kg can be used but more side effects are seen, i.e. sedation and constipation
- Gabapentin: 3–10 mg/kg orally q8h
- Amantadine: 3–5 mg/kg orally q24h.

The expectation with analgesia alone is approximately 3 months of palliation before either the pain is no longer manageable, or the affected bone suffers a pathological fracture.

Bisphosphonates: The use of this class of drugs has been derived from human medicine where they are used to treat post-menopausal bone loss, Paget's disease and bone pain associated with metastatic bone lesions, typically from breast and prostate cancer. They are toxic to osteoclasts and therefore reduce bone turnover, specifically resorption, thereby slowing bone destruction and improving bone quality in some dogs; in addition they specifically reduce bone pain. Experimentally, bisphosphonates have been shown to kill malignant osteoblasts. Long-lasting relief from bone pain using bisphosphonates alone can be seen in approximately a third of patients. Drugs commonly used include:

- Alendronate at a dose of 10 mg/dog once daily. The bioavailability of this drug in the dog is poor (10 times less than pamidronate and 100 times less than zoledronate) but it is the least expensive of the bisphosphonates
- Pamidronate at a dose of 1 mg/kg in 500 ml saline and given by intravenous infusion over 2 hours every 3–4 weeks
- Zoledronate at a dose of 0.1–0.25 mg/kg in 100 ml 0.9% saline (dogs) given intravenously over 15 minutes every 4–6 weeks (author's choice).

Checking renal function (creatinine, urea, urine specific gravity) is indicated prior to administration as they are renally excreted. In humans, side effects include transient bone aching and mandibular osteonecrosis, but these have not been reported in animals.

Bisphosphonates are rarely given alone for appendicular osteosarcoma. Instead, they are usually combined with supportive analgesia, chemotherapy or radiation therapy (see below). Euthanasia is eventually necessary due to intractable bone pain, or pathological fracture after 4–6 months.

Amputation alone: There is no faster, more efficient, economical, reliable and effective way of controlling bone pain than amputating the affected limb. This also eliminates the risk of pathological fracture. Mid-diaphyseal amputations are quicker, with smaller vessels being encountered, and they appear better cosmetically in the short term. However, the terminal muscles soon atrophy leaving a prominent stump, scapula or femoral trochanter. Depending on disease location, options include:

- **Radius** – mid to proximal humerus or full quarter amputation
- **Humerus** – full quarter amputation is necessary, i.e. including the scapula
- **Tibia** – mid-femoral amputation or coxofemoral disarticulation
- **Femur** – coxofemoral disarticulation is necessary.

Prognosis with amputation alone is approximately 3–4 months, with death resulting from metastatic disease which typically affects the lungs.

Palliative radiation (external beam): Radiation is very effective at controlling bone pain in some patients and can be delivered in a palliative or curative-intent setting (the latter is called stereotactic radiosurgery or stereotactic radiotherapy). Osteosarcoma is not very radiation-sensitive and so high doses are needed to sterilize malignant osteoblasts. Such high doses need complex delivery systems and advanced linear accelerators to spare local soft tissues, in anatomical locations where often the tumour is only a few millimetres beneath the skin. Therefore, radiation therapy is often prescribed in a palliative setting whereby the dose is not contoured as accurately to the tumour-bearing bone, so the surrounding soft tissue and skin receive more radiation and accordingly, a lesser dose can be given to minimize unwanted side effects.

Palliative protocols vary at the discretion of the oncologist, from doses delivered on day 1 and day 2 only, through to once weekly for 4 weeks. Each dose is typically 6–10 Gy, depending on the protocol, and delivered to the affected area with a broad margin of normal tissue. These doses are not effective at sterilizing neoplastic osteoblasts; instead the goal is to reduce bone pain. Improvements in gait may be seen within a few days to a week in most cases, but eventually pain returns, often after a few months. Side effects include whitening of the fur, some fur loss, and pathological fracture. Radiation can be combined with bisphosphonates and chemotherapy.

Recent work has shown the median survival of patients receiving palliative radiation and chemotherapy can be over 300 days (Oblak *et al.*, 2012).

Amputation and chemotherapy: Whereas amputation controls bone pain, it is chemotherapy that actually extends lifespan by targeting the micrometastatic disease in the patient. Chemotherapy agents commonly employed include:

- Carboplatin: 300 mg/m^2 intravenously every 3 weeks for four to six cycles
- Doxorubicin: 30 mg/m^2 intravenously every 3 weeks for five cycles.

Several studies have investigated single agent or alternating protocols of these and other drugs, but no protocol has been shown to be significantly better than others. Single agent carboplatin is therefore often chosen as it has a slightly better side-effect profile than doxorubicin and less tissue toxicity should extravasation occur during administration.

Median survival times reported for combined amputation and chemotherapy are in the 9–11 month range, with approximately 20% of dogs alive at 2 years. Dogs typically die from either lung metastasis or bone metastasis. Chemotherapy has not been shown to improve survival in dogs once detectable metastasis has occurred, although the author's group has had some anecdotal success in combining vinca alkaloids with doxorubicin in a gross-disease setting. However, once metastatic osteosarcoma has been diagnosed, the typical lifespan is 2–3 months at most.

Limb-sparing surgery and chemotherapy: Surgical attempts to preserve the affected limb are considered when it is believed by the clinician and/or the owner that amputation would be detrimental to the dog's quality of life, for example because of concurrent severe arthritis, obesity, neurological disease or myopathy. Alternatively, limb sparing can be considered if amputation and/or euthanasia are unreservedly refused for personal reasons. A wide range of limb-sparing techniques have been described. The choice of technique depends on which bone is affected, the familiarity of the surgeon with each technique, and the cost–benefit analysis for the patient. Choices for different locations include:

- **Ulna** – partial ulnectomy: for small well circumscribed tumours of the mid to distal ulna, the affected bone can be removed with a 1–3 cm margin either side and the limb functions normally. If distal, the styloid process

can be disarticulated without significant or noticeable change in lateral carpal stability (Figure 11.9). If the proximal osteotomy extends dorsal to the interosseus ligament, then the proximal ulna needs to be internally stabilized to the radius, typically with screws
- **Scapula** – partial or total scapulectomy: with a bone tumour of the scapula, it is possible to resect the mass, a margin of normal bone, and the overlying muscles. The scapular remnant is supported as well as possible by creating a muscle sling dorsal to the scapular osteotomy. Mechanical lameness is likely as the limb is now shorter than the contralateral limb and scapular support is lost, but function is deemed fair to excellent in most dogs (Montinaro *et al.*, 2013)
- **Radius** – selection criteria include tumours that involve less than 50% of the bone radiographically, no obvious metastasis, lack of pathological fracture, and that the dog is otherwise healthy. These mean that many patients are not suitable limb-spare candidates by the time of diagnosis or referral. If in doubt about the suitability of a patient for a limb-sparing procedure, making contact with a surgeon familiar with orthopaedic oncology is recommended at the earliest opportunity. If the primary clinician or the owners are considering limb-sparing, then any biopsy procedure should be withheld prior to consultation to avoid contaminating the surgical field with disseminated tumour cells which might increase the risk of local recurrence after surgery, or worse still rule out a surgical limb-spare completely. A number of surgical limb-sparing techniques of the radius have been reported.

- Endoprosthesis/allograft (Figure 11.10) – a cranial approach is made to the distal radius, working outside the expanded soft tissues surrounding the bone mass (the pseudocapsule) of the tumour. As much grossly normal tissue and skin overlying the mass as possible should be preserved to aid implant coverage and reduce the risk of infection. The radius is cut 3 cm proximal to radiographically abnormal bone and the distal section is disarticulated from the carpus and removed. If there is concern about the tumour invading or encroaching upon the ulna, the equivalent section of ulna is also resected. The bone defect is filled with either a metal spacer (endoprosthesis currently with two available lengths – 98 mm and 122 mm), or a section of sterile bone from a deceased donor

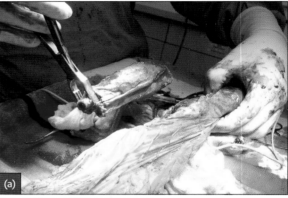

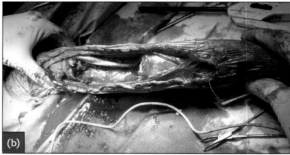

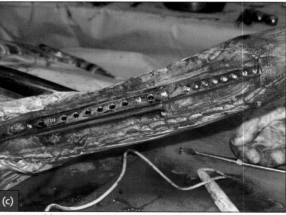

11.10 (a) The distal radius including the tumour is removed *en bloc* with the intimately attached distal ulna. The osteotomy is made 3 cm proximal to the radiographically and visibly abnormal bone. (b) The large tissue defect is evident between the ostectomized ends of the radius and ulna (left) and the proximal row of carpal bones (right). (c) A metal endoprosthesis is inserted into the defect and held in position with screws into the radius and third metacarpal bone. This effectively fuses the carpus in position, although a true arthrodesis is not expected to form as the carpal cartilage is not debrided, and a bone graft is not placed.

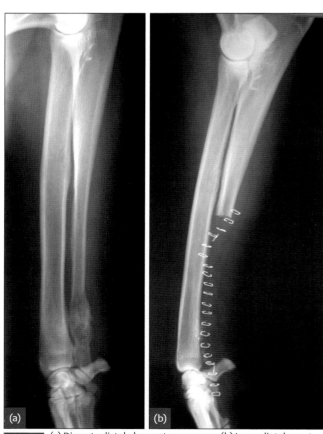

11.9 (a) Discrete distal ulnar osteosarcoma. (b) Immediately post partial ulnectomy; approximately the distal 50% of the ulna has been removed (the metal artefacts are skin staples). The limb is supported with a dressing for 10 days. The dog should be walking the day after surgery, with an excellent return to function expected.

(radius allograft). The endoprosthesis or bone graft is then held in position by a bone plate on the cranial aspect, extending from the proximal radius distally to the metacarpals, creating a carpal arthrodesis. In contrast to conventional carpal arthrodesis, no attempt is made to remove articular cartilage in the carpal joints and no bone graft is used. The lifespan of the patient (median survival 10–12 months with chemotherapy) means that bone union is not a priority, and no adverse effects of leaving the cartilage *in situ* and untouched have ever been reported. Complications include implant-related infection in 40–50%, local recurrence of the tumour in 7–28%, and implant failure (plate or screw loosening or breakage) in approximately 10% of cases. Chemotherapy is recommended.

- Plating *in situ* – a cranial approach to the radius is made without disturbing the pseudocapsule. A bone plate is contoured from the proximal radius, over the pseudocapsule and across the tumour mass and down the metacarpals: it is applied, with locking screws if possible to increase the strength of the construct, especially as accurate contouring over the irregular tumour and pseudocapsule rarely results in perfect plate–tissue contact in all areas. This technique provides analgesia by allowing the dog to walk on the implants and so avoid repeated stress on the neoplastic bone. Chemotherapy and bisphosphonates are recommended.

- Intramedullary Transcutaneous Amputation Prosthesis (ITAP) – distal limb amputation (for tumours of the distal radius) is followed by press-fit insertion of the ITAP into the medullary cavity of the ostectomized radius (Fitzpatrick *et al.*, 2011). The soft tissues, including skin, are attached directly to the ITAP, with dermal integration occurring over 3 weeks. Following ITAP, dogs reportedly walk pain-free by 8 weeks with a low risk of local recurrence. Systemic metastasis remains the life-limiting factor. Chemotherapy is recommended.

- Ulnar techniques – two procedures have been described. In **ulnar rollover**, the distal ulna is osteotomized, rolled into the radial defect and secured with a bone plate and screws. For **lateral manus translation**, once the radial segment is removed, the manus is moved laterally so the distal ulna buttresses against the radial carpal bone. Bone plates are applied to both the radius and ulna and down the third and fourth metacarpal bone respectively. Chemotherapy is recommended.

- Distraction osteogenesis – the tumour-bearing section of radius is removed, then circular external skeletal fixators are used to transport an intercalary segment of normal bone from the proximal radius distally to the radiocarpal bone, producing vascularized and viable regenerated bone which fills the bone defect. The frame is on the limb for approximately 90–350 days (typically 120 days for distraction from proximal to distal, then 70–80 days docked at the carpus for consolidation and healing). Chemotherapy is recommended.

- Stereotactic radiosurgery – a linear accelerator and advanced three-dimensional planning software is used to deliver a highly contoured dose of radiation to the tumour-affected bone. The cytotoxic dose kills both tumour and normal bone but the rapid drop-off of dose from the target means much normal tissue is spared, with often only minimal skin side effects. The advantage of this technique is that no resection of the tumour is needed, implant repair is not required, and almost any tumour in any long bone is treatable, unlike most limb-sparing techniques. Infection rate is close to zero, although approximately one-third of cases will fracture due to chronically weak cortices that have been further stressed by radiation necrosis. Internal fixation of such pathological fractures with reasonable function and survival time (364–897 days) has been reported (Covey *et al.*, 2014). In some tumours of the distal radius, where the cortices appear very thin and weakened, the surgical field and cancer can be sterilized by radiosurgery, and then a plate placed over the now irradiated tumour, to reduce the risk of the radius fracturing (Figure 11.11). Chemotherapy and bisphosphonates are recommended.

The median survival time for dogs treated with limb-sparing surgery and chemotherapy is not significantly different from amputation and chemotherapy and thus this option should not be chosen by owners believing it will give a longer lifespan. However, and somewhat paradoxically, if the limb-spare becomes infected, the dogs are expected to live significantly longer than those that remain uninfected, with reported median survival times of 480 days (infected) *versus* 228 days (non-infected). It is postulated that the infection acts as an immunostimulant that possibly upregulates anti-tumour immunity.

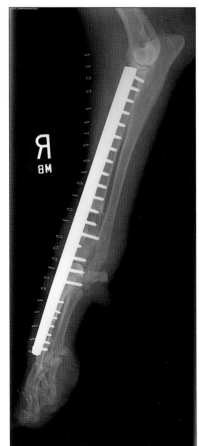

11.11 This Mastiff has undergone stereotactic radiosurgery for a distal radius osteosarcoma to sterilize the tumour. A bone plate has been applied to minimize the risks of post-radiation pathological fracture. The lytic bone in the radius and pre-existing ulnar pathological fracture can be seen beneath the bone plate.

Axial osteosarcoma: Axial osteosarcoma is as aggressive as appendicular osteosarcoma, except where the disease affects the mandible and maxilla.

Mandible/maxilla: Over 70% of dogs with mandibular osteosarcoma are alive and disease-free 12 months after mandibulectomy alone. The prognosis for both mandibular and maxillary osteosarcoma is dependent on achieving clean surgical margins. Maxillary tumours are often diagnosed in a caudal location in an advanced state, and the tumour can be difficult to excise cleanly. New surgical techniques are described that allow for a more aggressive surgery but maintain good function. For example, using the combined dorsolateral and intraoral approach (Lascelles *et al.*, 2003), previously untreatable tumours are now curable locally, with dogs now more likely to die from lung metastasis than local disease; the local recurrence rate is approximately 25%, with 50% dying from metastasis (Figure 11.12). Achieving tumour-free margins of excision in these dogs translates into a long disease-free life, compared to unresected ulcerated painful maxillary osteosarcoma.

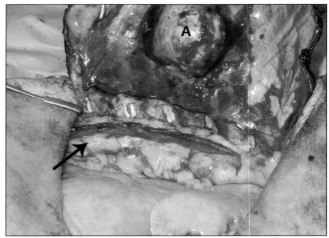

11.13 An intraoperative view of a chest wall resection for a rib osteosarcoma (A). Caudal is to the left; ventral at the top. The internal thoracic vessels can be seen running from caudal to cranial along the length of the surgical field (arrowed).

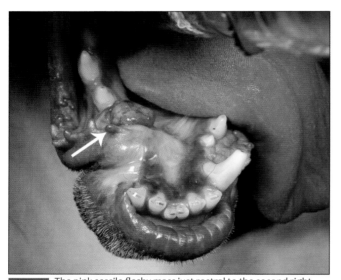

11.12 The pink sessile fleshy mass just rostral to the second right premolar (arrowed) is tumour recurrence following incomplete excision of a mandibular osteosarcoma.

Rib: Osteosarcoma of the canine rib is treated by chest wall resection of the affected ribs plus one unaffected rib either side (Figure 11.13). Median disease-free interval is 225–290 days, with 75% of cases dying from metastasis. Alkaline phosphatase has been shown to be a prognostic indicator for rib osteosarcoma post surgery; when it is normal, survival is 675 days compared to 210 days when it is elevated (Liptak *et al.*, 2008).

Pelvis: Osteosarcoma of the flat bones of the pelvis often requires a hemipelvectomy for local control, with removal of varying amounts of ilium, acetabulum, pubis and ischium to achieve a clean bone margin, depending on the origin and extent of the tumour. Functionally, these patients do well, following a similar pattern of recovery to coxofemoral disarticulation amputation. Given the complexity of the anatomy, local recurrence can be as high as 20% after surgery, with close to 50% metastasis. Median survival of osteosarcoma post hemipelvectomy with chemotherapy is 533 days.

Vertebrae: Osteosarcoma of the vertebrae is the most common axial tumour, accounting for 60% of cases in dogs. Patients present with back pain and variable clinical signs of neurological disease that depend on where and whether the tumour compresses the spinal cord (Figure 11.14). Like osteosarcoma in other locations, analgesia is a large part of therapy, with oral medications, palliative radiation and bisphosphonates all playing a role. Gross subtotal resection may be possible to decompress the spinal cord, but this would be working within the tumour (intra-lesional, or marginal at best) and therefore a careful discussion of risk–benefit assessment with the owner is vital. The role of chemotherapy is not known, as most cases are euthanased soon after diagnosis.

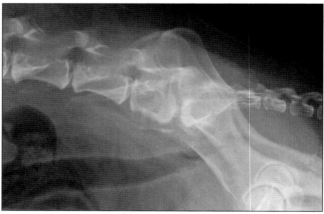

11.14 Osteosarcoma of the seventh lumbar vertebra in a dog assumed to have hindlimb weakness and stiffness due to non-neoplastic degenerative orthopaedic and neurological disease. Note the patchy ill defined lysis of the vertebral body of L7, with irregular poorly defined new bone along the ventral aspect and caudal endplate.

Feline osteosarcoma

Osteosarcoma can be located in the appendicular, axial and extraskeletal sites in the cat, with a roughly equal distribution between all three locations. The maxilla, mandible, digits, scapula, proximal humerus and tibia are the most frequently affected skeletal sites (Dimopoulou *et al.*, 2008). The high incidence in the subcutaneous tissues has been attributed to injection site sarcomas that produce osteoid.

Biological behaviour is very different to dogs, with only about 5–10% of feline osteosarcomas reported to metastasize. Amputation or wide local excision is the treatment of choice. Survival times of 12 months or longer are commonplace and chemotherapy has yet to be shown to significantly improve prognosis. It is reasonable to have a conversation with the owners about chemotherapy but there is no data to recommend it at this time.

Osteosarcoma of the feline mandible has an 83% survival at 2 years post mandibulectomy. The prognosis for the maxilla is not known but is likely worse, given the difficulty of achieving truly clean margins in the feline maxilla.

Chondrosarcoma
Clinical signs

Chondrosarcoma accounts for approximately 10% of all primary bone tumours in dogs. It has a very similar presentation to appendicular osteosarcoma, although it is more common in medium to large dogs rather than the giant breeds. In cats, 70% of chondrosarcomas arise in bone (63% are appendicular and 37% axial), and 30% arise in the subcutis, possibly associated with injection site sarcomas.

Diagnosis

Staging is the same as outlined for osteosarcoma, i.e. three thoracic radiographic views, complete blood count, biochemistry and urinalysis. Tissue diagnosis is made by fine-needle aspiration or Jamshidi™ needle biopsy. If chondrosarcoma is diagnosed or suspected after biopsy, no further body staging (bone scan, ultrasonography) is recommended.

Treatment and prognosis

Treatment options to manage bone pain are similar to those for appendicular osteosarcoma, including analgesia, bisphosphonates, radiation and surgery (amputation or limb-sparing if appropriate). The prognosis for appendicular chondrosarcoma is good following amputation alone as there is a relatively low metastatic rate. Survival times of 201–540 days without chemotherapy are described. Recently, it has been shown that survival is significantly linked with the grade of the primary tumour. It can be graded from 1–3 (low to high malignancy) and rates of pulmonary metastasis were 0% for grade 1, 31% for grade 2, and 50% for grade 3. Dogs with tumour grades of 1, 2 and 3 had median survival times of 6, 2.7 and 0.9 years, respectively, following amputation alone (Farese *et al.*, 2009).

Chondrosarcoma of the rib carries a good prognosis with a median survival time of over 1600 days reported following wide local excision.

Metastasis of chondrosarcomas is rare in cats. Radical excision of the primary tumour can result in a long-term control or cure.

Uncommon primary bone tumours
Fibrosarcoma

Clinical signs and diagnosis: Fibrosarcoma of the appendicular skeleton is an unusual malignancy and presents in a very similar way to primary osteosarcoma. It may not be possible to distinguish these two tumours on fine-needle aspiration alone and tissue histopathology following Jamshidi™ needle or open biopsy may be required.

Fibrosarcoma of the oral cavity is much more common than appendicular disease in dogs and cats. It usually presents with large ulcerated and bleeding masses affecting the mandible or maxilla. Diagnosis is by incisional or wedge biopsy as these tumours exfoliate poorly with fine-needle aspiration. Dental radiographs, skull radiographs, or CT of the head are all indicated for accurate surgical planning. Three radiographic views of the lungs are indicated.

Treatment and prognosis: The primary focus for treating appendicular fibrosarcoma is controlling bone pain. The metastatic rate of skeletal fibrosarcoma is not known, nor is it known whether the grading system used for fibrosarcomas of soft tissues is applicable to the skeleton (grade 1, least aggressive and metastatic, through to grade 3, most aggressive and metastatic). Little is known about the prognosis for appendicular fibrosarcoma post amputation.

Oral fibrosarcoma is best managed by wide local excision taking margins of normal bone of 1–3 cm, including associated and affected soft tissue. Depending on the location and extent of disease this might include a rostral mandibulectomy or maxillectomy, central or caudal mandibulectomies and maxillectomies, even hemimandibulectomies or unilateral maxillectomies, in both the dog and the cat. The median survival for oral fibrosarcoma in dogs following surgical excision is over 700 days with aggressive surgery. Approximately 25% recur and 25% metastasize. In cats with mandibular fibrosarcoma, 67% are still alive 2 years after surgery.

Multiple myeloma

Multiple myeloma is a systemic disease of malignant plasma cells and can present in a variety of ways, often due to a combination of hyperviscosity, hypercalcaemia and the presence of destructive bone lesions. Presenting signs include pain, polydipsia/polyuria, azotaemia, weakness, lethargy, heart failure and abnormal bleeding disorders. A complete blood count and biochemistry yield results consistent with a bone marrow disorder with decreased red cells, platelets and white cells. Hypergammaglobulinaemia is common and 16% have hypercalcaemia. The elevation in globulins is typically a monoclonal gammopathy and this is confirmed by protein electrophoresis. Bence-Jones proteins are present in the urine in 40% of patients. Osteolytic lesions are common, multiple, and are often seen in vertebral bodies, spinous processes and the pelvis. Pain and pathological fracture can be seen (Figure 11.15).

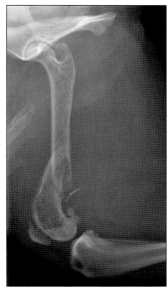

11.15 Pathological fracture of the femur secondary to diffuse bone lysis evident throughout the bone in a dog with multiple myeloma.

Treatment is with a combination of prednisolone and melphalan and a rapid response is expected. Melphalan should be started at 0.1 mg/kg once daily orally for 10 days, reducing to 0.05 mg/kg once daily thereafter until clinical signs worsen. Prednisolone should be started at 0.5 mg/kg once daily orally for 10 days, then reducing to every other day for 2–3 months. The prognosis is reasonable with median survival times of over 500 days expected. Negative prognostic indicators include multiple bone lesions with potential pathological fractures, hypercalcaemia and Bence-Jones proteinuria.

Solitary osseous plasmacytoma

Solitary osseous plasmacytoma is a discrete monostotic lytic bone lesion of plasma cells. This is a more typical primary bone lesion compared to multiple myeloma, and signs are more related to bone pain. Treatments include analgesics, radiation therapy and surgery. The role of adjunctive chemotherapy is not clear. It is possible this disease may progress to multiple myeloma but the incidence and natural history of that process is unknown. A survival of several years is reasonable if the lesion can be completely resected, for example in a digit or long bone.

Haemangiosarcoma

Clinical signs and diagnosis: Appendicular haemangiosarcoma arises from endothelial stem cells and displays very aggressive biological behaviour (Figure 11.16). It arises more often in the pelvic limb than the thoracic limb, and approximately 50% of cases affect the tibia. Smaller breeds of dog tend to be affected than is typical for osteosarcoma. Presenting signs include lameness, limb swelling and pain. It can be difficult histologically to differentiate from the uncommon vascular subvariant of osteosarcoma

called telangiectatic osteosarcoma, which occurs in 4–7% of osteosarcoma cases.

Thoracic radiographs reveal lung metastasis in 10% of cases at the time of presentation.

Treatment and prognosis: Treatment options are similar to osteosarcoma, with broadly similar outcomes. Median survival after amputation alone is 100 days, and this can increase to over 300 days with amputation and chemotherapy (doxorubicin, carboplatin or combinations). Substituting conventional chemotherapy with metronomic chemotherapy (continuous oral administration of low-dose chemotherapy) has been described for splenic haemangiosarcoma with similar survival times. The combination used is oral cyclophosphamide, etoposide and piroxicam (Lana *et al.*, 2007).

Multilobular tumour of bone/multilobular osteochondrosarcoma (MLO)

These are firm fixed bony tumours of middle-aged to older dogs that affect the flat bones of the skull, i.e. the calvarium, mandible and maxilla. They are very characteristic radiographically with a granular, coarse, stippled and mineralized appearance that often gives strong suspicion of the diagnosis even before biopsy (Figure 11.17). Although it may appear to have a clearly demarcated border on palpation and radiographs, CT often shows bone erosion away from the gross tumour edge and so is very useful in planning the resection. At least 1 cm of normal bone should be taken along with the mass. When involving the calvarium, this means exposing the brain and the bony defect is covered with local soft tissues or a moulded cement cap for protection. Prognosis depends on grade, location, and degree of excision. Mandibular MLOs have the best prognosis with a median survival post surgery close to 1500 days. In other locations, survival is 400 to 800 days. The metastatic rate of these tumours is nearly 50%, although metastasis tends to happen late in the course of the disease, and the secondary tumours often grow slowly. The role of chemotherapy in this disease is not clear, although it may have a role in the treatment of micrometastatic disease of grade 3 MLOs.

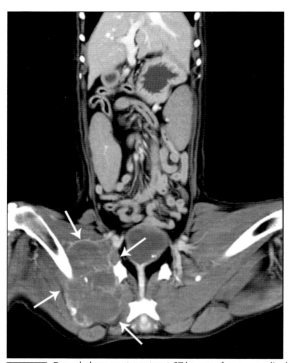

11.16 Dorsal plane post-contrast CT image of an appendicular haemangiosarcoma in the proximal femur of a German Shepherd Dog, with the soft tissue vascular component expanding along the ilium and into the obturator foramen (arrowed). This dog was treated with a hemipelvectomy, disarticulating the sacro-iliac joint and performing a midline pubic osteotomy.

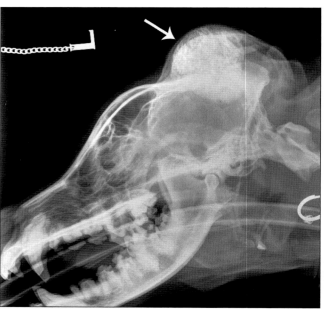

11.17 Classic appearance of a fixed multilobular tumour of bone on the calvarium of a dog.

Secondary/metastatic tumours of bone

Metastatic bone tumours are a differential diagnosis for any skeletal lesion. Typically they are found more in the diaphysis than the metaphysis of long bones, and they can be lytic or proliferative (Figure 11.18). The epithelial tumours most often associated with bone metastases include thyroid, lung, kidney, bladder, prostate and mammary. Apocrine gland tumours of the anal sac may also metastasize to the caudal lumbar vertebrae. Other tumours that can metastasize to bone include osteosarcoma and melanoma. Any bone lesion with an unusual presentation or suspicious radiographic appearance warrants fine-needle aspiration or bone biopsy; identification of epithelial cells demands a thorough search for the primary tumour.

Treatment options for metastatic bone tumours are primarily focused on palliation of bone pain. Surgery is rarely indicated due to the pre-existing tumour elsewhere; chemotherapy has no known benefit. Radiation would only be indicated in a palliative setting for analgesia.

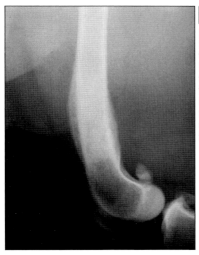

11.18 Radiograph showing a predominantly proliferative bone disease in the distal femoral diaphysis. Ultrasound-guided fine-needle aspirates from the area yielded malignant epithelial cells, later confirmed to be metastatic transitional cell carcinoma from the prostate.

Tumours of soft tissues

Synovial tumours

Clinical signs

Synovial tumours are rare but can affect a wide range of breeds and ages of dog. The most common synovial tumours are histiocytic sarcoma, synovial cell sarcoma and synovial myxoma. Animals often present with chronic lameness that is unresponsive to oral analgesia; the stifle is most commonly affected although in theory any joint can be affected. Soft tissue swelling can be seen later in the course of the disease. Up to 20% dogs will have metastasis at the time of presentation, and over 40% ultimately develop metastatic tumours.

Diagnosis

Radiographs may show often subtle bone lysis affecting both the subchondral bone of the joint and the adjacent epiphysis, although there may be no radiographic changes in some cases. These tumours will readily metastasize to draining lymph nodes so these should be palpated and aspirated as part of the initial investigation. Definitive diagnosis may be made on fine-needle aspiration, but an open biopsy is often needed to obtain tissue for histopathology and immunohistochemistry, if required. Synovial cell sarcomas tend to stain positive for cytokeratin on immunohistochemistry and histiocytic tumours are positive for CD18. Over 50% of synovial tumours are histiocytic in origin but only 15–25% are true synovial cell sarcomas. The rest are other mesenchymal malignancies. Given the marked difference in prognosis according to the cell type involved, definitive histopathological diagnosis should be pursued, including immunohistochemistry for cytokeratin, CD18 and smooth muscle actin. Histiocytic sarcoma is an aggressive malignancy that metastasizes widely, synovial cell sarcoma is locally aggressive and commonly metastasizes, and synovial myxoma is a benign but locally infiltrative lesion.

Treatment and prognosis

Oral analgesia will offer temporary pain relief. Amputation offers the best survival. Dogs with synovial sarcomas have been reported to have average survival times of 31.8 months for synovial sarcoma, 30.7 months for synovial myxoma, 5.3 months for histiocytic sarcoma, and 3.5 months for other sarcomas. Metastasis rates of 0% for myxoid sarcomas, 25% for synovial cell sarcoma, 91% for histiocytic sarcoma and 100% for other sarcomas are reported. The role of chemotherapy is not known. Histiocytic tumours have a worse prognosis with a median survival of less than 6 months, and over 90% metastasize to lymph nodes, lungs, liver and spleen. Radiation may play a role following cytoreductive surgery but insufficient data exist on this combination.

Haemangiosarcoma

Primary muscle (intramuscular) haemangiosarcoma is occasionally diagnosed as it can naturally occur in any tissue with blood vessels. It tends to have a high recurrence rate and incidence of metastasis. Often animals present with lameness or pain due to active bleeding within muscle fascia causing increased compartmental pressure (Figure 11.19). Staging requires a blood count and biochemistry, urinalysis, coagulation profile and then screening for metastasis: typically thoracic radiographs, abdominal ultrasonography ± echocardiogram.

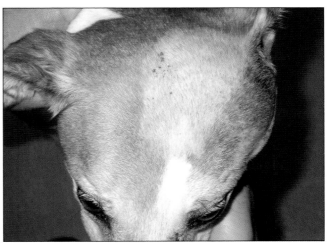

11.19 This dog presented with non-specific head pain and left-sided temporal swelling. Radiographs confirmed this was soft tissue swelling with no osseous reaction, later confirmed to be an intramuscular haemangiosarcoma of the temporal muscle.

Survival time is positively linked to smaller tumours (less than 4 cm diameter at diagnosis), absence of metastasis, and adequate local tumour control (often aggressive surgery plus radiation). Median survival time is 172 days. Chemotherapy can be considered although it has not yet been demonstrated to be effective at increasing life expectancy in these cases.

References and further reading

Britt T, Clifford C, Barger A *et al.* (2007) Diagnosing appendicular osteosarcoma with ultrasound-guided fine-needle aspiration: 36 cases. *Journal of Small Animal Practice* **48**, 145–150

Cooley DM, Beranek BC, Schlittler DL *et al.* (2002) Endogenous gonadal hormone exposure and bone sarcoma risk. *Cancer Epidemiology, Biomarkers and Prevention* **11**, 1434–1440

Covey JL, Farese JP, Bacon NJ *et al.* (2014) Stereotactic radiosurgery and fracture fixation in 6 dogs with appendicular osteosarcoma. *Veterinary Surgery* **43**, 174–181

Craig LE, Julian ME and Ferracone JD (2002) The diagnosis and prognosis of synovial tumours in dogs: 35 cases. *Veterinary Pathology* **39**, 66–73

Craig LE, Krimer PM and Cooley AJ (2010) Canine synovial myxoma. *Veterinary Pathology* **47**, 931–916

Dimopoulou M, Kirpensteijn J, Moens H and Kik M (2008) Histologic prognosticators in feline osteosarcoma: a comparison with phenotypically similar canine osteosarcoma. *Veterinary Surgery* **37**, 466–471

Dobson J and Lascelles D (2011) *BSAVA Manual of Canine and Feline Oncology, 3rd edn.* BSAVA Publications, Gloucester

Eberle N, Fork M, von Babo V, Nolte I and Simon D (2010) Comparison of examination of thoracic radiographs and thoracic computed tomography in dogs with appendicular osteosarcoma. *Veterinary and Comparative Oncology* **9**, 131–140

Enneking WF, Spanier SS and Goodman MA (1980) A system for the surgical staging of musculoskeletal sarcoma. *Clinical Orthopaedics and Related Research* **153**, 106–120

Farese JP, Kirpensteijn J, Kik M *et al.* (2009) Biologic behavior and clinical outcome of 25 dogs with appendicular chondrosarcoma treated by amputation: a Veterinary Society of Surgical Oncology retrospective study. *Veterinary Surgery* **38**, 914–919

Fitzpatrick N, Smith TJ, Pendegrass CJ *et al.* (2011) intraosseus transcutaneous amputation prosthesis (ITAP) for limb salvage in 4 dogs. *Veterinary Surgery* **40**, 909–925

Kirpensteijn J, Kik M, Rutteman GR and Teske E (2002) The prognostic significance of a new histologic grading system for canine osteosarcoma. *Veterinary Pathology* **39**, 240–246

Lana S, U'ren L, Plaza S *et al.* (2007) Continuous low-dose oral chemotherapy for adjuvant therapy of splenic hemangiosarcoma in dogs. *Journal of Veterinary Internal Medicine* **21**, 764–769

Lascelles BDX, Thomson MJ, Dernell WS *et al.* (2003) Combined dorsolateral and intraoral approach for the resection of tumors of the maxilla in the dog. *Journal of the American Animal Hospital Association* **39**, 294–305

Liptak JM, Kamstock DA, Dernell WS *et al.* (2008) Oncologic outcome after curative-intent treatment in 39 dogs with primary chest wall tumors (1992–1995). *Veterinary Surgery* **37**, 488–496

Lord LK, Yaissle JE, Marin L and Couto CG (2007) Results of a web-based health survey of retired racing Greyhounds. *Journal of Veterinary Internal Medicine* **21**, 1243–1250

Loukopoulos P and Robinson WF (2007) Clinicopathological relevance of tumour grading in canine osteosarcoma. *Journal of Comparative Pathology* **136**, 65–73

Montinaro V, Boston SE, Buracco P, Culp WT, Romanelli G, Straw R and Ryan S (2013) Clinical outcome of 42 dogs with scapular tumors treated by scapulectomy: a Veterinary Society of Surgical Oncology (VSSO) retrospective study (1995–2010). *Veterinary Surgery* **42**, 943–950

Oblak ML, Boston SE, Higginson G *et al.* (2012) The impact of pamidronate and chemotherapy on survival times in dogs with appendicular primary bone tumors treated with palliative radiation therapy. *Veterinary Surgery* **41**, 430–435

Chapter 12

Neurological causes of lameness

Sebastien Behr and Simona Tiziana Radaelli

Glossary

Ataxia:
- Incoordination
- Three types – general proprioceptive, vestibular (special proprioceptive) and cerebellar.

Paresis:
- Weakness can be defined as a deficit in the generation of the gait or the ability to bear weight
- Lower motor neuron (LMN) paresis is seen as an inability to support weight and the patient walks short-strided/lame
- Upper motor neuron (UMN) paresis is seen as a delay in the onset of protraction (the swing phase) and a longer stride.

Plegia:
- An absence of generation of gait (absence of voluntary movement).

Nociception:
- The patient's conscious perception of a noxious stimulus
- Because of the variation between animals in their response to noxious stimuli, the difference between the response to a mild and more severe noxious stimulus – referred to as superficial and deep pain – should be avoided and the term nociception should be used instead.

Proprioception:
- The patient's awareness of where the limbs are in space.

Introduction

Lameness is a common complaint in small animal practice and is usually associated with abnormal function or pain caused by an orthopaedic condition. Neurological conditions can, however, mimic orthopaedic disorders and lead to lameness as the main clinical sign. For example, in the case of a 'nerve root signature' (lameness due to nerve root compression), patients may be presented with lameness due to pain associated with nerve entrapment, often caused by lateralized foraminal stenosis or a peripheral nerve sheath tumour (Figure 12.1).

The term 'lameness' is rarely used when a patient presents with clinical signs that reflect a neurological disorder affecting one or more limbs; instead the terms *paresis* or *plegia* (with the prefix *mono-*, *para-*, *hemi-* or *tetra-* as

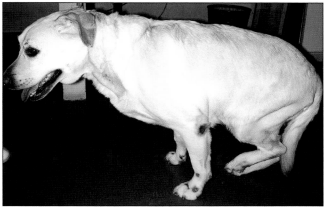

12.1 Labrador Retriever showing left pelvic limb nerve root signature caused by lumbosacral foraminal stenosis.
(© Sebastien Behr)

appropriate) or *ataxia* are more commonly used to describe the gait abnormality.

Paresis, or weakness, is defined as a deficiency in the generation of the gait or the ability to support the weight. The term plegia is used when paresis is so severe that the animal has lost any voluntary movement on the affected limb or limbs, even when well supported.

There are two types of paresis: upper motor neuron (UMN) and lower motor neuron (LMN):

- UMN paresis is characterized by a longer stride with a delay in the swing phase, and stiffness. UMN tracts, present in the spinal cord and caudal brainstem, run adjacent to the general proprioceptive (GP) tracts. Because of this anatomical localization, when a spinal cord lesion occurs, often the gait is the result of both UMN and GP deficits: paresis and ataxia. There is often also a variable degree of knuckling or scuffing
- LMN paresis is characterized by a short-striding gait, often with inability to support weight, especially if the radial nerve (thoracic limb) or the femoral nerve (pelvic limb) is involved. The LMNs that innervate the muscles of the limbs are located in the spinal intumescences (C6–T2 for the thoracic limb and L4–S1 for the pelvic limb). The cell bodies of the LMNs lie within the ventral horn of the spinal intumescences and they connect the spinal cord to the effector organs (the muscles). A lesion of LMNs affects the GP tracts but also the spinal reflexes (see spinal reflexes) and causes severe neurogenic muscle atrophy.

Ataxia or incoordination can be the result of:

- The loss of awareness of the position of the limbs (general proprioceptive ataxia)
- The loss of balance (vestibular ataxia)
- The loss of cerebellar 'control' of the gait (cerebellar ataxia).

The spinal cord can be divided into four regions and the neurological examination aims to determine which region is affected (Figures 12.2 and 12.3).

The three different types of axonal nerve injury and their prognoses are outlined in Figure 12.4.

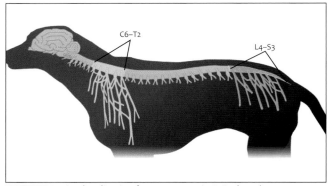

12.2	Lesion localization for monoparesis. Spinal cord segments C6–T2 and L4–S3 are highlighted.

Spinal cord segments	Neurological signs
C1–C5 Cranial cervical	UMN neurological deficits of both thoracic and pelvic limbs: gait abnormalities with proprioceptive deficits and normal or increased segmental spinal reflexes
C6–T2 Cervicothoracic intumescence	Reduced spinal reflexes in the thoracic limbs (LMN signs) with associated gait abnormalities and GP deficits Possible associated UMN signs in the pelvic limbs
T3–L3 Thoracolumbar	Thoracic limbs appear normal Pelvic limbs show UMN signs
L4–S1 Lumbosacral intumescence	The thoracic limbs appear normal Pelvic limbs show LMN signs

12.3	Relation of neurological signs to lesions of different spinal cord segments. LMN = lower motor neuron; UMN = upper motor neuron.

Axonal injury	Definition	Prognosis
Neurotmesis	Damage to the whole nerve, including axons, Schwann cells and surrounding connective tissue	Prognosis is very poor as regeneration of the nerve is almost impossible
Axonotmesis	Damage to the axon with preservation of the endoneurium and the surrounding myelin sheath (Schwann cells)	Axon can regenerate if the area damaged is not too extensive, but regeneration is very slow
Neurapraxia	Interruption of nerve conduction with no damage to the axon; usually caused by compression or transient lack of blood supply resulting in demyelination of undamaged axon	Recovery takes between 1 and 5 weeks

12.4	The three types of axonal injury and their prognosis.

Neurological examination

A thorough neurological examination should be performed whenever neurological disease is suspected. Gait abnormalities are more often caused by diseases affecting the spinal cord and/or peripheral nerves. However, intracranial diseases may also affect the gait.

Sensorium

Changes in the patient's sensorium (i.e. the entire sensory apparatus, including the reception and interpretation of stimuli) can range from dullness to coma and are often related to an intracranial disorder.

Owners might, in some cases, notice changes in the animal's behaviour due to pain: some animals tend to be withdrawn, while others might show signs of aggression.

Posture

The animal's posture at rest can be suggestive of pain or discomfort; low head carriage, for example, can be the sign of neck pain and kyphosis or lumbar hyperlordosis could be caused by thoracolumbar or lumbosacral discomfort.

Observing a patient's posture can also help to determine which limb the patient is reluctant to bear weight on.

Gait

The evaluation of the gait, best performed on a non-slippery surface, is a key part of the examination to determine which limb is affected, but it may not distinguish between orthopaedic and neurological lameness. The presence of scuffing, knuckling, dragging the limb or ataxia are suggestive of a neurological cause. Neurological lameness can affect either the thoracic limb, pelvic limb or both and can vary in severity from intermittent lameness to persistent non-weight-bearing lameness.

Palpation

Palpation of the muscles of the limbs helps to localize areas of focal muscle atrophy. Severe, rapid and selective muscle wastage of the lame limb suggests an underlying neurogenic cause to the lameness, whereas diffuse, slow and mild to moderate muscle wastage is more suggestive of the less aggressive atrophy associated with orthopaedic disease.

Palpation of the vertebral column may reveal focal areas of discomfort or anatomical abnormalities. Mobilization and flexion of the spine, especially of the cervical and of the lumbosacral areas, are used to detect pain and areas of restricted movement. When a lateralized caudal cervical lesion is present, flexion towards the site of the lesion is commonly resented.

In cases of thoracic limb lameness, palpation of the axillary area and caudal cervical spine are recommended to investigate areas of discomfort. In cases of pelvic limb lameness, palpation of the lumbosacral junction, including transrectal palpation, is recommended.

Postural reactions and segmental spinal reflexes

Thoracic limb lameness

Neurological thoracic limb lameness can be caused by diseases affecting:

- Spinal cord segments C6–T2
- The brachial plexus
- Peripheral nerves of the thoracic limb.

The most important peripheral nerves innervating the forelimb are the suprascapular, musculocutaneous, axillary, radial, median and ulnar nerves. The anatomy of the peripheral nerve supply to the thoracic limb is represented in Figure 12.5.

Detailed descriptions are given in Figures 12.6 and 12.7 of the most relevant nerves of the thoracic limb, including their segments of origin from the spinal cord, muscles innervated and localization of cutaneous innervation, together with the reflexes affected, loss of muscle function and the signs of dysfunction associated with lesions. This information can be used for specific neurolocalization of a lesion that affects only one or a few nerves.

Clinical signs that indicate a neurological cause of thoracic limb lameness are listed in Figure 12.8.

Pelvic limb lameness

Neurological pelvic limb lameness can be caused by diseases of:

- Spinal cord segments L4–S1
- The lumbosacral plexus
- Peripheral nerves of the pelvic limb.

The most important peripheral nerves innervating the pelvic limb are the femoral, obturator, sciatic, pelvic and pudendal nerves. At the level of the distal femur, the sciatic nerve separates into the common peroneal, tibial and cutaneous sural nerves. The anatomy of the peripheral nerve supply to the pelvic limb is shown in Figure 12.13.

Detailed descriptions are given in Figures 12.14 and 12.15 of the most relevant nerves of the pelvic limb, including their segments of origin from the spinal cord, muscles innervated and localization of cutaneous innervation, together with the reflexes affected, loss of muscle function and the signs of dysfunction associated with lesions.

Pelvic limb lameness is most commonly caused by a lesion of the femoral or the sciatic nerve. Clinical signs that indicate a neurological cause of pelvic limb lameness are listed in Figure 12.16.

Nociception

Nociception is the ability to feel pain. Nociception is composed of four physiological processes: transduction, transmission, modulation and perception. When testing a limb for presence of nociception, the clinician must look for a behavioural response from the animal. In other words, for a positive response, the patient should wince, yelp, pant or turn to bite. Withdrawal of the limb tested is NOT a sign of intact nociception; rather it is confirmation of an intact local segmental reflex.

Testing the presence or absence of nociception has an important prognostic value in the case of spinal cord or peripheral nerve injury: a positive nociceptive response is evidence of an intact neurological connection between the limb and brain and, therefore, a reasonable scope for recovery. Animals without apparent nociception show no such evidence of connection and this could represent complete and irreversible neurological injury.

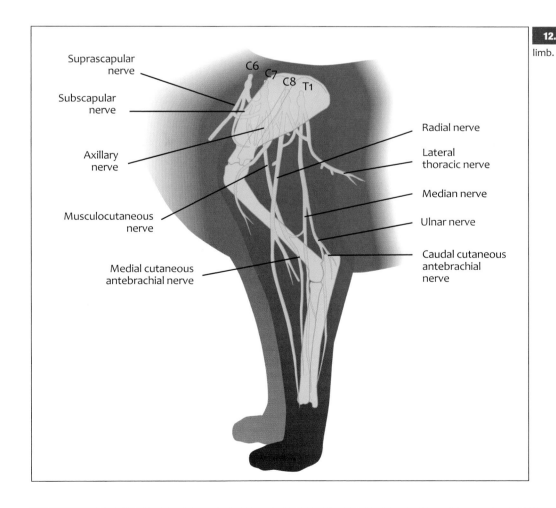

12.5 Anatomy of peripheral innervation of the thoracic limb.

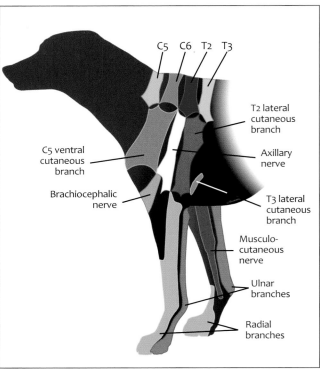

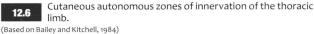

12.6 Cutaneous autonomous zones of innervation of the thoracic limb.
(Based on Bailey and Kitchell, 1984)

12.9 Miniature Schnauzer with thoracic limb monoparesis and proprioceptive deficit due to an ischaemic myelopathy. Note the knuckling of the right thoracic limb.
(© Sebastien Behr)

Nerve	Spinal cord segments	Muscles innervated	Reflexes affected	Muscle function loss	Cutaneous sensation	Signs of dysfunction
Suprascapular	C6–C7	Supraspinatus; infraspinatus		Shoulder extension	Shoulder	Little/limited gait abnormality ± shoulder abduction
Musculo-cutaneous	C6–C8	Biceps brachii; brachialis	Biceps; withdrawal (flexor)	Elbow flexion	Medial antebrachium and first digit	Little/limited gait abnormality; weak elbow flexion
Radial	C7–T2	Triceps brachii; extensor carpi radialis; digital extensors	Triceps; extensor carpi radialis	Elbow extension; carpus extension; digit extension	Cranial antebrachium and foot	Loss of weight-bearing; knuckling
Median and ulnar	C8–T2	Superficial and deep digital flexors; carpal flexors	Withdrawal (flexor)	Carpus flexion; digit flexion	Caudal antebrachium and foot; lateral aspect of the fifth digit	Little/limited gait abnormality; mild carpus hyperextension
Lateral thoracic	C8–T1	Cutaneous trunci	Cutaneous trunci	Cutaneous trunci		
Sympathetic nerves to head and neck	T1–T3	Dilator of pupil	Pupillary light	Pupil dilatation		Horner's syndrome (complete or partial with miosis only); ipsilateral peripheral vasodilatation causing elevated skin temperature

12.7 Origin and function of the peripheral nerves of the brachial plexus.

- Proprioceptive deficits of the affected thoracic limb (Figure 12.9) and eventually of the ipsilateral pelvic limb in the case of a lateralized lesion of the spinal cord
- Decreased flexor withdrawal reflex of the affected limb
- Absent cutaneous trunci (panniculus) reflex ipsilateral to the lameness. A brachial plexus lesion could cause this reflex to be absent along the whole length of the ipsilateral thoracolumbar spine, due to impairment of the motor efferent to the cutaneous trunci muscle (Figure 12.10)
- Horner's syndrome ipsilateral to the lameness (ptosis, miosis, enophthalmos with third eyelid protrusion) (Figure 12.11), due to a lesion of the sympathetic supply to the head that emerges from spinal cord segments T1–T3 (Figure 12.12)
- Neurogenic muscle atrophy of the affected limb

12.8 Clinical signs that indicate a neurological cause of thoracic limb lameness.

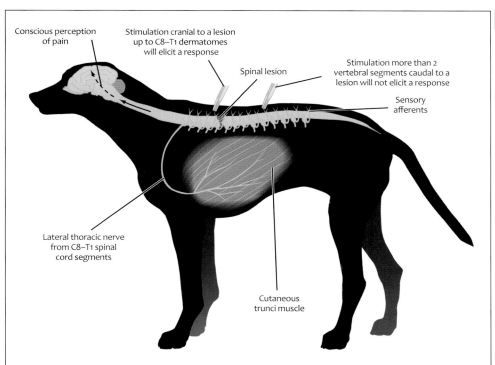

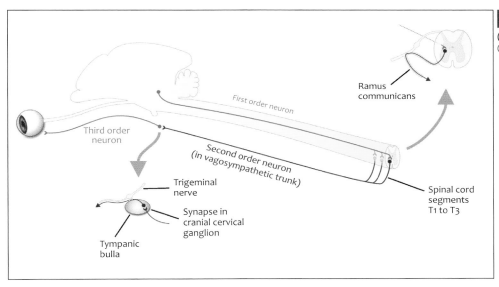

12.10 Neurological pathways of the cutaneous trunci reflex. Cutaneous stimulation along the thoracolumbar region often elicits a twitching of the skin. The twitching is due to confraction of the cutaneous trunci muscle.

12.11 Pathway of the sympathetic innervation of the eye (Horner's syndrome).
(© Jacques Penderis)

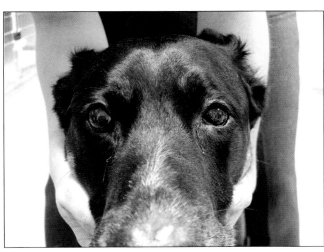

12.12 Dog with neurological thoracic limb lameness showing ipsilateral Horner's syndrome caused by a brachial plexus tumour.
(© Sebastien Behr)

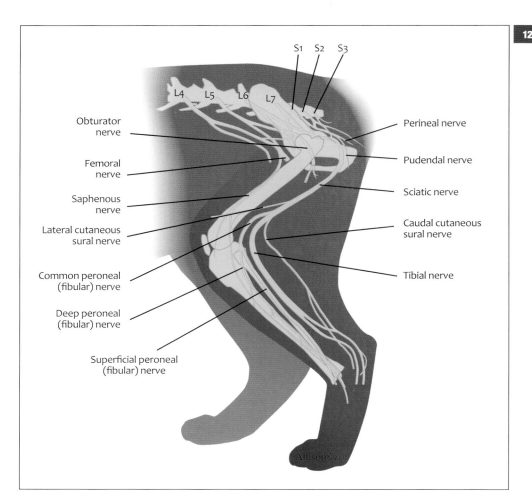

12.13 Anatomy of peripheral innervation of the pelvic limb.

S1 S2 S3

L4 L5 L6 L7

Obturator nerve

Femoral nerve

Saphenous nerve

Lateral cutaneous sural nerve

Common peroneal (fibular) nerve

Deep peroneal (fibular) nerve

Superficial peroneal (fibular) nerve

Perineal nerve

Pudendal nerve

Sciatic nerve

Caudal cutaneous sural nerve

Tibial nerve

Allison©20..

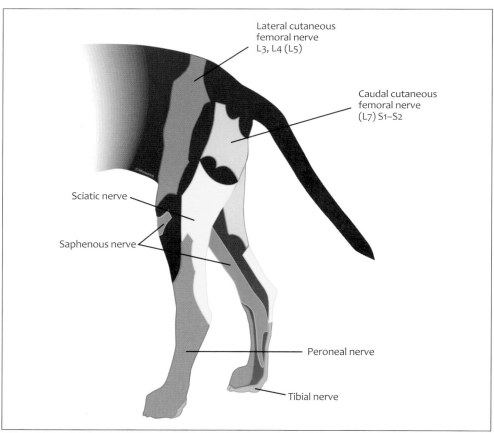

12.14 Cutaneous autonomous zones of innervation of the pelvic limb.
(Based on Bailey and Kitchell, 1987)

Lateral cutaneous femoral nerve L3, L4 (L5)

Caudal cutaneous femoral nerve (L7) S1–S2

Sciatic nerve

Saphenous nerve

Peroneal nerve

Tibial nerve

Nerve	Spinal cord segments	Muscles innervated	Reflexes affected	Muscle function loss	Cutaneous sensation	Signs of dysfunction
Obturator	L4–L6	Pectineus; gracilis		Hip adduction		Little/limited gait abnormality
Femoral	L4–L6	Quadriceps group; psoas group	Patellar	Stifle extension; hip flexion	Medial surface of limb and first digit	Loss of weight-bearing
Sciatic	L6–S2	Biceps femoris; semimembranosus; semitendinosus; cranial tibial; gastrocnemius	Withdrawal (flexor); cranial tibial; gastrocnemius	Hip extension; stifle flexion; hock flexion and extension; digit flexion and extension	Entire limb, except medial aspect and first digit	Knuckling of paws but weight-bearing present
Peroneal	L6–S2	Cranial tibial	Cranial tibial	Hock flexion; digit extension	Craniolateral surface of limb, distal to stifle	Hyperextended hock; knuckled paw
Tibial	L6–S2	Gastrocnemius	Gastrocnemius	Hock extension; digit flexion	Caudal surface of limb, distal to stifle	Dropped hock

12.15 Origin and function of the peripheral nerves of the lumbosacral plexus.

- Proprioceptive deficits of the affected limb
- Decreased flexor withdrawal reflex of the affected limb
- Decreased patellar reflex. Note that:
  - The patellar reflex can be physiologically decreased in older animals
  - A decreased patellar reflex with associated decreased extensor tone is likely to be clinically significant
  - The patellar reflex can also be decreased as a result of orthopaedic disease affecting the stifle, but when this is associated with a proprioceptive deficit, it is more suggestive of a femoral nerve neuropathy
- Focal pain on palpation of the lumbar spine
- Selective neurogenic muscle atrophy of the affected limb

12.16 Clinical signs that indicate a neurological cause of pelvic limb lameness.

Diagnostic procedures

In cases of suspected neurological lameness a minimum database (haematology and biochemistry and chest radiographs in patients over 8 years old) is recommended before considering more specific investigations that often are carried out under general anaesthesia.

Electrodiagnostic testing

The use of electrodiagnostic testing is recommended when the findings of the clinical examination are equivocal between a neurological and an orthopaedic lameness. If the duration of the clinical signs is greater than 1 week, electromyography can confirm a neurological lameness should spontaneous electrical activity be recorded in the muscles of the affected limb (Figure 12.17), regardless of the specific aetiology.

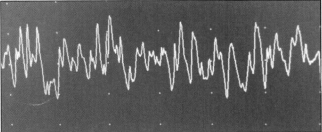

12.17 Electromyogram of the cranial tibial muscle in a dog recorded under general anaesthesia showing fibrillation potentials due to denervation.
(© Sebastien Behr)

When a neurological lameness is suspected, electrodiagnostic testing can provide further information on the site of the lesion (peripheral nerve, neuromuscular junction, muscle) and its distribution.

In veterinary medicine, electrodiagnostic testing can be divided into electromyography, motor nerve conduction velocity studies, repetitive motor nerve stimulation and F-waves. These procedures have to be carried out under general anaesthesia to allow sufficient muscle relaxation for the electromyography, and analgesia for motor nerve conduction studies. Further details on electrodiagnostic testing can be found in the *BSAVA Manual of Canine and Feline Neurology*.

Electromyography

Electromyography (EMG) is performed with a concentric needle that enables recording of the electrical activity of the muscle. Normal striated muscle is electrically silent under general anaesthesia, however, when the needle is inserted into the muscle, brief electrical activity occurs and insertion potentials can be recorded. Each muscle should be sampled at different locations and depths, as the concentric needle only samples a small volume of muscle in close vicinity to the tip of the needle. EMG should include recordings from the appendicular muscles of the limbs, epaxial muscles and masticatory muscles; in some cases further recordings can be obtained from the laryngeal, tongue, tail and anal sphincter muscles. The presence of spontaneous electric activity in a muscle (fibrillation potentials and/or positive sharp waves) occurs either due to a primary myopathy or secondary to denervation (see Figure 12.17). EMG alone cannot differentiate between the two conditions.

Motor nerve conduction studies

Motor nerve conduction studies are performed to further investigate peripheral neuropathy. Results of these studies are normal in cases of myopathy and/or junctionopathy. The recording involves stimulating a peripheral nerve at a minimum of two distinct sites and recording the compound muscle action potential (CMAP) distally. This enables the morphological analysis of the CMAP, its amplitude, duration and latency, as well as the evaluation of the conduction velocity of the nerve tested. For the thoracic limb, the most commonly tested nerve is the ulnar nerve. For the pelvic limb the most commonly tested nerve is the sciatic nerve. Nerve conduction studies can enable differentiation between axonopathy and demyelination.

Repetitive stimulation

This testing modality is useful when a junctionopathy such as myasthenia gravis is suspected. The set-up is similar to the one used for the motor nerve conduction studies but in this case ten consecutive stimulations and recordings are performed at low frequency (3 Hz). If the amplitude of the CMAP decreases by more then 10% after the third stimulation, a junctionopathy is strongly suspected.

F-waves

F-waves are later latency, lower amplitude waves compared with CMAP. F-waves are recorded after antidromic conduction along the axon of the peripheral nerve following electrical stimulation. Recording of F-waves enables the evaluation of the most proximal part of the peripheral nerve including the nerve roots. This can be useful in cases of suspected foraminal stenosis, trauma to the plexus and in cases of polyradiculoneuritis.

Imaging
Radiographs

Survey radiographs of the spine can be acquired to investigate for caudal cervical spondylomyelopathy, degenerative lumbosacral stenosis, discospondylitis, spinal trauma or spinal neoplasia as differentials of neurological lameness. Survey radiographs may or may not be diagnostic, therefore advanced imaging is often necessary to confirm the diagnosis. Contrast radiography (myelogram and/or epidurogram) is of limited diagnostic value in cases of suspected neurological lameness.

Computed tomography and magnetic resonance imaging

Computed tomography (CT) and magnetic resonance imaging (MRI) are the imaging modalities of choice to investigate neurological lameness, especially if foraminal stenosis or peripheral nerve sheath tumours are suspected. Both enable the production of three-dimensional images. MRI is superior to CT for the evaluation of intramedullary lesions, such as ischaemic myelopathy or intramedullary extension of a peripheral nerve sheath tumour. MRI gives better resolution of the soft tissue compared with CT, thus enabling better visualization of the nerve roots and peripheral nerves, especially when volumetric acquisitions are used. MRI sequences, such as STIR (short tau inversion recovery, a fat suppression sequence) can be very useful to detect an abnormal peripheral nerve, nerve root or plexus (Figure 12.18). An MRI study requires general anaesthesia and is more time-consuming and costly than a CT scan. MRI is also susceptible to artefact, should any metal be in the vicinity of the area imaged (e.g. microchip, metallic surgical implant).

Differential diagnoses

The most common neurological conditions presenting as lameness or monoparesis are:

- Trauma:
  - Brachial plexus avulsion
  - Sciatic nerve injury
  - Femoral nerve injury
  - Obturator nerve injury.

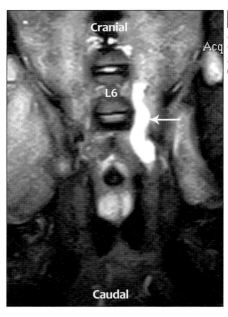

12.18 Dorsal STIR MR image of a lumbar plexus tumour (arrowed) in a dog.
(© Sebastien Behr)

- Vascular:
  - Ischaemic myelopathy and acute non-compressive nucleus pulposus extrusion
  - Aortic thromboembolism.
- Degenerative:
  - Foraminal stenosis.
- Neoplasia:
  - Nerve sheath tumours
  - Spinal tumours.
- Inflammatory:
  - Neuritis (immune-mediated, neosporosis, toxoplasmosis)
  - Discospondylitis.
- Toxic (tetanus).

Traumatic nerve injury

In cases of traumatic nerve injury, testing the nociception of the affected limb has a very important prognostic value. The presence of nociception indicates an intact neurological pathway between spinal cord and distal limb and hence a reasonable prognosis for recovery. The absence of nociception indicates a severely disrupted pathway between spinal cord and distal limb which carries a much more guarded prognosis; this is because recovery is not possible if neurotmesis has occurred (complete nerve avulsion/transection), as is usually the case with brachial plexus injury. Recovery is theoretically possible if axonotmesis or neurapraxia have occurred (see Figure 12.4).

Brachial plexus avulsion

The most common cause of acute neurological thoracic limb lameness and monoparesis is avulsion of the brachial plexus due to a traumatic injury. Often, this is caused by road traffic accidents or a fall from a height. The injury causes forced abduction of the limb which places abnormal avulsion traction forces on the nerve roots of the brachial plexus and causes damage. If the abduction is severe, the spinal cord can also be damaged which causes UMN signs in the ipsilateral pelvic limb.

Clinical signs

Clinical signs reflect the nerve roots affected. Onset is usually peracute. Clinical signs can be divided into three types depending on the nerve root affected (Figure 12.19).

The presence or absence of nociception (deep pain sensation) at the level of the digits is very important as a prognostic indicator in these types of traumatic lesions. A detailed map of the cutaneous sensory loss with brachial plexus avulsion can be found in Figure 12.20.

Diagnosis

The diagnosis is based on the history of a traumatic incident and on the clinical and neurological examinations (neurological presentation as indicated above and no other orthopaedic disease).

EMG can be performed 7–10 days after the trauma, by which time denervation changes will be detectable in the affected muscles. Nerve conduction studies may be performed on the radial and ulnar nerves to help determine the severity of the injury.

MRI and contrast CT (Figure 12.21) of the affected area may be used to evaluate the degree of soft tissue and nerve trauma and might help rule out associated vertebral

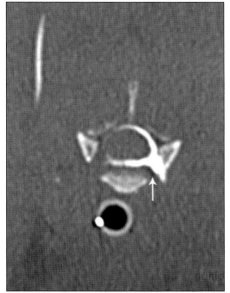

12.21 Transverse CT myelogram of a cat with a brachial plexus avulsion injury. Contrast medium can be seen escaping from the dura at the level of the intervertebral foramen (arrowed).

Type of brachial plexus avulsion	Neurological signs
Complete avulsion of C6–T2 nerve roots	• The animal cannot bear weight on the affected limb • The limb is flaccid and without any cutaneous sensation • Spinal reflexes and postural reactions are absent • The cutaneous trunci reflex is lost ipsilaterally • The animal may show signs of Horner's syndrome that is either complete, or partial with only miosis
Caudal avulsion of only the C8–T2 nerve roots	This disrupts the innervation to the triceps brachii; therefore: • The animal cannot maintain elbow extension • The animal cannot bear weight on the affected limb • Flexor function of the elbow and shoulder is unaffected; therefore, the limb may be held flexed into the body and kept off the floor • Cutaneous sensation is lost at the level of the caudolateral aspect of the antebrachium and distal to the elbow
Cranial avulsion of only the C6–C7 nerve roots	This is a rare injury: • The animal can bear weight on the affected limb • There is loss of shoulder movement and elbow flexion • Cutaneous sensation is lost at the level of the craniomedial aspect of the antebrachium • Muscle atrophy specifically affects the supraspinatus and infraspinatus muscles

12.19 Neurological signs of brachial plexus avulsion.

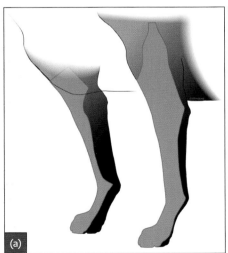 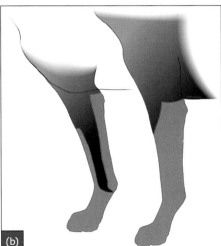 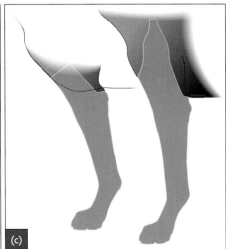

12.20 Sensory loss associated with brachial plexus avulsion. Shaded zones are dermatomes that lack sensation. (a) Cranial plexus avulsion. (b) Caudal plexus avulsion. (c) Complete plexus avulsion.
(Based on Bailey et al., 1984)

and spinal cord injuries (e.g. fracture, luxation, epidural haematoma), but are usually not necessary as the history and clinical presentation are highly suggestive, and the neurological examination confirms the diagnosis.

Treatment

Treatment of this injury is initially conservative. The severity of the damage to the nerve roots influences the recovery and the prognosis.

Aggressive physiotherapy plays a key role in recovery, especially in cases where nociception is still present. Gabapentin (10–20 mg/kg orally q8h) can be given in cases of paraesthesia that could lead to self mutilation.

Tendon transplantation or carpal arthrodesis can be performed to recover joint function and the ability to bear weight on the limb. This is only possible in cases where the proximal branches of the radial and musculocutaneous nerves are intact, to allow flexion of the elbow and the use of the extensor muscles. EMG is very important and is used to select the appropriate patients for these surgeries; the patient needs to have undamaged elbow extensor muscles for transplantation.

If the neurological damage is too severe and the animal develops self mutilation, joint contractures or damage of the distal limb due to paraesthesia and dragging, there is little option but to amputate. This is normally performed a minimum of 2–3 months after the initial injury to allow recovery of neurological function, should it be possible.

Prognosis

Cranial brachial plexus avulsion has a good prognosis if the animal can bear weight and has normal distal sensation.

In cases of caudal plexus or total avulsions with neurotmesis, the prognosis is poor to hopeless for recovery of function. In cases of neurapraxia the prognosis is good, but this is rare and functional recovery can take up to 4 months, as the axon regeneration rate in dogs is 1–3 mm/day.

The most reliable prognostic factor is the presence or absence of nociception. The presence of nociception is a good indicator that recovery may be possible and therefore supportive treatment should be offered. However, if there is no sign of improvement within the first 4 weeks, the chance of recovery becomes slim. If there are signs of improvement within the first 4 weeks (either clinically or on electrodiagnostic studies), the animal should be given at least 3–4 months to allow the nerves to recover to their full potential.

Radial nerve damage

Fractures of the first rib can damage the radial nerve proximally, while fractures of the humerus can damage it distally.

Clinical signs

Proximal lesions of the radial nerve present with lack of ability to extend the elbow, carpus and digits. The animal walks with a 'dropped' flexed elbow and carpus and digits knuckled over.

Distal lesions spare the function of the triceps muscle and therefore the animal can extend the elbow, but the carpus and digits are knuckled over.

Damage to the radial nerve normally has a good prognosis as it is usually caused by neurapraxia resulting from adjacent trauma. However, if neurotmesis occurs and the animal loses nociception in the lateral digit and cutaneous sensation in the cranial aspect of the limb distal to the injury, the prognosis is poor.

Treatment

Appropriate treatment of the fracture when indicated and supportive treatment of the nerve damage, with physiotherapy when possible, are recommended.

Sciatic nerve injury

The sciatic nerve originates from spinal segments L6–S2 and runs caudally in the spinal canal to reach the corresponding intervertebral foramina. Sciatic nerve injury is often the consequence of trauma to the lumbosacral plexus and can be caused by:

- Fracture of L6 or L7
- Fracture of the ilium, ischium or acetabulum
- Iatrogenic injury associated with pelvic fracture repair
- Fracture/luxation of the sacroiliac area
- Femoral fracture or hip surgery
- Surgery of the coxofemoral joint or triple pelvic osteotomy
- Intramedullary pinning of the femur
- Intramuscular injection erroneously performed on the caudal thigh.

The sciatic nerve can be damaged directly by the trauma, from the sharp ends of fractured bones, from inadvertent manipulation or damage at the time of surgery, or by the constrictive formation of scar tissue postoperatively.

Intramuscular injections to the caudal thigh can damage the sciatic nerve by direct laceration by the needle, or by secondary injury due to the drug injected. Such injections should be avoided.

Clinical signs

Proximal sciatic nerve injury presents with severe LMN signs. The animal is able to bear weight as the femoral nerve is still intact and therefore most hip movement and stifle extension is intact, but walks with the paw knuckled over and is unable to flex the stifle and to flex or extend the tarsus or digits. The withdrawal reflex is severely affected and cutaneous sensation is lost over the whole limb except for the medial aspect. With severe sciatic nerve lesion, loss of nociception can occur in all digits except the medial digit (which is innervated by the femoral nerve).

> **PRACTICAL TIP**
>
> Care should be taken when assessing sciatic nerve function because although it innervates most of the pelvic limb, this does not include the medial aspect, including digit 2, and the stifle extensors and hip flexors: these are innervated by the femoral nerve (see below). In other words, testing nociception on digit 2, or witnessing withdrawal that features hip flexion without stifle or hock flexion, confirms integrity of the femoral nerve, but not the sciatic nerve

In the presence of concurrent orthopaedic fractures, the animal can be difficult to assess neurologically due to the presence of pain and the mechanical inability to move the leg appropriately.

Treatment

Management of the orthopaedic fractures or scar tissue is recommended to relieve the pressure on the sciatic nerve.

Supportive treatment is recommended in all circumstances, to help the nerve in the recovery process and to minimize disuse muscle atrophy; aggressive physiotherapy should be started as soon as is allowed by the concurrent fractures.

In cases of neurotmesis with loss of nociception, or if no significant improvement is seen within 3–4 months, the prognosis is poor and there is little realistic alternative to limb amputation.

Obturator nerve injury

Obturator nerve injury is rare, but it can be a consequence of pelvic fractures. It causes impairment of pelvic limb adduction. On clinical examination the animal usually shows abduction of the affected limb when walking and pain at the medial surface of the left thigh. EMG can show denervation in the adductor muscles of the pelvic limb.

Femoral nerve injury

The femoral nerve is often damaged by L4–L6 spinal cord lesions, or femoral nerve root damage due to spinal disorders (neoplasia, disc disease, discospondylitis, trauma, vascular conditions). In these circumstances the clinical signs may be bilateral.

Isolated unilateral femoral injury is uncommon, as the nerve is protected by the sublumbar muscles. However, unilateral femoral nerve damage can occur associated with retroperitoneal disease (abscess, haematoma, neoplasia), trauma and iliopsoas myopathies.

Clinical signs

Gait abnormalities are quite severe with femoral nerve damage as there is a significant decrease in the extensor tone of the limb. The animal cannot bear weight on the affected limb and carries it with the stifle flexed, and cannot extend the stifle or flex the hip. The patellar reflex is severely reduced or absent, and cutaneous sensation of the medial aspect of the limb and the medial digit (digit 2) is lost. Nociception of the medial digit should be tested to check femoral nerve integrity. The quadriceps muscle rapidly develops neurogenic atrophy.

Diagnosis

History and clinical signs, as noted above, raise suspicion of femoral nerve damage; this can be then confirmed by EMG. In cases of retroperitoneal disease and suspicion of associated compression of the femoral nerve, an MRI study can be performed.

Treatment

Extensive physiotherapy and measures to protect the foot from abrasions are important to support nerve recovery.

If indicated, exploratory surgery can be performed to evaluate the degree of nerve damage and to attempt a repair via a neurorrhaphy (anastomosis) or neurolysis (debridement of the inflammatory adhesions from the entrapped nerve).

Prognosis

The prognosis depends on the severity of nerve damage. Neurapraxic lesions recover within few weeks, while axonotmetic lesions might take longer and have a higher chance of recovery if they are closer to the muscle to be reinnervated.

Repeated neurological examinations and EMG help with follow-up and establishing a prognosis as they allow early subtle signs of recovery to be documented. If there is no improvement within 3–4 months, the prognosis is poor and amputation should be considered.

Peroneal nerve injuries

The peroneal nerve can be damaged by traumatic injuries at the level of the lateral stifle. Common causes of trauma at this level are:

* Iatrogenic – orthopaedic surgery of the stifle, usually lateral fabellar suture placement
* Intramuscular injections
* Pressure from orthopaedic casts.

The animal shows proprioceptive deficits and weak flexion of the tarsus, together with reduced sensation on the dorsal aspect of the paw.

Treatment involves the removal of the cause (e.g. lateral fabellar/extracapsular suture) when possible and physiotherapy. The prognosis is often good, but it depends on the degree of nerve damage.

Tibial nerve injuries

The tibial nerve can be damaged by a traumatic lesion or by intramuscular injection.

Clinical signs include loss of ability to extend the tarsus, proprioceptive deficits and loss of sensation of the plantar aspect of the paw.

Conservative management is recommended in the first instance. If recovery does not occur within a few months and the inability to maintain hock extension is debilitating then pantarsal arthrodesis can be considered, so long as the lack of plantar cutaneous sensation is not causing skin wounds. The prognosis depends on the severity of nerve damage.

Vascular disease

Ischaemic myelopathy and acute non-compressive nucleus pulposus extrusion

Ischaemic myelopathy (also called fibrocartilaginous embolism) and acute non-compressive nucleus pulposus extrusion (also called type III disc herniation and low volume high velocity disc herniation) have a very similar clinical presentation, with peracute lateralized signs of spinal cord injury, which are non-progressive 24–48 hours after onset unless myelomalacia develops. Median age at onset is around 6 years with males overrepresented in acute non-compressive nucleus pulposus extrusion.

Ischaemic myelopathy is the result of an embolism of fibrocartilage that blocks afferent blood vessels and disrupts blood flow to the spinal cord, causing acute spinal cord infarction. The fibrocartilage has the same composition as the nucleus pulposus of intervertebral discs, but the exact pathophysiological mechanism of embolization has not been elucidated: different theories exist. Non-chondrodystrophic breeds are predisposed and cats can also be affected.

Acute non-compressive nucleus pulposus extrusion relates to the extrusion of hydrated nucleus pulposus secondary to a rapid increase in the intradiscal pressure during vigorous exercise or trauma. The spinal cord injury is due to contusion of the parenchyma with the small volume of extruded nucleus pulposus causing minimal to no spinal cord compression.

Clinical signs

Owners often report that animals show clinical signs acutely during or just after vigorous exercise. A very acute episode of pain may be reported, e.g. a single yelp. Progression of neurological signs typically stabilizes within 24 to 48 hours. In cases of ischaemic myelopathy, no spinal hyperalgesia is noticed 24–48 hours after onset of the condition, but in cases of acute non-compressive nucleus pulposus extrusion, this can remain present for longer. Clinical signs are often asymmetrical for both conditions (in around 60–70% of cases). In animals with a thoracolumbar lesion, a Schiff–Sherrington posture is common with this type of spinal cord injury due to the acuteness of the signs but this does not mean a poorer prognosis. Loss of nociception carries a very poor prognosis.

Diagnosis

History and clinical signs (acute, asymmetrical, associated with exercise) can be strongly indicative of an ischaemic myelopathy or an acute non-compressive nucleus pulposus extrusion. However, definitive diagnosis can only be made based on MRI, which enables observation of the intramedullary changes and differentiation between the two conditions whenever possible (Figure 12.22).

Treatment and prognosis

Treatment for both conditions involves physiotherapy, hydrotherapy and nursing care during the recovery process. Complete clinical recovery or partial recovery compatible with a good quality of life can be achieved in 80% of cases that receive necessary supportive care.

The prognosis depends, in particular, on the extent of the spinal cord damage and the presence/absence of nociception in the affected limb. If the animal recovers some function within 2 weeks, it has a better prognosis, although the recovery of normal limb function might not be complete. In one study (Gandini *et al.*, 2003), dogs regained the ability to ambulate without assistance 2 weeks after the onset of the signs in two out of three cases. Absence of nociception, LMN signs and symmetrical neurological signs are negative prognostic factors. Faecal incontinence is five times more likely in dogs with presumptive acute non-compressive nucleus polposus extrusion (23%) compared with presumptive ischemic myelopathy (7.5%) (Mari *et al.*, 2017).

Aortic thromboembolism

Aortic thromboembolism affects cats much more frequently than dogs and is most commonly associated with hypertrophic cardiomyopathy in cats. The vascular obstruction of the aortic or iliac arteries causes a lack of blood supply and the release of vasoactive substances that cause ischaemia of the sciatic nerve and pelvic limb muscles.

Clinical signs

Cats typically show acute onset of asymmetrical pelvic limb gait abnormalities. Weakness and eventually loss of nociception are common signs. The affected pelvic limbs are cold and the nail beds can be cyanotic. The arterial pulse is lacking in the affected limb. The condition is very painful, especially on palpation of the caudal abdomen and of the pelvic limb muscles. Cats can show signs of tachypnoea, hypothermia, arrhythmias and congestive heart failure.

In dogs, the clinical presentation differs from cats as the aortic thrombus tends to cause a partial occlusion resulting in more progressive signs of exercise-induced weakness in the pelvic limbs and intermittent mono/paraparesis. In dogs the most common causes are protein-losing nephropathy or enteropathy leading to a loss of antithrombin III.

Diagnosis

Acoustic Doppler ultrasonography of the metatarsal pulses can be used to evaluate the integrity of blood flow to the distal limb. Colour flow Doppler ultrasonography of the aorta and its trifurcation can document blood flow and show the presence of the thrombus (Figure 12.23). Echocardiography and thoracic radiographs are used to confirm the underlying cardiac disease. Blood haematology and biochemistry and urine analysis can help to identify other underlying causes.

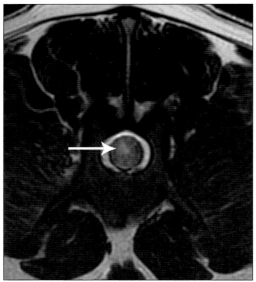

12.22 Transverse T2-weighted MR image at the level of L3 in a dog with an ischaemic myelopathy. Note the well demarcated hyperintensity within the spinal cord (arrowed).
(© Sebastien Behr)

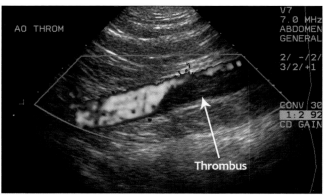

12.23 Doppler ultrasonogram of an aortic thrombus in a Greyhound with intermittent progressive paraparesis and exercise intolerance. Note the obstruction of the blood flow in the aorta (orange) due to the thrombus (arrowed), leading to hypoperfusion of the hindlimbs.
(© Sebastien Behr)

Treatment

The initial treatment aims at treating the primary cause, supportive care and prevention of further thrombus formation (aspirin at 10 mg/kg orally q12h or clopidogrel at 2–4 mg/kg orally q24h). Pain relief with opioids is recommended as part of the treatment of this condition. At present, no treatment (medical or surgical) of the aortic thromboembolism produces a significantly better recovery than no therapy. Use of thrombolytic agents to dissolve the embolus awaits clinical trials. Recovery can be achieved in 40–45% of cases, but recurrence is likely (around 60%) especially if the underlying cause is not treated.

Degenerative disease

Foraminal stenosis

Foraminal stenosis can happen all along the vertebral column, but it causes neurological lameness only if it occurs at the level of the caudal cervical, caudal lumbar or lumbosacral veretebral column segments. Should foraminal stenosis occur elsewhere in the vertebral column such as in the cranial cervical or thoracolumbar regions, the clinical signs will be pain rather than lameness. Foraminal stenosis can occur at the level of the entrance, the middle and the exit zone of the neuroforamen. The most common site of foraminal stenosis is the lumbosacral intervertebral foramen.

Pathogenesis

The disease processes causing foraminal stenosis are lateralized foraminal disc extrusion (Figure 12.24) or protrusion, articular facet osteoproliferation, vertebral malformations, and juxta-facet cysts (Figure 12.25), such as synovial cysts and perineural cysts (also called Tarlov cysts).

Clinical signs

The clinical signs most commonly encountered in cases of foraminal stenosis are ipsilateral lameness with associated nerve root signature, spontaneous pain or pain on palpation and mobilization of the affected limb, paraesthesia with excessive grooming/licking of the affected limb and LMN signs of the affected limb.

In cases of lumbosacral foraminal stenosis, discomfort on lumbosacral palpation (preferably performed in lateral recumbency to reduce false-positives associated with hip pain caused by concurrent hip loading) and decreased hock flexion are often encountered before obvious proprioceptive deficits are appreciated. In more severe cases, proprioceptive deficits and reduced or absent flexor withdrawal and tibial cranial reflexes can also be seen. In such cases, the patellar reflex can appear to be increased; this is referred to as pseudo-hyperreflexia and results from decreased tone of the muscles that antagonize stifle extension. Muscle atrophy, especially of the cranial tibial muscle, can be present.

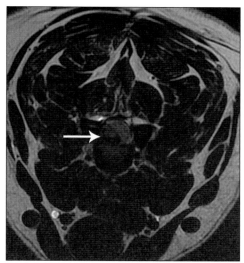

12.24 Transverse T2-weighted MR image of a lateralized cervical disc extrusion (Hansen type I) at C5 in a dog causing severe ventrolateral compression of the spinal cord and nerve root (arrow showing the lateralized disc extrusion).
(© Sebastien Behr)

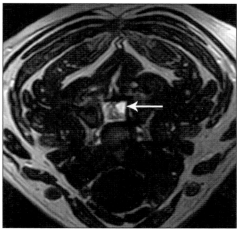

12.25 Transverse T2-weighted MR image of a cervical juxta-facet cyst at C5–C6 in a dog causing dorsolateral compression of the spinal cord and nerve root (arrow showing the juxta-facet cyst).
(© Sebastien Behr)

Diagnosis

- EMG can confirm the neurological aetiology of the lameness.
- Survey radiographs obtained under sedation or anaesthesia may be unremarkable but can sometimes show foraminal opacification (in cases of lateralized calcified disc extrusion), reduced size of the intervertebral disc space, osteoproliferative changes of the articular facets (Figure 12.26) or spondylosis deformans.
- Advanced imaging with cross-sectional images is the modality of choice to investigate foraminal stenosis. CT enables good visualization of the vertebral foramen and can identify bony proliferations (Figure 12.27) or calcified disc extrusions, but is less likely to identify soft tissue proliferation. MRI is the imaging modality of choice (Figures 12.28 and 12.29) to investigate soft tissue proliferation or secondary enlargement of the affected spinal nerve proximal to the level of stenosis, especially on STIR sequences.

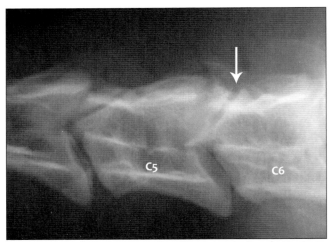

12.26 Lateral survey radiographs of the cervical spine of a Great Dane. Note the articular facet hypertrophy (arrowed) at the level of C5–C6.
(© Sebastien Behr)

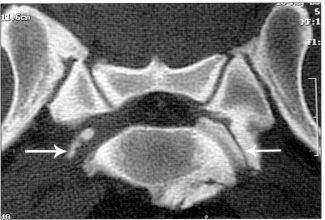

12.27 CT scan of a dog showing bilateral lumbosacral foraminal stenosis due to lateralized spondylosis and osteoproliferation (arrowed).
(© Sebastien Behr)

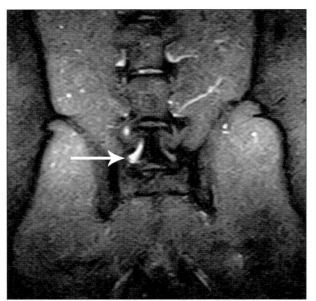

12.28 Dorsal STIR MR image of the lumbar spine in a dog. Note the thickened and hyperintense L7 nerve root (arrowed), within the vertebral canal secondary to foraminal stenosis.
(© Sebastien Behr)

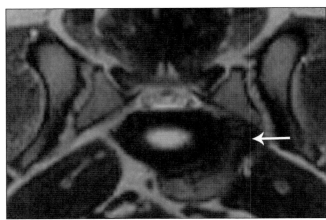

12.29 Transverse T2-weighted MR image of a severe and lateralized lumbosacral foraminal stenosis due to lateralized spondylosis (arrowed) in a 2-year-old dog, causing pelvic limb lameness.
(© Sebastien Behr)

Treatment

Medical management: Indications for initial medical management include patients for whom pain, lameness or neurological gait abnormalities are not that severe, and consists of analgesia and an extended period of rest for at least 6 to 12 weeks. Figure 12.30 summarizes the options for medical management of neuropathic pain.

- Non-steroidal anti-inflammatory drugs (minimum course of 2 weeks) are recommended initially, in association with gabapentin (10–20 mg/kg orally q8h for 4 weeks then q12h for 8 weeks)
- If non-steroidal anti-inflammatory drugs cannot be used, substitute with paracetamol (0.5–1 mg/kg orally q12h; **do not use in cats**)
- Replace gabapentin with pregabalin (2–4 mg/kg orally q12h) should the side effects of gabapentin (sedation and weakness) be excessive
- Add amitriptyline (1–2 mg/kg orally q12h) if clinical response is not satisfactory after 2 weeks

12.30 Medical management of neuropathic pain.

For lumbosacral stenosis some authors have recommended epidural injection of methylprednisolone actetate, which has a good short-term outcome; further studies are required to evaluate long-term benefit.

Surgical management: Indications for surgical management include failure of medical management, patients that are in severe pain or have severe neurological abnormalities, or patients that are deteriorating neurologically.

Cervical foraminal stenosis:

- **Lateralized cervical disc extrusion.** Surgical management of lateralized cervical disc extrusion with associated foraminal stenosis is usually best addressed using a dorsolateral approach (lateral to the vertebral spinous process) and cervical hemilaminectomy. This allows better and more complete decompression of the foramen than via a ventral slot, but it risks relapse (i.e. further extrusion), as fenestration of the affected disc space cannot be safely performed via a dorsolateral approach. Alternatively, a ventral slot can be performed as a compromise; for example, if the main site of stenosis is at the entrance zone of the foramen.

- **Juxta-facet cysts.** Surgical management of juxta-facet cysts is usually performed via dorsal laminectomy and is associated with a good outcome in most cases.
- **Caudal cervical foraminal stenosis due to articular facet osteoproliferation.** This causes mainly dorsolateral compression and surgery is usually performed via dorsal laminectomy. Often several sites are affected, necessitating continuous dorsal laminectomy over several disc spaces. Improvement in clinical signs following a ventral distraction and stabilization technique, without the need for direct decompression, has been reported.
- **Caudal cervical stenosis due to disc-associated caudal cervical spondylomyelopathy** (Figure 12.31). This requires distraction of the disc space, which concurrently achieves enlargement of the intervertebral foramina. Distraction can be achieved by a variety of different surgical techniques including the use of spacers, a cement plug (polymethylmethacrylate), vertebral screws and polymethylmethacrylate, or a tantalum cage with bone grafting. Intervertebral disc replacement (cervical disc arthroplasty) is now possible; this aims to preserve some motion of the affected disc spaces and enables multiple disc spaces to be treated more easily. Only preliminary results are available and larger studies are required to evaluate the long-term benefit of such implants. Complication rates (around 20%) appear similar regardless of the technique used, the most common ones being subsidence and adjacent segment syndrome.

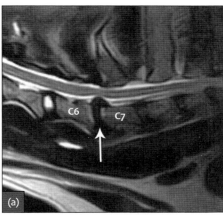
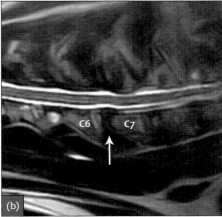

12.31 Sagittal T2-weighted MR images of the caudal cervical vertebral column (arrowed) (a) before and (b) after traction. The ventral compression of the spinal cord at the level of the C6–C7 intervertebral disc almost completely resolves on the traction image consistent with a traction-responsive disc-associated lesion at C6–C7.
(© Sebastien Behr)

Lumbosacral foraminal stenosis: Surgical management of lumbosacral foraminal stenosis aims to decompress the affected nerve root, either by dorsal laminectomy and/or foraminotomy, or by distraction/stabilization techniques. This depends on whether the maximum level of stenosis is at the entrance, middle or exit zone of the foramen. Alternatively, a facetectomy can be performed but this requires dorsal stabilization with pedicles screws and bone cement (polymethylmethacrylate) or rods, or a dorsal locking plate system.

Detailed consideration of surgical techniques is beyond the scope of this chapter but further information can be found in the *BSAVA Manual of Canine and Feline Neurology.*

Inflammatory diseases

Neurological lameness can be caused by inflammatory diseases that affect the spinal cord (myelitis, or meningo-myelitis if the meninges are also involved) or the peripheral nerves (brachial plexus neuritis).

Brachial plexus neuritis

Brachial plexus neuritis is a rare immunoallergic condition that affects the thoracic limbs of dogs and cats. It can be caused by administration of some vaccines (rabies) and specific viral infections.

Clinical signs

Affected animals present with severe shoulder and upper limb pain, with LMN signs of the thoracic limb.

Diagnosis

MRI findings can help to confirm the suspicion of neuritis. MRI appearance can be similar to a peripheral nerve sheath tumour affecting the brachial plexus; however, brachial plexus neuritis tends to affect younger animals, is more rapid in onset and can be bilateral, which can help to differentiate it from a brachial plexus tumour. Definitive diagnosis requires biopsy of the affected peripheral nerves and histopathological confirmation.

Treatment

Supportive treatment (physiotherapy and hydrotherapy) and the use of an immunosuppressive dose of cortico-steroids are recommended. Gabapentin can be used for pain management (10–20 mg/kg orally q8h). Prognosis is guarded as recovery can be very slow or absent.

Toxoplasmosis and neosporosis

Toxoplasmosis can affect dogs and cats. It commonly causes generalized infection but can lead to neurological signs. Canine toxoplasmosis has similar presenting signs to neosporosis and the two conditions have previously been confused. *Toxoplasma gondii* infection is acquired via the ingestion of infected intermediate hosts, or trans-placentally. *Neospora caninum* can also be transmitted vertically *in utero*, or it can be acquired through the ingestion of infected faeces in the environment or the ingestion of infected muscles of intermediate hosts. Toxoplasmosis is more common in cats, and neosporosis in dogs.

Clinical signs

Toxoplasmosis leads to neurological signs in fewer than 10% of affected cats. The neurological signs will depend on the site of the lesion and include ataxia, paresis, circling, tremors and seizures. It rarely occurs in dogs but it can cause signs of myositis with stiffness and muscle wastage.

Protozoal radiculitis is commonly caused by *N. caninum*, and rarely by *T. gondii*. In young dogs, *N. caninum* tends to affect the lumbar spinal nerve roots, the spinal cord segments and the pelvic limb muscles, whereas in older dogs it has a predilection for the cerebellum. A characteristic early sign of neosporosis is progressive rigidity of the limb due to neuritis and myositis. In the puppy, neurogenic muscle atrophy can develop rapidly and lead to muscle fibrosis and contracture, while the young bones continue to grow leading to arthrogryposis (joint contractures) and deformity of the distal pelvic limbs. The clinical findings are characteristic of a diffuse neuromuscular disease with LMN neurological signs in the pelvic limbs. Neosporosis in adult dogs can cause cerebellar signs resulting in ataxia and hypermetria that affect all four limbs but can also cause multifocal neurological signs.

Diagnosis

Both toxoplasmosis and neosporosis are diagnosed most reliably by measuring serum and cerebrospinal fluid (CSF) antibody titres by immunofluorescence; in particular, the demonstration of increasing titres is convincing evidence of infection. Polymerase chain reaction (PCR) on the CSF or a sample of muscle can be performed to try to confirm the diagnosis.

Serology for *T. gondii* should include measurement of both IgM and IgG. Active infection usually results in a high IgM titre, or an increase in IgG titre four-fold or greater. IgG elevation alone indicates exposure only and is not diagnostic of an active infection.

Serology is considered to be diagnostic of neosporosis when positive at a dilution of 1/800. Antibodies to *Neospora* do not cross-react with those to *Toxoplasma*.

CSF analysis can demonstrate pleocytosis with an increased number of neutrophils, the presence of large mononuclear cells and sometimes, eosinophils. CSF total protein level is usually elevated. PCR for the detection of *T. gondii* or *N. caninum* can be performed on CSF but false-negative results are possible.

Muscle and nerve biopsy samples can help to identify the presence of microorganisms but immunochemical stains are required to differentiate the two species.

Treatment

It is recommended that antiprotozoal treatment is started immediately when either toxoplasmosis or neosporosis is suspected. The use of clindamycin (15–20 mg/kg orally q12h) and trimethoprim/sulphonamide (15–20 mg/kg orally q12h) is recommended for an initial duration of 4 to 8 weeks and discontinuation is guided by return to normal serum titres.

The prognosis is favourable if therapy is initiated early, but in puppies with neosporosis and arthrogryposis leading to limb deformities, improvement is unlikely.

Prevention of toxoplasmosis involves measures to reduce the incidence of feline infections (e.g. avoiding feeding cats with raw meat). For neosporosis, it involves controlling breeding from *Neospora*-infected bitches since repetitive transmission can occur to successive litters.

Discospondylitis

Discospondylitis is caused by bacterial or fungal infection of the vertebral endplates and the intervertebral disc. The most common agent causing discospondylitis is coagulase-positive *Staphylococcus*. The infection originates from haematogenous spread from distant foci of infection, penetrating wounds, internal migration of plant material or surgery.

The most common spinal segments affected are L7–S1, caudal cervical and mid-thoracic to thoracolumbar. In cases of L7–S1 discospondylitis, associated inflammation and infection of the surrounding soft tissue, including the L7 nerve, can contribute to nerve root signature.

Clinical signs

Discospondylitis affects mainly large-breed dogs, often young intact males. A predominant clinical sign is pain with concurrent lameness. If compression of the spinal cord occurs due to instability or empyema, ataxia and paresis may be present. Affected dogs can also show signs of pyrexia and weight loss.

Diagnosis

Radiographic changes of the spine only become apparent 2–4 weeks after the onset of discospondylitis infection (Figure 12.32). Irregularity of the vertebral endplates with narrowing of the intervertebral disc space is a typical finding. CT imaging is superior to radiography as the three-dimensional images are easier to interpret, osseous changes are more detailed and it may enable identification of a migrating foreign body, if present. MRI gives superior detail of soft tissue, including the paraspinal tissues, nervous system and epidural space. Ultrasound-guided aspiration of the disc space can be performed and samples submitted for cytology, culture and sensitivity. Surgical biopsy can be performed if the patient fails to respond to antibiotic therapy.

Blood and urine culture should be performed when discospondylitis is suspected. Sampling should occur prior to the start of antibiotic therapy to minimize the chance of a false-negative result. A complete work-up to investigate primary foci of infection is recommended, including abdominal ultrasonography, thoracic radiographs or thoracic and abdominal CT imaging.

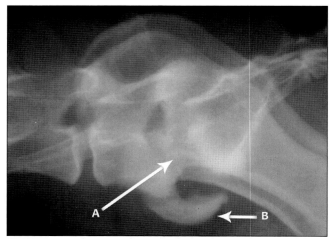

12.32 Lateral survey radiograph of a dog showing discospondylitis (A) and lumbosacral ventral spondylosis (B). Note the irregular endplates at L7–S1 consistent with osteolysis.
(© Sebastien Behr)

Treatment

Antibiotic treatment targeted against *Staphylococcus pseudintermedius* should be started (using high doses of antibiotics, such as cefalexin or co-amoxiclav, unless the culture and sensitivity result recommends a different antibiotic). Concurrent analgesia and cage rest are recommended. Clinical signs should improve markedly within 5 days but complete neurological resolution may take up to 5 months and reoccurrence is possible.

Surgical treatment is rarely performed and should only be considered in refractory cases with associated neurological signs.

The prognosis is good unless there is a fungal infection or the animal suffers from complications such as endocarditis, vertebral fractures or subluxations.

Neoplasia

Neoplastic disease of the vertebrae, spinal cord or meninges can cause LMN signs in the thoracic or pelvic limbs, particularly if the pathology is lateralized.

Malignant nerve sheath neoplasms

Malignant nerve sheath neoplasms are the most common peripheral nerve tumours in dogs. They arise from the cells surrounding the axons and are usually located in the spinal nerves and their roots; therefore, they can also compress the spinal cord.

Malignant nerve sheath neoplasms often originate from the caudal cervical and cranial thoracic spinal nerves (C6–T2). These tumours spread locally and slowly, so by the time the diagnosis is made, there are usually several nerves involved.

Clinical signs

Common clinical signs are initial episodes of pain followed by progressive lameness and paresis with noticeable muscle atrophy of the affected limb (Figure 12.33). Pain may be elicited on palpation of the axillary region and a mass can sometimes be palpated in this area.

If the mass extends up to the vertebral canal and compresses or infiltrates the spinal cord, UMN signs (e.g proprioceptive deficits) can develop in the ipsilateral pelvic limb. When the cranial thoracic spinal nerves or spinal cord are involved, Horner's syndrome may develop and the ipsilateral cutaneous trunci reflex may be absent (C8–T1).

Diagnosis

MRI is the procedure of choice to investigate the spinal canal and the area of the brachial or lumbar plexus involved when a nerve sheath tumour is suspected (Figure 12.34). The study should include post-contrast images and STIR images (Figure 12.35) of the spinal cord and the plexus. MRI is best suited to determine the proximal extension of the tumour, i.e. into the cervical spine and, possibly, intramedullary invasion. If the disease is at a very early stage, then MRI may not reveal any abnormality; if the index of clinical suspicion is high, follow-up MRI may have to be scheduled. CT scans (pre- and post-contrast) can also identify peripheral nerve neoplasia and enable visualization of the enlargement of the neural foramen (Figure 12.36).

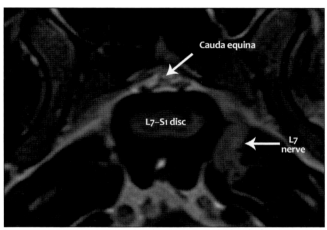

12.34 Transverse T2-weighted MR image at the level of L7–S1 in a dog showing an L7 peripheral nerve sheath tumour (arrowed).
(© Sebastien Behr)

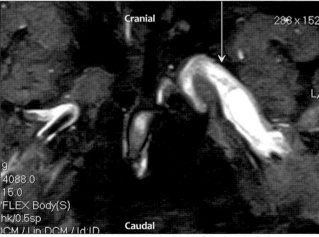

12.35 Dorsal STIR MR image at the level of the brachial plexus in a dog (ventral to the vertebral column). Note the enlargement of the brachial plexus on the left (arrowed) due to a brachial plexus tumour.
(© Sebastien Behr)

12.33 A 9-year-old Yorkshire Terrier with right forelimb lameness and muscle atrophy due to a peripheral nerve sheath tumour.
(© Sebastien Behr)

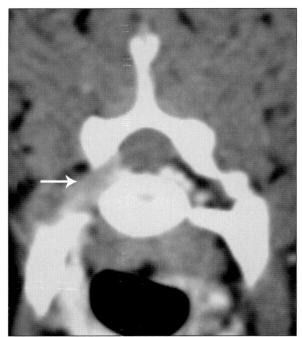

12.36 Transverse post-contrast CT scan showing contrast uptake by and enlargement of peripheral nerve C8 (arrowed), as well as associated foraminal enlargement, in a dog.
(© Sebastien Behr)

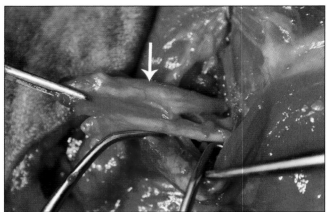

12.37 Intraoperative view during thoracic limb amputation as treatment for confirmed malignant peripheral nerve sheath tumour affecting the radial nerve (arrowed) in a dog. Tumour excision was complete according to histopathology.
(© Sebastien Behr and Rob White)

Electrodiagnostic studies can help to confirm that neurological disease is present. In cases of peripheral nerve sheath tumours in dogs, such studies can also have a prognostic value as epaxial electromyographic abnormalities appear to be predictive of intervertebral or vertebral canal invasion by the tumour.

A full systemic work-up to investigate the presence of primary neoplasia or metastasis should ideally be performed because, although unlikely, peripheral nerve neoplasia can be related to lymphoma or adenocarcinoma. This should include either thoracic radiographs and abdominal ultrasonography, or CT imaging of both the thorax and abdomen.

Ultrasound-guided aspirates of the suspected nerve sheath tumour can be performed if the lesion is large enough to allow sampling, but this procedure can be non-diagnostic and mainly aimed at ruling out other differentials, such as lymphoma and neuritis. Surgical biopsy can also be considered to confirm the diagnosis prior to making further therapeutic decisions.

Treatment

Palliative treatment with prednisolone (0.5 mg/kg orally q12–24h) and gabapentin (10–20 mg/kg orally q8–12h) is recommended if the owners opt against amputation, or should signs of nerve root or spinal cord involvement be apparent on advanced imaging.

Surgery (limb amputation) is the treatment of choice if no evidence of proximal extension within the foramina, vertebral canal or spinal cord can be identified on advanced imaging, and if no evidence of primary or metastatic tumour is identified. Surgery can be curative if the surgical margin is clean, but this can only be confirmed by histopathological inspection of the margin of the excised nerve root (Figure 12.37). If excision is incomplete, local reoccurrence is to be expected. Peripheral nerve sheath tumours are poorly responsive to adjunctive chemotherapy and/or radiotherapy.

Lymphoma

Lymphoma is the most common spinal cord tumour in the cat and it can occasionally infiltrate the peripheral nerves. Lymphoma has been associated with feline leukaemia virus and affected cats are often less than 2 years old.

Clinical signs are progressive and reflect the location of the lymphoma within the spinal cord and the peripheral nerves. Spinal lymphoma is most commonly extradural and can be diagnosed by combined imaging (myelography, CT-myelography or MRI) and CSF analysis. CSF analysis can reveal malignant lymphocytic pleocytosis. Diagnosis can also be confirmed by surgical biopsy or presence of lymphoma in another organ (abdominal, thoracic or bone marrow). Commonly, a single diffuse extradural lesion that is amenable to surgical resection is present but intraparenchymal lesions can also be encountered. Treatment can include surgical resection of the tumour (after dorsal laminectomy or hemilaminectomy) if spinal cord compression is identified. Adjunctive treatment with chemotherapy and/or radiotherapy is recommended following histopathological confirmation. A combination of surgery and chemotherapy has led to prolonged remission in cats.

Prognosis is usually guarded but depends on the grade and stage of the tumour, the clinical signs and the response to treatment.

Neurological conitions caused by toxins

Tetanus

Tetanus is caused by the toxin tetanospasmin produced by the anaerobic organism *Clostridium tetani*. The spores are typically introduced via a penetrating wound and produce toxins when they germinate. The toxin tetanospasmin reaches the central nervous system by retrograde intra-axonal transport.

Clinical signs are often generalized (muscle stiffness and *risus sardonicus*), but in some cases, especially in cats, a focal form can be present. In the focal form, the signs are limited to the site of infection; therefore, in the case of a distal limb injury, the animal can present with monoparesis and limb rigidity.

Tetanus is diagnosed on the basis of clinical presentation and treated symptomatically and medically (penicillin G, antitoxin, metronidazole). Recovery is very slow but the outcome is favourable if treatment is initiated early.

Lameness caused by generalized neuromuscular disorders

Detailed consideration of neuromuscular diseases is beyond the scope of this chapter but further information can be found in Chapter 10 and in the *BSAVA Manual of Canine and Feline Neurology*.

Intermittent lameness

Both orthopaedic and neurological lameness can be episodic, for example patellar luxation or nerve root signature due to foraminal stenosis. Sometimes both the orthopaedic and neurological examinations are unremarkable and no abnormalities or pain can be elicited on assessment. In these cases, it is recommended to ask the owners to provide a video of the episodes of paroxysmal or episodic lameness. History should include occurrence, duration, possible trigger, number of limbs affected and relation with duration of exercise.

Intermittent lameness can sometimes be related to a movement disorder, such as paroxysmal dystonia and dyskinesia. The term dyskinesia refers to movements of the body that are involuntary. Dystonia occurs when opposing muscles are contracting simultaneously. These conditions are rare but increased awareness of them may enable better detection. In such cases, there is involuntary, usually repetitive, contraction of a group of muscles without alteration of the level of consciousness. These episodes can be triggered by excitement, stress or exercise but they can also sometimes happen at rest (non-kinesogenic) or after sudden initiation of a voluntary movement (kinesogenic). It can be difficult to differentiate them from partial seizures but their duration will commonly be longer than that of a partial seizure, and certain triggers, such as exercise, can sometimes initiate them. Most of these movement disorders are inherited and are related to a suspected channelopathy, i.e a genetic mutation affecting ion channels of the neuron cell membrane. Precise classification and aetiology of these movement disorders does not exist to date in veterinary medicine, but certain breeds have been identified as affected by such movement disorders. In some cases a genetic test is available. Results of diagnostic investigations, such as an MRI study, EMG and cerebrospinal fluid analysis, are within normal ranges; these are useful to rule out other underlying causes.

Scotty cramp

Scottish Terriers from 6 months to 3 years of age can be affected by episodes of paroxysmal dystonia, often related to excitement and exercise. Scotty cramp is an inherited autosomal disorder but no genetic testing is available at the moment and a presumptive diagnosis can be made based on video recording of the episodes, clinical signs and signalment. Clinical examination undertaken between episodes is normal, and diagnostic investigations are unremarkable. Treatment is palliative, consisting of modification of the exercise regimen, and treatment of the most severe episodes with either acepromazine (0.1–0.75 mg/kg q12h) or diazepam (0.5 mg/kg q8h). The condition is non-progressive and acceptable quality of life is achieved in most dogs. Similar conditions have been described in other breeds, such as the Border Terrier (also called Spike's disease or epileptoid cramping syndrome in this breed), Cocker Spaniel and Norwich Terrier.

Episodic falling in the Cavalier King Charles Spaniel

This condition is also called episodic hypertonicity syndrome, or collapsing Cavalier King Charles Spaniel. The signs tend to occur in young dogs from 3 to 7 months of age and are typically present before one year of age. The episodes are mostly triggered by exercise. Signs include stiffness in the pelvic limbs with a repetitive movement of abduction of the pelvic limb (sometimes only in one pelvic limb). It is an inherited condition in the Cavalier King Charles Spaniel with around 13% of dogs being carriers. A genetic test is available that can be performed on blood (EDTA sample) or buccal mucosal swabs. Treatment is either clonazepam (0.5 mg/kg orally q8h) or acetazolamide (4–8 mg/kg orally q8–12h). Tolerance to clonazepam can develop with time.

Stiff Labrador syndrome

This progressive non-painful disease affects young male Labrador Retrievers from 2 to 40 months of age and leads to generalized paroxysmal stiffness and bradykinesia. As the disease progresses, limited range of motion of the limbs occurs and the animal may not be able to rise unaided. An X-linked hereditary disorder is suspected but no genetic test is currently available. No treatment has been shown to limit the progression of the disease; the most severely affected dogs are usually euthanased due to poor quality of life.

References and further reading

Anor S (2014) Monoparesis. In: *BSAVA Manual of Canine and Feline Neurology*, 4th edn, pp. 328–341. BSAVA Publications, Gloucester

Bailey CS and Kitchell EL (1984) Clinical evaluation of the cutaneous innervations of the canine thoracic limb. *Journal of the American Animal Hospital Association* **20**, 939–950

Bailey CS and Kitchell RL (1987) Cutaneous sensory testing in the dog. *Journal of Veterinary Internal Medicine* **1**, 128–135

Bailey CS, Kitchell RL, Haghighi SS and Johnson RD (1984) Cutaneous innervation of the thorax and abdomen of the dog. *American Journal of Veterinary Research* **45**, 1689–1698

Bailey CS, Kitchell RL, Haghighi SS and Johnson RD (1988) Spinal nerve root origins of the cutaneous nerves of the canine pelvic limb. *American Journal of Veterinary Research* **49**, 115–119

Bailey CS, Kitchell RL and Johnson RD (1982) Spinal nerve root origins of the cutaneous nerves arising from the canine brachial plexus. *American Journal of Veteterinary Research* **43**, 820–825

Cauzinille L (2000) Fibrocartilaginous embolism in dogs. *Veterinary Clinics of North America: Small Animal Practice* **30**, 155–167

Cummings JF, Lorenz MD, De Lahunta A, Washington LD (1975) Canine brachial plexus neuritis: a syndrome resembling serum neuritis in man. *The Cornell Veterinarian* **63**, 589–617

da Costa RC, Parent JM, Dobson H *et al.* (2008) Ultrasound-guided fine needle aspiration in the diagnosis of peripheral nerve sheath tumors in 4 dogs. *Canine Veterinary Journal* **49**, 77–81

da Costa RC, Parent JM, Holmberg DL, Sinclair D and Monteith G (2008) Outcome of medical and surgical treatment in dogs with cervical spondylomyelopathy: 104 cases (1988–2004). *Journal of the American Veterinary Medical Association* **233**, 1284–1290

De Lahunta (2001) *A Clinical Neurology. Small Animals – Localization, Diagnosis and Treatment*. International Veterinary Information Service, New York, USA

De Risio L and Platt SR (2010) Fibrocartilaginous embolic myelopathy in small animals. *Veterinary Clinics of North America: Small Animal Practice* **40**, 859–869

Dickinson PJ, Sturges BK, Berry WL *et al.* (2001) Extradural spinal synovial cysts in nine dogs. *Journal of Small Animal Practice* **42**, 502–509

Fadda A, Lang J and Forterre F (2013) Far lateral lumbar disc extrusion: MRI findings and surgical treatment. *Veterinary and Comparative Orthopaedics and Traumatology* **26**, 318–322

Gandini G, Cizinauskas S, Lang J *et al.* (2003) Fibrocartilaginous embolism in 75 dogs: clinical findings and factors influencing the recovery rate. *Journal of Small Animal Practice* **44**, 76–80

Gemmill T and McKee M (2012) Monoparesis and neurological causes of lameness. In: *Small Animal Neurological Emergencies*, pp. 299–315. Manson, London

Gill JL, Tsai KL, Krey C *et al.* (2012) A canine BCAN microdeletion associated with episodic falling syndrome. *Neurobiology of Disease* **45**, 130–136

Gödde T and Steffen F (2007) Surgical treatment of lumbosacral foraminal stenosis using a lateral approach in twenty dogs with degenerative lumbosacral stenosis. *Veterinary Surgery* **36**, 705–713

Haghighi SS, Kitchell RL, Johnson RD, Bailey CS and Spurgeon TL (1991) Electrophysiologic studies of the cutaneous innervation of the pelvic limb of male dogs. *American Journal of Veterinary Research* **52**, 352–362

Kitchell RL, Whalen LR, Bailey CS and Lohse CL (1980) Electrophysiologic studies of cutaneous nerves of the thoracic limb of the dog. *American Journal of Veterinary Research* **41**, 61–76

Kraft S, Ehrhart EJ, Gall D *et al.* (2007) Magnetic resonance imaging characteristics of peripheral nerve sheath tumors of the canine brachial plexus in 18 dogs. *Veterinary Radiology and Ultrasound* **48**, 1–7

le Chevoir M, Thibaud JL, Labruyère J *et al.* (2012) Electrophysiological features in dogs with peripheral nerve sheath tumors: 51 cases (1993–2010). *Journal of the American Veterinary Medical Association* **241**, 1194–1201

Lewis M, Olby NJ, Sharp NY and Early P (2013) Long-term effect of cervical distraction and stabilization on neurological status and imaging findings in giant breed dogs with cervical stenotic myelopathy. *Veterinary Surgery* **42**, 701–709

Mari L, Behr S, Shea A *et al.* (2017). Outcome comparison in dogs with a presumptive diagnosis of thoracolumbar fibrocartilaginous embolic myelopathy and acute non-compressive nucleus polposus extrusion. *Veterinary Record* **181(11)**, 293

McKee M (2007) Lameness and weakness in dogs: is it orthopaedic or neurological? *In Practice* **29**, 434–444

Platt S and Olby N (2013) *BSAVA Manual of Canine and Feline Neurology, 4th edn.* BSAVA Publications, Gloucester

Sale CS and Smith KC (2007) Extradural spinal juxtafacet (synovial) cysts in three dogs. *Journal of Small Animal Practice* **48**, 116–119

Sharp JW, Bailey CS, Johnson RD and Kitchell RL (1990) Spinal nerve root origin of the median, ulnar and musculocutaneous nerves and their muscle branches to the canine forelimb. *Anatomia Histologia Embryologia* **19**, 359–368

Vanhaesebrouck AE, Shelton GD, Garosi L *et al.* (2011) A novel movement disorder in related male Labrador Retrievers characterized by extreme generalized muscular stiffness. *Journal of Veterinary Internal Medicine* **25**, 1089–1096

Vanhaesebrouck AE, Van Soens I, Poncelet L, Duchateau L *et al.* (2010) Clinical and electrophysiological characterization of myokymia and neuromyotonia in Jack Russell Terriers. *Journal of Veterinary Internal Medicine* **24**, 882–889

Vite CH (2002) Myotonia and disorders of altered muscle cell membrane excitability. *Veterinary Clinics of North America: Small Animal Practice* **32**, 169–187

Walmsley G, Scurrell E, Summers B *et al.* (2009) Foreign body induced neuritis masquerading as a canine brachial plexus nerve sheath tumour. *Veterinary and Comparative Orthopaedics and Traumatology* **22**, 427–429

Chapter 13

Principles of orthopaedic surgery

Rob Pettitt

Introduction

For any animal, motion is required for it to function and enjoy a reasonable quality of life; the aim of orthopaedic surgery is to restore this function with minimal associated pain. For joint surgery, a pain-free joint with normal range of movement is the ideal outcome but, as in the case of arthrodeses, mobility may have to be compromised to achieve pain-free function. For non-articular fractures (see the *BSAVA Manual of Canine and Feline Fracture Repair and Management*), limb alignment and length are the primary aims. As for all surgeries, a few basic rules need to be followed in order to maximize success. Dr William Halsted devised a list of surgical principles to improve surgical technique over 100 years ago, and they still remain valid today (Figure 13.1). Failure to apply these principles increases the risk of complications associated with any surgical procedure, and thus risks poor outcomes.

- Atraumatic tissue handling
- Meticulous haemostasis
- Strict aseptic technique
- Preservation of blood supply
- Elimination of dead space
- Accurate apposition of tissues
- Minimal tension on sutures

13.1 Halsted's principles of surgery.

Patient assessment

It is essential to fully assess the patient before surgery. A number of orthopaedic conditions are bilateral so careful assessment of the contralateral limb is important to avoid inadvertently missing concomitant pathologies that may affect the outcome. A full history should be obtained first, to identify potential confounding issues that may have an effect on the outcome of the orthopaedic problem. Concurrent medical disease, previous responses to treatment and signalment of the animal may all influence the outcome of any treatment undertaken. The history is supported by a full orthopaedic and, if indicated, neurological examination of the patient. If the history has indicated concurrent pathologies then these should also be explored prior to any surgical decisions being made, for example in cases where joint replacement is being considered but the animal has an active infectious skin condition or neurological deficits. Routine preoperative

blood tests are not performed by the author in most cases unless the history and examination highlight any need to do so. In trauma cases, extra vigilance is needed to evaluate any possible life-threatening conditions, such as thoracic trauma or rupture of the urinary tract, before addressing the orthopaedic issues.

The decision to elect for surgical *versus* conservative management is not always straightforward; if conservative management was improving the condition then is surgery necessary? This can be a balancing act that requires education and careful communication with the owner. Some conditions, such as hip dysplasia, may settle with time and not require surgery. Equally these conditions can cause reduced quality of life and the need for long-term medication (and costs) and so may be better addressed by surgical means, e.g. total hip replacement. Careful history taking, discussion of all options with the owner and a realistic expectation of outcomes need to be addressed before the decision for surgery is taken. Once the decision for surgery has been made then multiple factors need to be considered.

Clinical decision-making

Once fully evaluated, then appropriate management of the orthopaedic problem can be decided upon. The decision to elect for surgery instead of conservative management is not always straightforward. It may be that conservative management may work just as well but take slightly longer to reach those levels (Vasseur, 1984; Barr *et al.*, 1987) or conservative options may lead to a reduced quality of life and potential increased costs that may be better addressed surgically (Farrell *et al.*, 2007).

Preoperative planning

Planning for surgery is discussed further in the joint-specific chapters and in the *BSAVA Manual of Canine and Feline Fracture Repair and Management*. Time spent preoperatively in planning the approach, implant sizes, potential pitfalls and back-up plans, is time well spent and can help reduce surgical time. This is certainly the case where an unfamiliar surgery is being performed or when the surgeon has limited orthopaedic experience.

Initial planning is usually based upon the radiographs. An acetate tracing can help the surgeon to visualize the surgery; the acetate can be taken into theatre and used as an *aide mémoire* during the surgery. Surgical approaches need to be carefully thought out using available texts to ensure adequate exposure of the desired location is achieved with minimal iatrogenic trauma. Failure to adhere to a standard approach may lead to increased difficulty during surgery and potentially poorer postoperative recovery, so access to textbooks detailing these approaches is essential.

For fractures, a tracing of the fracture fragments can help formulate a plan. Measurement of potential screw lengths can also be useful to give an indication of the possible screw lengths required. The flaw with this is that unless the drill hole is in the same plane as the radiograph, the actual screw length may vary from that initially measured on the radiograph.

Surgical principles

Asepsis

Aseptic techniques should be applied for all surgical procedures, but for orthopaedics this is particularly important. The physical act of placing foreign material, such as orthopaedic implants, increases the risk of infection and, therefore, strict attention must be paid to aseptic techniques. Predisposing factors to surgical site infections include:

- Avascular tissue
- Presence of foreign material
- Increased surgical time
- Implants
- Poor theatre practice
- Contamination from hair/skin of the patient or the surgeon.

A clean surgical environment is required for orthopaedic surgery. A hospital level theatre suite is not available in many practices, but certain principles and standards need to be adhered to if orthopaedic surgeries are to be considered.

- The operating theatre should not be in a general thoroughfare to minimize the risk of airborne bacterial contamination, i.e. it should be a dedicated room and not a corridor.
- All staff in the theatre should wear dedicated surgical clothing. Operating staff should wear sterile operating attire (e.g. gloves and gowns).
- Clipping and preparation of the animal should be performed outside the theatre with a final scrub performed after transfer of the patient to the operating table.
- If required, placement of a purse string suture and/or evacuation of the patient's rectum or colon can be performed.
- Positive pressure ventilation of clean filtered air allows flow of air down on to the patient, away to the extremities of the room and on to less clean areas, reducing bacterial contamination.
- Consideration should be given to the organization of the theatre; surgical checklists are very useful to ensure important aspects of theatre set-up are not overlooked (Figure 13.2).
- Distractive noise, general conversation and disturbance should be minimized.
- Devise and adhere to strict theatre cleaning protocols at the end of each session.

Surgical technique can also play a role in minimizing the risk of infection. As well as abiding by Halsted's principles, it is important to maintain a moist surgical environment to prevent desiccation of the exposed tissues. Significant heat is generated by power tools when drilling or sawing bone, so constant lavage (approximately one drop of saline per second from a 20 ml syringe is a useful guide) should be applied to the cutting piece throughout its use. Finally, prior to closure, the wound should be copiously lavaged and the excess fluid removed using suction in order to reduce any bacterial load. Necrotic tissue caused as a result of desiccation or thermal insult will act as a nidus for bacteria, increasing the risk of infection.

Surgeons and scrubbed assistants in appropriate theatre attire should scrub their hands and arms in an aseptic manner using recognized techniques. Povidone–iodine and chlorhexidine have historically been the surgical scrubs of choice; recent evidence shows that in both the human and veterinary fields, an alcohol-based preparation is more effective, e.g. Sterilium. In trials, hydro-alcoholic rub and chlorhexidine solutions had similar immediate effects but the alcohol rub had a much improved sustained effect. Povidone–iodine had significantly lower immediate and sustained effects (Verwilghen *et al.*, 2011). Scrub solutions such as chlorhexidine should be in contact with the skin for at least 5 minutes prior to gowning but this time may be reduced to as little as 1.5 minutes for some of the modern hydro-alcohol rubs (Kampf and Widmer, 2011; Verwilghen *et al.*, 2011). Once the hands and forearms have been aseptically prepared and are air-dried, a sterile gown and gloves should be donned in an aseptic manner, i.e. avoiding skin contact with the front of the gown and the outside of the gloves. Single use gowns and gloves are preferable to ensure sterility.

Surgical equipment

Lighting

Good lighting, ideally from two separate theatre lights with handles that can be sterilized and used to adjust the direction of lighting (Figure 13.3), is preferable for orthopaedic surgery. The bidirectional light facilitates adequate inspection of deep structures such as joints accessed through small approaches. The sterile handles allow the surgeon to directly adjust the lighting as required. A head lamp can be used (Figure 13.4) to supplement overhead lighting as necessary and can be particularly useful for focal deep inspection.

Operating table

The operating table should be adjustable in both height and tilt in order to maximize surgeon comfort and facilitate appropriate patient positioning. The table should also have a soft cover and facilitate patient warming devices.

Sterilization of instruments

All surgical instruments must be sterilized; an autoclave is suitable for most instrumentation and models with variable capacities and capabilities are available. Instruments with sharp points should have the tips protected with small autoclavable plastic covers to prevent inadvertent penetration through the sterile bags. All instruments should be double-wrapped and clearly marked with a sterilization expiry date (Figure 13.5). Large instruments and some orthopaedic instrument sets will not fit into a standard

Theatre checklist

Before induction	Before 1st incision	Before leaving theatre
Sign IN	**Time out**	**Sign OUT**
Have the following been confirmed? ☐ • Patient identification • Site of surgery • Procedure • Consent **Is the pink sheet and file with the patient?** ☐	**People new to theatre introduce themselves** ☐ **Verbally confirm patient identification, site of surgery and procedure** ☐	**Verbal confirmation of:** • Swab and equipment counts ☐ • Sharps removed ☐ • Specimens labelled ☐ • Equipment problems to be addressed ☐
Is the surgical site marked? ☐ (yes/not applicable)	**Anticipated critical events** **Surgeons** Anticipated blood loss, special equipment needed, critical points ☐ **Anaesthetists** Specific concerns, equipment needed ☐ **Nurses** Has sterility been confirmed, any equipment issues ☐	**Surgeons and anaesthetists review key concerns for recovery** ☐
Has the anaesthetic machine been checked? ☐ (prep and theatre)	**Have antibiotics been given within 60 minutes?** ☐ (yes/not required) **Is any essential imaging displayed?** ☐ (yes/not required)	Date:... Procedure:... .... Patient name:..................................... .... Owner:.. .... Number:..
Does the patient have a known allergy? No ☐ Yes ☐ **Difficult airway/aspiration risk?** No ☐ Yes ☐ **Risk of >15% blood loss?** No ☐ Yes ☐ **Current medications checked?** ☐		

Recovery checklist

	Postoperative complications
Date:... Procedure:... .... Patient name:... .... Owner:.. .... Number:..	**Anticipated complications:** **Discussed with ICU/ward nurse** ☐

Analgesia plan	Surgeon's initials:
Anaesthetist's initials:	**Inform surgeon/anaesthetist if**
Medications:	Temp ↑ ↓
	HR ↑ ↓
CRIs:	RR ↑ ↓
	BP ↑ ↓
Discussed with ICU/ward nurse ☐	Other

13.2 Example of a theatre checklist used for orthopaedic surgeries at the Small Animal Teaching Hospital, University of Liverpool. These lists are routinely used in human hospitals and provide important safety checks to minimize mistakes relating to patients undergoing surgical procedures. BP = blood pressure; CRI = constant rate infusion; HR = heart rate; ICU = intensive care unit; RR = respiratory rate; Temp = temperature.

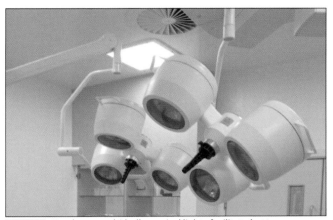

13.3 Two large, multi-bulb surgical lights facilitate better illumination of the surgical site.

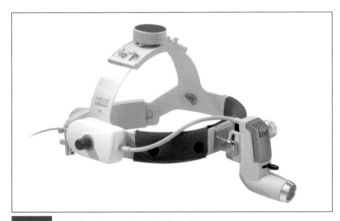

13.4 Headband-mounted LED headlamp.

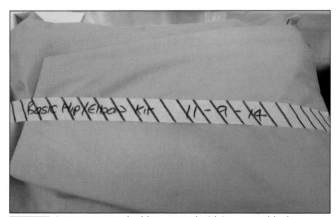

13.5 Instrument set double-wrapped with impermeable drapes and clearly identified, along with a sterilization expiry date.

autoclave so some form of external sterilizing service may have to be sought. Sterilization of orthopaedic equipment by soaking in sterilizing solutions can be ineffective and is not advisable (Rutala and Weber, 2008).

Drills and other electrical devices, e.g. burrs and saws, arthroscopy fibre-optic lighting and camera cables, may not be suitable for autoclave sterilization so alternative methods are necessary. These may include gas sterilization by ethylene oxide, or covering the non-sterile device with a specific instrument surgical drape (Figure 13.6); however, this is not an ideal compromise as contamination of the surgical site can occur.

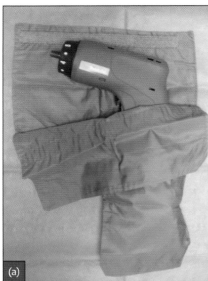
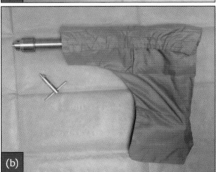

13.6 Large non-autoclavable instruments may be used in a sterile manner by shrouding in a sterile, custom-made drape. (a) In this case, an orthopaedic drill is enclosed in a drill-specific shroud which, along with the removable chuck, has been autoclaved separately. (b) The chuck is connected after enclosing the drill in the shroud. The shroud can be secured to the protruding chuck by gently wrapping with sterile Vetrap or similar.
(Courtesy of Richard Hewitt, Helen McCrorie and Cat Burdett)

Orthopaedic equipment should be kept in a dedicated store room or cupboard (Figure 13.7). This should not be overloaded, to prevent accidental damage to the sterilized instrument bags. Instruments should be handed aseptically to the surgeon and placed on a fully draped trolley. The patient should be fully draped prior to laying out the majority of instruments to minimize the risk of airborne contamination emanating from its coat. The trolley should be sited close to the surgeon, ideally with no gap between trolley and surgical table.

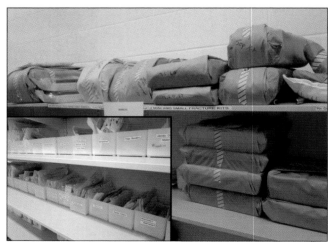

13.7 Instrument store room with ample space to prevent inadvertent damage to sterile covers due to overloading. Inset: smaller individual instruments can be stored in sterile double autoclavable bags.

Use of antibiotics

Perioperative antibiotics

Perioperative antibiotic therapy is defined as antibiotics given immediately preoperatively and then continuously either until the end of the surgical procedure, or up until 24 hours postoperatively. Most orthopaedic surgeries are classified as clean wounds, with the exception of grade 2 and 3 open fractures. Reported infection rates for surgeries on clean wounds are 2.0–4.8%. Perioperative antibiotics are recommended when one or more of the following criteria are met:

- Clean contaminated or worse procedure
- Surgery duration is greater than 90 minutes
- An implant is placed and remains *in situ*
- Presence of traumatized/devascularized tissue
- Where subsequent surgical site infection would have a disastrous consequence.

These factors all result in a reduction in the patient's defence mechanisms and increase the risk of infection. Most orthopaedic surgeries, with the possible exception of arthroscopies where no implants are placed, fit these criteria and so perioperative antibiotics are routinely administered. The use of perioperative antibiotics for orthopaedic procedures has been shown to be clinically beneficial (Whittem *et al.*, 1999) but postoperative antibiotic therapy is more controversial. It may be more justifiable in those patients that have an increased risk of infection due to concomitant disease (e.g. hyperadrenocorticism) or in those cases where the risk of infection could be catastrophic such as joint replacements. Antibiotics should not be used to justify or compensate for poor aseptic technique, atraumatic tissue handling or inadequate haemostasis.

Postoperative antibiotics

For general orthopaedic surgery the evidence supporting the use of prophylactic postoperative antibiotics is poor. The current recommendation is that postoperative antibiotics are not required in most elective orthopaedic cases, unless a breakdown of asepsis is noted at surgery. However, Fitzpatrick and Solano (2010) evaluated 1000 consecutive tibial plateau levelling osteotomy (TPLO) surgeries and found a significant reduction in infection rates in patients prescribed 14 days of postoperative antibiotics. A recent prospective study of 93 dogs undergoing routine plate application demonstrated a protective benefit from a 7-day course of antibiotics (either a cephalosporin or co-amoxiclav) compared with no antibiotics at all (Pratesi *et al.*, 2015). Further work is needed to confirm these findings in other groups of patients, but these studies suggest there may be an indication for prophylactic postoperative antibiotics in small animal orthopaedic surgery.

It is important that the clinician chooses appropriate antibiotics based on the likely bacterial contamination, and ensures the drug will be present at the surgical site before the first incision. The most common source of contamination is from the patient's skin; expected bacteria are likely to be Gram-positive commensals, especially *Staphylococcus* species. When selecting an antibiotic it is important to consider a number of factors:

- Appropriate spectrum of activity
- Pharmacokinetics of the drug
- Bioavailability

- Route of administration – intravenous preferred for preoperative use
- Toxicity
- Compliance with the Cascade system for prescribing non-licensed drugs.

Given these considerations, beta-lactam antibiotics, such as cephalosporins (e.g. cefuroxime) or co-amoxiclav are appropriate for most orthopaedic procedures. The aim is to have maximum plasma concentrations at the surgical site when surgery commences, so the drug should be administered intravenously 30–60 minutes before the first incision (Weese and Halling, 2006) and repeated every 90 minutes throughout surgery. The author uses doses of 10–15 mg/kg for cephalosporins and 20 mg/kg for co-amoxiclav. Although there is no direct evidence in the literature, the variable rate of uptake into the plasma that occurs with depot preparations makes them unsuitable for perioperative use. If antibiotics are continued post surgery, they should be of a similar class to that given during surgery. Surgical site infections should be swabbed before commencing broad-spectrum antibiotics as described above and the therapy should subsequently be tailored depending upon the results of the culture. In the absence of culture results, administration of multiple antibiotics should be avoided as this will tend to select for resistance; instead a suitable broad-spectrum antibiotic is chosen.

Analgesia

Orthopaedic surgery is inherently painful and appropriate analgesia before, during and following surgery is essential. A balanced multimodal approach is preferable. Readers are also referred to the *BSAVA Manual of Canine and Feline Analgesia and Anaesthesia,* for further information.

Bandages may be appropriate for fracture patients, as this can help reduce the associated pain. Distal limb fractures (below the elbow and stifle) are very amenable to a well applied dressing, which can be utilized prior to any surgery. For fractures of the humerus or femur, there is a risk a bandage may slip below the fracture site and increase instability by acting as a pendulum; this could increase discomfort and soft tissue trauma. Therefore for most proximal limb fractures, bandaging is not routinely recommended.

Preoperative analgesia

Preoperative pain should be managed using a combination of non-steroidal anti-inflammatory drugs (NSAIDs), pure opioid agonist analgesics, such as methadone, morphine or pethidine, or mixed action opioid agonists, e.g. buprenorphine. Studies have shown that methadone is superior to buprenorphine in dogs undergoing orthopaedic surgeries (Hunt *et al.*, 2013); in cats it has been shown that buprenorphine (0.01 mg/kg) provides superior analgesia to morphine (0.1 mg/kg) and with a longer duration of activity when given by intramuscular injection (Stanway *et al.*, 2002) but not so when given subcutaneously (Steagall *et al.*, 2006). Although both methadone and morphine have been shown to be suitable analgesics when administered subcutaneously, and superior to subcutaneous buprenorphine (Steagall *et al.*, 2006), early indications from studies yet to be published show methadone to be superior to both buprenorphine and morphine. Appropriate doses of opioids should not be a problem in the majority of cats and they are only 'sensitive' to inappropriate doses of opioids. Partial agonists will competitively inhibit the action of pure agonists.

NSAIDs should be incorporated into a balanced approach to analgesia provided there is no pre-existing renal impairment, history of gastrointestinal disease, or prior intolerance. Care should be taken in the perioperative period as anaesthesia may result in a decrease in blood pressure. Supportive treatments, such as intravenous fluid therapy, will help maintain blood pressure and reduce the risks associated with decreased renal perfusion. Figure 13.8 lists the currently available NSAIDs, their licensed formulations and the species for which they can be used. For dose rates, readers are referred to the *BSAVA Small Animal Formulary*.

In patients who are unremittingly painful and fail to respond to routine analgesia, other techniques can be considered such as constant rate intravenous infusions of single or multiple analgesic drugs, e.g. medetomidine or morphine–lidocaine–ketamine. Longer acting preparations such as transdermal fentanyl patches (off licence) or depot spot-on for dogs (Recuvyra) are available. Finally, perioperative local analgesia in the form of extradural and nerve blocks can be very effective (see Chapter 17 and *BSAVA Manual of Canine and Feline Anaesthesia and Analgesia*).

Postoperative analgesia

Opioid analgesia should be continued for as long as necessary post surgery. Most orthopaedic patients require opioid analgesia for 12 to 48 hours. A flexible, pre-emptive approach to analgesia should be adopted with regular examinations to assess the efficacy of pain management. A summary of the currently available opioids is provided in Figure 13.9. There are various pain scoring systems available (e.g. Glasgow Composite Pain Score) that offer clinicians a reliable, albeit somewhat subjective, assessment of their patients. Patients should be discharged when comfortable and when analgesia is adequate using only oral medication.

Tramadol is popular amongst veterinary surgeons, although there is little evidence of its efficacy and the drug is not licensed for use in dogs or cats in the United Kingdom. It has recently been reclassified as a Schedule 3 Controlled Drug. Tramadol itself is metabolized into eight substrates of which only one is active in the dog, and that is only for a short (1–2 hour) period.

NSAIDs are generally continued in the immediate postoperative period and are the mainstay of pain relief programmes for orthopaedic cases. The duration for which NSAIDs are required for postoperative analgesia is casedependent but in most patients should not be more than 2–4 weeks. Animals exhibiting significant signs of pain beyond this time should be carefully reassessed. There is a multitude of NSAIDs available for dogs but at the time of publication, only three NSAIDs are licensed in cats, one of which (meloxicam) is licensed for long-term use. Preference for which NSAID to use is normally down to the experience of individual surgeons as most modern NSAIDs are licensed based on similar, rather than increased, levels of safety and efficacy.

Drug generic name	Trade name	Licensed formulation	Species
Carprofen	Carprodyl	20, 50 and 100 mg tablets	Dogs
	Rimadyl	50 mg/ml solution	Dogs/cats
	Rimadyl	20, 50 and 100 mg tablets	Dogs
	Dolagis	50 mg tablet and 120 mg chewable tablet	Dogs
Cimicoxib	Cimalgex	8, 30 and 80 mg chewable tablets	Dogs
Cinchophen	PLT	200 mg (plus 1 mg prednisolone)	Dogs
Firocoxib	Previcox	57 and 227 mg chewable tablets	Dogs
Ketoprofen	Ketofen	5 and 20 mg tablets	Dogs
	Ketofen	1% solution	Dogs
Mavacoxib	Trocoxil	6, 20, 30, 75 and 95 mg chewable tablets	Dogs
Meloxicam	Meloxidyl	5 mg/ml injection	Dogs/cats
	Meloxidyl	1.5 mg/ml suspension	Dogs
	Meloxidyl	0.5 mg/ml	Cats
	Metacam	1 and 2.5 mg chewable tablets	Dogs
	Metacam	5 mg/ml solution	Dogs/cats
	Metacam	1.5 mg/ml suspension	Dogs
	Metacam	0.5 mg/ml suspension	Cats
	RevitaCAM	5 mg/ml oromucosal spray	Dogs
	Inflacam	1.5 mg/ml oral suspension	Dogs
	Inflacam	1 and 2.5 mg chewable tablets	Dogs
	Meloxivet	0.5 and 1.5 mg/ml oral suspension	Dogs
Phenylbutazone	Phenylbutazone	200 mg tablets	Dogs
Robenacoxib	Onsior	6 mg flavoured tablets	Cats
	Onsior	5, 10, 20 and 40 mg flavoured tablets	Dogs
	Onsior	20 mg/ml solution	Dogs/cats
Tolfenamic acid	Tolfedine	4% injection	Dogs/cats
	Tolfedine	6, 20, 60 mg tablets	Dogs/cats

13.8 Summary of the currently available non-steroidal anti-inflammatory drugs (NSAIDS) that are licensed in the UK. (Courtesy of Briony Alderson)

Drug	Species licensed	Dose rate	Route of administration	Duration of action	Comments
Buprenorphine	Dogs and cats	0.01–0.02 mg/kg	i.m., i.v., s.c., oral transmucosally	6–12 hours	May provide poor analgesia via the s.c. route Oral transmucosal route more reliable in cats than dogs
Butorphanol	Dogs and cats	0.1–0.5 mg/kg	i.m., s.c., i.v.	1–4 hours	Little/no analgesia, good sedation
Fentanyl	Dogs	1–5 µg/kg	i.v.	10–20 mins	Not licensed in cats, but can be used in this species Transdermal solution requires training before use
		2.6 mg/kg	Transdermally	4 days	
Methadone	Dogs and cats	0.1–1.0 mg/kg	i.m., s.c., i.v., extradurally	3–6 hours	Licensed dose of 0.5–1.0 mg/kg is higher than the commonly used doses
Morphine	None	0.1–0.5 mg/kg	i.m., s.c., slow i.v., extradurally	3–5 hours	May cause histamine release on rapid i.v. injection More suitable for prolonged infusions than methadone More commonly used via the extradural route
Pethidine	Dogs and cats	3–5 mg/kg	i.m.	30 mins–2 hours	Not to be used i.v. as it is likely to cause histamine release

13.9 Summary of opioids in common use in veterinary medicine and surgery. (Courtesy of Briony Alderson)

Although it is well documented that NSAIDs can prevent heterotrophic ossification in humans, controversy remains regarding the clinical effects of NSAIDs on fracture healing. Only a handful of prospective studies exist in humans and most show no adverse effect (Barry, 2010). Research using rodents and rabbits has indicated that NSAIDs can negatively affect bone healing but whether these effects are clinically significant in small animals remains controversial and unproven. It should be borne in mind that early patient mobilization is facilitated by appropriate analgesia, and the benefits of mobilization are likely to outweigh any marginal negative effects of NSAIDs.

Other analgesics can be used in addition to NSAIDs if required, although their use becomes off licence. Pardale V (paracetamol/codeine) is licensed in dogs for treatment of acute pain of traumatic origin and postoperative analgesia. The licence is only for 5 days and at a dose rate of 33.33 mg/kg (paracetamol) q8h. Paracetamol alone is not licensed but the recommended dose is 10 mg/kg paracetamol q12h. Pardale V may be useful in cases where NSAID intolerance has been reported or in cases where patients are already on steroid therapy. It is the author's preference to use Pardale V in conjunction with a NSAID (in the same way as humans now use paracetamol and a NSAID concurrently) although this indication is off licence and owners must be made aware of this. The course can be extended for longer than 5 days but this is again an off licence indication. Paracetamol should never be used in cats.

Preparation for surgery

Patient preparation

A wide surgical margin should be clipped for almost all orthopaedic surgical procedures. In practice, this usually means the complete limb, from the dorsal midline to just proximal to the foot, is clipped. For distal limb surgeries, such as digit amputation or fractures of the manus and pes, the clip should start proximal to the elbow or stifle, respectively, and should be sufficiently distal to allow adequate draping. If necessary, complete clipping of the foot should be performed. Clipping should be undertaken immediately prior to surgery, as clipping more than 4 hours before surgery has been shown to be associated with an increased risk of surgical site infection. The limb should be surgically scrubbed and prepared, using a scrub solution of 4% chlorhexidine and water in equal parts, before the patient is moved to theatre. The scrubbed area should be covered with a sterile drape before moving; the drape is then removed once the animal is positioned. Once the patient is correctly positioned on the operating table, a final preparation using either a sterile, single use applicator containing a solution of 2% chlorhexidine gluconate and 70% isopropyl alcohol (Adams et al., 2005) or lint free gauze swabs in chlorhexidine followed by an alcohol-based spray, is performed.

Draping

It is important to have an impermeable layer when draping, to prevent wicking of fluid and bacteria from underneath the drapes into the surgical site. Cloth drapes can be used as the initial layer but then a disposable impermeable layer should be used superficially. There are various ways to aseptically drape a patient for surgery and one method is described in Figure 13.10. Whichever option is performed it is essential that a number of rules are adhered to:

- Non-sterile parts of the patient and assistants should not be above the sterile field
- Drapes must always be moved from sterile towards non-sterile fields and not *vice versa*
- The sterile area should be sufficiently large to allow for assessment of whole limb alignment if appropriate to the procedure and manipulation of the limb without contaminating the surgical field through inadvertent exposure of non-sterile areas of the patient.

The limb should be draped in a four-quarter manner (Figure 13.10a–d). The paw should be protected with a cohesive dressing such as Vetrap. It should be transferred from non-sterile assistant to sterile surgeon in an aseptic fashion, i.e. the surgeon takes the foot in either a small surgical drape or in a hand that is double-gloved; the second glove is then taken off the surgeon's hand down to cover the paw. A final layer of sterile cohesive bandage is placed, e.g. sterile Vetrap. Ideally a further large drape covering the four quarter drapes should be placed to expand the sterile surgical field (Figure 13.10e). The use of adhesive incise drapes has not been demonstrated to significantly reduce contamination of the surgical wound in dogs undergoing ovariohysterectomy or stifle arthrotomy (Owen et al., 2009). However, adhesive drapes may have a place in ultra-clean procedures such as total joint replacement. If adhesive

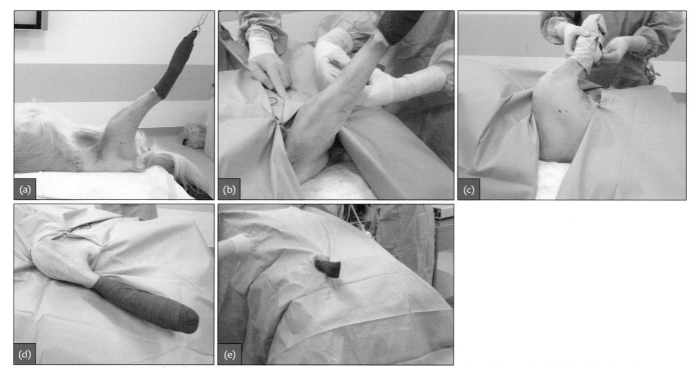

13.10 Four-quarter draping of the limb with the limb supported to prevent inadvertent contamination of the sterile field. (a) The limb can be draped in a four-quarter manner with the limb suspended to allow all around access. The paw should be protected with a cohesive dressing such as Vetrap. (b) After partial draping, (c) the paw can be transferred from a non-sterile assistant to a sterile surgeon in an aseptic fashion, i.e. the surgeon takes the foot in either a small surgical drape or in a hand that is double-gloved. (d) A final layer of sterile cohesive bandage (e.g. sterile Vetrap) and the fourth 'quarter' drape can then be placed. (e) Ideally a further large drape covering the four quarter drapes can be placed to expand the sterile surgical field. In some cases it is suitable to use a single large drape alone without the need for four-quarter draping.

drapes are used, iodine-impregnated drapes are preferred. They can be further attached to the edges of the surgical wound using staples or continuous sutures to prevent loss of adherence during surgery (Figure 13.11).

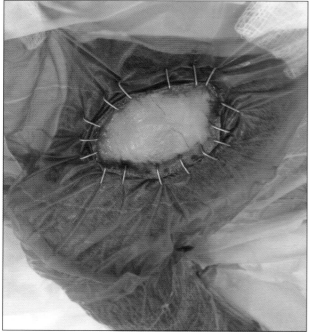

13.11 An adhesive drape can be further secured to the skin using either skin staples or monofilament suture material to prevent inadvertent lifting of the drape and exposure of the adjacent skin.

Articular surgeries

Articular surgeries, especially for fractures, offer unique challenges to the surgeon, particularly in light of the inevitable subsequent osteoarthritis and the potential need to manage its effects long after the primary injury has been addressed. There are many reasons that articular surgery is performed but they can be broadly summarized as one, or a combination of, the following:

- Diagnosis
- Prevention
- Therapy
- Palliation
- Stabilization
- Salvage.

Diagnosis

Radiographs frequently allow a diagnosis to be reached when the bone is affected (e.g. by incongruity, fracture or degenerative joint disease), but soft tissue involvement and some bone pathology is not well evaluated by radiography. Other imaging modalities, such as ultrasonography, computed tomography (CT) and magnetic resonance imaging (MRI), offer benefits over radiography, although interpreting the images requires a high degree of skill and experience (see respective joint chapters for more information).

Arthroscopy (see Chapter 15) allows for greater magnification of lesions and inspection of the joint in a more normal environment, i.e. tissues bathed in fluid. Arthroscopy is the modality of choice for surgical diagnostic purposes as it is less invasive and more rapid than arthrotomy (with experienced and proficient surgeons) and allows for a more rapid recovery. Examination of intra-articular structures, such as cartilage and ligaments, is possible with both techniques, and biopsy samples can be obtained for histopathological examination simultaneously. Culture of the synovium can be considered following biopsy, but studies have shown conflicting results in terms of the benefits of this compared with synovial fluid culture (Fink *et al.*, 2008; Cross *et al.*, 2014). Stifle arthroscopy has been shown to have less associated morbidity when compared with arthrotomy, and is the gold standard in human orthopaedics (Hoelzler *et al.*, 2004). However, arthroscopy requires expensive equipment and is technically challenging to perform, especially in the stifle. Arthrotomy offers a cheaper alternative and is quicker if the surgeon is not experienced with arthroscopy or does not have the required equipment. However, greater morbidity is associated with the former and a balance should be made between the various pros and cons when deciding on the modality to be used.

Prevention/retardation of osteoarthritis

Some surgical techniques are designed to prevent or retard the development of joint disease and associated signs as opposed to attempting to resolve them. The effect of these surgeries is at the joint, although the actual surgery may be periarticular, or even at a distance from the joint, e.g. pelvic osteotomy techniques and juvenile pelvic symphysiodesis for the management of hip dysplasia. Some other techniques are designed to ameliorate clinical signs by altering the location and magnitude of the forces within the joint (e.g. sliding humeral osteotomy).

Therapy

Management of articular fractures or luxations, if successful, can lead to complete resolution of clinical signs and a full return to function, at least in the short term. Accurate alignment of fragments and rigid internal stabilization are key aims in the management of articular fractures (see the *BSAVA Manual of Canine and Feline Fracture Repair and Management*). However, osteoarthritis is an inevitable sequel to articular fracture, irrespective of the accuracy of postoperative articular alignment, and management of this may be necessary long term (Anderson *et al.*, 1990). The requirement for surgical management of joint sepsis from the outset is controversial, as there is no evidence to support it unless gross contamination is present. The author would consider arthroscopic lavage of any appropriately sized joint that fails to respond to initial and appropriate medical management.

Palliation

Some conditions (e.g. osteochondrosis, cranial cruciate disease) cannot often be completely resolved surgically as inflammation, instability and osteoarthritis persist. Surgery in these cases helps to palliate the clinical signs and allow the animal to lead an acceptable quality of life. If the clinical signs continue to worsen, then further salvage surgery such as total joint replacement or arthrodesis should help to ameliorate the ongoing pain and lameness.

Stabilization

Stabilization is the most common reason for performing articular surgery, in particular for the management of cranial cruciate disease. This subject is discussed comprehensively in Chapter 23.

Joints are normally restrained in their range of motion by anatomical conformation, the joint capsule, menisci, ligaments, tendons and muscles. Trauma or chronic degeneration of these tissues leads to increased laxity (and in extreme cases subluxation/luxation), which excessively loads the joint. Stabilization of the joint may be achieved directly using ligament reconstruction either primarily or with a prosthesis, secondarily by temporary immobilization such as a transarticular external fixator, or indirectly by arthrodesing the joint. The management and outcomes for these surgeries are discussed elsewhere in the joint-specific chapters.

Salvage

When a joint is irreversibly damaged, there is often associated intractable pain. This leads to a loss of function of that joint and limb resulting in muscle atrophy, fibrosis and an abnormal range of motion. Depending upon the joint in question, salvage procedures consist of:

* Total joint replacement
* Excision arthroplasty
* Arthrodesis.

As the name suggests, these surgeries are reserved for when all other attempts to restore joint function have either failed or are not an option.

Arthrotomy

An arthrotomy is defined as a surgical incision into a joint. In dogs and cats, the stifle is the most common joint to be subject to an arthrotomy. As for all surgical approaches, any arthrotomy should be performed as atraumatically as possible, using recognized surgical approaches. A thorough working knowledge of joint anatomy is essential; for less experienced surgeons, there are textbooks available that accurately describe the approaches to the bones and joints, and these should be referred to when necessary. The standard surgical approaches aim for the best access to the joint, while causing the least possible damage to the adjacent soft tissue and neurovascular structures, and allow for simple and stable closure. Failure to follow these approaches is likely to make the surgery more complicated, as exposure of the required area may be decreased and morbidity increased.

Surgical approaches

As mentioned above, these are detailed in a number of textbooks along with the indications for each approach and should be regularly referred to. With familiarity, less reference is needed but the author still refreshes his knowledge of unfamiliar approaches or approaches that have not been performed in a while. Approaches to the joint tend to be via muscle separation only or via osteotomy/tenotomy techniques or a combination of both. Whatever approach is chosen, it is important to stabilize and accurately suture the tissues when closing in order to ensure adequate joint stability and not create a further problem (e.g. osteoarthritis as a result of iatrogenic joint instability). The aim of osteotomy/tenotomy techniques is to increase the exposure of a joint to facilitate surgery but a balance needs to be made between increased exposure and increased risk of complications. Osteotomies need to be carefully planned and executed in order to prevent too small a fragment being created to allow adequate stabilization. Conversely, too large an osteotomy may result in iatrogenic fractures or increased postoperative morbidity and complications (Suess *et al.*, 1994; Tobias *et al.*, 1994).

> **WARNING**
>
> Osteotomies performed to reflect a ligament are likely to involve iatrogenic trauma to the articular surface resulting in postoperative complications, whereas those used to reflect a tendon tend to be extra-articular and, with care, healing should be relatively uncomplicated

Osteophyte removal

Controversy surrounds the removal of osteophytes at the time of surgery. In humans, there is no indication to remove them during knee arthroscopy (Mayr *et al.*, 2013), although short-term positive outcomes, particularly reduced pain and increased range of motion, have been documented for osteophyte removal associated with elbow surgeries (Yan *et al.*, 2011). In experimental dogs, osteophytes return to 60% of pre-removal levels within 24–48 weeks and there is evidence to show no significant difference between treated and untreated dogs (Nesbitt, 1982). Conversely, where osteophytes are impinging on the free running of the joint, their removal should reduce pain even if just in the short term (e.g. osteophytosis of the proximal trochlear sulcus of the femur interfering with the gliding of the patella). Large osteophytes are often removed during total joint arthoplasties for the same reason as they often limit movement of the prosthesis, particularly in the elbow, although osteophyte recurrence may be less likely due to normalized joint movement afforded by the arthroplasty.

Ligament repair

This is covered comprehensively in Chapter 9 but in summary, the method of repair needs to oppose the traction forces acting on it. The aim must be to restore the stability of the joint and careful assessment post repair is essential. Surgical repair of a ligament, whether the injury be iatrogenic as part of the surgical approach, or traumatic, can either be via a primary suture repair, prosthetic replacement or indirect stabilization of the joint using a transarticular external skeletal fixator to allow healing by fibrosis. Spiked washers can be used to give increased purchase of the soft tissues and increase the stability of the repair of the joint; careful assessment of stability and range of movement post repair is essential.

Closure

As for any surgical wound, accurate tension-free closure of the individual layers is required in all cases. Complete closure of the joint capsule is preferable, although where this is not possible synovial fluid leakage through small defects is minimal as the synovium rapidly seals the joint.

Suture materials and patterns are at the discretion of the surgeon and depend on the procedure and joint being operated on. Consideration needs to be given to the expected duration of healing and the degree of load on the tissues. For fibrous retinacular tissues, especially around the stifle, a relatively long half-life monofilament material such as polydioxanone, is recommended as

complete healing times can be relatively long. This can be placed in either an interrupted or continuous suture pattern but it is important to choose the appropriate size for the case (cats: 2 metric (3/0 USP), small dogs: 3 metric (2/0 USP) and large dogs: 3.5–4 metric (0–1/0 USP)). A range of Triclosan-coated suture materials is available with evidence that their use is associated with a significant reduction in surgical site infection rates.

Arthroscopy

With the advent of smaller, high-definition cameras and, in particular, smaller instrumentation, the role of arthroscopy is increasing. It is commonplace in most advanced veterinary practices and is the gold standard for investigations and treatment of joint disease in dogs, although there is a necessity for appropriate instrumentation and a steep learning curve for the surgeon. The general principles of arthroscopy are described in Chapter 15.

The main advantages of arthroscopy are greater magnification of lesions and less postoperative morbidity (Hoelzler *et al.*, 2004). Fluid flow is critical to facilitate a satisfactory surgery. Too low a pressure does not distend the joint sufficiently to allow insertion of the instruments or to observe any lesions. It may also not be enough to allow adequate haemostasis. Conversely, too high a pressure leads to extravasation of the fluid which in turn leads to collapse of the joint space. In the extreme this may lead to the surgery requiring conversion to arthrotomy, or aborting and rescheduling.

Patient preparation and surgical approaches

As for arthrotomies, there are well described approaches to the various joints (see the *BSAVA Manual of Canine and Feline Endoscopy and Endosurgery*). Patient preparation depends on the likelihood of successful arthroscopy without the need to convert to an arthrotomy. For the inexperienced arthroscopist a full clip, in anticipation of a conversion, is preferable and the patient is draped as for an arthrotomy. As the surgeon becomes more proficient, the clip can be made smaller although care should be taken not to increase the risk of breakdown of asepsis by employing too small a clipped area. A margin of 10 cm around the intended surgical approach is usually sufficient. The site can be four-quarter draped or a single large drape can be used with a fenestration cut over the index joint. Once the surgical field is draped and the arthroscope inserted into the joint, the lights should be dimmed in order to maximize the clarity of the image on the monitor.

For arthroscopic surgery, perioperative antibiotics are not indicated unless the duration of surgery is expected to be long. If implants are not placed into the joints, then even arthroscopies where the lesions are treated do not warrant antibiotic therapy.

Arthrodesis

Arthrodesis is the surgical fusion of two bones at a functional angle across a joint. The arthrodesis angle corresponds to the normal standing angle and is described for various joints in Figure 13.12. Arthrodesis is a salvage procedure and is indicated in the following situations:

- Intractable pain or instability
- Non-reconstructable articular fracture
- Chronic recurrent sepsis or sepsis that fails to respond to medical therapy

Joint	Dogs (degrees)	Cats (degrees)
Shoulder	105–110	110
Elbow	120–145	100–135
Carpus	5–10	10
Stifle	135–140	120–125
Tarsus	135–145	115–125

13.12 Suggested angles for arthrodesis; the appropriate angle in each case should be determined by assessing the animal preoperatively in a weight-bearing position.

- Injuries to the carpus and tarsus resulting in a palmigrade or plantigrade stance, respectively
- Neoplasia and limb-sparing surgery.

Most joints in the body, with the exception of the coxofemoral joint, can be arthrodesed. In general the distal joints, except those of the digits themselves, respond better to arthrodesis and careful consideration should be given to the pros and cons of surgically fusing a joint as opposed to alternative salvage via amputation. Elbow and stifle arthrodeses, while giving pain-free ambulation, give rise to significant gait abnormalities and are technically very challenging to perform. If there are concerns with the ability of the contralateral limb to support the animal, as may be the case where the disease process is bilateral (e.g. elbow dysplasia) or, if the owner does not wish amputation, then arthrodesis is a viable alternative (Figure 13.13).

Principles of arthrodesis

The main principles of arthrodesis are shown in Figure 13.14. To be successful it is important to fuse the joint at an appropriate angle to facilitate weight-bearing without creating iatrogenic valgus, varus or torsional deformity.

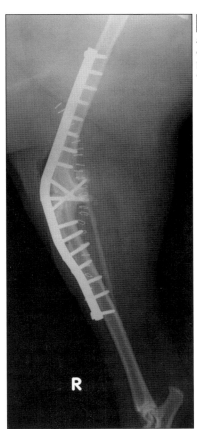

13.13 Stifle arthrodesis performed as an alternative to amputation due to severe concurrent pathology of the contralateral pelvic limb.

- Careful preoperative planning
- Complete removal of articular cartilage from the area to be arthrodesed
- Close apposition and rigid fixation of the opposing surfaces
- Stabilization at an appropriate angle for weight-bearing
- Addition of a cancellous bone graft or demineralized bone matrix to promote healing

13.14 Principles of arthrodesis.

The range of angles for most joints is described in Figure 13.12; preoperative planning should include measurements of the same joint on the contralateral limb to aid in planning. For most of the commonly performed arthrodesis procedures, there are specific plates available and these have been designed with an appropriate preset angle (e.g. pancarpal and pantarsal arthrodesis plates). However, where no such plates exist, the surgeon needs to assess the angle intraoperatively to ensure it is appropriate. A goniometer can be used for this although the author prefers a pre-bent Steinmann pin that is then autoclaved as this is more useful during surgery. In surgeries where a significant amount of bone needs resecting (e.g. stifle/shoulder arthrodesis), the limb should be fused at a slightly more extended angle than the contralateral joint in order to compensate for the loss in limb length caused by the resection.

Technique

Wide-margin draping of the limb is important to allow for accurate alignment of the limb following surgery. Extending the clip to include the entire foot will allow for the whole of the distal limb to be assessed in order to reduce the risk of inducing a deformity. If the limb is hidden by a double layer of sterile draping, it is very hard to assess alignment and mistakes can easily be made. To avoid this, the limb can instead be draped using a transparent sterile adhesive dressing to facilitate better assessment of alignment (Figure 13.15).

As for all orthopaedic surgery, it is important to use the appropriate surgical approach to expose the joint but minimize trauma to the adjacent tissues. Distal limb surgeries tend to bleed disproportionately, which hinders the surgery. Accurate dissection with careful use of diathermy can significantly reduce bleeding. In addition, bleeding can be reduced further by careful use of a tourniquet. This can be in the form of an Esmarch bandage or, as is the author's preference, a cohesive bandage can be used (Figure 13.16). The recommendation in human orthopaedic surgery is that the duration of tourniquet application does not exceed 2 hours, and the absolute maximum is 3 hours (Kutty and McElwain, 2002). Such guidelines have not been defined in cats and dogs, but it is reasonable to assume a similar duration is appropriate.

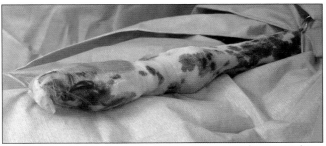

13.15 Application of a sterile adhesive transparent dressing to the foot allows correction of angulation or rotation prior to performing a carpal arthrodesis.

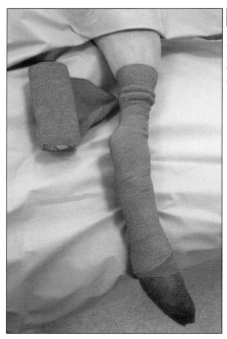

13.16 A sterile cohesive bandage used as a tourniquet to minimize bleeding at the surgical site for distal limb surgery.

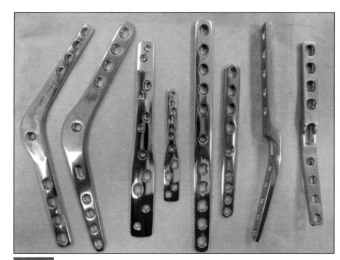

13.17 A small selection of joint-specific arthrodesis plates.

Removal of the articular cartilage is essential in order for the adjacent bones to adequately fuse. This removal can be achieved with Rongeurs or scalpel blades, but a high speed burr or a drill is more appropriate as it is rapid and achieves a more comprehensive debridement of the cartilage surface than the other techniques. Care must be taken not to remove too much subchondral bone, as this will cause inadvertent shortening or angulation of the limb.

Bone grafts are considered to be an essential part of the procedure and can either be harvested from the animal (autograft or from pre-prepared commercial sources (allograft)). The advantages of the latter are speed and availability, although there is an associated cost, and in human orthopaedic surgery, at least, they are somewhat unproven. The gold standard in human surgery is still autograft plus or minus the addition of an allograft. Donor site morbidity following the harvesting of bone grafts is a significant problem for human patients, but this appears to be much less so for dogs and cats. Fracture following harvesting is reported but rare. For further information, see the *BSAVA Manual of Canine and Feline Fracture Repair and Management*.

Rigid fixation and compression of the adjacent bone surfaces is required for arthrodesis to occur and, in most cases, this is achieved with internal fixation using compression plates. There is now a plethora of custom-made plates designed for arthrodeses, each offering their own advantages (Figure 13.17). Reports exist in the literature detailing the use of crossed pins for carpal arthrodesis (Haburjak *et al.*, 2003; Calvo *et al.*, 2009), and external skeletal fixators (Okrasinski *et al.*, 1991). For partial tarsal arthrodesis, lateral plating has been shown to have a lower complication rate than lag screws or pin and tension-band wire (Barnes *et al.*, 2013). External skeletal fixators can be used particularly for achieving arthrodesis when concurrently managing open wounds.

PRACTICAL TIP

A useful tip for arthrodesis is to use Kirschner wires to temporarily stabilize a very unstable joint in the correct alignment prior to applying the plate

A bandage is applied following tarsal or carpal arthrodesis for 24–48 hours to control postoperative swelling. Complications associated with casts and bandages can be severe and even, in extreme circumstances, life/limb-threatening (Meeson *et al.*, 2012). Unless very close and adequate attention can be given to the bandage both by the surgeon and the owner, it may be preferable not to use one after discharge from hospital as major complications can occur in a very short space of time. Biomechanical studies have shown that plates designed for use without supplementary casts have no superior strength to hybrid plates, with both types unlikely to suffer from fatigue failure, and for pancarpal arthrodesis, that there is no demonstrable benefit to adjunctive coaptation (Bristow *et al.*, 2015). Based on this, the author does not use bandages for arthrodeses except in exceptional circumstances.

References and further reading

Adams D, Quayum M, Worthington T, Lambert P and Elliott T (2005) Evaluation of a 2% chlorhexidine gluconate in 70% isopropyl alcohol skin disinfectant. *Journal of Hospital Infection* **61**, 287–290

Anderson TJ, Carmichael S and Miller A (1990) Intercondylar humeral fracture in the dog: a review of 20 cases. *Journal of Small Animal Practice* **31**, 437–442

Barnes DC, Knudsen CS, Gosling M *et al.* (2013) Complications of lateral plate fixation compared with tension-band wiring and pin or lag screw fixation for calcaneoquartal arthrodesis. Treatment of proximal intertarsal subluxation occurring secondary to non-traumatic plantar tarsal ligament disruption in dogs. *Veterinary and Comparative Orthopaedics and Traumatology* **26**, 445–452

Barr ARS, Denny HR and Gibbs C (1987) Clinical hip dysplasia in growing dogs: the long-term results of conservative management. *Journal of Small Animal Practice* **28**, 243–252

Barry S (2010) Non-steroidal anti-inflammatory drugs inhibit bone healing: a review. *Veterinary and Comparative Orthopaedics and Traumatology* **23**, 385–392

Bristow P, Meeson R, Thorne R *et al.* (2015) Clinical comparison of the hybrid dynamic compression plate and the castless plate for pancarpal arthrodesis in 219 dogs. *Veterinary Surgery* **44**, 70–77

Calvo I, Farrell M, Chase D *et al.* (2009) Carpal arthrodesis in cats. Long-term functional outcome. *Veterinary and Comparative Orthopaedics and Traumatology* **22**, 498–504

Cross MC, Kransdorf M, Chivers FS *et al.* (2014) Utility of percutaneous joint aspiration and synovial biopsy in identifying culture-positive infected hip arthroplasty. *Skeletal Radiology* **43**, 165–168

Duke-Novakovski T, de Vries M and Seymour C (2016) *BSAVA Manual of Canine and Feline Anaesthesia and Analgesia, 3rd edn.* BSAVA Publications, Gloucester

Farrell M, Clements DN, Mellor D *et al.* (2007) Retrospective evaluation of the long-term outcome of non-surgical management of 74 dogs with clinical hip dysplasia. *Veterinary Record* **160**, 506–511

Fink B, Makowiak C, Fuerst M *et al.* (2008) The value of synovial biopsy, joint aspiration and C-reactive protein in the diagnosis of late peri-prosthetic infection of total knee replacements. *Journal of Bone and Joint Surgery: British Volume* **90**, 874–878

Fitzpatrick N and Solano MA (2010) Predictive variables for complications after TPLO with stifle inspection by arthrotomy in 1000 consecutive dogs. *Veterinary Surgery* **39**, 460–474

Gemmill T and Clements D (2016) *BSAVA Manual of Canine and Feline Fracture Repair and Management, 2nd edn*. BSAVA Publications, Gloucester

Haburjak JJ, Lenehan TM, Davidson CD *et al.* (2003) Treatment of carpometacarpal and middle carpal joint hyperextension injuries with partial carpal arthrodesis using a cross pin technique: 21 cases. *Veterinary and Comparative Orthopaedics and Traumatology* **16**, 105–111

Hoelzler MG, Millis DL, Francis DA and Weigel JP (2004) Results of arthroscopic versus open arthrotomy for surgical management of cranial cruciate ligament deficiency in dogs. *Veterinary Surgery* **33**, 146–153

Hunt JR, Attenburrow PM, Slingsby LS and Murrell JC (2013) Comparison of premedication with buprenorphine or methadone with meloxicam for postoperative analgesia in dogs undergoing orthopaedic surgery. *Journal of Small Animal Practice* **54**, 418–424

Kampf G and Widmer AF (2011) Scrub or rub? What is best practice for hand hygiene before surgery? *Veterinary Journal* **190**, 307–308

Kutty S and McElwain JP (2002) Padding under tourniquets in tourniquet controlled surgery: Bruner's ten rules revisited. *Injury: International Journal of the Care of the Injured* **33**, 75–75

Lhermette P and Sobel D (2008) *BSAVA Manual of Canine and Feline Endoscopy and Endosurgery*. BSAVA Publications, Gloucester

Mayr HO, Rueschenschmidt M, Seil R *et al.* (2013) Indications for and results of arthroscopy in the arthritic knee: a European survey. *International Orthopaedics* **37**, 1263–1271

Meeson RL, Goodship AE and Arthurs GI (2012) A biomechanical evaluation of a hybrid dynamic compression plate and a castless arthrodesis plate for pancarpal arthrodesis in dogs. *Veterinary Surgery* **41**, 738–744

Nesbitt T (1982) The effects of osteophyte debridement in osteoarthrosis. *Proceedings of the 17th Annual Meeting of the American College of Veterinary Surgeons,* San Diego

Okrasinski EB, Pardo AM and Graehler RA (1991) Biomechanical evaluation of acrylic external skeletal fixation in dogs and cats. *Journal of the American Veterinary Medical Association* **199**, 1590–1593

Owen LJ, Gines JA, Knowles TG and Holt PE (2009) Efficacy of adhesive incise drapes in preventing bacterial contamination of clean canine surgical wounds. *Veterinary Surgery* **38**, 732–737

Pratesi A, Moores AP, Grierson J, Downes C and Maddox TW (2015) Efficacy of postoperative antimicrobial use for clean orthopedic implant surgery in dogs: a prospective randomized study in 100 consecutive cases. *Veterinary Surgery* **44**, 653–660

Ramsey I (2017) *BSAVA Small Animal Formulary, 9th edn – Part A: Canine and Feline*. BSAVA Publications, Gloucester

Rutala W and Weber D (2008) *Guideline for disinfection and sterilization in healthcare facilities*. Centers for Disease Control and Prevention, Augusta, Georgia

Stanway GW, Taylor PM and Brodbelt DC (2002) A preliminary investigation comparing pre-operative morphine and buprenorphine for postoperative analgesia and sedation in cats. *Veterinary Anaesthesia and Analgesia* **29**, 29–35

Steagall PVM, Carnicelli P, Taylor PM *et al.* (2006) Effects of subcutaneous methadone, morphine, buprenorphine or saline on thermal and pressure thresholds in cats. *Journal of Veterinary Pharmacology and Therapeutics* **29**, 531–537

Suess RP, Trotter EJ, Konieczynski D *et al.* (1994) Exposure and postoperative stability of 3 medial surgical approaches to the canine elbow. *Veterinary Surgery* **23**, 87–93

Tobias TA, Miyabayashi T, Olmstead ML and Hedrick LA (1994) Surgical removal of fragmented medial coronoid process in the dog – comparative effects of surgical approach and age at time of surgery. *Journal of the American Animal Hospital Association* **30**, 360–368

Vasseur PB (1984) Clinical results following nonoperative management for rupture of the cranial cruciate ligaments in dogs. *Veterinary Surgery* **13**, 243–246

Verwilghen DR, Mainil J, Mastrocicco E *et al.* (2011) Surgical hand antisepsis in veterinary practice: Evaluation of soap scrubs and alcohol based rub techniques. *Veterinary Journal* **190**, 372–377

Weese JS and Halling KB (2006) Perioperative administration of antimicrobials associated with elective surgery for cranial cruciate ligament rupture in dogs: 83 cases (2003–2005). *Journal of the American Veterinary Medical Association* **229**, 92–95

Whittem TL, Johnson AL, Smith CW *et al.* (1999) Effect of perioperative prophylactic antimicrobial treatment in dogs undergoing elective orthopedic surgery. *Journal of the American Veterinary Medical Association* **215**, 212–216

Yan H, Cui GQ, Wang JQ, Yin Y and Ao YF (2011) Arthroscopic debridement of osteoarthritic elbow in professional athletes. *Chinese Medical Journal* **124**, 4223–4228

Chapter 14

Surgical instruments and implants

John Lapish and David Strong

The bones and joints of the dog and cat vary significantly in size and amount of overlying soft tissue, and surgical accessibility depends on anatomical location. Combining correct technique with selection of appropriate instrumentation will help optimize access to, and observation of, the anatomical structures within the surgical site. Additional instruments may be required to treat specific lesions. The aim of this chapter is to broadly cover the instrumentation most commonly used in small animal orthopaedics as well as a selection of widely used basic implants. Instrumentation specific to arthroscopy is also included in this chapter but the reader is referred to the *BSAVA Manual of Canine and Feline Fracture Repair and Management* for implants relating to that topic.

Basic surgical kit

The components of a basic kit for orthopaedic surgery will be determined, at least to a degree, by personal preferences and patient size, but should contain as a minimum the elements shown in Figure 14.1.

Towel clamps

A minimum of four towel clamps is required, with six being preferable for secure draping. Additional draping will require extra towel clamps. Backhaus towel clamps are the most popular design.

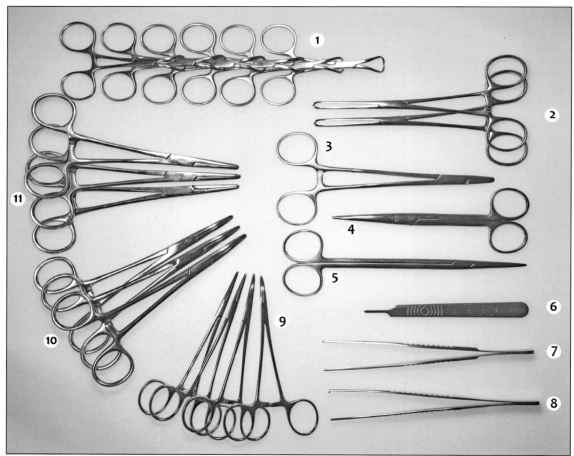

14.1 Basic joint surgery instruments.
1 = Backhaus towel clamps; 2 = Allis tissue forceps; 3 = Mayo–Hegar needle holders; 4 = straight Mayo scissors; 5 = straight Metzenbaum scissors; 6 = No. 3 scalpel handle; 7 = DeBakey dissecting forceps; 8 = rat-toothed dissecting forceps; 9 = Halsted artery forceps; 10 = curved Spencer Wells artery forceps; 11 = straight Spencer Wells artery forceps.

Scalpels

A fresh scalpel blade makes the cleanest cut with a minimum of trauma. At the microscopic level, even the sharpest of scissors cut tissue with a crushing action. Where sharp dissection is required, use of the scalpel is considered less traumatic. A No. 10 or 15 blade is suitable for incising the skin and superficial soft tissues in small animals; both fit the No. 3 scalpel handle. The No. 15 blade is the smaller blade. The sharp-pointed No. 11 can be useful when used for either stab incision into soft tissue structures, e.g. the joint capsule, or for sharp dissection of soft tissue away from bone, (Figure 14.2). It is preferable to use a separate scalpel blade for the skin incision to prevent contamination of deeper tissues.

For intra-articular procedures, small Beaver-type blades are helpful. Fitting into a Beaver-type handle, the 65 and 65a blades work as mini No. 11 blades. The tip of the 64 Beaver blade is rounded and cuts along its tip, ventral and dorsal surfaces. Being end-cutting, it cuts as it pushes through structures, which allows for more precise control. Both blades allow for accurate blade control in a confined space, e.g. when performing meniscal surgery.

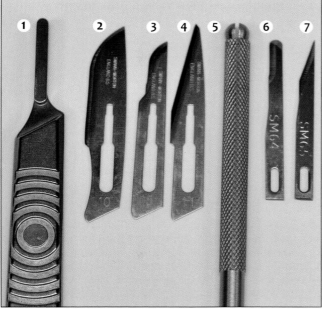

14.2 Scalpels. 1 = No. 3 handle; 2 = No. 10 blade; 3 = No. 15 blade; 4 = No. 11 blade; 5 = Beaver-type handle; 6 = No. 64 blade; 7 = No. 65 blade.

Surgical scissors

Mayo and Metzenbaum (see Figure 14.1) are the most commonly used surgical scissors. A standard surgical kit would typically contain a pair of 14 cm Mayo scissors and a pair of 18 cm Metzenbaum scissors. A 14.5 cm version of the latter is available for smaller hands.

The more delicate Metzenbaums are preferred for fine work in surgery, but when dealing with tougher fibrous tissues, they may become overloaded and damaged. For this reason, when cutting tougher tissues with scissors, Metzenbaum scissors should not be used; either Mayo or dedicated connective tissue scissors should be used instead.

Mayo scissors are less well suited to delicate work than Metzenbaum scissors due to their physical bulk, but since the geometry of their cutting edges and material specification is typically the same, the cut quality of Mayo scissors should be equal to the Metzenbaum if properly maintained. Mayo scissors are the instrument of choice for heavier scissor cuts.

Tungsten carbide-edged scissors are available. Tungsten carbide is a very hard material, but more brittle than stainless steel. Scissors with tungsten carbide edges are more expensive than their all-steel counterparts, but stay sharper for longer. For most procedures, straight scissors will be the surgeon's first choice, but many surgeons like the flexibility of having both straight and curved scissors in their kits.

Suture scissors

Cutting suture material can prematurely blunt scissors such that they do not cut tissues as cleanly. It is good practice to have separate, dedicated suture scissors in the surgical pack. These should be identified as separate from tissue scissors and only used for cutting sutures. These may be older scissors no longer suitable for cutting tissues, or scissors specifically designed and purchased for cutting sutures. Some suture materials, such as high-tensile braids used in ligament reconstruction, are particularly hard to cut and the use of dedicated scissors with tungsten carbide edges may be preferable in the long term.

Dissecting forceps

A pair of rat-toothed forceps (e.g. Adson or Treves), usually with one-into-two teeth and between 12.5 cm and 15 cm long, provide a secure grip for the skin and are occasionally used for other tough tissues. Dressing forceps with a serrated jaw or, better still, atraumatic gripping forceps with a DeBakey tooth pattern are normally used for more delicate tissues. Adson or Adson–Brown style forceps offer an intermediate jaw shape that is good for delicate tissue but less traumatic than rat-toothed forceps, while providing a much better grip than a DeBakey tooth pattern. These are especially useful for connective tissues (Figure 14.3).

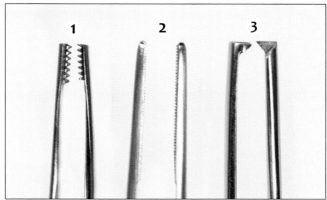

14.3 Tissue forceps showing different tips. 1 = Adson–Brown forceps; 2 = DeBakey; 3 = rat-toothed.

Artery forceps

Many patterns are available, but a combination of Spencer Wells and the much finer Halsted mosquito forceps will assist appropriate haemostasis for the range of blood vessels likely to be encountered in articular surgery. A combination of curved and straight forceps, 12.5 cm and 15 cm long, is useful.

Tissue forceps

Allis tissue forceps are the most commonly used tissue forceps in general surgery. Their jaws are traumatic, so they should only be used on tissues that are to be excised. Their typical uses include securing electrocautery cables, air hoses, and suction and drainage tubes indirectly to the surgical drape without puncturing it. All examples of this type of forceps have the same basic pattern but vary according to how many teeth are found along the tips. A broad grip of four or five teeth is most popular. Babcock forceps are less traumatic and can be used on skin margins as the weight of the instrument alone will create some retraction. If the forceps are held by an assistant the retraction is greater and directional.

Needle holders

Repair of fascial and joint capsule incisions, tenotomies, ligament repairs and closure of dead space and skin invariably require the use of suture material with a needle that is held and handled by needle holders. Locking designs with narrow jaws offer maximum control. There are a number of different locking mechanisms available, but typically they are ratcheted (Figure 14.4). If correctly weighted, these mechanisms should be comfortable to engage and disengage without the need for excessive force, and should lock securely.

Jaws with tungsten carbide inserts are highly desirable as the very hard tungsten carbide bites into the relatively soft steel of the needle minimizing slippage, improving efficiency and reducing surgeon frustration. Suitable locking designs with fine jaws include patterns such as the industry standard Mayo–Hegar or the narrower jawed DeBakey, which was originally developed for vascular surgery.

Combination-type needle holders, such as the Olsen–Hegar and Gillies, incorporate suture cutting scissors and needle-holding jaws. This helps improve workflow by avoiding the need to change instruments, but the combination of needle holder and scissors brings compromise. The scissor part can be difficult to use in areas with limited access as it is set quite far back from the tips, and the needle-holding action is not as secure as dedicated needle holders as the jaws are set further away from the instrument's pivot pin, reducing the mechanical advantage. Combination-type needle holders also have the disadvantage that the suture material may be cut inadvertently when the user is intending to grasp the needle. The working tips of Mayo–Hegar, DeBakey and Olsen–Hegar needle holders are shown in Figure 14.5.

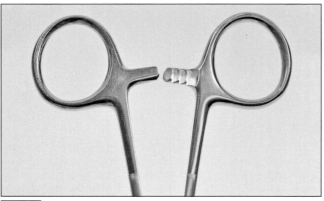

14.4 Ratchets on a pair of needle holders.

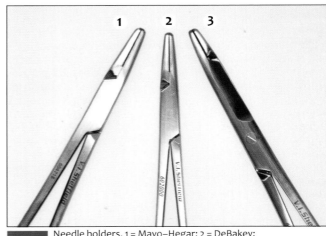

14.5 Needle holders. 1 = Mayo–Hegar; 2 = DeBakey; 3 = Olsen–Hegar.

The most common sizes of needle holder for small animal joint surgery are 16.25 cm, but they are available in a wide range of sizes to suit all hand sizes and situations. If using Mayo–Hegar or DeBakey-type needle holders, suture scissors should be included in the surgical pack.

Retractors

Adequate retraction of overlying soft tissues is essential to facilitate inspection and surgical intervention of deeper structures. Instrumentation should be selected to maximize exposure while minimizing trauma to the tissues. Care must be taken to protect arteries, veins and particularly nerves adjacent to the surgical field. Optimal retraction also minimizes direct handling of skin and wound margins, thereby satisfying one of Halsted's principles of surgery.

Self-retaining retractors

Many veterinary surgeons work with minimal assistance; thus, self-retaining retractors, which maintain distraction of tissues using some kind of self-locking system, are invaluable. Self-retaining retractors are available in a large range of sizes and types covering the large variation in size of veterinary patients. In general terms, the more superficial the need for retraction, the more prongs and the wider the 'spread' the retractor needs to have. At the level of the joint capsule, retractors with single prongs are used to maintain a window for observation or to allow greater access.

Multipronged retractors

These are illustrated in Figure 14.6.

- **Travers:** the multiple prongs and long flat arms create a wide aperture, making this type of instrument ideal for skin and superficial connective tissue. This style of retractor is available in a range of sizes from 9.5 cm (4.3 cm spread) to 20 cm (9 cm spread).
- **Weitlander:** very similar to the Travers, but proportioned slightly differently: 14 cm long with a 6 cm spread.
- **West:** 14 cm long, similar to the Weitlander but with curved arms that can sit more neatly on smaller veterinary patients. Both Weitlander and West retractors may be used in conjunction with the bigger Travers in larger patients to retract deeper layers.

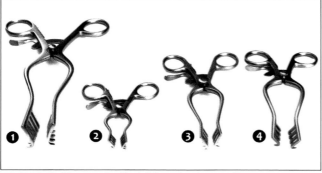

14.6 Multipronged self-retaining retractors. 1 = Travers 20cm; 2 = Travers 9.5cm; 3 = Weitlander; 4 = West.

Gelpi-type retractors

The Gelpi was originally developed as a human vulval retractor; the long sharp tips on the standard human models makes introduction into small spaces difficult and generally impractical for veterinary use. The veterinary versions have shorter tips that are either blunt or pointed, and provide excellent focal retraction, which can be invaluable at the level of the joint capsule. These retractors are also useful to retract small muscle bellies, tendons and ligaments, either for access or tissue protection. Used in pairs at right angles to each other, they can create a very useful window through which to work.

This family of retractors (Figure 14.7) has evolved over the years and is now available in many variations of design and size making them very versatile. Small and miniature sizes with small tips and lighter handles are ideal for mini-arthrotomies of the more superficial joints and for use with smaller patients. Gelpis with smaller teeth on the ratchet offer better control of retraction.

Odd leg Gelpis (Figure 14.8), with one leg longer than the other are more typically used for spinal surgery, but can be very useful for achieving the desired distraction in some cases where eccentric distraction is required. They are handed, so are sold in pairs.

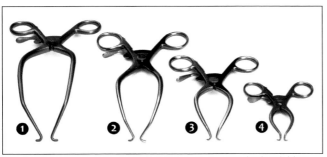

14.7 Gelpi-type retractors. 1 = long reach; 2 = standard with blunt tips; 3 = small; 4 = mini 9.5 cm.

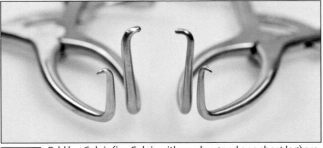

14.8 Odd leg Gelpis (i.e. Gelpis with one long and one short leg) are useful for eccentric distraction.

Hand-held retractors

Where assistance is available, hand-held retractors can provide excellent and flexible retraction, particularly of muscle bellies (Figure 14.9). Langenbeck single-blade retractors are most commonly used and are available in a range of sizes. The 6 mm and 13 mm blade widths are the most useful. Meyerdings are heavier and usually used for deep tissue retraction during total hip replacement surgery in dogs. The Senn retractor is a smaller, double-ended instrument. One end is similar to a small Langenbeck, the other is sharp and multipronged and is often referred to as a 'cat's paw' retractor. It is commonly used to retract the stifle fat pad.

As part of the handle design, some retractors, occasionally referred to as finger retractors, have a single loop similar in size and appearance to the finger loops of scissors. This provides a very practical and comfortable means of holding the instrument (Figure 14.10).

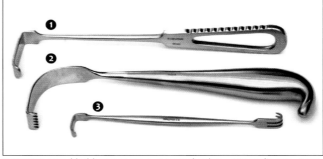

14.9 Hand-held retractors. 1 = Langenbeck; 2 = Meyerding; 3 = Senn 'cat's paw'.

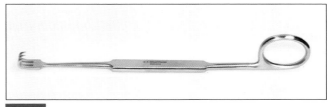

14.10 Cat's paw finger retractor.

Hohmann retractors

This is a large family of retractors with over 20 variants. The instrument is designed as a combined retractor and elevator (Figure 14.11). The tip is used to elevate a bone or bone fragment by depressing and levering the wider blade portion of the instrument against a body of muscle. Thus, the skeletal element in question is elevated relative to surrounding muscles. These roles make the Hohmann particularly useful in exposing articular surfaces.

The most useful sizes for general small animal joint surgery are the short-tipped 12 and 18 mm versions. The 18 mm version with the short tip is the standard 'Hohmann' and where the term 'Hohmann' is used in a veterinary orthopaedic text, it is generally referring to this instrument. Common applications for Hohmann retractors include exposure of the caudal tibial plateau during stifle arthrotomy for investigation of cranial cruciate ligament disease, exposure of the fabella by retraction of the biceps femoris, and the exposure of the femoral head and neck for femoral head and/or neck excision ostectomy surgery. Many variants exist for special applications.

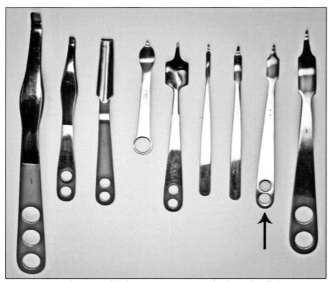

14.11 A selection of Hohmann retractors; the 'standard' 18 mm version with short tip is indicated by the arrow.

Penrose drains

Latex rubber Penrose drains, although not technically instruments, are very useful for gently retracting and maintaining the identification of nerves and other vital structures with minimal trauma. The drain is passed around the nerve, and the drain ends are clamped together using a pair of artery forceps or Allis tissue forceps. The weight of the forceps sitting on the drape is usually sufficient to maintain gentle retraction. Penrose drains are available in different widths with 6 mm (¼ inch) or 12 mm (½ inch) widths being the most common.

Specialist orthopaedic instruments

Graft passers

Graft passers are used to pull grafts, implants or suture material through joints or bone tunnels. Straight graft passers are used for bone tunnels. A range of diameters, varying between 2 cm and 8 cm, is available to suit most breeds.

Femoral head disarticulators

Disarticulation of the femoral head can be challenging if the joint capsule is very thickened and the round ligament of the femoral head is intact. The process can be much simplified using a specialist instrument. Two types of instrument are available. The disarticulator has a curved end with a sharp cutting edge in between two forks; this is designed to trap and sharply cut the round ligament. Alternatively the Hatt spoon is a deep spoon with a sharp cutting edge that is introduced into the hip and pushed around the femoral head cutting the round ligament and all adjacent soft tissue in the process (Figure 14.12).

Stifle joint distractors

Examination and effective management of the intra-articular structures of the stifle is arguably the most challenging part of routine stifle surgery. Without appropriate distraction it is impossible to completely examine and

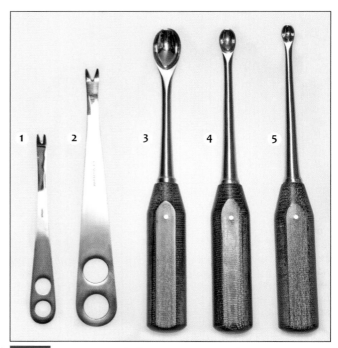

14.12 Disarticulators (1–2) and Hatt spoons (3–5) in various sizes.

treat the medial meniscus. Intra-articular stifle distractors (Figure 14.13) work on the same principle as self-retaining retractors. As the handles are closed together, the working tips spread apart. Moving the hinge closer to the working tips increases the leverage of the distractor, which is important as separation of the femur and tibia in a large dog can require substantial force.

Overlapping of the tips in the closed position allows for easier insertion into tight spaces and minimizes articular cartilage trauma on insertion and removal. Distractor tips must securely engage both the proximal tibia and distal femur in non-load-bearing areas to avoid cartilage damage; they must not slip. Care must be taken with their use to avoid iatrogenic damage to the cartilage, menisci and other intra-articular structures. Distractors enable parallel distraction of joint surfaces. The distracted joint is maintained in the open position, allowing inspection and treatment of meniscal and other lesions. Smaller versions of stifle distractors are similar to small Gelpis, and can also be used as such; their overlapping tips allow insertion into very restricted areas to create small windows. (Figure 14.13 insert). An example of their use is the creation of a joint capsule window during medial elbow arthrotomy.

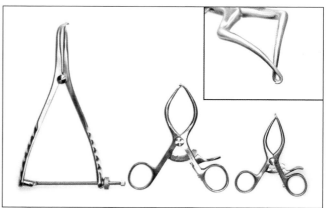

14.13 Stifle distractors. Note the crossing tips for insertion into the joint (insert).

Extra-articular stifle distractors avoid the need for insertion of a distraction device into the joint, reducing clutter in the surgical field and minimizing intra-articular trauma. They are particularly well suited to arthroscopy or arthrotomy in smaller and tighter stifles where space is limited. The use of extra-articular stifle distractors requires pins to be driven into the proximal tibia and the distal femur. The device clamps on to these pins and a distraction screw forces the two bones and their articular surfaces apart (Figure 14.14).

Hohmann retractors may also be used for stifle distraction. These do not separate the joint surfaces in the same proximodistal manner as stifle distractors; instead they displace the tibial plateau cranially relative to the femur. This can achieve excellent exposure of the menisci. The use of a Hohmann ideally requires an assistant to maintain distraction while the surgical procedure, e.g. partial meniscectomy, is being performed. Stifle levers are purpose-designed Hohmann retractors. Their blades are longer, stronger and narrower than standard Hohmann retractors. The blade is less traumatic to the articular trochlea and is less obstructive when viewing the menisci. Versions exist for both open and arthroscopic use.

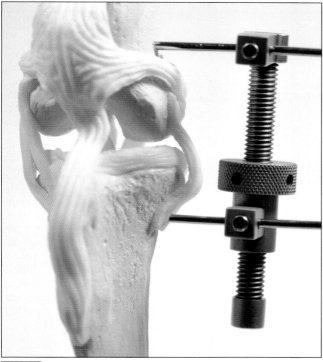

14.14 Extra-articular stifle distractor applied to bone model.

Hand saws

Hand saw blades vary with respect to blade thickness, tooth size and flexibility (Figure 14.15). The tooth size dictates the depth of cut created with each pass of the blade. Smaller toothed blades offer better control, but cut more slowly. The degree of 'saw set' (how much the tooth protrudes from the blade) dictates how wide the cut is and how much bone is removed.

Small industrial hacksaw blades are still widely used in veterinary surgery. They are normally made from high carbon steel which does not resist corrosion, i.e. they rust quickly. Standard hacksaw handles support the blade at each end; this prevents the blade from being useful in confined spaces.

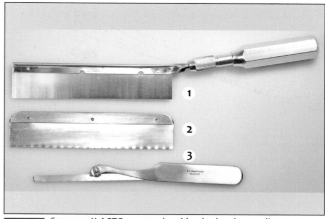

14.15 Saws. 1 = X-ACTO saw; 2 = hard-backed orthopaedic saw; 3 = adjustable bone saw.

Hard chrome-plated surgical blades are available in the hacksaw style. The hard chrome plating makes these blades more resistant to corrosion than industrial blades, so they will last much longer. They are intended for cutting bone and not metal and are designed so that they can be inserted into dedicated stainless steel handles, supporting the blade at just one end. This makes them much more versatile than blades supported at both ends, allowing them to be used in more confined areas, and they are useful for procedures such as tibial tuberosity transposition. Being supported at just one end, this type of saw lacks some directional control over its more industrial counterparts and bends easily so it is best used to cut on the pull stroke.

To increase control, some surgical saw blades are stiffened along their length by adding a metal spine to the top edge. This allows the blade itself to be made much thinner but the depth of cut is limited to the depth of the thinner portion of the blade before this spine. Hard-backed saws are available in both stainless and non-stainless forms, with a range of tooth sizes. It is the preferred instrument for femoral wedge sulcoplasty and the initial cuts on block sulcoplasty, where control over angle and direction of cut is important.

X-ACTO saw blades have a loyal following amongst many orthopaedic surgeons, especially for femoral wedge or block sulcoplasty. They have very thin blades and very fine teeth. They are manufactured from high carbon steel, so will rust quickly, especially when exposed to body fluids or put through steam autoclaves, so are best viewed as single use instruments.

Gigli wire saw

The Gigli wire saw (Figure 14.16) is a cutting wire and is particularly useful where access is restricted. The saw may be threaded through very small spaces, and cuts only when placed under tension. Examples of use include proximal ulnar osteotomy and the ischial cut in the triple pelvic osteotomy procedure. Gigli saws always cut towards the hands of the operator and can slip against the surface of the bone. This can cause problems, such as in femoral head and neck excision where the Gigli saw can slip proximally, leaving a distal spur of femoral neck. Gigli saws must be used with care, as they are inclined to catch tissues and can produce significant heat. They should also only be used with dedicated handles to avoid trauma to the operator.

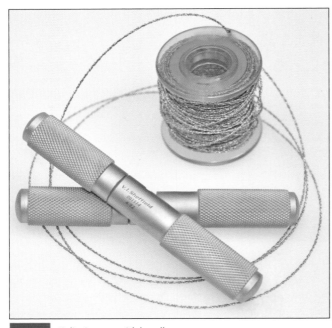

14.16 Gigli wire saw with handles.

Osteotomes

Osteotomes have a slim, sharp blade symmetrically sharpened from both sides. They drive straight and are designed to slice through bone so they are generally preferred for joint surgery (Figure 14.17); in comparison, chisels have a much heavier blade sharpened from just one side and are designed for more aggressive work elsewhere in orthopaedics. Being sharpened on just one side, chisels can be more of a challenge to use when attempting to make straight, accurate cuts in most orthopaedic applications. Osteotomes can be very effective in detaching bone associated with ligamentous and tendinous attachments, for example the greater trochanter of the femur. No bone is lost, compared with sawing, which causes bone loss equivalent to the width of the cut. If reattachment is anticipated, pre-placement of Kirschner wire or screw holes is recommended prior to cutting.

The osteotome width should be appropriate for the task, e.g. 6 mm for a small malleolus increasing to 20 mm for a femoral head and neck excision in a large dog. When using an osteotome or chisel, the bone will sometimes fissure in unexpected directions and it can also be difficult to adjust the cut angulation mid-cut; the use of an osteotome and mallet therefore requires both confidence and experience. Bone can be surprisingly hard and the cutting

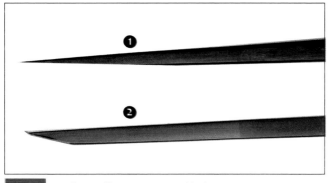

14.17 1 = edge profile osteotom; 2 = chisel.

edge of osteotomes must be maintained for optimal performance. Care must be taken with brittle bone not to cause splintering. Primarily used for femoral block sulcoplasty in veterinary orthopaedics, modular osteotomes (Figure 14.18) have replaceable blades in a variety of widths. The blades are thinner than standard osteotomes, such that they are less likely to damage the block.

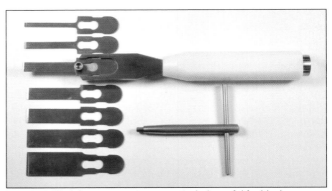

14.18 Modular osteotomes are particularly useful for block sulcoplasties of the femoral trochlea in patellar luxation surgeries.

Rongeurs

Rongeurs (Figure 14.19) are designed to nibble bone incrementally. The spoon-type jaws enclose the bone or cartilage fragment to be removed, which is withdrawn from the operative site. A large range is available, varying in bite size, jaw angle, instrument size and general design. They may be of a regular single action pattern, a double action pattern or of a 'tubular' design such as Kerrisons. Double action rongeurs offer increased mechanical advantage for a more powerful cut, but at the expense of a narrower jaw opening. Rongeurs have varied applications in orthopaedic and spinal surgery. For most small animal joint applications, a combination of a 5 mm angled bite and a 2.5 mm straight bite (e.g. Lempert) is sufficient.

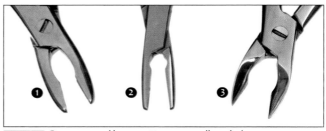

14.19 Rongeurs and bone cutters. 1 = small-angled rongeurs; 2 = straight Lempert rongeurs; 3 = small-angled cutters 15 mm jaw.

Bone cutters

The jaws of bone cutters are designed to section and separate bone fragments (Figure 14.20). In some situations, they can offer better control than osteotomes and are widely used. They are less sharp than osteotomes and tend to crush as well as cut. As the jaws close, they can sometimes skid down the bone to the narrowest part. Great care must be taken in brittle bone not to cause splintering. Bone cutters with fine angled tips are best suited to most veterinary applications as they offer better access and visibility as a cut is made. They are particularly useful in small and miniature breeds for performing femoral head and neck excision and to detach tibial tuberosities during

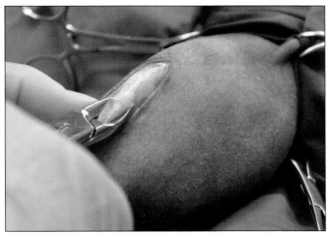

14.20 The use of notched small-angled cutters during tibial tuberosity transposition in a cat.

the correction of patella luxation (Figure 14.20). The addition of a notch in the blades near the hinge improves visibility further and allows distal periosteal attachments to be more easily preserved when cutting from distally to proximally during tibial tuberosity transposition. Powered sagittal, oscillating or reciprocating saws can offer greater control over bone cutters in cases where heavy cuts or cuts in dense bone are being performed.

Bone rasps

Rasps (Figure 14.21) are available in flat, curved and tapering designs. They are useful for removing osteophytes, adjusting femoral sulcoplasty and for tidying up osteotomies, i.e. removing rough edges. They are appropriate for the removal of bone spurs, particularly with procedures such as femoral head and neck excision, but are not appropriate for major debulking of bone. The bone debris created should be carefully flushed away prior to closure.

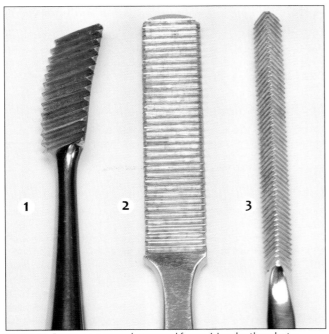

14.21 Rasps. 1 = a curved rasp used for excisional arthroplasty; 2 = a flat rasp used in block sulcoplasty; 3 = a tapered rasp used in wedge sulcoplasty.

Bone scoops and curettes

Bone scoops are useful for the collection of cancellous bone for grafting (Figure 14.22). Small scoops (up to 5–6 mm) are typically the more useful for veterinary applications. They can be used for the removal of cartilage in arthrodesis of large joints, but a power burr is much more effective.

A purpose-designed curette is available for the treatment of osteochondritis dissecans (OCD) lesions in the shoulder (Figure 14.22). Small dental curettes and scalers have been used with success in the probing and treatment of OCD lesions in the elbow.

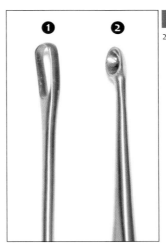

14.22 Bone scoops and curettes. 1 = OCD curette; 2 = Volkmann bone scoop.

Periosteal elevators

A periosteal elevator is used to elevate soft tissue and periosteum from the surface of bones for the application of plates, screws and wires. A variety of different shapes and sizes are available, with either curved or square ends (Figure 14.23); periosteal elevators must have sharp edges to be effective. The AO-type periosteal elevator is the archetypal periosteal elevator and is single-ended with a chunky handle and a choice of either curved or square-ended tips. The Freer periosteal elevator and the modified Howarth dissector are arguably more versatile, being double-ended with a rounded tip at one end and a square tip at the other. The Freer has finer tips and is particularly well suited to spinal work and smaller patients.

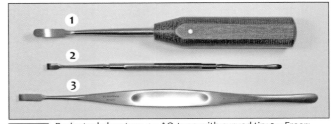

14.23 Periosteal elevators. 1 = AO-type with curved tip; 2 = Freer; 3 = modified Howarth.

Powered instruments

Many surgical procedures are made easier by using powered instruments to create osteotomies, to drive pins or to drill holes for suture anchors, screws or bone tunnels. Power instrumentation typically enables a quicker, more precisely controlled procedure with less error from factors such as hand wobble when compared with hand instruments.

Several saw types exist including reciprocal saws, oscillating saws, sagittal saws and tibial plateau levelling osteotomy (TPLO) saws. When choosing a saw it is necessary to ensure that an appropriate range of blades is available; for example, closing wedge tibial plateau levelling procedures may require blades of 40 mm or longer.

Battery-powered units

Produced in very high volumes, industrial-type battery-powered units are the most economical (Figure 14.24). High quality industrial units can offer very good reliability and often come with high torque motors and variable speed. Although they can be sterilized using ethylene oxide, most surgeons opt to use them non-sterile, enclosed in steam-sterilized fabric shrouds from which steam-sterilized extensions protrude. Shrouding these units helps to keep them clean as they have numerous gaps and vents within their bodywork which would otherwise be impractical to keep clean from biological debris. The airflow from the fans in industrial units has the potential to compromise sterility and many are quite bulky for surgical purposes.

Dedicated orthopaedic battery-powered units (Figure 14.25) are becoming increasingly popular. They are steam autoclavable (not the batteries) and take the form of either a stand-alone drill and saw or a modular system (Figure 14.25). Modular systems comprise a hand piece with interchangeable attachments; these usually include a chuck

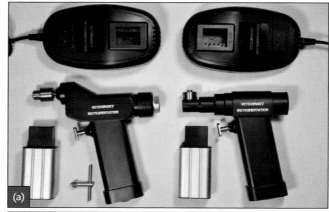

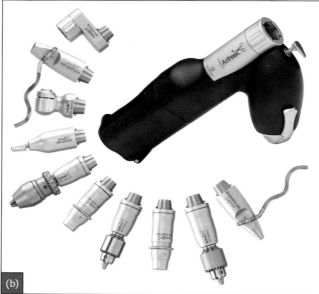

14.25 Autoclavable orthopaedic power tools. (a) Autoclavable stand-alone surgical battery drill and battery saw – VI Black Series shown. (b) Modular autoclavable surgical battery system – Arthrex V300 system shown.
(b, © Arthrex GmbH)

for drilling, an oscillating saw and a wire driver. Some of the more expensive units feature an oscillating mode which can be useful for minimizing the wrapping of soft tissues during pin insertion.

Air-powered tools

Air-powered tools have been around for longer than battery-powered units. Having simple internal mechanisms, they tend to be lighter than battery units and offer excellent longevity and serviceability. Long term, air tools can prove very economical. Their use requires a hose connected to either a compressor or a cylinder of medical air. The hoses of modern units have two lumens, so that the waste gases pass back down the hose and away from the operation site. The hoses, cylinders and compressors can get in the way and many surgeons find battery power to be more convenient. Most air tools require a pressure of 7 bar. Small, high-speed pencil grip handpieces are almost all air-powered, providing excellent power to weight ratios. The use of a high-speed burr is an effective means of stripping articular cartilage prior to joint arthrodesis and they are also used for spinal surgery. Side-cutting burrs are more efficient than round burrs and better suited to arthrodesis. A selection of air-powered tools is shown (Figure 14.26).

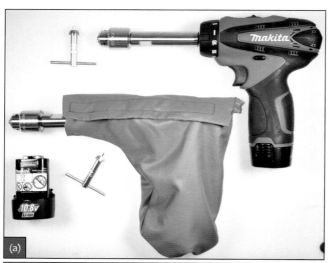

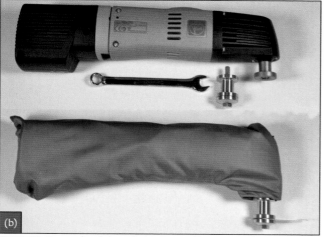

14.24 Exposed and shrouded orthopaedic power tools. (a) Industrial-type battery drill – Makita shown. (b) Industrial-type battery saw – Fein Multimaster shown.

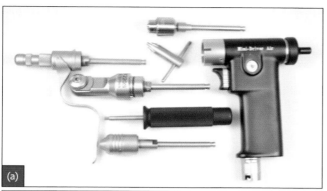

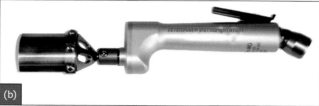

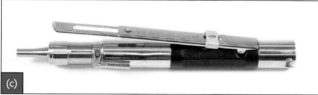

14.26 Air-powered tools. (a) Modular autoclavable air system – Mini Driver shown. (b) Air-driven TPLO saw – Whittemore shown. (c) Pencil grip high speed burr – Minos shown.

Periarticular implants

Tissue anchors, suture anchors, interference screws, buttons and toggles

Anchoring devices are used to reattach ligaments and tendons, or to attach prosthetic suture material.

Tissue anchors

Ligaments and tendons can be directly reattached using either staples with a toothed under-surface or a spiked washer secured with a screw (Figure 14.27).

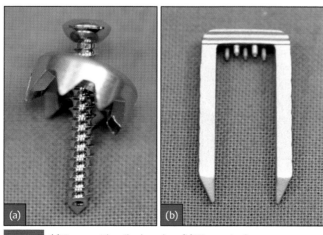

14.27 (a) Screw with spiked washer. (b) Tissue staple.

Suture screws and anchors

Suture screws have a modified protruding head that has a hole for passing a suture through it (Figure 14.28). These are largely replacing the more basic approach of using screws in combination with an orthopaedic washer to trap the suture in place, as they typically provide better suture security.

With the exception of 'suture anchor pins' with their 'snap-off' shaft, screw-type anchors require dedicated drivers. The shaft of the suture anchor pin is gripped in a standard three-jaw chuck for driving the suture anchor into the bone under power, but can then be snapped off from the anchor device at a pre-determined weak area.

Some suture anchors come pre-loaded with suture material and are placed below the bone surface where they cause minimal interference with overlying soft tissues. The anchors may be self-drilling and self-tapping, or require a pilot hole to be pre-drilled. In some cases, additional pre-tapping may be required.

Interference screws

Interference screws are popular in human surgery and becoming more popular for veterinary use. A hole is pre-drilled and the suture material is inserted into the hole. Insertion of the interference screw into the hole afterwards traps the suture in place. The headless varieties of these devices provide a very low profile (Figure 14.29).

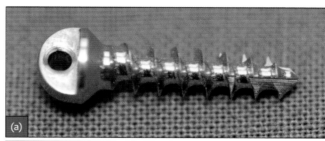

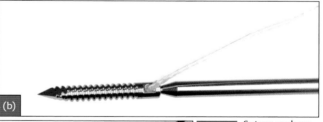

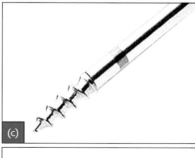

14.28 Suture anchors. (a) Suture screw. (b) Suture anchor pin. (c–d) Arthrex FASTak® anchor in insertion tool and deployed. (c–d © Arthrex GmbH)

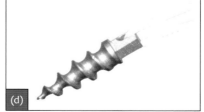

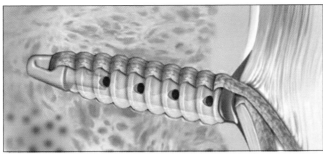

14.29 Arthrex SwiveLock®, a modified headless interference screw. (© Arthrex GmbH)

Buttons and toggles

Buttons and toggles provide an alternative method of suture anchorage (Figure 14.30). Toggles have one or more central holes and the suture is pre-placed on to the toggle before the toggle is pushed through a bone tunnel. The orientation of the toggle changes when it is pushed through the trans-cortex of the bone, so that it presents a larger cross-section than the hole diameter and will no longer fit back through the hole. They are particularly useful where access to the far side of the bone is impractical or would provide significant additional trauma, for example in the management of hip luxation.

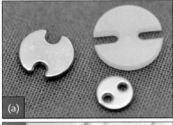

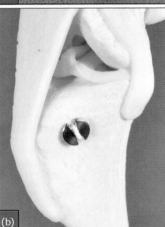

14.30 Buttons and a toggle:. (a) An 'Ormrod' button made of ultra-high molecular weight polyethylene (UHMWPE) (top right) alongside two titanium buttons. (b) A titanium button used to anchor a braided UHMWPE suture in a modification of the lateral suture technique for cranial cruciate ligament insufficiency. (c) The medial wall of an acetabulum showing a hip toggle *in situ* as used in the management of hip luxation.

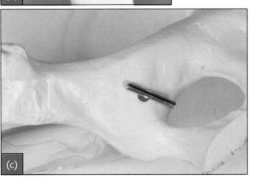

When access to the far side of the bone can easily be achieved, buttons that are much larger than the bone tunnel can be used; these are stronger and dissipate forces better than toggles. For example, a button can be placed medial to the tibial tuberosity to secure an extracapsular lateral fabellar suture for stifle stabilization. Buttons can be slotted or have holes. Slotted buttons are often easier to use as they can be slid under a loop of suture rather than having to be threaded on to the end of the suture.

When working with bone tunnels, aiming devices and push–pull suture passers can be very useful.

Kirschner and arthrodesis wires

Arthrodesis wires (A-wires) have a relatively short trocar tip at one or both ends (effectively mini Steinmann pins) which both cut and deform bone as they are placed (Figure 14.31). Kirschner wires (K-wires) have a long spatulated tip which cuts more efficiently than A-wires, but only in a clockwise direction (the same as conventional drill bits).

Most surgeons prefer the use of arthrodesis wires as they can be driven into the bone both clockwise and anti-clockwise, can engage with the bone at a much shallower angle of inclination and find a path past other previously placed implants more easily than K-wires.

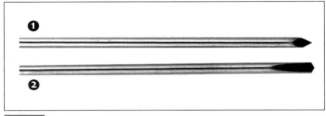

14.31 1 = arthrodesis wire; 2 = Kirschner wire.

Insertion is best accomplished using a low-speed drill rather than a hand chuck. When drilling such wires, the exposed portion should be as short as possible to minimize bending and wobble. Dedicated wire drivers are best, either stand-alone or as part of a modular system, as they facilitate the incremental insertion of wires without having to adjust the chuck. The wire is effectively fed through the cannulated driver into the bone.

Wires should be cut, when necessary, with dedicated pin cutters rather than sawn with hacksaw blades. The latter will cause metal debris to be seeded into the surgical site, whereas pin cutters produce a clean, debris-free cut. If it is desirable that the cut end of the wire should be under the bone surface (e.g. at an articular surface), the wire is scored using hard wire cutters and then driven into the bone such that the scored portion is just beneath the bone surface. The protruding wire is bent at right angles to the score line. The wire will harden and become brittle at this partial cut before snapping. It is not necessary to bend the wire aggressively, which may disrupt the repair. Alternatively, the wire may be cut at the bone surface and driven deeper using a pin punch. This technique is more traumatic to articular cartilage.

In non-articular areas, or where the wires are to be used as anchorage for tension-band wires, the wires are deliberately cut long and bent over. This minimizes soft tissue irritation and prevents the wire from working its way forward throughout the bone. It is important that the wire bends at, or close to, the bone surface. Bending below the bone surface will tend to open the osteotomy or fracture site; dedicated wire benders focus the bending forces at the bone surface, minimizing disruption of the repair (Figure 14.32). The wire benders are used in one of two ways:

- The single bend technique – concentrating forces at the bend in the wire and not at the bone. The wire may need to be worked deeper after the bend is created. Best for delicate fragments
- The two bend technique – putting the bone under greater force, but ensuring the bend is right at the bone surface.

Both Kirschner and arthrodesis wires are made from high-tensile stainless steel (grade 316LVM) or titanium alloy and require hard wire cutters to cut them, typically with tungsten carbide inserts. Cutters designed to only cut soft wire such as orthopaedic wire (see below) or bone will be damaged if used to cut hard wires.

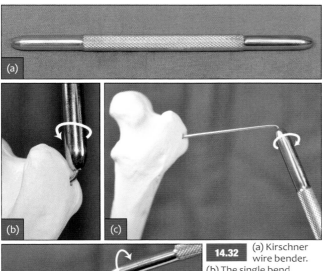

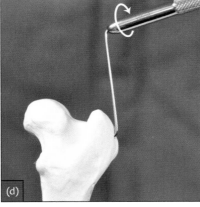

| 14.32 | (a) Kirschner wire bender. |

(b) The single bend technique. (c–d) The two bend technique. The arrows suggest the direction in which the instrument should be moved.

Orthopaedic wire

More malleable orthopaedic wire (also stainless steel grade 316LVM) is used for cerclage wiring and for the tension-band wiring used to repair osteotomies and avulsion fractures. The required size is dependent on a number of factors such as anatomical location, but typical sizes are shown in Figure 14.33.

Orthopaedic wire may be supplied in long rolls or in shorter lengths with an eyelet at one end (Figure 14.34). Malleable orthopaedic wire is much softer than the wire used for Kirschner and arthrodesis wires and can be cut using most implant cutters.

Patient bodyweight (kg)	Suggested wire diameter (mm)
2–5 kg	0.4–0.7 mm
5–10 kg	0.5–0.8 mm
10–15 kg	0.7–1.0 mm
15–20 kg	0.8–1.2 mm
20–30 kg+	1.0–1.5 mm

| 14.33 | Typical orthopaedic wire diameter based on patient weight.

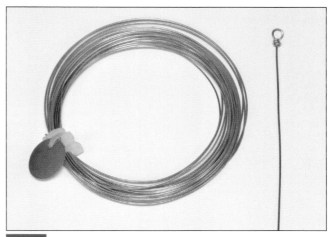

| 14.34 | Coiled orthopaedic wire (left) and eyed wire (right).

Wire tightening may be accomplished in one of a number of ways. Wires without eyelets are most frequently tightened by twisting the wire ends evenly around each other to create an even twist (Figure 14.35). An uneven twist will not only make the failure of one of the two ends of the wire more likely as it is tightened, but will also allow one end of the wire to slip relative to the other. An even twist wraps each wire around each other providing excellent security. There are several devices available to help generate an even twist.

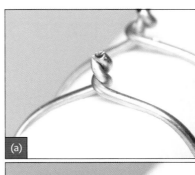

| 14.35 | (a) Good twist – both wire strands wrap around each other. (b) Bad twist – one wire wraps around the other, which may allow the central wire to slip through.

Ideally, the twisted end of the wire should be left standing proud in order to maintain maximum tension. Sometimes this will cause unacceptable interference with overlying soft tissues. Rather than push the twist sideways after cutting it short (which may lose tension), the wire can be rotated sideways while continuing to twist and this will result in a twist that lies flatter to the bone without appreciable loss in tension (Figure 14.36).

When used in tension-band wiring, the wire is bent through an acute angle and even tensioning cannot be achieved by tightening on one side only. Tightening is achieved by creating a twist on both sides of the wire loop and tightening each in turn until the desired tension is reached (Figure 14.37).

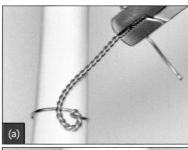
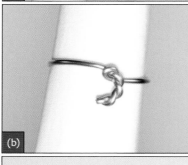
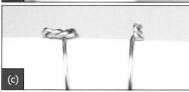

14.36 (a–b) Once the wire is tight, continuing to twist while pushing down and sideways will flatten the twist against the bone with minimal loss in tension. The tail can then be trimmed to the appropriate length. (c) Flattened twist (left) and proud twist (right).

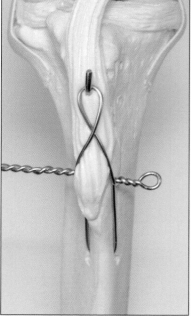

14.37 Twisting both sides of the tension-band wire will provide symmetrical tension.

Wires with eyelets are used exclusively for cerclage and require a special instrument to tighten them. The free end of the wire is fed through the eyelet and into the tightener. The crank handle is turned until the desired tension is achieved before bending the wire back on itself (Figure 14.38). The wire is then bent back and forth a few millimetres from the eyelet until it cycles to failure. A similar effect can be created by passing a double wire and feeding both free ends through the loop created.

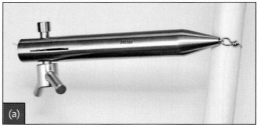
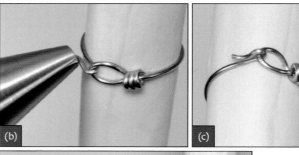
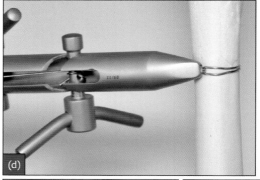
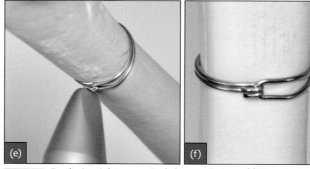

14.38 Eyed wire-tightener – single loop technique. (a) The wire is fed around the bone, through the eyelet, through the tip of the device and through a hole in the shaft of the crank. The crank is turned until the desired tension is achieved and then folded back on itself away from the eyelet. (b) The crank is loosened, exposing more wire before bending upwards. (c) The wire is cut leaving a 0.5–1.0 cm return. (d) The double loop technique using the double crank. The wire is folded to create a loop. This is passed around the bone and both free ends are passed through the loop, through the tip of the double wire-tightener and through the holes in the shafts of the cranks. The cranks are turned separately to take up the slack and then turned simultaneously to create equal tension in both free ends of the wire. The wires are folded back on themselves. (e–f) The cranks are loosened and the free ends bent upwards at a suitable length as per the single loop technique.

Cerclage wires placed with the twisting method should be placed with extra care as the twisting action can cause the wire to become oblique rather than perpendicular to the long axis of the bone. Without additional means to keep them in position, oblique wires will loosen very quickly (Figure 14.39). Eyed wires and wires placed using the double loop technique are less likely to be placed obliquely compared with wires tightened using a twisting technique.

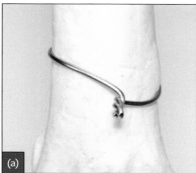
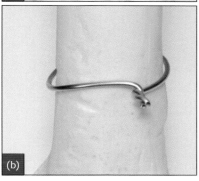

14.39 (a) An obliquely placed wire feels tight with twisting in one direction only. (b) A small rotation in the other direction as may occur under normal load-bearing leaves the wire loose.

Electrosurgery

Electrosurgery involves the passage of radiofrequency (500–3300 Hz) alternating current through body tissues to produce cutting and/or coagulation. The electrosurgical effect is varied by adjusting voltage and the pulse rate of the electrical energy. Continuous low voltage creates a cutting effect; pulsed high voltage will cause coagulation; and blends of the two types will create intermediate effects. The different modes are selected from the control panel of the electrosurgical unit.

Settings should be adjusted appropriately to achieve adequate haemostasis but avoid tissue damage and burning. Proper haemostasis is one of Halsted's principles of surgery and is essential as it gives excellent surgical visibility that is not obscured by bleeding, in addition to minimizing loss of blood.

Monopolar units, such as that shown in Figure 14.40a, create heat at a single point as the electrical energy passes from the probe tip through the body to a large earth plate under the patient. The electrical energy, thus, affects a relatively large area until fully dissipated. If the patient is poorly grounded, i.e. if there is only minimal contact between the patient and the ground plate, serious tissue burns may occur at the grounding point, distant from the surgical site. Bipolar units (Figure 14.40b) create heat as electrical energy passes between the similar sized tips or edges of bipolar instruments, so that the effect of the electrical pulse is very localized. The use of bipolar rather than monopolar equipment is recommended in the vicinity of nerves.

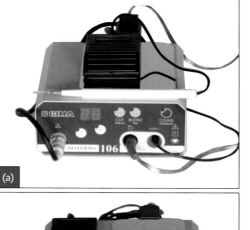
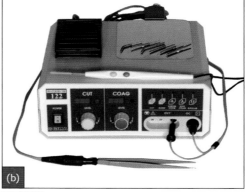

14.40 Electrosurgical machines. (a) Monopolar; (b) Bipolar.

Suction

Use of suction greatly aids visibility as it allows excessive fluids such as blood or surgical irrigation fluids to be removed efficiently. Frazier and Adson suction tips are used most frequently in veterinary orthopaedics. The Frazier suction tips are typically around 2.6 mm in diameter and the Adson suction tips around 4 mm, enabling focal suction to be achieved (Figure 14.41). These are generally better suited to work in and around the joints than larger devices.

The larger Yankauer suction tip and certain disposable suction tips are, however, occasionally employed in and around the hip when larger fluid volumes may be used. Suction control is typically provided by controls on the main suction unit that houses the motor and via a small finger port on the suction tip that provides suction at the working tip when occluded.

New suction units are generally supplied with a short silicone tube for attachment to a long disposable suction tube and tip.

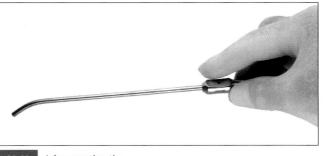

14.41 Adson suction tip.

Lighting

Without appropriate lighting, surgery with even the best approach will be more challenging and visibility significantly impaired: good quality surgical lighting is recommended for all orthopaedic surgery.

Auxillary stand- or ceiling-mounted point lighting that brings in light from just one direction is very economical and is particularly useful for superficial surgeries. However, it can be counterproductive when working down narrow or deep corridors of dissection as excessive light/dark contrast is created, exaggerating shadows and making visualization difficult. High quality ambient lighting often provides better visibility as this high contrast effect is less pronounced.

For ceiling- and stand-mounted lighting, generally the bigger the better. Large light sources that can be focused bring in light from a wide area, casting less shadow. These units are highly desirable, but can be very expensive.

Keeping radiant heat to a minimum helps reduce tissue desiccation, which can be surprisingly rapid under theatre lighting. Dedicated theatre lighting described as 'cool lighting' generates low radiant heat, keeping desiccation to a minimum. LED lighting generates very little heat and is highly desirable, but not all LEDs provide the same light quality and this may influence the appearance of tissues and materials. If hot lights are used, additional attention should be paid to appropriate irrigation of the tissues throughout the procedure to prevent desiccation.

Head-mounted point lighting can be very useful for narrow dissection corridors since it brings in light from a direction very close to the surgeon's line of sight, reducing shadow casting to a minimum.

Arthroscopy equipment

Positioning aids and distraction devices

Good patient positioning is vital for arthroscopy, especially when it comes to stifle arthroscopy. Positioning aids such as the VI multi-arm greatly facilitate this. Hanging limb techniques, sandbags used as a fulcrum and arthroscopic distractors can all be used to help open joint compartments and improve access.

Arthroscope

A typical arthroscope with blunt and sharp trocars is shown in Figure 14.42. Arthroscopes are a form of rigid endoscope. The fragile fibre optic core is protected to an extent by an integral metal jacket. This jacket also permits the mounting of an objective lens, a light post for connecting a light-source connection and an eyepiece or snap coupling. The working end of the arthroscope is slid within an outer metal arthroscope sheath. These sheaths permit insertion and simplify manoeuvring of the arthroscope, whilst offering added protection to the lens and shaft; many feature a stopcock for fluid control. For insertion into the joint, a correctly sized sharp or blunt trocar is placed in the sheath. Once this is introduced into the joint, the sheath is maintained in position, the trocar is removed and the arthroscope itself is placed in the sheath. The arthroscope is secured/locked in position in the sheath by a rotating collar at the operator's end of the sheath.

The small size of small animal joints necessitates small diameter arthroscopes:

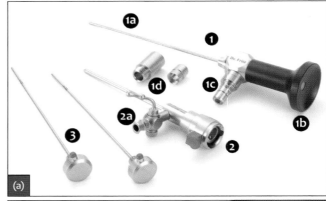

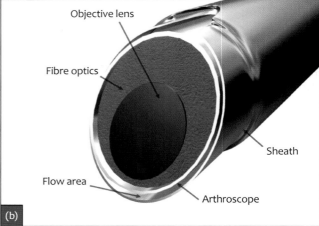

14.42 (a) Components of an artroscope. 1 = arthroscope; 1a = shaft; 1b = eyepiece; 1c = light-post; 1d = adaptors for light-post; 2 = arthroscopic sheath; 2a = flushing port and stopcock; 3 = sharp and blunt obturators. (b) Objective end of an arthroscope.

- 1.9 mm arthroscopes are well suited to the elbow, tarsus and several joints in cats and small-breed dogs. This size tends to be fragile and must be handled with particular care
- 2.3/2.4 mm arthroscopes are perhaps the most versatile and commonly used in small animal arthroscopy with uses across a range of joints and patient sizes. This size is typically used in particular for elbow arthroscopy of medium sized dogs
- 2.7 mm endoscopes are very popular, though not quite as versatile as 2.4 mm endoscopes
- 4 mm endoscopes are ideal for stifle arthroscopy in most medium- to large-breed dogs, but are used rarely in small animal orthopaedics.

The shape and angulation of the objective lens dictates the field of view and viewing angle (Figure 14.43). The viewing angle of veterinary arthroscopes is typically 30 degrees from the long axis of the shaft; 0 degrees and 70 degrees arthroscopes are also available. Smaller diameter endoscopes tend to offer a narrower field of view and poorer light transmission.

Unlike flexible endoscopes, most arthroscopes can be sterilized in an autoclave, although this will reduce the expected working life of the arthroscope. Ethylene oxide sterilization is preferred, but cold sterilization in a sterilization liquid is also possible. For further information the reader is recommended to read the manufacturers' recommendations.

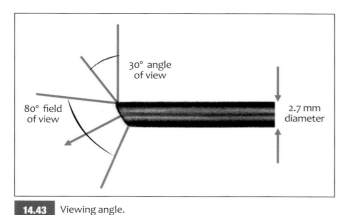

14.43 Viewing angle.

Camera, monitors and recording equipment

In theory, it is possible to use eyepieces directly without the need for a camera. This is not a sterile technique. It is also very limited in terms of convenience and comfort. The use of a camera to project the images on to a screen at magnification is considered essential as:

- Surgical asepsis is preserved
- Image magnification may permit more accurate diagnosis
- Surgeon posture may be greatly improved
- Surgeon comfort looking straight at a monitor is much better
- Instrumentation and arthroscope can be simultaneously handled more easily whilst maintaining sterility and good observation of intra-articular structures
- Images can be shared immediately, locally and remotely engaging the surgical team
- With the aid of image and video capture, the case can be documented and images and videos used for case discussion with the owner and colleagues.

A number of different camera technologies are available and these can be broadly broken down into four categories:

- Single chip – A single charge-coupled device (CCD) sensor chip is used. Efficiencies in manufacture make this an economical choice, but at the expense of resolution. The single chip must resolve red, green and blue, meaning that only every third sensor element is used for each colour. Newer 'high definition' CCD chips are available offering increased resolution with attractive pricing
- Three chip – Three chip cameras feature a colour separation prism, splitting the light into separate red, green and blue. Using the same sensor element density per CCD chip as for single chip cameras, but across three chips, with each chip dedicated to a colour results in much higher resolution with typically better colour rendition
- Three chip HD – Advances in chip technology offer higher definition. High-definition flat panel monitors typically offer a much larger viewable area for their weight and expense *versus* their equivalent cathode ray tube (CRT) predecessors, and take full advantage of HD camera technology
- Three chip HD high resolution (1920 x 1080 pixel resolution or higher) – Advances in chip technology

continue to increase sensor density of sensor elements on CCD chips permitting ever higher resolutions. As with HD cameras, using a monitor of sufficient resolution to take advantage of the full camera resolution is indicated.

The camera and cable can be prepared for surgery in two ways: either sterilized in the autoclave (only specific models designed as such), or using ethylene oxide, or placed and handled in a sterile flexible sheath that obviates the need for direct sterilization (Figure 14.44). Some cameras are now wireless which means that a camera cable is no longer necessary.

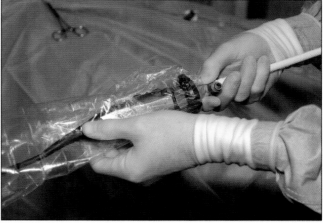

14.44 A sterile plastic sheath used to enclose the camera in a sterile manner.

Light source

Illumination of the joint space and accurate colour rendition requires light of the right quality to be introduced through the arthroscope and into the joint. A mains operated light source is the usual solution and is connected to the light post on the arthroscope via a sterilizable fibre optic light cable. Light sources of this type allow the brightness to be accurately controlled and the light quality to be maintained.

The two most popular light source technologies currently available are xenon and LED. Xenon lamps provide excellent brightness and colour rendition, but the bulbs are prone to sudden failure, such that a spare should be kept available. LED lamps have advanced tremendously over the last few years, becoming brighter with ever improving colour quality, whilst generating very little heat. The service life of new LED systems is often quoted as tens of thousands of hours, amounting to many years of heavy use without the need for replacement.

Battery units that connect directly to the light post are becoming available and may offer some convenience to the operator, however, they typically lack control of brightness, the light quality may be lacking and battery life may be limited. As technologies advance, these drawbacks may all be overcome.

Irrigation

Access to most joints is greatly facilitated by introducing fluid under pressure; this makes insertion of larger scopes possible whilst limiting the risk of iatrogenic trauma to the cartilage surfaces. Adequate irrigation to maintain a clear field of view and for flushing blood and debris from the joint may require considerable volumes. Delivering these fluids can be achieved using a fluid bag surrounded by a pressure cuff. These may be manually or automatically operated to maintain appropriate pressures as the fluids empty. Greater control and consistency can be achieved by means of dedicated arthroscopy irrigation pumps. Three-way taps and extension tubing can also be used to control pressure and delivery of fluid.

Needles and obturators

Hypodermic-type needles are used for the initial introduction of fluids into the joint and may be suitable for use throughout the procedure.

Arthroscopic sheaths should be placed with an obturator fitted to limit damage/coring of soft tissues and permit joint puncture. Obturators are available as sharp, semi-sharp and blunt, although a blunt one is preferable to minimize iatrogenic trauma to the articular surfaces (Figure 14.45).

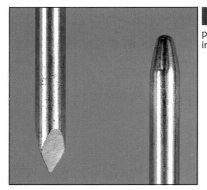

14.45 A blunt (right) and sharp (left) trocar point used to insert cannulae into the joint.

Hand instrumentation

A wide range of hand instrumentation is available for arthroscopy. It is typically smaller than similar instrumentation used for open arthrotomy. The small size makes it fragile, necessitating the use of specially selected high-grade materials and very careful attention to the manufacturing tolerances. Regardless, such instrumentation is delicate and must be handled carefully. Some surgeons prefer to use instrumentation with a matt or dark finish to reduce glare and improve contrast between tissues and the instrumentation.

Alternatively, if open portals are used for elbow and, to a lesser extent, shoulder arthroscopy, fine straight haemostats can be used for fragment manipulation and retrieval. Although more bulky, a standard haemostat is also more robust.

Probes

Arthroscopic probes are used for a variety of purposes, including the manipulation of tissues (e.g. cartilage flaps in OCD) and assessing the integrity of ligaments and menisci. Many arthroscopic probes feature an etched scale on the tip (Figure 14.46).

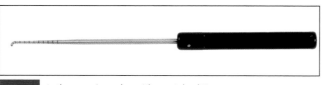

14.46 Arthroscopic probe with an etched tip.

Cutting instruments (hooks, smiley, banana knife, osteotomes)

The often limited access achieved with arthroscopy necessitates the use of dedicated cutting instrumentation. Hook knives, smiley knives and banana knives (Figure 14.47) are used extensively in arthroscopic meniscal surgery. The main application of osteotomes in small animal arthroscopy is medial coronoid resection in elbow surgery (Figure 14.48).

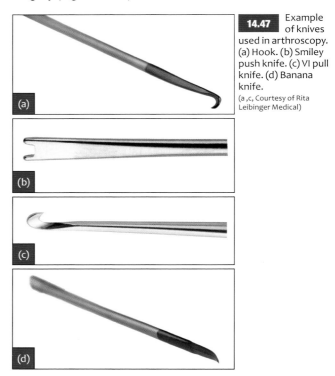

14.47 Example of knives used in arthroscopy. (a) Hook. (b) Smiley push knife. (c) VI pull knife. (d) Banana knife.
(a ,c, Courtesy of Rita Leibinger Medical)

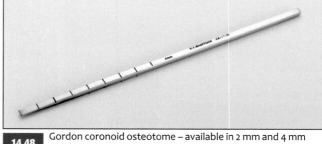

14.48 Gordon coronoid osteotome – available in 2 mm and 4 mm widths.

Punches, scissors, biopsy forceps and grasping instrumentation

The arthroscopic versions of these instruments have a cylindrical shaft, the diameter of which makes up part of the product description. The moving parts of these instruments can be very small.

These cylindrical shafts can be very useful for the management of meniscal tears, for grasping small fragments and for the biopsy of cartilage, synovium and other tissues. These instruments are sold in a range of tip angles to enable approach to tissues at a suitable angle through limited access. In addition, the shafts of several designs can be rotated, to present the tips at the most useful angles. The working ends of a selection of arthroscopic punches, scissors, biopsy and grasping forceps are shown in Figure 14.49.

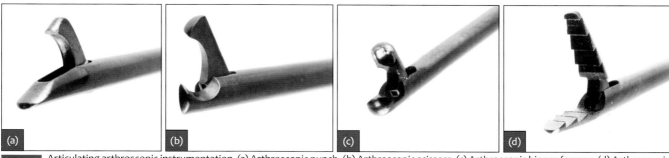

14.49 Articulating arthroscopic instrumentation. (a) Arthroscopic punch. (b) Arthroscopic scissors. (c) Arthroscopic biopsy forceps. (d) Arthroscopic grasping forceps.
(© Arthrex GmbH)

At the time of writing, the smallest of these instrument lines in common use are 2.0 mm, calling for extremely precise manufacture. It is easy to forget how small and potentially fragile these instruments are when viewed on a monitor at high magnification. Naturally, the larger the instrument, the more robust it will be, but this may limit application.

Failure of the smaller components of these instruments may be by acute overload, but it will be greatly accelerated by the accumulation of biological debris and by corrosion. Many of these instruments incorporate flushing portals to help reduce contamination on their inner mechanisms, permit lubrication and extend longevity.

Curettes, hand mills and picks

Curettes and hand mills are used to remove hard tissues, such as cartilage and bone. Picks are typically used to freshen areas of chondromalacia with the hope of stimulating fibrocartilaginous infill of defects. They are frequently employed in the management of OCD. A selection of curettes, a hand mill and a pick are shown in Figure 14.50.

Shaver units

Shaver units are powered units that can be used in much the same way as hand mills. A number of different tips are available, of which the most common are burrs and shavers of different sizes and designs, such that they can be used for debridement not just of hard tissues, but soft tissues as well (e.g. cranial cruciate ligament (CCL) remnants, hypertrophied villi, etc.). A shaver unit is shown in Figure 14.51a with an example of a soft-tissue resection blade in Figure 14.51b. As powered units, they work more quickly, accurately and easily than hand mills. As the rotating end piece is protected by a sheath, there is less chance of iatrogenic damage of adjacent structures, but this also has the tendency of producing microscopic metal debris in the joint from metal-on-metal contact. An added advantage is that all the debris they generate is evacuated through their tubular shaft along with irrigation fluid.

Ablation

Radiofrequency ablation wands are available and require their own console unit. They work by desiccating the tissues and are useful for the combined rapid ablation and cautery of villus hypertrophy and ligamentous structures.

Aiming guides

Arthroscopic aiming guides connect the arthroscopic sheath housing an arthroscope to an arthroscopic sheath

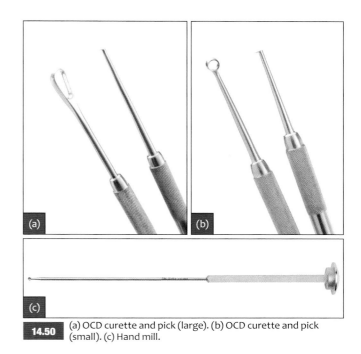

14.50 (a) OCD curette and pick (large). (b) OCD curette and pick (small). (c) Hand mill.

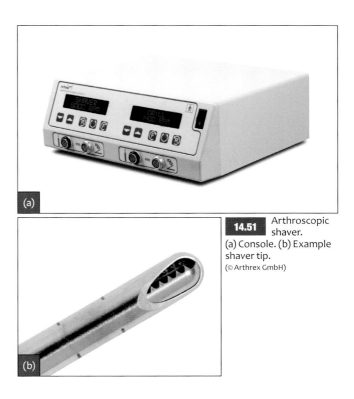

14.51 Arthroscopic shaver.
(a) Console. (b) Example shaver tip.
(© Arthrex GmbH)

for an instrument portal. The triangulation ensures the tip of the arthroscope and instrument are suitably approximated for optimum function. Their main application is in shoulder surgery, a popular example is shown in Figure 14.52.

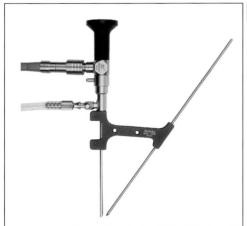

14.52
Fritz triangulator, commonly used in shoulder arthroscopy.
(Courtesy of Dr Fritz)

Arthroscopy towers

With the crossover from the human market, almost all arthroscopy set-ups can be integrated into a dedicated, semi-portable tower system. Tower systems keep all of the major pieces of arthroscopy equipment secure, together and ready for use. A tower system is shown in Figure 14.53. This example incorporates a monitor, light source, image/video capture, irrigation pump, shaver unit and radiofrequency ablation.

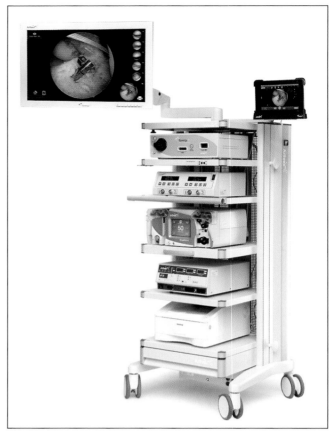

14.53 Tower system incorporating monitor, light source, image/video capture, irrigation pump and shaver unit.
(© Arthrex GmbH)

Impervious drapes/fluid collection

Arthroscopy can generate a lot of free fluid. Impervious drapes are essential for preventing strike-through and keeping the patient dry. A means of fluid collection is also indicated to reduce slip hazards. Special arthroscopy drapes are available with fluid collection pouches. These function well for small volumes, but where larger volumes are collected, they make the drapes heavy such that they may become displaced unless very firmly attached, and there is also the risk of fluid overflow. Other solutions include covering flooring with adequate absorbent material or matting and/or the use of suction pumps with special connectors for removing free fluid from the floor.

References and further reading

Gemmil T and Clements D (2016) *BSAVA Manual of Canine and Feline Fracture Repair and Management, 2nd edn.* BSAVA Publications, Gloucester

Chapter 15

Arthroscopy

Bernadette Van Ryssen and John Lapish

Introduction

Arthroscopy is a minimally invasive technique used in the diagnosis and treatment of many joint disorders. Since its introduction in the 1960s, the use of arthroscopy has become commonplace in human medicine. Increasing use of industrial endoscopy to allow the internal inspection of machinery and aircraft without dismantling and the desire to improve the capabilities of medical arthroscopy have both driven continuous development and improvements in instrumentation (especially the arthroscope and its light source). This has led to the development of new advanced techniques and applications in human medicine, such as osteochondral grafting, laser surgery, and arthroscopically assisted joint replacement.

Arthroscopy has been used in horses and in dogs since the 1970s. In the horse, it is now a well established technique that has replaced most arthrotomies. In the dog, much progress has been made although the subject is still developing. Most specialized centres offer arthroscopy as a routine diagnostic and surgical technique.

Arthroscopy is an advanced technique that should not be self taught. Participation at basic and then more advanced courses augmented by increasing experience, starting with the technically less demanding joints, such as the shoulder and elbow, is advised.

General indications for diagnostic arthroscopy

Arthroscopy is particularly useful in those cases where lameness is associated with little or no clinical or radiographic evidence of pathology. Lesions involving articular cartilage, synovial membrane and intra-articular ligaments or tendons may be identified and described by direct visualization via the arthroscope, whereas they are only outlined or not directly visible with other imaging modalities. Arthroscopy can also be used to confirm suspected lesions, such as a fragmented coronoid process or a partial rupture of the cranial cruciate ligament. Arthroscopic findings can be used to refine a prognosis, as in severe or chronic cases of osteoarthritis, or to evaluate the status of a previously treated joint, e.g. in the evaluation of tissue ingrowth.

Other indications include joint lavage for refractory cases of septic arthritis and synovial biopsy.

The success of arthroscopy can be explained by its several advantages over other diagnostic and surgical modalities. These advantages include:

- The minimally invasive nature of the technique, which enables quick recovery and minimizes scar tissue formation
- Visibility within the joint is substantially improved. The detailed view, the magnification of the intra-articular structures and lesions and the extended field of view obtained by repositioning the arthroscope (e.g. in various compartments) increases the diagnostic possibilities. Discrete lesions are seen arthroscopically, as well as early lesions that cannot be detected radiographically. By positioning the arthroscope in different joint compartments, areas and structures are visible which would not be possible during arthrotomy without major surgical trauma. In cases of bilateral disease, the prognosis for the contralateral side can be estimated by arthroscopic inspection of the opposite limb at the time of the original surgery and, if necessary, a bilateral treatment can be performed
- A second look by arthroscopy in previously treated joints provides valuable data in some cases. However, second-look arthroscopy must be justified in terms of potential benefit to the patient. It is not acceptable to perform it merely for scientific curiosity, even if the owner's consent is obtained. Nevertheless, it can be extremely useful to investigate why recovery is progressing more slowly than anticipated, or in formulating the next step in the management protocol.

Studies that objectively show evidence in favour of arthroscopy are scarce. In human medicine, a study comparing different surgical interventions for a specific type of shoulder problem could not demonstrate any difference in outcome between the arthroscopic and the open treatment method (Tashjian, 2013). In veterinary medicine, only one study has analyzed three different treatment methods for elbow medial compartment disease. The conclusion was that arthroscopy was superior to arthrotomy (Evans et al., 2008). Nevertheless, the minimally invasive nature of the procedure and the superior view are irrefutable advantages.

Disadvantages of arthroscopy include:

- A steep and long learning curve that can easily discourage the learning surgeon

- The challenge of gaining familiarity with the instruments and technique
- Difficulty in interpreting the significance of observed lesions
- Consequential potential difficulty in making the correct treatment decisions
- Technical problems such as failure to insert the instruments correctly, disorientation within the joint, unintentional ejection from the joint, breakage of instruments, iatrogenic damage and impatience of the surgical team
- Extravasation of fluid, which can be troublesome, if there is need to convert to an open arthrotomy.

Nevertheless, the advantages of the technique, particularly for orthopaedic surgery, make it well worth persevering.

Not all joints can be approached arthroscopically. In small-breed dogs and cats, it may be difficult, or even impossible, to insert the instruments, with the exception of the shoulder and stifle joints. Because of the size and anatomy of the tarsus, it is difficult to perform arthroscopy of the talocrural joint, even in large- to giant-breed dogs.

Arthroscopy should always be preceded by a thorough lameness evaluation, including clinical and radiographic examination, and should never replace this. A thorough appreciation of the clinical presentation and current evidence base is mandatory if correct treatment decisions are to be made. Care should be taken to avoid overuse, disuse or abuse of arthroscopy. Arthroscopy can be used in certain cases as a diagnostic tool in place of imaging modalities, such as radiography or computed tomography (CT). Where financial constraints exist, and in certain clinical scenarios, it might be preferable to proceed straight to arthroscopy to determine the diagnosis (e.g. 10-month-old Labrador Retriever with elbow effusions).

The surgical team

Arthroscopy is a demanding procedure, not only because of the learning curve, but also because of the need for a well trained team. Although some surgeons prefer to work alone, it is very helpful to have an assistant to hold the camera or the limb. Movements can be more controlled and an extra hand can open up the joint space to facilitate the procedure. The surgeon should be patient and gentle and show ability for precise surgery. The operating team should be receptive to new techniques and willing to invest time. During the learning phase, the team should also encourage the surgeon who, however experienced he or she is in surgery, will be confronted with failures and prolonged operation times.

Patient preparation

Anaesthesia

Small animal arthroscopy requires general anaesthesia for complete relaxation and full patient cooperation without undesirable movements that would make arthroscopic surgery impossible. Although the puncture wounds are small, intra-articular treatment of painful joints requires anaesthesia that is sufficiently deep, not only for the welfare of the animal and the surgeon, but also to avoid instrument breakage by unexpected movements.

Positioning

Manipulation of arthroscopes and instrumentation inside a joint via an image on a monitor screen can be very challenging; therefore careful and accurate positioning of the patient and the surgeon is essential. An operating table, fully adjustable for height and tilt, is a prerequisite for good arthroscopy.

The position of the patient depends on the joint being examined and the planned approach. For example, elbow arthroscopy is performed with the dog in lateral or dorsal recumbency with the joint being treated resting on the table, suspended free, or rigidly fixed in a brace/limb stand (Figure 15.1). Shoulder arthroscopy may either be performed with the patient in lateral recumbency with the treated joint uppermost, or by a hanging limb technique. Stifle arthroscopy is performed with the patient in dorsal recumbency and for hip arthroscopy the patient should be in lateral recumbency. For tarsal arthroscopy, different positions are possible.

Once fully draped, orientation around a limb can be difficult. Full use should be made of channels, ties and sandbags to fix the overall position of the patient. A leg holder or support is useful to hold the leg in a fixed position and to distract the joint or apply forces to it. Distraction devices are widely utilized in human arthroscopy. Their employment in the dog has been reported (Schulz *et al.*, 2004), but their use would appear to be less widespread. A multi-arm positioning device is available to provide multiple fixed positioning during an investigation; when attached between the distal limb and the table, it may be locked into a range of positions (Figure 15.2). This optional accessory allows the stifle or elbow to be positioned accurately for investigation.

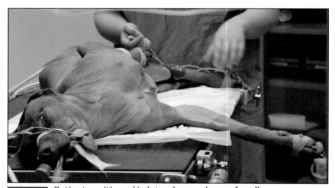

15.1 Patient positioned in lateral recumbency for elbow arthroscopy. The medial side of the elbow is clipped and is positioned near the edge of the table to allow rotation and abduction.

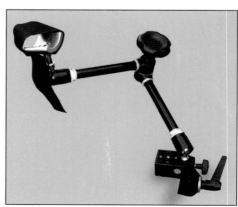

15.2 Multi-arm positioning device used to immobilize the limb and hold it in position.
(Courtesy of Dr Fritz)

Preparation of the operative field

Clipping, scrubbing and surgical asepsis are standard and are as important as for any surgical procedure (see Chapter 13). Several methods can be used to drape the surgical field. General principles dictate that the draping should be impermeable and allow sufficient mobility of the limb (Figure 15.3). A simple and quick system is the use of an adherent operating drape that is either self-adherent (i.e. it has an adherent window) or is applied with the use of a sterile spray (Figure 15.4). If an adherent drape is used, the surgical field should be dried well before applying the drape or spray. In this way, only a limited field needs to be prepared while good mobility of the limb is maintained. However, this may not be sufficient if the arthroscopic procedure has to be converted into an arthrotomy; if progression to an arthrotomy is likely then sufficient clipping and preparation should be performed to facilitate this.

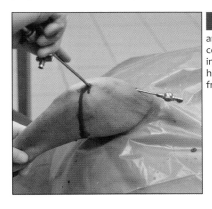

15.3 Preparation of a patient for stifle arthroscopy. The dog is covered with an impermeable sheath with a hole for the limb to allow free mobility.

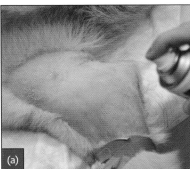

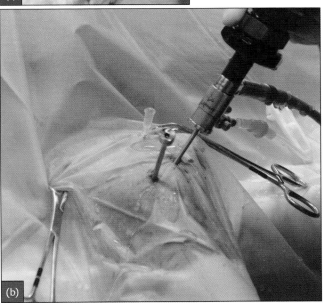

15.4 Arthroscopy of a left elbow joint. (a) A plastic sheath is attached to the clipped elbow region. (b) Insertion of instruments through the cover and manipulation of the limb with the cover in place are possible.

General arthroscopic procedure

An arthroscopic procedure consists of three steps, which may vary from joint to joint and from surgeon to surgeon.

1. A needle is inserted into the joint to aspirate synovial fluid and to inject irrigation fluid. Thus, the joint capsule is distended, which facilitates the next step of the procedure. In the carpus, there is no need to distend the joint capsule prior to insertion of the arthroscope cannula.
2. To determine its correct position and direction for arthroscope insertion, a needle is inserted in the joint where the arthroscope will be positioned. The needle is positioned correctly if it has the expected inclination (direction) and depth, and if irrigation fluid exits from it. Insertion of a needle prior to insertion of the arthroscopic sleeve helps to localize the most advantageous position and to prevent iatrogenic damage. The arthroscopic sheath is inserted into the joint via a stab incision along the line of the needle. Depending on the type of joint and the preference of the surgeon, the stab incision can be limited to the skin or it may puncture the joint capsule. A sharp or blunt trocar is contained within the arthroscopic sheath during its insertion. Once correct intra-articular placement is verified, the trocar is removed from the sheath and replaced by the arthroscope.
3. The operating instrument or instrument cannula is inserted. The puncture site and direction are determined with a needle under arthroscopic guidance (similar to step 2 above). The instrument is inserted directly into the joint via a stab incision (open portal) or via the instrument cannula.

Postoperative care

A local anaesthetic, such as mepivacaine, can be injected into the joint through the egress needle or via the stopcock of the arthroscopic sleeve prior to its removal at the end of the procedure. The wounds are routinely sutured and a light bandage can be applied to reduce swelling and bleeding. Most animals can be discharged on the same day if required. Postoperative care generally consists of anti-inflammatory treatment with a non-steroidal anti-inflammatory drug and exercise control (for further details, the reader is referred to individual chapters and procedures).

The arthroscopic image

Image quality depends on several factors and each element of the arthroscopy system should function optimally to obtain the best result. These elements include the arthroscope, its light cable, the light source, camera and monitor. The view obtained of the joint will also depend on joint irrigation, the degree of haemorrhage and the intra-articular position of the arthroscope. If one of the elements is inadequate, observation, orientation, interpretation and surgery will be either difficult or impossible (Figure 15.5). Optimizing the system is part of the learning curve.

The video cart, patient and surgeon should ideally be in one line (Figure 15.6). This helps hand/eye coordination and right/left control. The camera should be kept in a fixed position towards the animal to maintain the correct orientation. This means that the structures seen left and right on the screen are also localized left and right to the arthroscope. The arthroscope can be rotated around its axis by moving the light post (Figure 15.7).

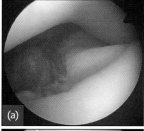
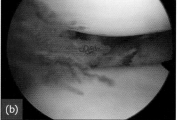
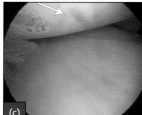

15.5 Causes of inadequate arthroscopic visibility. (a) Fogging of the eyepiece of the arthroscope. (b) Poor positioning of the arthroscope such that the view is obstructed by synovium. (c) Scratch on the lens (arrowed).

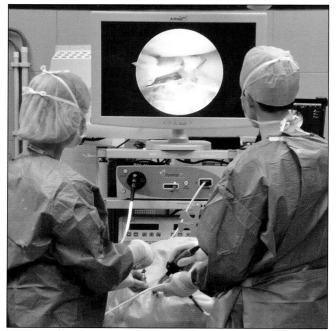

15.6 The monitor, patient and surgical team are in line, which facilitates a comfortable operating position with ease of instrument manipulation and a good view of the monitor.

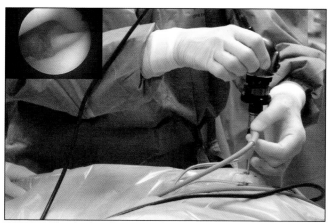

15.7 The viewing direction is altered by rotating the light post. The camera remains in a fixed position with the top pointing dorsally/cranially depending on the joint being examined. Note the notch on the border of the image (insert), which highlights the direction in which the arthroscope is pointing.

Visible intra-articular structures and their appearance

Cartilage

Normal cartilage has a smooth, white and glistening surface (Figure 15.8).

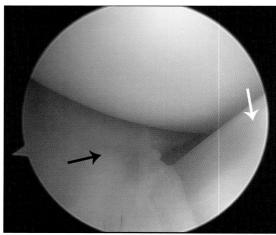

15.8 Normal canine stifle joint showing normal smooth cartilage of the femoral condyle, part of the cranial cruciate ligament (white arrow) and part of the medial meniscus (black arrow).

Primary lesions

The most important primary lesions of cartilage are those of osteochondral and cartilage fragments in cases of elbow dysplasia and osteochondritis dissecans (OCD) of the shoulder, stifle and hock joints (Figure 15.9). A flap, fissure, chondromalacia (seen as soft discoloured irregular cartilage often covering abnormal subchondral bone), or one or more bony fragments containing subchondral bone, may be seen.

Secondary lesions

Secondary lesions of cartilage (Figure 15.10) may be caused by pressure from a fragment, by repetitive altered loading due to limb deformity or joint incongruency or by chronic synovitis altering the composition of the synovial fluid and, thus, its nutritional capacity. Secondary changes can be limited to a small zone or may extend over a large area. They can be seen as rough zones, discoloration of the cartilage (more yellow), fibrillation (which may be very discrete to extensive) (Figure 15.10a), small fissures, 'cracks' and erosions. Erosions may be superficial or full thickness (Figure 15.10b). The latter may appear as stripes, patches, nude bone, irregular bone or as broad tracks (Figure 15.10; see also Subchondral bone, below). Secondary cartilage lesions can be graded as part of the routine examination, using the modified Outerbridge scoring system (Figure 15.11).

> Iatrogenic cartilage lesions can be created during the insertion of needles, arthroscope and instruments and during manipulation of the surgical instruments, in particular with powered instruments. A careful approach with the smallest possible instruments and the use of a blunt obturator instead of a sharp trocar prevents damage to the sound cartilage surface

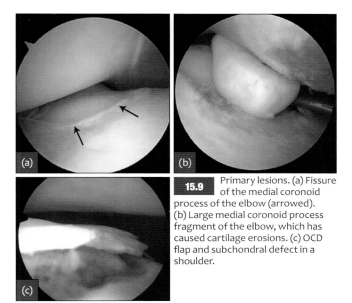

15.9 Primary lesions. (a) Fissure of the medial coronoid process of the elbow (arrowed). (b) Large medial coronoid process fragment of the elbow, which has caused cartilage erosions. (c) OCD flap and subchondral defect in a shoulder.

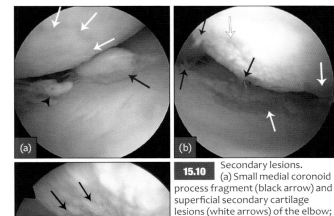

15.10 Secondary lesions. (a) Small medial coronoid process fragment (black arrow) and superficial secondary cartilage lesions (white arrows) of the elbow; cartilage pitting due to fibrillation. A hyperplastic synovial villus (arrowhead) is visible protruding into the joint space. (b) Fibrillation (black arrows) and focal full thickness cartilage lesions (white arrows). (c) Severe erosions with multiple small islands of fibrocartilage (arrowed).

Modified Outerbridge classification	Description of gross cartilage findings
0	Normal cartilage
1	Chondromalacia (cartilage with softening and swelling)
2	Superficial fibrillation. Superficial cartilage lesions with pitting or a 'cobblestone' appearance. Lesions that do not reach subchondral bone
3	Deep cartilage lesion that does not reach the subchondral bone. Deep fibrillation
4	Full thickness cartilage loss with exposure of the subchondral bone
5	Eburnated bone

15.11 The modified Outerbridge system used to classify cartilage lesions.
(Vermote et al., 2010)

Findings that may be clinically insignificant

Not all arthroscopic findings are significant; experience may be required to determine which are incidental findings and which represent significant pathology. For instance, the synovial membrane, originating at the transition zone of cartilage to bone, is often seen as an indistinct margin, creating zones without cartilage but covered with synovial membrane. This can be the case in both normal and diseased joints. These zones may look like aggressive lesions when the synovial membrane is inflamed, particularly in the elbow, shoulder and stifle (Figure 15.12).

Pannus may be seen as hypervascular tissue covering cartilage, menisci, ligaments or tendons secondary to joint incongruency and severe inflammation.

Osteophytes

In osteoarthritis, osteophytes are visible at the border of the cartilage. They originate at the transition between cartilage and synovial membrane and appear as irregular new bone covered with cartilage. Particularly in the shoulder, this irregularity is often misinterpreted as a cartilage lesion at the caudodistal border of the humeral head. Other typical sites for osteophytes are the caudal rim of the glenoid cavity in the shoulder, the lateral border of the humeral condyle in the elbow and along the femoral condyles in the stifle (Figure 15.13).

Synovial membrane

The extent of the synovial membrane that can be inspected is limited, but changes usually affect the entire membrane and are seen all over the joint. In normal joints, the number of synovial villi is limited and they are thin and short; in particular, the normal shoulder joint has a rim of synovial villi at the proximal aspect of the biceps tendon (Figure 15.14). The number of villi is not equally distributed; typically, some areas in the joint have more villi than others. Pathological changes include:

- Increase in the number of villi
- Alteration of colour of villi (red, orange or white)
- Changes in vascularization of villi (avascular or hypervascular)
- Differing forms of villi (elongated, thickened or 'branches') (Figure 15.15).

Small red villi indicate acute inflammation, while hyperplastic large white villi suggest a chronic process. Often a mixture of different forms is found.

Primary pathology of the synovial membrane are evident in cases of capsular neoplasia where increased numbers of thickened discoloured villi can easily be observed (Figure 15.15a). In the acute stage of infection, the villi are hypertrophic and hyperaemic. In chronic cases, these villi develop a more hyperplastic appearance (Figure 15.15b). Often fibrin rafts adhere to the joint capsule and cross the joint space. Autoimmune disorders present as a severe inflammation, but are not characterized by specific changes.

Secondary changes are seen in association with other primary processes such as osteochondritis, ligamentous problems, (micro)trauma, etc. The changes always involve the entire joint, but may be more prominent in the proximity of the primary problem.

During the arthroscopic procedure, the appearance of the synovium changes quite quickly as joint distension and intra-articular manipulation causes hyperaemia of the villi.

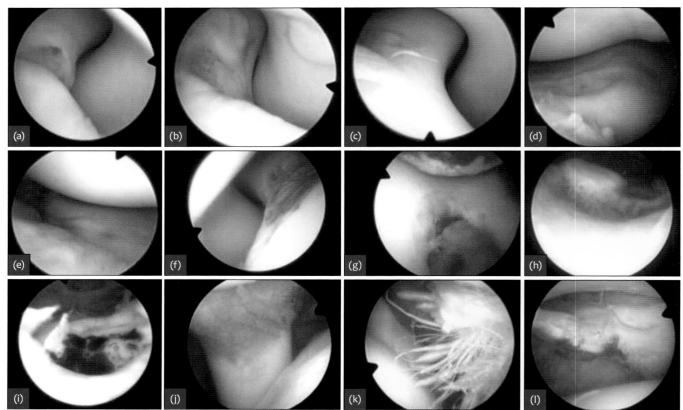

15.12 Secondary and concomitant pathological changes that do not require treatment. (a) Elbow diagnosed with moderate incongruity and medial coronoid fragmentation: the trochlear notch shows a depression without cartilage, filled with a small amount of pannus. (b) Elbow diagnosed with severe incongruity and medial coronoid fragmentation: the trochlear notch shows a deep depression without cartilage, covered with hypervascular pannus. (c) Sound elbow: the trochlear notch is covered with normal smooth cartilage. (d) Elbow diagnosed with moderate incongruity and medial coronoid disease: pannus and irregular cartilage covering the radial head. (e) Elbow diagnosed with moderate incongruity and medial coronoid disease: pannus and irregular cartilage covering the step. (f) Elbow with medial coronoid disease: pannus with clear blood vessels covering the medial part of the trochlear notch of the ulna. (g) Stifle diagnosed with a partial rupture of the cranial cruciate ligament: red, inflamed synovial membrane at the distal pole of the patella. (h) Stifle diagnosed with a partial rupture of the cranial cruciate ligament, transition of synovial membrane to cartilage at the proximal site of the patellar groove: zones covered with pannus. (i) Stifle with a partial cruciate ligament showing severe inflammation and local hypertrophic synovial membrane. (j) Shoulder diagnosed with OCD: biceps tendon covered with hypertrophic synovial membrane. (k) Shoulder diagnosed with a calcified body at the caudal edge of the glenoid: chronic inflammation caused fibrillation of the joint capsule and intracapsular ligaments. (l) Shoulder with chronic osteoarthritis: partial tear of the medial glenohumeral ligament.

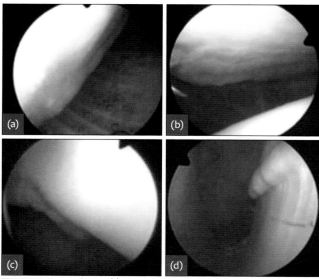

15.13 Osteophytes. (a) Shoulder: caudodistal part of the humeral head. (b) Shoulder: caudal border of the glenoid cavity. (c) Elbow: lateral ridge of the humeral condyle. (d) Stifle: lateral ridge of the femoral condyle.

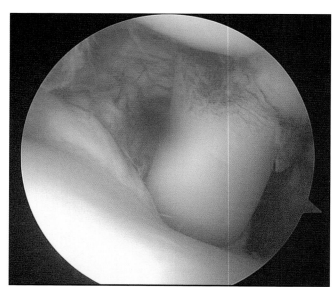

15.14 View of a normal right shoulder showing normal synovial membrane surrounding a small part of the biceps tendon: normal blood vessels run in the synovial membrane and the synovial villi are small.

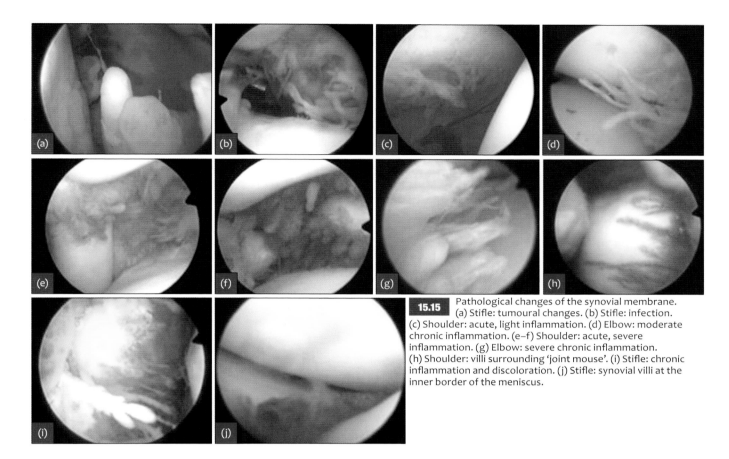

15.15 Pathological changes of the synovial membrane. (a) Stifle: tumoural changes. (b) Stifle: infection. (c) Shoulder: acute, light inflammation. (d) Elbow: moderate chronic inflammation. (e–f) Shoulder: acute, severe inflammation. (g) Elbow: severe chronic inflammation. (h) Shoulder: villi surrounding 'joint mouse'. (i) Stifle: chronic inflammation and discoloration. (j) Stifle: synovial villi at the inner border of the meniscus.

Ligaments and tendons

Several ligaments and tendons are intracapsular and are surrounded by the synovial membrane; these can easily be inspected arthroscopically. The biceps tendon, subscapularis tendon, lateral and medial glenohumeral ligaments can be inspected in the shoulder; the medial collateral ligament, annular ligament (medial and lateral part) and the proximal part of the distal biceps tendon in the elbow; the cruciate ligaments, meniscal ligaments and long digital extensor tendon in the stifle; the deep flexor tendon in the hock joint; the teres ligament in the hip joint; and several ligaments within the carpus (Figure 15.16).

The normal appearance of a tendon or ligament is smooth, white and glistening. Primary and secondary lesions appear similar and present as thickening, discoloration, fibrillation and partial or complete ruptures with hypertrophy and calcification of the remnants. Only rarely can haemorrhage be seen in a ruptured tendon. In the author's [BVR] experience, primary ligamentous lesions are frequently accompanied by a severe secondary synovitis. Common primary disorders include partial or complete

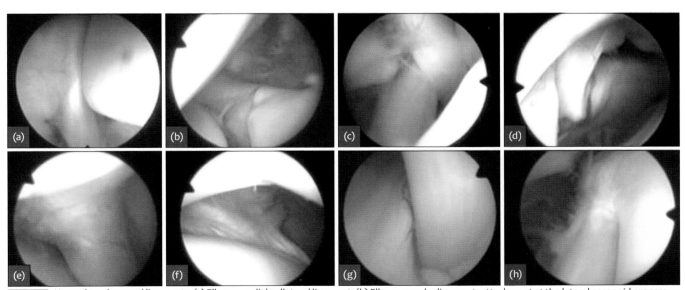

15.16 Normal tendons and ligaments. (a) Elbow: medial collateral ligament. (b) Elbow: annular ligament, attachment at the lateral coronoid process. (c) Elbow: crossing of the medial collateral ligament and distal part of the biceps tendon. (d) Carpus: intra-articular ligaments. (e) Shoulder: biceps tendon. (f) Shoulder: medial glenohumeral ligament. (g) Stifle: cruciate ligaments. (h) Stifle: origin of the long digital extensor tendon.

rupture of the cranial cruciate ligament and partial or complete rupture of the biceps tendon. A controversial subject is shoulder instability in which fibrillation and partial or complete rupture of the medial glenohumeral ligament and/ or subscapularis tendon is involved (see Chapter 18).

In recent years, flexor enthesopathy has been recognized as a cause of elbow lameness. A normal enthesis is visible as a short and smooth tendinous structure attaching at the medial epicondyle in the proximal part of the elbow. In affected joints, the enthesis of the flexor muscles (most commonly the flexor carpi ulnaris muscle) is fibrillated and partially ruptured. Fibres and ruptured parts of the enthesis protrude into the joint, because the covering synovial membrane is damaged simultaneously (Figure 15.17).

In chronic inflammation, intra-articular ligaments and the joint capsule may show light to severe secondary fibrillation. These secondary lesions should not be confused with a rupture.

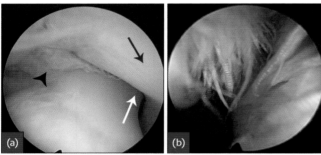

15.17 Images of flexor enthesopathy in a left elbow. (a) Medial compartment of the elbow showing an affected enthesis of the flexor muscle (arrowhead); visible normal structures are: part of the medial epicondyle (white arrow) and the anconeal process (black arrow). (b) Fibrillation and partial rupture of the enthesis.

Subchondral bone

Subchondral bone is not visible in normal joints as it is covered by articular cartilage. It is only seen when there is damage to the overlying cartilage as a result of fragmentation, flap development or erosion (Figure 15.18).

Bone can also be visible as a part of a fragment. Most often this bone has a different colour, being more yellow or white in colour. It is of a softer consistency when compared with normal subchondral bone. The bone associated with a fragment or delineated by a fissure is often not vascularized, but in some cases it bleeds during removal, which indicates healing potential. In the authors' experience, in several cases with large fragments in the elbow, larger fragments were vascularized while the smaller ones were not. After removal of an OCD flap or fragment, the underlying subchondral bone becomes visible. Usually the bone just underneath the fragment is soft, granular and easily detachable. In some cases of shoulder OCD, several brown spots are visible in the subchondral bone. After removal of the fragment and superficial curettage of the defect, normal bone is visible as pink and relatively hard. In young dogs, subchondral bone bleeds easily after curettage.

Nude subchondral bone in connection with kissing lesions and end-stage erosive degenerative joint disease is often pink and hard (Figure 15.18fg). These kissing lesions occur at the site opposite the lesion, or can surround a lesion. In the author's [BVR] experience, bleeding barely occurs even when this type of lesion is foraged. The appearance of these kissing lesions can differ. Usually there is one smooth surface, but some lesions are covered with white foci, and in other cases, tracks are visible.

Menisci

The stifle menisci are fibrocartilaginous structures that are not visible on plain radiographs unless they are mineralized; this is a rare finding in the dog, although a more common finding in cats. Primary tears occur in different forms and locations but it is most commonly the medial meniscus that is affected as a consequence of cranial cruciate ligament degeneration and associated joint instability. Both menisci may also show secondary changes as a result of inflammation or microtrauma. These secondary changes are fibrillation or thickening of the axial border, synovial growth on the abaxial and axial borders or an irregular, striated surface (Figure 15.19). The arthroscopic

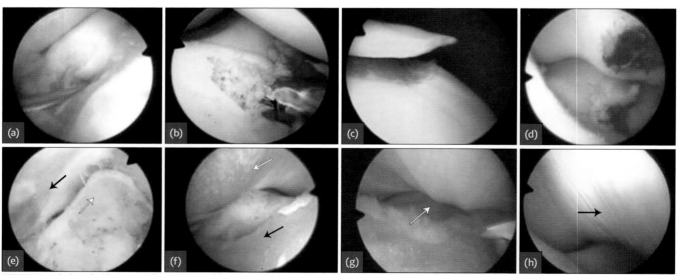

15.18 Subchondral bone in different joints. (a) Displaced fragment of the medial coronoid process: yellow subchondral bone covered by white cartilage. (b) Soft bone visible during motorized shaving of a coronoid fragment. (c) OCD of the shoulder: subchondral bone is visible underneath the cartilage flap. (d) OCD of the elbow: large bleeding defect of the medial humeral condyle. (e) Defect of talus after removal of large fragment (white arrow) with concurrent erosion of the distal tibia (black arrow). (f) Complete cartilage erosion of the medial compartment of the elbow joint. A fragment is visible in the middle of the image, between the medial condyle (white arrow) and the remaining part of the medial coronoid process (black arrow). (g) Severe kissing lesions of the medial condyle (arrowed). (h) Superficial cartilage lesions of the medial condyle (arrowed).

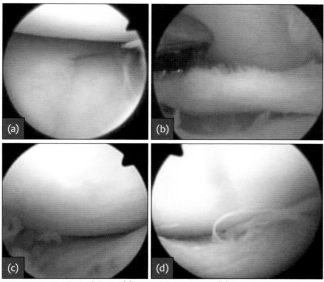

15.19 Menisci of dogs. (a) Normal meniscus. (b) Luxated bucket handle tear of the medial meniscus with cranial displacement. A small grasper is approaching it. (c) Synovial villi covering the axial border of the medial meniscus. (d) Fibrillation of the axial border of the lateral meniscus.

diagnosis of meniscal lesions is not always easy because the view of them may be obstructed by synovial villi and remnants of a ruptured cruciate ligament and because of the narrow joint space between the medial femoral condyle and the caudal part of the tibial plateau. The use of a 2 mm probe to assess the integrity of the menisci has been shown to significantly increase the detection of meniscal pathology (Pozzi et al., 2008).

Indications for diagnostic and surgical arthroscopy of specific joints

Shoulder

The most important indication for shoulder arthroscopy is OCD: the arthroscopic detection and removal of cartilage flaps is a rewarding procedure. Triangulation can be challenging because of the large muscular layer and relatively deep location of the lesion (see Chapter 18 for further details).

In shoulders with suspected biceps tendon pathology, arthroscopy enables the detection through direct observation and probing of a partial or complete rupture of the biceps. It is useful to gently flex and extend the shoulder while observing the tendon to assess its structural integrity. Tenotomy or transection of the remnants can be performed via arthroscopy but may be impeded by haemorrhage, or because the tendon is difficult to access with instruments.

Arthroscopy allows the detection and removal of caudal glenoid mineralized bodies although the fragments may be difficult to remove because of their position or size. Shoulder instability may be diagnosed based on the partially ruptured glenohumeral ligaments and subscapularis tendons. A technically demanding arthroscopically-guided suturing of the joint capsule has been described (Franklin et al., 2013).

Elbow

Arthroscopy of the elbow is usually performed to investigate and treat elbow dysplasia. In joints affected by medial coronoid disease, arthroscopy can be used to diagnose the primary lesion (fissure, chondromalacia or fragment) and to assess joint incongruity and secondary cartilage damage. Diagnosis may be difficult when lesions are very discrete and the arthroscopic findings should be complemented by other imaging findings (radiography and computed tomography) (Moores et al., 2008). Arthroscopic treatment is challenging for large fragments or when the lesion is hard to access because of a narrow joint space or cranial displacement (see Chapter 19 for further details).

OCD lesions of the elbow can be diagnosed when the arthroscope is directed medially, although hypertrophic synovial villi may obstruct the view. Treatment may be impeded by the close proximity of the joint capsule which makes insertion of instruments more challenging.

In cases of an ununited anconeal process, arthroscopic inspection allows an estimation of the stability and displacement of the anconeal fragment. Additionally, the medial coronoid process can be inspected for a concomitant fissure or fragment. The arthroscopic removal of those fragments requires a strong large grasper and is impeded by the large size of the fragment and the strong connection to the joint capsule. A small caudomedial or caudolateral arthrotomy may be preferable in cases where the anconeal process requires removal, although removal is associated with a poorer prognosis.

In cases of medial compartment disease, other lesions may be detected or excluded as a cause of lameness. There is no efficient arthroscopic treatment for this problem.

In joints affected by flexor enthesopathy, it is important to determine whether it is the only lesion (primary flexor enthesopathy) or whether there is also another elbow disorder (concomitant flexor enthesopathy).

In cases of discrete medial coronoid disease, arthroscopic diagnosis is challenging.

Carpal joint

Diagnosis of cartilage lesions and ligament injuries is feasible but indications are rare.

Coxofemoral joint

Hip dysplasia is the most important indication for hip arthroscopy. The approach to this joint is quite simple but because of the deep localization it may be difficult to define the joint space. In young dogs, the arthroscopic findings may influence the choice of treatment, based on the presence of degenerative cartilage lesions, e.g. whether joint preserving techniques, such as triple or double pelvic osteotomy may be appropriate or not (see Chapter 22).

Stifle joint

Stifle arthroscopy is an advanced procedure because of the difficult orientation and visibility within the joint, largely due to the obstructive presence of the infrapatellar fat pad. Diagnostic arthroscopy of the stifle joint is usually performed to assess cranial cruciate ligament and meniscal lesions. In cases of a partial cranial cruciate ligament rupture with minimal instability, arthroscopy enables an accurate diagnosis which may not be possible by more invasive conventional means, and without necessitating an arthrotomy. The arthroscopic treatment of cranial cruciate ligament lesions has been described but this is an advanced procedure that has been almost completely discarded due to the difficulty of finding suitable implants, and the preference for osteotomy techniques, such as tibial plateau levelling osteotomy and tibial tuberosity advancement. Meniscal tears may be diagnosed and treated prior to joint stabilization. In cases of recurrent lameness following stifle surgery, arthroscopy allows the investigation and treatment of 'late' meniscal lesions. Arthroscopic removal of meniscal tears is technically demanding and may be impeded by the narrow joint space. The arthroscopic suturing of menisci has been described recently; this challenging procedure is only indicated in selected cases (Pozzi et al., 2008).

OCD of the stifle is a rare condition, which can be accurately treated arthroscopically.

Tarsal joint

OCD of the medial trochlear ridge is the most common indication for arthroscopy of the tarsus. Diagnosis may be impeded by the presence of chronically inflamed villi. Observation of large fragments may be difficult because of the small joint space and the close proximity to the arthroscope. Ideally CT should precede arthroscopy of the tarsus in order to fully determine the extent of the lesions. The arthroscopic treatment of OCD is only feasible in a limited number of cases; often the fragment is large, firmly attached and difficult to reach via a stab incision. Alternatively, treatment can be performed under arthroscopic guidance via a mini-arthrotomy.

Complications and problems

Arthroscopy in small animals is a challenging procedure and even an experienced surgeon will encounter problems from time to time. There are two reasons why small animal arthroscopy is difficult. Firstly, the joints are very small compared with human or equine joints, so the introduction of instruments alongside the arthroscope is challenging. Secondly, the most frequently affected joints in the dog have specific anatomical difficulties:

- The shoulder is surrounded by large muscles
- The elbow has a narrow joint space
- Observation of intra-articular structures in the stifle is hampered by the fat pad, synovial villi and ligamentous remnants
- The tarsal joint has a very small joint space, which easily collapses.

In addition to the specific difficulties associated with each joint, there are several general problems or complications that can cause a delay or even failure of the intervention. The most common problems are related to technique. These include:

- Difficulties with accurate instrument insertion (triangulation)
- Poor positioning of the arthroscope, resulting in limited mobility and decreased field of vision
- Collapse of the joint space due to periarticular fluid accumulation
- Dislodgement of the arthroscope from the joint
- Instrument breakage
- Obstruction of the view due to intra-articular pathology such as synovial villi.

Although these problems can occur at any time, most will be resolved with experience.

The most frequent complication is iatrogenic cartilage damage. This is caused during insertion of the instruments and their subsequent manipulation. Small iatrogenic lesions do not have any clinical consequences but they should be avoided as much as possible. Expansion of the joint by fluid injection helps to minimize iatrogenic trauma but particular care must be taken when attempting to insert the cannulae. Blunt obturators should be used in preference to sharper ones, which will inevitably cause more trauma. Other complications include fluid extravasation into the periarticular tissues, haemorrhage and loss of an osteochondral fragment. Care should be taken to minimize the extravasation of fluid as it can prevent introduction of the arthroscope and, in severe cases, lead to the postponement of the surgery. Haemorrhage during surgery can be overcome by increasing the fluid flow rate in order to maintain a clear image. Following surgery, a pressure bandage can be used to control the haemorrhage, although this is rarely encountered. The incidence of postoperative sepsis and neurovascular injuries is negligible. As for any surgery, the more experienced the surgeon becomes, the less frequently complications will occur. The incidence rate of complications following a case series of 750 elbow arthroscopies was recently reported (Perry and Li, 2014).

References and further reading

Beale B, Hulse D, Schulz K and Whitney W (2003) Small Animal Arthroscopy. WB Saunders, Philadelphia

Cook JL and Cook CR (2009) Bilateral shoulder and elbow arthroscopy in dogs with forelimb lameness: diagnostic findings and treatment outcomes. Veterinary Surgery 38, 224–232

Devitt CM, Neely MR and Vanvechten BJ (2007) Relationship of physical examination test of shoulder instability to arthroscopic findings in dogs. Veterinary Surgery 36, 661–668

Evans RB, Gordon-Evans WJ and Conzemius MG (2008). Comparison of three methods for the management of fragmented medial coronoid process in the dog. A systematic review and meta-analysis. Veterinary and Comparative Orthopaedics and Traumatology 21, 106–109

Franklin SP, Devitt CM, Ogawa J et al. (2013). Outcomes associated with treatments for medial, lateral, and multidirectional shoulder instability in dogs. Veterinary Surgery 42, 361–364

Kivumbi CW and Bennett D (1981) Arthroscopy of the canine stifle joint. Veterinary Record 109, 241–249

Lewis DD, Goring RL, Parker RB et al. (1987) A comparison of diagnostic methods used in the evaluation of early degenerative joint disease in the dog. Journal of the American Animal Hospital Association 23, 305–315

McGinty JB (1996) Preface. In: Operative Arthroscopy, 2nd edn. Lippincott–Raven, Philadelphia

Miller CW and Presnell KR (1985) Examination of the canine stifle: arthroscopy versus arthrotomy. Journal of the American Animal Hospital Association 21, 623–629

Moores AP, Benigni L and Lamb CR (2008) Computed tomography versus arthroscopy for detection of canine elbow dysplasia lesions. Veterinary Surgery 37, 390–398

Perry KP and Li L (2014) A retrospective study of the short-term complication rate following 750 elective arthroscopies. Veterinary and Comparative Orthopaedics and Traumatology 27, 68–73

Person MW (1985) A procedure for arthroscopic examination of the canine stifle joint. Journal of the American Animal Hospital Association 21, 179–186

Person MW (1986) Arthroscopy of the canine shoulder joint. Compendium on Continuing Education for the Practicing Veterinarian 8, 537–546

Person MW (1989) Arthroscopic treatment of osteochondritis dissecans in the canine shoulder. Veterinary Surgery 18, 175–190

Person MW (1989) Arthroscopy of the canine coxofemoral joint. Compendium on Continuing Education for the Practicing Veterinarian 1, 930–935

Pozzi A, Hildreth BE and Rajala-Schultz PJ (2008) Comparison of arthroscopy and arthrotomy for diagnosis of medial meniscal pathology: an ex vivo study. Veterinary Surgery 37, 749–755.

Rodriguez-Quiros J, Rovesti GL, Devesa V et al. (2014) Evaluation of a joint distractor to facilitate arthroscopy of the tibio-tarsal joint in dogs. Journal of Small Animal Practice 55, 213–218

Schulz KS, Holsworth IG and Hornof WJ (2004) Self-retaining braces for canine arthroscopy. *Veterinary Surgery* **33**, 77–82

Siemering GB (1978) Arthroscopy of dogs. *Journal of the American Veterinary Medical Association* **172**, 575–577

Tashjian RZ (2013) Is there evidence in favor of surgical interventions for the subacromial impingement syndrome? *Clinical Journal of Sport Medicine* **23**, 406–407

Van Ryssen B, de Bakker E, Beaumtin Y *et al.* (2012) Primary flexor enthesopathy of the canine elbow: imaging and arthroscopic findings in eight dogs with discrete radiographic changes. *Veterinary and Comparative Orthopaedics and Traumatology* **25**, 239–245

Van Ryssen B and van Bree H (1992) Arthroscopic evaluation of osteochondrosis lesions in the canine hock joint: a review of two cases. *Journal of the American Animal Hospital Association* **28**, 295–299

Van Ryssen B and van Bree H (1997) Arthroscopic findings in 100 dogs with elbow lameness. *Veterinary Record* **40**, 360–362

Van Ryssen B and van Bree H (1997) Diagnostic and surgical arthroscopy in osteochondrosis lesions. *Veterinary Clinics of North America: Small Animal Practice* **28**, 161–189

Van Ryssen B, van Bree H and Missinne S (1993) Successful arthroscopic treatment of shoulder osteochondrosis in the dog. *Journal of Small Animal Practice* **34**, 521–528

Van Ryssen B, van Bree H and Simoens P (1993) Elbow arthroscopy in clinically normal dogs. *American Journal of Veterinary Research* **54**, 191–198

Van Ryssen B, van Bree H and Vyt P (1993) Arthroscopy of the canine hock joint. *Journal of the American Animal Hospital Association* **29**, 107–115

Van Ryssen B, van Bree H and Vyt P (1993) Arthroscopy of the shoulder joint in the dog. *Journal of the American Animal Hospital Association* **29**, 101–105

Vermote K, Bergenhuyzen A, Gieben I *et al.* (2010) Elbow lameness in dogs of six years and older: arthroscopic and imaging findings of medial coronoid disease in 51 dogs. *Veterinary and Comparative Orthopaedics and Traumatology* **23**, 43–50

Chapter 16

Complications of orthopaedic surgery

Simon Roch

Orthopaedic surgery is undertaken to improve function and relieve musculoskeletal discomfort. However, complications can occur which have the potential to significantly affect both short-term and long-term outcomes (Figure 16.1). The risk of complication should be recognized and discussed with the client preoperatively. While complications may occur that are outwith the control of the surgeon, the majority are foreseeable and, to an extent, avoidable. By following the fundamental principles of surgery as laid down by Halsted, basic orthopaedic principles and sound planning, it is possible to keep complications to a minimum. Early recognition and appropriate intervention when complications arise may mitigate the long-term sequelae that might otherwise occur. It is vital that surgeons recognize their own technical limits and any limits imposed by the equipment, facilities and professional assistance available.

Halsted's principles of surgery
- Atraumatic tissue handling
- Meticulous haemostasis
- Strict aseptic technique
- Preservation of blood supply
- Elimination of dead space
- Accurate apposition of tissues
- Minimal tension on sutures

Complication	Notes
Surgical site infection	
Vascular injury or compromise	
Nerve injury	
Implant-related problems	Breakage, loosening or impingement
Subluxation or persistent joint instability	
Luxation	
Fracture	Re-fracture
Bone healing complications	Delayed union, malunion or non-union
Dressing-related problems	Pressure sores, vascular compromise, necrosis
Infarction	Pulmonary, cerebral
Adverse drug reaction	Gastrointestinal disturbance or renal compromise following non-steroidal anti-inflammatory drug (NSAID) administration
Death	

16.1 Potential postoperative complications.

Defining complications

A complication is defined as a deviation in the postoperative course of events from that which is normally expected. In the literature, complications are often categorized as major or minor; however, the difference between these two groups is sometimes difficult to define clearly. Efforts have been made to standardize the reporting of complications in clinical studies. Cook *et al.* (2010) suggested that complications may be divided into three groups:

- Catastrophic: where the complication or associated morbidity causes permanent unacceptable function, is directly related to death, or is cause for euthanasia
- Major: where the complication or associated morbidity requires further treatment based on current standards of care; further subdivided into complications where resolution requires surgical treatment and those that require medical treatment
- Minor: not requiring additional surgical or medical treatment to resolve (e.g. bruising, seroma, minor incision problems).

Prevention and minimization of complications

The prevention of complications is preferable to retrospective treatment in the face of a deteriorating patient. While it is impossible to completely eliminate complications, many can be anticipated and prevented by strict attention to detail (Figure 16.2). By starting with an accurate diagnosis, detailed preoperative planning, appropriate instrumentation, meticulous aseptic technique, gentle tissue handling and diligent postoperative care, it is possible to substantially reduce the incidence of complications. The use of a presurgical checklist can help to prepare for each case; an example is given in Figure 13.2.

Before embarking on a surgical procedure, surgeons must consider carefully whether they are sufficiently experienced and capable of dealing with the case, or whether referral to a more experienced colleague would offer the patient a greater chance of a successful outcome. It is better to be frank and honest with the animal's owner from the outset regarding how many similar procedures you have performed and offer referral to them as an option, than to have to offer a defence when facing litigation

Patient factors

- Ascites
- Chronic inflammation
- Corticosteroid therapy (controversial)
- Obesity
- Diabetes
- Extremes of age
- Hypocholesterolaemia
- Hypoxaemia
- Peripheral vascular disease
- Postoperative anaemia
- Prior site irradiation
- Recent operation
- Remote infection
- Skin carriage of staphylococci
- Skin disease in the area of incision
- Undernutrition

Environmental factors

- Contaminated medications
- Inadequate disinfection/sterilization
- Inadequate skin antisepsis
- Inadequate ventilation

Treatment factors

- Drains
- Emergency procedure
- Hypothermia
- Inadequate antibiotic prophylaxis
- Oxygenation (controversial)
- Prolonged preoperative hospitalization
- Prolonged operative time

16.2 Factors that may contribute to the development of surgical site infection.

following an overly ambitious surgical procedure! If there is any doubt regarding the difficulty of a procedure, the attending clinician should contact an experienced referral surgeon to discuss the optimal strategy for management of the case.

Signs of complications

Following surgery, it is important that the surgeon and client are aware of what progress should be made, in order to identify and treat complications early and efficiently. Failure to improve and progress adequately in the postoperative period should prompt the clinician to undertake further diagnostic evaluations to identify and treat the cause of problems.

The most common indicator that complications have occurred following orthopaedic surgery is that limb function deteriorates, or remains persistently poor following surgery. Prompt reassessment is indicated to detect signs of inflammation (heat, pain, redness and swelling) and to evaluate the limb for deformity, crepitus, pain, altered range of motion or instability. As time progresses, the range of motion of affected joints may become abnormal and articular cartilage may degenerate, resulting in joint pain; significant muscle atrophy may develop. Failure of implants or alterations in normal limb growth as a result of the initial injury or surgical intervention may lead to abnormal limb angulation. Neurological dysfunction can occur as a consequence of intraoperative iatrogenic nerve injury or as a part of muscle compartment syndrome. Other complications may seem less directly related to the orthopaedic surgery itself and may include renal compromise following prolonged hypotension, gastrointestinal ulceration secondary to the use of non-steroidal anti-inflammatory drugs, and thromboembolic disease. Complications that are not directly related to the musculoskeletal surgery itself are outwith the scope of this manual and readers are referred elsewhere for more information.

Types of complications

Postsurgical complications may occur for many reasons. A list of potential causes is given in Figure 16.1.

Surgical site infection

Bacterial infection is a commonly encountered complication that is reported to occur in 0.8% to 18.1% of small animal surgical procedures (Nelson, 2011). Significant variation in rates of surgical site infection (SSI) is seen between types of surgery. Morbidity associated with SSI has the potential to vary in severity from mild to limb- or life-threatening. The risk of SSI occurring depends on the magnitude of contamination and the virulence of the organism, which may be mitigated by the ability of the host to fight infection. Host resistance is in part determined by the presence of concomitant disease but may also be strongly influenced by procedural or environmental conditions that prevail during surgery, including the duration of anaesthesia, the adequacy of analgesia, surgeon experience, the number of observers present during surgery and the duration of hospitalization (Eugster et al., 2004). A list of factors that may contribute to the development of SSI is found in Figure 16.2.

Infection around implants

Infection around metallic or non-absorbable implants can be especially difficult to treat, due to the formation of bacterial biofilm on the implant surface. This multi-layered glycocalyx film resists antibiotic and antibody penetration, thereby protecting the bacteria and leading to persistence of viable bacteria and the recurrence of infection, despite prolonged therapy. A typical pattern is that while antibiotics are given, bacterial numbers are controlled and clinical signs wane; when antibiotics are discontinued, bacteria proliferate and clinical signs recur, often within 2 weeks of ceasing antimicrobial therapy. Different implant materials have differing susceptibility to biofilm formation; titanium appears to be less susceptible than stainless steel. In view of this observation, titanium may be preferable where implantation in potentially infected environments is necessary.

Fractures and osteotomies will heal in the face of ongoing infection as long as the bone is vascularized and stable. Antibiotics should be given until the bone has healed and once osseous union has been achieved, removal of the infected implant is often necessary. After implant removal, a prolonged course of antibiotics is often given; however, the necessity for this has been questioned (Savicky et al., 2013). Implants should be submitted for culture following removal. Consideration may be given to the application of antibiotic-impregnated materials within the surgical site at the time of implant removal, including antibiotic-impregnated collagen sponges (e.g. Collatamp G, Tribute Pharmaceuticals) or antibiotic-impregnated polymethylmethacrylate beads.

Where permanent implants are essential to the patient, for example following an infected pancarpal arthrodesis in an active large-breed dog, a two-stage revision is generally performed. This involves implant removal, debridement and lavage, followed by a prolonged period of aggressive antibiotic therapy. A second surgery to replace with new implants may be performed following resolution of infection. In the human field, single-stage revision has been proposed following infected joint replacements (Wolf *et al.*, 2014). This involves removal and the immediate replacement of the infected implants during a single surgery. This has obvious advantages to the patient; however, the superiority of single *versus* two-stage revision remains unclear.

Minimizing the incidence of surgical site infection

It is preferable to take all necessary steps to prevent infection rather than deal with an established infection following surgery but, despite attempts to prevent them, infections inevitably occur in some cases. Infection of the tissues surrounding non-absorbable implants can be particularly problematic.

Contamination of a surgical field with bacteria may occur preoperatively, intraoperatively or postoperatively.

Preoperative infection may occur as a result of established infection affecting the joint, surrounding soft tissues, overlying skin or other tissues distant to the joint. Otitis externa, dental disease and pyoderma (Figure 16.3) are the most commonly encountered conditions that can result in direct transfer or haematogenous spread of pathogens into the surgical site; other conditions such as urinary tract infection or endocarditis may be encountered less frequently. If pre-existing infection is identified prior to surgery, empirical broad-spectrum antibiotics may be started pending culture and sensitivity testing. Elective surgery should be postponed until complete resolution of the infection. In some situations, e.g. the treatment of an infected open joint injury, it may be necessary to perform surgery despite the presence of infection. In these cases, definitive surgery may be postponed to allow management of the contaminated tissues, and modification of the surgical technique can be considered to reduce the use of permanent implants, particularly braided non-absorbable suture materials, or to facilitate staged implant removal if persistent infection develops.

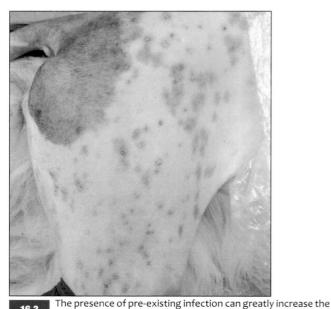

16.3 The presence of pre-existing infection can greatly increase the risk of surgical site infection. This dog was presented for total hip replacement but pyoderma was noted after clipping of the hair coat. In this circumstance, antibiotic therapy should be started and elective surgery postponed until the pyoderma is resolved.

The prophylactic use of antibiotics remains a contentious issue. The rationale is to reduce the incidence of infection following a surgical procedure by ensuring therapeutic antibiotic concentrations are present throughout surgery. Commonly used antibiotics include potentiated amoxicillin or first generation cephalosporins. These are ideally given intravenously immediately after induction. Procedures of short duration do not require antibiotic cover but prophylaxis is indicated when the duration of anaesthesia is likely to exceed 60 minutes, or when permanent implants are placed (see Chapter 13). Current recommendations suggest there is little benefit in the continuation of antimicrobials for more than several hours after surgery; however, some studies have shown reduced rates of SSI in dogs that received postoperative antibiotic therapy following stifle surgery (Fitzpatrick and Solano, 2010; Nazarali A *et al.*, 2014; Pratesi *et al.*, 2015).

Degree of wound contamination

Classification of wound types as clean, clean-contaminated, contaminated and infected has been shown to be useful in predicting the degree of wound contamination that is likely to be present. The incidence of SSI for different wound grades is listed in Figure 16.4.

The potential for intraoperative contamination of the surgical field can be reduced by correct patient preparation, strict adherence to aseptic principles by the surgical team (see Chapter 13), minimizing tissue trauma and reducing operative time. The reader is directed to the *BSAVA Manual of Canine and Feline Surgical Principles: A Foundation Manual* for more detailed information.

In veterinary patients there is significant potential for postoperative contamination of the surgical incision. Contamination may occur by direct transfer of bacteria from adjacent surfaces (e.g. tables, radiographic plates, kennels, bedding) or following contamination of the wound by substances such as mud, faeces and dirty water. In the author's opinion, animals licking at the wound following surgery commonly results in superficial infection of the surgical site; this can often be prevented by the use of sterile adhesive dressings such as Primapore (Smith & Nephew, UK) and Elizabethan collars. Contamination of the wound is most likely to occur due to self-trauma breaking the fibrin seal, or bacteria being seeded into the wound within the first 24 hours before the fibrin seal is formed, due to poor wound management. By taking relatively simple precautions it is possible to reduce the chance of postoperative contamination occurring (Figure 16.5).

Classification of wound	Incidence of SSI %
Clean	2.0–4.9
Clean-contaminated	3.5–4.5
Contaminated	4.6–9.1
Dirty	6.7–17.8

16.4 The incidence of surgical site infection (SSI) in relation to the degree of wound contamination (Eugster *et al.*, 2004).

- Cover the surgical wound using a sterile adhesive wound dressing under aseptic conditions
- Reduce the likelihood of self-trauma by using a neat subcuticular skin closure, applying wound or limb dressings and by the diligent use of Elizabethan collars
- Provide antibiotic cover as indicated by the clinical situation
- On discharge, carefully counsel the owners regarding the importance of strict wound hygiene and the avoidance of self-trauma

16.5 Simple steps that may be taken to reduce postoperative wound contamination.

Diagnosis of surgical site infection

Sepsis should be considered in all cases where limb function deteriorates following surgery, or where function remains persistently poorer than expected. Frequently encountered clinical signs include pain, lameness and heat on palpation around the surgical site. Discharging sinuses may form where extra-articular sepsis is present but are rare where the infection is confined to the joint.

> Animals with joint sepsis are often not pyrexic: normal rectal temperature does not rule out infection

Diagnosis of joint sepsis is made by aspiration of fluid from the joint. Infected synovial fluid is likely to have reduced viscosity and may be turbid. It is useful to prepare and stain a smear for immediate in-house cytology. Septic joint fluid contains increased numbers of polymorphs (neutrophils), consistent with an inflammatory arthropathy, rather than the mononuclear cell populations that are found in normal joint fluid (see also Chapters 4 and 6). The presence of intracellular bacteria within neutrophils is unequivocally diagnostic of joint sepsis but bacteria are not commonly observed. Although the history and clinical signs are most likely to be consistent with sepsis, consideration should be given to other causes of inflammatory arthropathy such as immune-mediated joint disease and Lyme disease. These generally cause a polyarthropathy rather than a monoarthropathy, although the latter is possible. Culture of the aspirated fluid should be performed in all cases where inflammatory arthropathy has been identified. Submission of fluid in blood culture broth is considered more reliable than use of a charcoal swab. Such broth can usually be obtained via a commercial laboratory. **A negative culture does not eliminate sepsis as a positive culture is only achieved in about 50% of septic joints.**

It is important to keep detailed records of SSI cases to monitor the incidence of surgical cases, and to allow clinical audit to identify the source of the infection (Weese, 2012).

Treatment of surgical site infection

Antibiotic therapy should be started immediately upon confirmation of an inflammatory cytological picture. The choice of antibiotics is initially empirical, pending culture and sensitivity testing, and should be broad-spectrum and bactericidal. The author most commonly uses potentiated amoxicillin as a first-line treatment where sepsis is suspected, although first or second generation cephalosporins can also be prescribed. Therapy can then be adjusted if needed, based on the results of culture and sensitivity testing.

For joint sepsis, clinical improvement is usually apparent within 5 days of starting an appropriate antibiotic and should usually be continued for at least 6 weeks. Towards the end of this period, repeat synovial fluid analysis is indicated to confirm resolution of the inflammatory arthropathy prior to cessation of antibiotic therapy.

In cases of suspected joint sepsis that do not respond to initial antibiotic therapy, joint lavage may be performed under sedation using aseptically placed wide-bore needles via an ingress–egress system. Several litres of sterile isotonic fluid are lavaged through the joint. While the long-term benefits of joint lavage remain unproven, in the author's experience many cases will show rapid improvement, presumably due to reduction in both bacterial numbers and the concentration of intra-articular inflammatory mediators. Fibrin clots present in the infected joint can block the needles and may not be removed from the joint. If arthroscopy is available then this is an excellent modality for flushing as it facilitates wide-bore egress, high pressures and rapid passage of large amounts of fluid while allowing visual inspection of the intra-articular environment.

Osteomyelitis can commonly be successfully treated by a prolonged course of appropriate antibiotics providing there is stability and a sufficient blood supply. If the response to empirical antibiotic therapy is poor then the collection of bone biopsy samples for histopathology and culture should be considered. The presence of infected, devitalized bone can lead to sequestrum formation. These typically require debridement and complete removal of the necrotic bone before the infection will resolve. Sequestrum formation is uncommon in small animals, especially compared to equine patients.

Implant failure

Many orthopaedic surgeries involve the application of implants. These implants interface with the bone to form a construct that must be considered as a unit. The structural properties of implant–bone constructs vary widely depending on the implants used, the manner in which they are applied and the ability of the reconstructed bone to share load (the forces of weight-bearing) with the implant. For example, a simple transverse fracture or osteotomy that has been anatomically repaired using a dynamic compression plate will share load between the bone plate and the reconstructed bone, whereas in a non-reconstructed fracture or open-wedge ostectomy, the bone takes little or no load and the implant alone must resist all the forces generated during weight-bearing and ambulation. The surgeon must carefully consider the choice and size of implants and the most appropriate mode of application before a surgery is undertaken. Errors in implant selection or an inappropriate application technique may lead to failure of the construct or inhibit healing following surgery. Critical appraisal of postoperative radiographs is mandatory following almost all orthopaedic surgeries to identify any technical shortcomings that may predispose to implant failure. Immediate revision of fixation should be performed where indicated; this may involve adjustment of the existing implants or the application of supplementary fixation.

Failure of implants generally occurs at the weakest point in the construct. Implant breakage may occur acutely or, more commonly, as a result of cyclic loading over an extended period of time.

Single load to failure

Acute failure of implants most commonly occurs after a single event where a force of large magnitude has been applied to the implant system; for example, after a fall or following sudden explosive activity such as jumping, or where normal forces are applied to undersized or inadequately strong implants. The type of failure can differ depending on the physical characteristics of the implant–bone construct. Acute failure of less rigid metallic implants is likely to occur by bending of the implants, whereas excessively stiff implant systems tend to fail by screw pullout (bone–implant interface failure) or by bone fracture around the implants (Figure 16.6). Non-metallic implants such as nylon leader line may stretch, snap or pull through anchorage points.

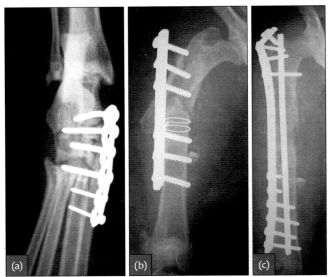

16.6 (a) Bending of the proximal bone screws applied during a partial tarsal arthrodesis procedure in a cat. Acute overload resulted in implant deformation and lateral deviation at the level of the tarsometatarsal joint. (b) Pull-out of the bone screws (bone–implant interface failure) from the proximal femur that occurred as a result of an excessively stiff bone plate for this animal (2.7 mm dynamic compression plate) in combination with excessive lever arm bending due to too short a plate. (c) This was subsequently revised using a longer and less rigid bone plate (2.0 mm veterinary cuttable plate) supported by an intramedullary pin.

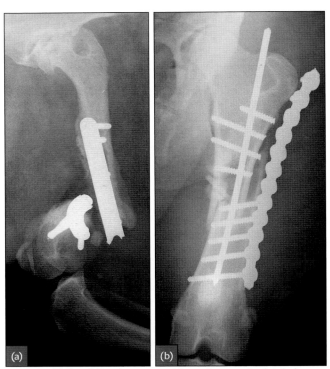

16.7 (a) Plate failure has occurred through an empty plate hole following cyclic loading, i.e. repetitive loading with low magnitude forces. Stresses concentrate within the metal, resulting in work hardening, fissuring and crack propagation. (b) Screw breakage following locking plate fixation using a String of Pearls bone plate combined with an intramedullary pin. This occurred as a result of stress concentration at the interface between the screws and the plate.

Cyclic loading to failure

Chronic failure generally occurs due to implant fatigue when a material is subjected to cyclical loading and unloading. If the magnitude of the load exceeds a critical threshold, microscopic cracks begin to form at areas of stress concentration, such as screw holes, corners or flaws in the implant surface. Eventually a crack reaches a critical size and will propagate, leading to implant breakage (Figure 16.7a).

The popularity of locking plates is increasing with an ever-expanding range of implants now available. Locking implants are advantageous in reducing the need for meticulous plate contouring and are of proven value in certain situations, such as during tibial plateau levelling osteotomy (Leitner *et al.*, 2008; Kowaleski *et al.*, 2013). However, locking systems also have disadvantages that must be recognized before use. With locking plate fixation, the weakest point of the construct may become the interface between screw thread and bone. With repetitive loading, screw breakage at the bone surface can occur (Figure 16.7b). This mode of failure is exacerbated with some implant designs, such as the String of Pearls plate (SOP, Orthomed), that use standard cortical screws with a smaller core diameter which are less resistant to bending than dedicated locking screws with their larger core diameter (Figure 16.8). In order to avoid screw breakage, it may be prudent to consider using a larger size locking plate system, using a locking plate system with screws of a larger core diameter, using a combination of implants to better share the load, e.g. plate-rod or double plating, or placing greater numbers of locking screws than usual in each fragment.

Implant loosening

The interface between bone and surgical implants is vitally important to the long-term security of orthopaedic implants. Care must be taken to preserve the viability of the

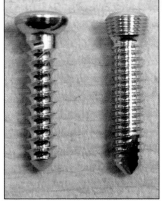

16.8 The 3.5 mm non-locking cortical bone screw shown on the left (Synthes) has a 2.4 mm diameter core, whereas the 3.5 mm locking screw on the right (Synthes) has a larger 2.9 mm core diameter. As the resistance (R) to bending is proportional to the radius (r) of the screw ($R = r^4$), the 21% increase in core diameter results in a substantial but disproportionate 213% increase in bending strength and resistance to fatigue failure.

bone–implant junction by minimizing damage to the bone caused by thermal necrosis. Use of a sharp drill bit and low-speed drilling with constant lavage are recommended; careless drilling where oversized holes may be created should be avoided. By preserving the soft tissue attachments to bone and therefore preserving blood supply, bone healing is likely to progress in a normal time frame.

Bone constantly remodels in response to stresses placed on it, in accordance with Wolff's law. An excessively stiff implant can cause a reduction of stress transmitted through the bone, which in turn induces osteopenia. The application of moderate stress to the bone may result in sclerosis, whereas the application of excessive stress may cause microfracture, bone resorption and premature implant loosening.

Postoperative fracture

Fracture of the bone around implants or drill holes is a recognized complication. This typically occurs as a result of excessive stress concentration at a site of insufficient bone strength. Bone can fracture because of weakness created by holes for implants, bone resorption caused by implant loosening, or overall reduction in bone strength caused, for example, by metabolic bone disease such as rickets or nutritional hyperparathyroidism. In the author's experience, the tibia is a relatively common bone where fractures may be seen postoperatively following surgery such as tibial tuberosity transposition or tibial tuberosity advancement via the modified maquet procedure (MMP) technique (Figure 16.9) (De Sousa et al., 2017). These fractures occur at a point where stress concentrates as the bone tapers at the distal extent of the tibial crest, particularly where a (Maquet) hole may weaken the cranial cortex. In order to reduce the potential for such tibial fractures, extreme care must be taken when drilling holes in the region of the distal tibial tuberosity: i.e. prepare holes away from the tibial tuberosity–shaft junction and avoid compromising the integrity of the cranial cortex. Bone plates can be applied to bridge areas of stress concentration if the surgeon is concerned and this may reduce the chance of fracture occurring. Care must equally be exercised if multiple drill holes are made close together in any bone as the strength of the bone may be adversely affected.

Postoperative fracture can also occur where short stiff implants are applied for the treatment of long bone fractures, particularly where a long section of bone is left unsupported. During load-bearing following internal fixation, lever arm bending forces are concentrated towards the end of the bone plate, or at the most proximal or distal external fixator pins, which may lead to fracture through an adjacent screw hole (Figure 16.10). The chance of fractures occurring is reduced by spanning the whole length of bone with fixation of rigidity appropriate to the clinical situation.

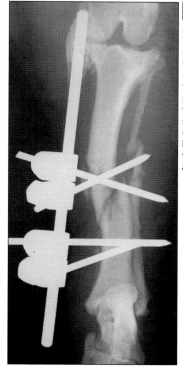

16.10 An external fixator has been applied in an attempt to treat a tibial fracture. The principles of external fixator application have not been followed: the fixation pins are concentrated around the fracture and the two proximal pins cross in the diaphyseal bone very close to the fracture. Long sections of diaphyseal bone are unsupported creating excessive lever arm forces at the level of the implants, resulting in fracture at the proximal pin tract.

PRACTICAL TIP

Implants can be too flexible or too rigid and both may result in complications such as implant failure or fracture. Try to match the implant stiffness to the clinical situation.

Always try to span the whole length of the bone with implants where possible

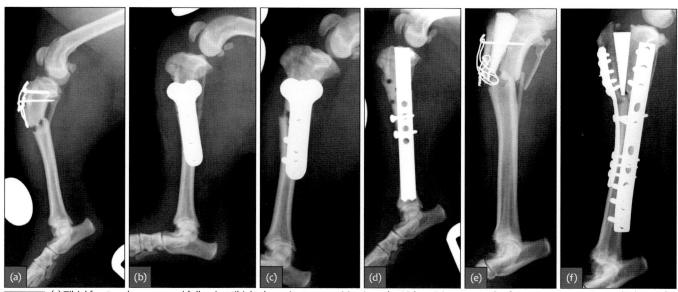

16.9 (a) Tibial fracture has occurred following tibial tuberosity transposition in a 5 kg Bichon Frise as a result of stress concentration at the base of the tibial tuberosity. (b) The fracture was initially revised by application of an excessively large and rigid implant that did not span the length of the bone, which (c) subsequently refractured. (d) This was revised by placing a less rigid veterinary cuttable bone plate (Synthes) that spanned the whole of the tibial diaphysis. (e) A similar fracture that occurred 5 days after tibial tuberosity advancement surgery using the MMP technique in an English Springer Spaniel. (f) Orthogonal bone plates were applied to stabilize the fracture and maintain tibial tuberosity advancement.

Complications of bone healing

Osseous healing is the goal following fracture repair, arthrodesis and elective osteotomy. In simple terms, successful bone healing needs the bone fragments to be adequately apposed, stabilized and well vascularized. Failure to achieve one or more of these factors may result in delayed union, non-union or malunion. The duration for bone healing may be influenced by many factors including the age of the patient, the anatomical region affected, and the presence of concomitant injuries or illness, the degree of bone apposition and the relative stability of the fracture or osteotomy gap. The presence of devitalized tissue and infection can also adversely affect bone healing and should be considered in all cases where poor bone healing is apparent; where this is suspected, thorough debridement and culture of tissue samples is indicated. Careful appraisal of the radiographic appearance of the bone may suggest which of these factors are inhibiting bone healing. Readers are referred to the *BSAVA Manual of Canine and Feline Fracture Repair and Management* for more details.

Delayed union

Delayed union is where bone takes longer than expected to heal; the exact timing of this will vary depending upon the signalment and concomitant pathologies of each patient. Importantly, the bone is continuing to heal, and this can be seen on sequential radiographs. Most cases of delayed bone union will eventually progress to bone union given enough time, providing no other complications such as implant loosening occur.

Non-union

Where there is no prospect of bone healing occurring without further intervention, non-union has occurred. Unfortunately, determining when delayed union has become non-union can be difficult. In humans, non-union is considered to be present when there is failure to show progressive change in the radiographic appearance of the fracture for at least 3 months after the period of time during which normal fracture union would be expected to have occurred (Mora *et al.*, 2006).

Non-unions are classified as biologically active (viable) or biologically inactive (non-viable).

Viable non-union: There are three types of biologically active non-union:

- Hypertrophic
- Eutrophic
- Oligotrophic.

Hypertrophic non-union is characterized by exuberant callus formation (elephant's foot callus). This suggests an adequate cellular response and vascular supply with inadequate interfragmentary stability. Such cases are often the most straightforward of non-unions to treat, as the application of supplementary fixation, for example using an additional external fixator or bone plate to stabilize the fracture, plus optional bone graft, usually results in union occurring. Resection of bone is not generally necessary in the presence of a hypertrophic non-union.

Eutrophic non-union has a small amount of callus formation present.

Oligotrophic non-union is characterized by bone ends that are quiescent with little or no evidence of callus formation (making it very difficult to differentiate from an inactive non-union). Eutrophic and oligotrophic non-union may develop following poor bone apposition, the application of excessively stiff fixation (particularly where the bone ends have not been compressed), or with inadequate stability (in particular in cases where poorly applied cerclage wires have been used and the implants are loose) in combination with poor vascularity or cellular response.

Excessive injury to the soft tissue envelope surrounding the fracture (caused by initial injury or following excessive periosteal stripping at surgery) may slow bone healing and contribute to non-union. Careful assessment of the biological and mechanical factors is necessary to plan the most appropriate revision strategy. Options include altering the stiffness of the fixation or achieving interfragmentary compression with or without bone resection. Placement of bone grafts, either allograft or autogenous, is recommended in the management of these types of non-union. Extracorporeal shock wave therapy has been used with some success for the treatment of non-union in humans and animals. This uses pulsed sound waves that release energy at the bone surface to induce neo-angiogenesis, osteogenesis and stimulate bone formation through stem cell stimulation (Johannes *et al.*, 1994; Schaden *et al.*, 2001; D'Agostino *et al.*, 2016).

Non-viable non-union: There are four types of non-viable non-union:

- Dystrophic (avascular) – associated with poor vascularization on either side of the gap
- Necrotic – devitalized (possibly infected) bone is present and not incorporated
- Defect – bone loss with excessive fracture gap filled with fibrous tissue or muscle
- Atrophic – end stage to the other forms of non-viable non-union, characterized by loss of vascularity, resorption, rounding and sealing of the bone ends from the fracture site with loss of the medullary canal, and osteopenia.

The treatment of non-viable non-union cases involves:

- Debridement of the bone ends
- Removal of dead or poorly vascularized tissues
- Restoration and opening of the medullary canal
- Application of bone graft to the freshened fracture ends
- Reduction and compression of the fracture and stabilization, ideally compression with lag screws or a dynamic compression plate

---

There are various different types of bone graft available (autograft, allograft, cortical, cancellous) in addition to synthetic bone graft products and materials with osteopromotive properties. Readers are directed to the *BSAVA Manual of Canine and Feline Fracture Repair and Management* for further information on bone grafts and substitutes.

It is important to remember that bone resection may cause loss of bone length, which can cause functional deficit. An alternative but more complex strategy to avoid limb shortening involves the gradual transport of a vascularized bone segment across the defect using a circular external skeletal fixator. This induces regenerate bone formation in the wake of the transported bone segment, which ultimately remodels and fills the defect. The transported segment is brought into contact and eventually 'docks' and achieves osseous union with the distal bone segment.

Pseudoarthrosis (false joint) formation can be a deliberate intention in some cases (e.g. femoral head and neck excision) but this can also develop as a complication following fracture non-union and results in undesirable motion at the fracture site. In some situations pseudoarthrosis may cause relatively minor functional impairment, while in other cases serious disability can occur. When function is poor, surgical intervention is indicated, including resection of poorly vascularized bone, interfragmentary compression, the application of bone graft and rigid interfragmentary fixation.

Malunion

Malunion occurs where a fracture or osteotomy heals but there is malalignment. This may result in angular or torsional malalignment of the adjacent joints and/or abnormal bone length (Figure 16.11). Malunion may be functional or non-functional. Functional malunion occurs where the animal is able to adequately compensate for the deformity and there is no permanent lameness or disability. Where non-functional malunion occurs, corrective surgery is indicated to restore normal limb length and alignment. Surgery to correct malunion typically involves corrective osteotomy, of which there are many types. Such procedures require meticulous planning and are frequently very challenging to perform.

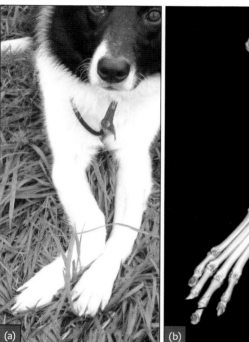 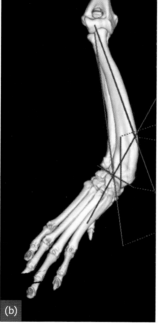

16.11　(a) A 2-year-old Border Collie with a non-functional malunion following antebrachial fracture sustained as a puppy. (b) A volume rendered three-dimensional computed tomography (CT) reconstruction of the bone was used to plan a corrective osteotomy.

Soft tissue complications

Changes in the surrounding soft tissues can occur as a complication of surgery when the vascularity of the tissues has been adversely affected, where excessive soft tissue tension remains or where postoperative swelling is excessive. Overly tight dressings may also contribute to these problems. Incisional dehiscence is the most common manifestation of perioperative soft tissue compromise; however, in some situations, severe and extensive tissue

necrosis can develop where prolonged ischaemia is present. This is more common with surgeries of the distal limb, particularly where extensive surgical approaches are made and large bone plates are applied, such as for carpal or tarsal arthrodesis. Most commonly it involves dehiscence of the skin incision overlying implants (Figure 16.12). In many cases wound healing will occur and granulation tissue grows to cover the implant. Implant-associated sepsis is highly likely to occur and implant removal may be necessary in some cases if skin closure cannot be obtained by other means. However, it is normally not possible to remove the implants until the bone has healed. Severe plantar necrosis has been specifically reported as a complication of tarsal arthrodesis surgery (Figure 16.13). While this is likely to be multifactorial in origin, plantar

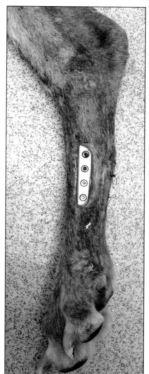

16.12　Exposure of the bone plate has occurred following a pantarsal arthrodesis procedure. This is likely to have resulted from excessive wound tension, self-trauma or postoperative swelling. Granulation and epithelialization will often occur around the margins of the viable soft tissue; however, it can be difficult or impossible to completely close the skin defect. Implant removal after osseous union has occurred will frequently allow soft tissue healing; however, re-fracture or breakdown of arthrodesis at one or more levels are possible consequences.

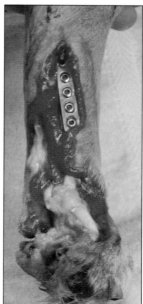

16.13　Plantar necrosis has occurred following partial tarsal arthrodesis. The cause of such severe loss of tissue is likely to be multifactorial. Excessive tissue swelling and overly tight dressing application probably contribute to this catastrophic complication. Injury to the perforating metatarsal artery during medial plate application or debridement of the tarsometatarsal joints has also been suggested as a possible cause. While some dogs will regain functional limb use following extensive and prolonged wound management, the prognosis is poor.

necrosis appeared to occur more frequently following medial bone plate application and following debridement of the tarsometatarsal joint. An association with injury to the perforating metatarsal artery has been suggested (Roch et al., 2008).

Persistent discharging sinuses may form after surgery that remain refractory to medical management. In these cases the presence of an infected implant leads to the persistence of infection within biofilms and warrants implant removal along with any other foreign material. The surrounding tissues should be debrided and lavaged before closure (Figure 16.14).

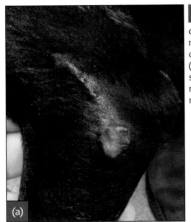

16.14 (a) This dog developed a discharging sinus several months after the stabilization of a humeral condylar fracture. (b) Surgical exploration of the sinus was performed and resulted in the excision of the nylon suture.

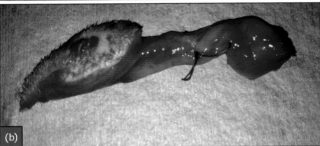

Complications associated with casts, dressings and splints

External coaptation is commonly used for the treatment of many orthopaedic conditions; however, the degree of stability conferred to the underlying tissues is often less than intended. This is due to the inevitable motion between the dressing materials and the compression of adjacent soft tissues. Soft dressings such as the Robert Jones dressing are useful as a first aid measure to control swelling, protect the wound from further damage, and provide temporary support where fracture or severe ligamentous injury has occurred. Unfortunately, the inappropriate application of soft or more rigid dressings can result in severe complications that may be of greater significance than the original injury (Meeson et al., 2011).

The use of inappropriately tight dressings can readily impair the vascular supply to the limb and result in pain, oedema and in some cases severe soft tissue necrosis (Figure 16.15) (Anderson and White, 2000). If an over-tight dressing has been applied then immediate removal is necessary. Assessment of vascularity and sensation are useful indicators of viability; however, the decision to perform radical treatment should be delayed for several days until the extent of tissue necrosis has been determined.

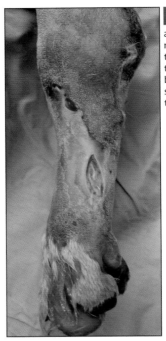

16.15 An excessively tight distal limb dressing had been applied several days earlier, resulting in progressive necrosis of the paw. There was no sensation to the distal limb and no active bleeding was evident after making small incisions into the affected tissues. Amputation was necessary.

Where dressings are applied to the distal limb, it is important that the dressing includes the digits. A small window can be left distally to allow palpation of the distal phalanges and visual assessment of the claws and adjacent soft tissues to monitor for signs of vascular compromise (Figure 16.16), but the digits should not be readily visible. A properly applied dressing should always be comfortable for the patient.

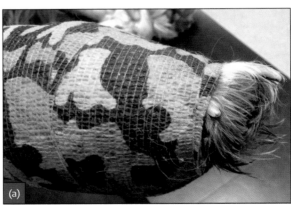

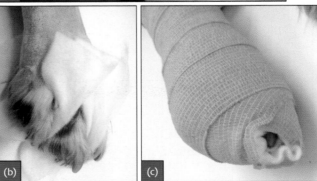

16.16 (a) Swelling of the distal extremities frequently occurs if the digits are not enclosed within the dressing. (b) The incidence of complications, such as rubbing between the digits, may be reduced by placing padding between the digits and enclosing the toes. (c) A small gap can be left at the end of the dressing to allow assessment of perfusion to the claws and digits.

Prolonged external coaptation of bones and the adjacent joints prevents early weight-bearing and joint mobilization. This has numerous adverse effects, which have been termed fracture disease. These include potentially permanent joint stiffness, disuse osteopenia, induction of irreversible cartilage degradation and muscle atrophy.

Other less severe complications are also commonly encountered following external coaptation, such as the development of pressure sores and rubs (Figure 16.17). Where these occur, removal of the dressing remains the simplest and often most effective means of treatment. Where dressing removal is not possible, modification of the dressing or splint to reduce pressure over the ulcerated tissues may be necessary.

Extreme care should also be taken when applying dressings to skeletally immature animals as osteopenia and joint laxity can develop alarmingly quickly, often within 5 to 7 days (Figure 16.18). Treatment involves the re-establishment of weight-bearing function using alternative methods of coaptation, no dressings, or application of an external fixator if necessary. In most cases the laxity will resolve and bone density will improve spontaneously.

Muscle contracture

Muscle contracture is the shortening of a muscle not associated with active contraction. Clinical signs include lameness, pain, weakness, decreased range of joint motion, a firm muscle texture, and often a characteristically abnormal gait. Predisposing factors for the development of muscle contracture include trauma, fracture, compartment syndrome, infection, repetitive strains, infectious disease, immune-mediated disease, neoplasia and ischaemia. Contracture occurs where progressive and irreversible fibrosis affects the whole muscle belly. In general, muscle contractures affecting the hindlimb are less well tolerated than those affecting the forelimb.

The most significant muscle contracture that occurs as a postsurgical complication is quadriceps muscle contracture (Bardet and Hohn, 1983). The condition typically affects young dogs following femoral fracture, particularly where osteomyelitis, quadriceps muscle injury or stifle joint immobilization have occurred. Hyperextension of the stifle joint

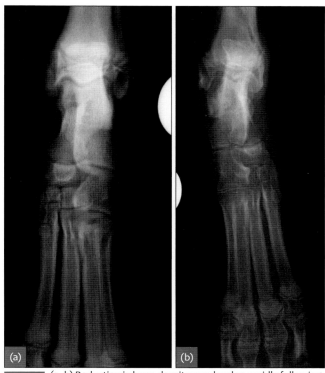

16.18 (a–b) Reduction in bone density can develop rapidly following external coaptation in young animals. Note the reduction in bone density between the two images that was associated with external coaptation of only 1 week's duration.

and marked muscle atrophy are the typical signs and secondary patellar luxation, genu recurvatum and hip luxation can occur. The condition is caused by the formation of firm fibrous adhesions between the vastus muscle belly and femur, together with irreversible muscle fibre necrosis. Once fibrosis has occurred, the prognosis is guarded. Attempts at treatment have been reported and usually involve the surgical release of adhesions followed by intensive physiotherapy, or the application of a stifle flexion device (Figure 16.19) (Moores, 2009). However, muscle fibrosis is irreversible, the prognosis is guarded and the outcome of treatment is usually suboptimal, particularly in long-standing cases. In the majority of fracture cases, quadriceps contracture can be readily avoided by appropriate fracture management plus the prompt institution of passive range of motion exercises within a few days of femoral/stifle surgery.

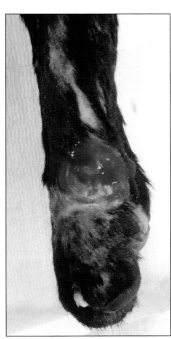

16.17 A severe full thickness pressure sore on the lateral aspect of a cat's paw following prolonged dressing application. Cast sores and rubs are common following the prolonged use of external coaptation. It is important to relieve pressure over the sore and prevent further abrasion from occurring. Often removal of the dressing is the most expedient way of treating dressing-related injuries.

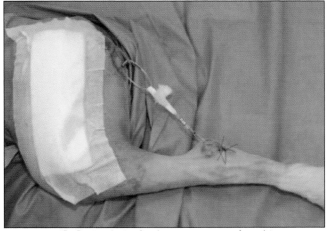

16.19 Stifle flexion device for the management of quadriceps contracture.
(Courtesy of A Moores)

References and further reading

Anderson DM and White RA (2000) Ischemic bandage injuries: a case series and review of the literature. *Veterinary Surgery* **29**, 488–498

Baines S, Lipscomb V and Hutchinson T (2012) *BSAVA Manual of Canine and Feline Surgical Principles: A Foundation Manual*. BSAVA Publications, Gloucester

Bardet JF and Hohn RB (1983) Quadriceps contracture in dogs. *Journal of the American Veterinary Medical Association* **183**, 680–685

Cook JL, Evans R, Conzemius MG *et al.* (2010) Proposed definitions and criteria for reporting time frame, outcome, and complications for clinical orthopedic studies in veterinary medicine. *Veterinary Surgery* **39**, 905–908

D'Agostino MC, Frairia R, Romeo P *et al.* (2016) Extracorporeal shockwaves as regenerative therapy in orthopedic traumatology: a narrative review from basic research to clinical practice. *Journal of Biological Regulators and Homeostatic Agents* **30**, 323–332

De Sousa R, Egan P, Parsons K *et al.* (2017) Treatment of tibial diaphyseal fractures following plateless tibial tuberosity advancement to manage cranial cruciate disease. *The Journal of Small Animal Practice* **58**, 372–379

Eugster S, Schawalder P, Gaschen F and Boerlin P (2004) A prospective study of postoperative surgical site infections in dogs and cats. *Veterinary Surgery* **33**, 542–550

Fitzpatrick N and Solano MA (2010) Predictive variables for complications after TPLO with stifle inspection by arthrotomy in 1000 consecutive dogs. *Veterinary Surgery* **39**, 460–474

Gemmill T and Clements D (2016) *BSAVA Manual of Canine and Feline Fracture Repair and Management, 2nd edn*. BSAVA Publications, Gloucester

Johannes EJ, Kaulesar Sukul DM and Matura E (1994) High-energy shock waves for the treatment of nonunions: an experiment on dogs. *Journal of Surgical Research* **57**, 246–252

Kowaleski MP, Boudrieau RJ, Beale BS *et al.* (2013) Radiographic outcome and complications of tibial plateau levelling osteotomy stabilized with an anatomically contoured locking bone plate. *Veterinary Surgery* **42**, 847–852

Leitner M, Pearce SG, Windolf M *et al.* (2008) Comparison of locking and conventional screws for maintenance of tibial plateau positioning and biomechanical stability after locking tibial plateau levelling osteotomy plate fixation. *Veterinary Surgery* **37**, 357–365

Meeson RL, Davidson C and Arthurs GI (2011) Soft-tissue injuries associated with cast application for distal limb orthopaedic conditions. A retrospective study of sixty dogs and cats. *Veterinary and Comparative Orthopaedics and Traumatology* **24**, 126–131

Moores A (2009) Management of quadriceps contracture in a dog using a static flexion apparatus and physiotherapy. *Journal of Small Animal Practice* **50**, 251–254

Mora R, Pedrotti L and Galli GB (2006) Failure of Union. *Non-union of the Long Bones: Diagnosis and Treatment with Compression-Distraction Techniques*, pp. 27–37. Springer, Milano

Nazarali A, Singh A and Weese JS (2014) Perioperative administration of antimicrobials during tibial plateau levelling osteotomy. *Veterinary Surgery* **43**, 966–971

Nelson L (2011) Surgical site infections in small animal surgery. *Veterinary Clinics of North America: Small Animal Practice* **41**, 1041–1056

Pratesi A, Moores AP, Downes C, Grierson J and Maddox TW (2015) Efficacy of postoperative antimicrobial use for clean orthopedic implant surgery in dogs: a prospective randomized study in 100 consecutive cases. *Veterinary Surgery* **44**, 653–660

Roch SP, Clements DN, Mitchell RAS *et al.* (2008) Complications following tarsal arthrodesis using bone plate fixation in dogs. *Journal of Small Animal Practice* **49**, 117–126

Savicky R, Beale B, Murtaugh R, Swiderski-Hazlett J and Unis M (2013) Outcome following removal of TPLO implants with surgical site infection. *Veterinary and Comparative Orthopaedics and Traumatology* **26**, 260–265

Schaden W, Fischer A and Sailler A (2001) Extracorporeal shock wave therapy of nonunion or delayed osseous union. *Clinical Orthopaedics and Related Research* **387**, 90–94

Weese S (2012) Monitoring for surgical infection. In: *Veterinary Surgery: Small Animal, Volume 1*, ed KM Tobias and SA Johnston, pp. 170–179. Elsevier Saunders, St Louis

Wolf M, Clar H, Friesenbichler J *et al.* (2014) Prosthetic joint infection following total hip replacement: results of one stage versus two stage exchange. *International Orthopaedics* **38**, 1363–1368

Chapter 17

Postoperative management and rehabilitation

Briony Alderson, Rob Pettitt and Louise Dale

The aim of orthopaedic surgery is to improve the quality of life of the patient to a level where it can lead as normal a life as possible. The postoperative period is as important as the surgery itself in terms of analgesia and rehabilitation and depends on a team approach involving everyone including the surgeon, registered veterinary nurses, animal care staff and owners. This chapter will discuss most of the key aspects of this period but for further information, the reader is referred to the *BSAVA Manual of Canine and Feline Rehabilitation, Supportive and Palliative Care*.

Analgesia

It is important to ensure adequate analgesia, particularly before attempting any form of therapeutic exercises in the postoperative orthopaedic patient. Analgesia in the post-operative period is essential for patient welfare and to maximize the use of the affected limb and early return to normal function. An appropriate analgesia protocol that is regularly assessed needs to be part of the daily care plan. Pain scoring can be a useful way of providing a more objective evaluation of the patient's analgesia in the postoperative period and can be continued through into the follow-up assessments. This can be done with an *ad hoc* scale that has been developed in house, or by using previously developed systems such as:

- The Glasgow Composite Pain Scale for cats and dogs (http://www.newmetrica.com/acute-painmeasurement/)
- The Colorado scale for cats and dogs http://www.vasg.org/pdfs/CSV_Acute_Pain_Scale_kitten.pdf and http://www.vasg.org/pdfs/CSV_Acute_Pain_Scale_Canine.pdf

Analgesic medications are usually required preoperatively in orthopaedic cases and pre-emptive multimodal analgesia is ideal; there are many different analgesics available to the veterinary practitioner and each patient should have an individualized analgesia plan that is constantly monitored and adjusted.

Non-steroidal anti-inflammatory drugs (NSAIDs) are usually indicated in orthopaedic cases as they act on the initial transduction of the pain pathway where the tissue damage first occurs, in addition to reducing inflammation and swelling at the surgical site. However, each individual patient should be assessed for their risk of developing side

effects; where there is a history of gastrointestinal sensitivity, NSAIDs should be avoided or used judiciuously, such as in combination with gastroprotectants. Many licensed products are available and selection is often based on personal preference. If one NSAID causes unacceptable side effects in a patient such as vomiting or a poorer than expected level of analgesia, another product may have greater efficacy with fewer side effects in that patient. NSAIDs often have a cumulative effect so it is worth giving extended courses of the drug as further improvement is noted with time (Innes *et al.*, 2010).

Opioids are used in the perioperative period to provide analgesia for the orthopaedic patient. Methadone is licensed in dogs and cats and can be carried on in the immediate postoperative period. Alternatively, infusions of shorter acting agents, such as fentanyl, can be used and titrated to effect, therefore potentially reducing side effects (for example sedation). It is usual to 'stage down' to buprenorphine the day after surgery if the animal is comfortable enough to warrant this. Alternatively, tramadol is often used, although it is unlicensed and studies have shown mixed, often limited, efficacy. Pain scoring should be used to assess requirements and the analgesia plan adjusted accordingly.

Loco-regional analgesia techniques should be employed where possible as these will reduce intra- and postoperative anaesthesia and analgesia requirements. A well performed loco-regional technique can provide excellent short duration postoperative analgesia and aid in the ability to perform physiotherapy in the early postoperative period. Pain scoring can be employed to assess the need for additional analgesia when these techniques are performed. The most common loco-regional analgesic techniques are:

- Epidural analgesia
- Femoral and sciatic nerve block
- Lumbar plexus nerve block
- Brachial plexus nerve block
- RUMM (radial, ulnar, musculocutaneous and median) nerve block.

The duration and onset of action of a loco-regional technique will depend on the choice of local anaesthetic drugs used. The individual patient requirements and the length and type of surgery should be taken into consideration when choosing the local anaesthetic. For example, lidocaine has a quick onset of action but a short duration of action of approximately 4 hours, whereas bupivacaine has a duration of action of approximately 8 hours but a longer onset of action. It may be important that the patient is able to walk within a short period after the surgery in order to prevent recumbency or gait abnormalities and the subsequent complications that could occur, but also to enable meaningful postoperative gait evaluation and prevent any unnecessary immobilization of the joints.

Ketamine is useful in the perioperative period and can be continued as an infusion into the immediate post-operative period, especially in cases with chronic pain. Paracetamol can also be given to dogs (NOT cats) in the postoperative period; although the data sheet warns against concurrent use of paracetamol and NSAIDs, in the authors' practice it has been used in many cases in combination with NSAIDs or steroids with no known ill effects.

Other drugs that are to be used longer term should also be started as soon as possible following (or even prior to) surgery. Many of these alternatives, e.g. gabapentin, tramadol and amantadine, are not licensed, and informed owner consent should be sought prior to use. Use of such drugs preoperatively and intraoperatively would be un-usual for orthopaedic patients.

It is preferable to use multimodal analgesia where possible; this also includes non-pharmacological interventions. The acronym NOLAN (P) is useful when considering analgesia at all points along the pain pathway. Where:

N = NSAIDs: reduce inflammation at the surgical site (e.g. meloxicam, firocoxib)

O = opioids: e.g. fentanyl – short action, quick onset, causes respiratory depression; methadone – licensed in both dogs and cats, longer acting

L = local anaesthetics: e.g. lidocaine – quick onset, short duration, approximately 4 hours; bupivacaine – longer duration of action, potential for cardiac toxicity if accidentally administered intravenously

A = alpha-2 adrenoceptor agonists: e.g. medetomidine – causes reflex bradycardia through vasocon-striction, provides analgesia, good sedation

N = NMDA antagonists: e.g. ketamine – good for chronic pain, analgesic dose is smaller than anaesthetic dose

P = paracetamol: mode of action unclear. Do not use in cats

It is imperative that medication is given correctly and at the required frequency. Medications given in food should be monitored to ensure that they are taken and not rejected; ideally place the medication in one piece of food and feed this first to ensure the patient receives it. Detailed hospital sheets, daily care plans and discharge instruc-tions help to ensure all instructions for medications are followed correctly.

Non-pharmacological methods of pain reduction may also be employed if feasible and thought to be of benefit; for example, acupuncture and the use of therapeutic exer-cises. Evidence suggests that acupuncture may help to manage chronic pain by interrupting/re-setting the pain pathway, although it is not frequently used. Reduction of chronic pain could be useful prior to surgical intervention to help prevent 'wind-up' that can occur pre-, intra- or postoperatively.

Further information is available in Chapter 13 of this manual and in the *BSAVA Manual of Canine and Feline Anaesthesia and Analgesia*. The above section is only intended as an overview.

Immediate postoperative nursing care

Wound care

Every surgical wound should have a protective covering applied immediately postoperatively in order to help reduce the incidence of self-trauma and surgical site infec-tions (Figure 17.1). Non-woven adhesive wound dressings, e.g. Primapore, can be applied aseptically while the patient is still in theatre prior to moving to radiography or recovery. These dressings should remain on the patient for 2–3 days and be changed when necessary, for example if there is excessive strike-through or loss of adhesion of the dress-ing. In the event of a small amount of dry strike-through, a further dressing can be applied on top of the original one, to prevent damage of the fibrin seal caused by removal of the dressing. Too frequent dressing changes could lead to an increased risk of wound infection if aseptic technique is not used. Dressing changes may be uncomfortable for the patient and subsequent dressings may not adhere as well, so unnecessary changes should be avoided.

A topical skin adhesive can be used with intradermal skin sutures to provide a protective seal in the postopera-tive period (e.g Dermabond Advanced® or Histoacryl®). Studies have shown that following application of Dermabond Advanced®, a barrier is created that reduces microbial filtration into the healing wound (Bhende *et al.*, 2002) (Figure 17.2). The skin adhesive is completely water-proof for the first 48–72 hours, although excessive bathing of patients should be avoided. There is no requirement to

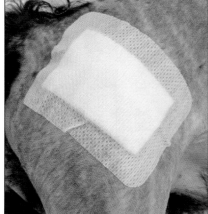

17.1 Application of a protective non-adhesive dressing immediately postoperatively to protect the wound.

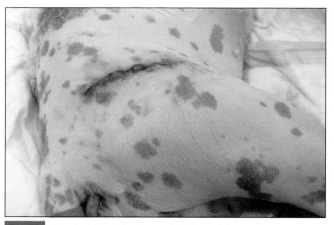

17.2 A topical skin adhesive used in place of skin sutures or staples.

cover these wounds with an additional non-adhesive dressing but, as with any wound, patient interference must be prevented and Elizabethan collars must always be applied for patients that interfere with the wound or dressing. Soft Elizabethan collars (Figure 17.3) can be useful and less stressful for the patient but care should be taken to make sure that the patient cannot get access to the wound/dressing. The collars should be regularly washed.

Discharging wounds should be cleaned and swabbed if infection is suspected (i.e. if there is pain, redness and/or swelling), in order to isolate the pathogenic bacteria involved and select the appropriate antibiotic therapy based on culture and sensitivity testing. Swabs should be taken from deep within the wound if possible so that the culture result is representative and does not simply represent contamination from skin commensals. If this is not possible, a fine–needle aspirate from within the wound is preferable. If a multidrug resistant isolate is identified, appropriate practice protocols should be in place to minimize contamination and spread of the bacteria. Regular environmental swabbing can help to ensure kennels, wards and theatre areas are not harbouring any multidrug resistant bacteria (Readers are referred to Surgical site infections in Chapter 16 for further information).

may be beneficial to reduce motion of the shoulder joint or to prevent weight-bearing on a thoracic limb. Although both of these prevent weight-bearing on a thoracic limb, the carpal flexion bandage, in contrast to the Velpeau sling, permits motion in the proximal joints and is preferable to prevent complications associated with immobilization. As an alternative, a custom-made jacket can be used to act in a similar fashion to a Velpeau sling (Figure 17.4). The advantage of this is that it can easily be removed to allow range-of-motion exercises to be performed, if appropriate, on a daily basis. It is also an opportunity to check the health of the tissues beneath the dressing.

An Ehmer sling can be used to prevent weight-bearing on a pelvic limb; its main indication is the management of hip luxation. (Figure 17.5).

When bandaging, plenty of padding should be applied around any bony prominences and any wounds should be appropriately covered. Care should be taken to ensure that materials used do not rub against the skin and create wounds. Correct technique (see Operative Technique 17.1) should be used when applying conforming bandage to ensure circulation is not compromised. Ideally, unless applying a pressure bandage, at least the tips of the the digits should be accessible in order to assess distal limb

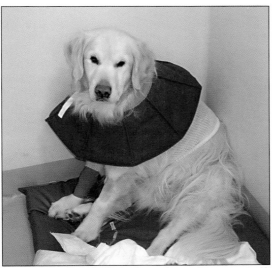

17.3 A soft cloth Elizabethan collar used to prevent self-trauma of wounds or inadvertent removal of indwelling catheters/drains.

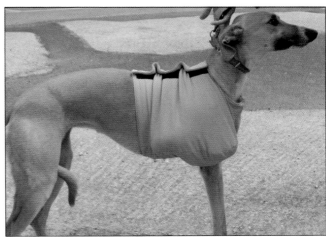

17.4 A custom-made jacket used as a Velpeau sling to restrict motion and prevent weight-bearing on a thoracic limb.

Bandaging

Bandaging can be useful in the early postoperative period to help support tissues, restrict joint motion and help to reduce and prevent oedema and swelling. However, care must be taken to ensure bandages are applied correctly (see Operative Technique 17.1) and applied only when it will provide benefit.

Following tibial plateau levelling osteotomy surgery, bandaging has been shown to be ineffective in reducing postoperative swelling (Unis *et al.*, 2010). There may be some merit in applying a modified Robert Jones bandage in order to reduce wound trauma and potential infection within the first 24–48 hours while the wound seals, but this has not been demonstrated and is not routine in the authors' practice.

There are a number of functionally specific bandages that can be considered in appropriate situations. A carpal flexion bandage is used to prevent weight-bearing, for example in the management of accessory carpal bone fractures and luxation (see Chapter 20). A Velpeau sling

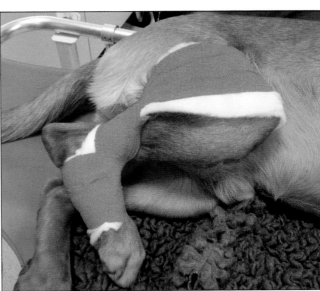

17.5 Use of an Ehmer sling to prevent weight-bearing on a pelvic limb.

temperature, superficial skin sensation and swelling. The digits should be assessed on a daily basis as a minimum and these checks should be included in the patient's daily care plan. Dressings should be changed at least once weekly or if they slip, become dirty or wet, or there is concern over the circulation or health of the limb (see Operative Technique 17.1). A waterproof covering should be used to protect the bandage whenever the animal goes outside. Necessary measures such as Elizabethan collars, constant supervision or cage confinement should be taken to prevent the animal from interfering with the bandage. It should be noted that bandages and casts are not benign and care must be taken when they are used. An inappropriately tight dressing can impair the vascular supply to the limb and result in pain, oedema and in some cases severe soft tissue necrosis (Meeson et al., 2011).

Complications of bandage use include:
- Rub wounds/sores
- Reduced circulation to the affected limb; this can cause extensive tissue damage including irreversible necrosis and tissue death
- Wound dehiscence
- Swelling ± oedema of the toes
- Unnecessary pain or discomfort for the patient
- Increased financial cost to the client
- Increased hospitalization time for the patient

Prolonged use of a bandage or limb sling may result in contraction, stiffness and atrophy of the surrounding muscles and tissues. In puppies, it typically leads to laxity of soft tissues which results in excessive joint movement, for example hyperextension of the carpus or digits. Once the bandage or sling is removed the patient may require further physiotherapy to help combat this.

Grooming

Grooming can be a source of stimulation for the patient. For long-haired breeds regular grooming is important during hospitalization, in order to prevent matting of the fur and contamination with faeces, saliva or food especially around the eyes, face or anus.

Nutrition

Adequate nutrition has been shown to aid recovery in the postoperative patient (Arnold and Barbul, 2006). If possible the patient's normal diet should be used during the hospitalized period. If this is not available then highly digestible diets are preferred as there is less risk of gastrointestinal upset. Protein is important for muscle and tissue repair but carbohydrates should be reduced during the hospitalization period due to a reduction in activity of the patient. Many hospitalized patients have a reduced appetite, so it is important to use a diet that is highly palatable. For example, Hill's Prescription Diet A/D Critical Care has increased levels of potassium and highly digestible proteins, as well as highly digestible and palatable nutrients, and is designed to support cats and dogs after serious injury, illness or surgery. Other diets that are suitable include Royal Canin Veterinary Diet Recovery or Gastrointestinal, Purina Convalescence or Eukanuba Veterinary Diet Intestinal.

Patients who lack interest in food need to be carefully assessed for pain or other possible causes of inappetence. It may be necessary to tempt animals by hand-feeding or

heating the food gently which may help to stimulate the appetite. This is particularly so with cats. A balanced diet should be fed; the addition of tempting foods such as chicken may be helpful to encourage inappetent animals to eat, but this should be kept to a minimum. Feeding too often may make the patient appear inappetant, and patients that are usually fed only once a day may not want to eat more frequently than this within a hospital environment, which may be misinterpreted as anorexia or inappetence. It is useful to gather information on feeding habits from owners prior to admission, or during recovery if inappetence appears to be a problem. Patients should be weighed daily to ensure sufficient energy intake and so that negative energy balance is avoided. Updated weights should be clearly visible on the daily care plan.

Any signs of reaction/aversions to any medication, including diarrhoea or gastrointestinal disturbance, should be communicated and if appropriate dealt with immediately. Any medications that the patient may already be on at home must also be included in the care plan with the appropriate timings.

Husbandry

Stressed or anxious patients should be housed in an appropriate area of the hospital. If possible these patients should be kennelled in a quiet area away from noisy or aggressive patients. Ideally cats should be hospitalized in a separate area to dogs. The kennel should be big enough to allow some movement yet small enough to prevent unwanted or unrestricted movement. Some patients may be recumbent or have reduced ability to move or turn over in the kennel; therefore this should be lined with absorbent material such as kennel liners or VetBed that will allow fluid to soak through leaving the patient dry (Figure 17.6). Regular checks of the kennel should be incorporated into the daily care plan. Mattresses should be lifted and the whole kennel thoroughly cleaned from top to bottom at least once daily, and cleaned regionally as necessary should the animal pass urine or faeces in it. Padding to prevent pressure sores is very important for breeds with bony prominences and poor soft tissue cover such as Greyhounds and for recumbent animals. Barrier creams such as Cavilon™ (3M Health Care, UK) can be applied to help prevent urine scalding. Recumbent patients can benefit from an indwelling urinary catheter in the first few days until some mobility has returned; however, the associated risks (such as urinary tract infection) mean that this should only be done when deemed in the best interest of the patient (Figure 17.7).

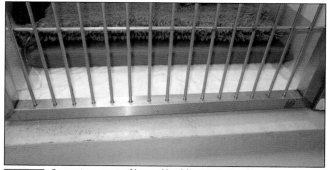

17.6 Correct amount of kennel bedding organized to prevent inadvertent soaking of the patient while allowing suitable padding for recumbent patients. Incontinence pads are placed in contact with the floor; on top of these is a waterproof padded mattress and on top of this is a soft padded layer, such as VetBed, on which the patient would lie.

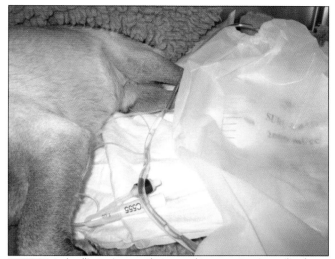

17.7 Indwelling urinary catheter used to manage urine soiling/scalding in recumbent patients until some degree of mobility has returned.

Regular opportunities to urinate and defaecate in an appropriate area away from the kennel should be incorporated into the daily care plan, and notes detailing when this occurs should be kept. Patients may need encouragement to urinate in the first few days after surgery, especially if their pain is not managed adequately, or following epidural techniques (especially those involving opioids) (see *BSAVA Manual of Canine and Feline Anaesthesia and Analgesia*). Urine output and water intake should be monitored regularly and the bladder should be checked/expressed when and if necessary. In particular, male dogs that have received an epidural anaesthetic may not urinate and should be monitored closely for failure to pass urine or signs of overflow. Harnesses and slings can be used to help the patient move to a suitable area in which to urinate and defaecate. Care should be taken to ensure the patient does not tire, fall or twist on the affected limb and this may require two people to ensure adequate support (Figure 17.8). Physiotherapy can be performed while on a 'toilet trip' outside to help mentally stimulate the patient.

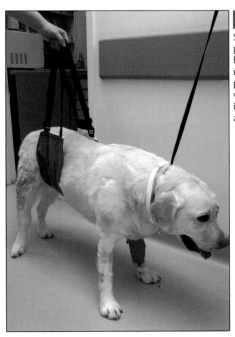

17.8

Slings are particularly useful to help move paretic or non-ambulatory patients safely and without risking injuries to the animal.

Physiotherapy/rehabilitation

Rehabilitation is defined as a return to function, but function will mean different things to different individuals and owners. Physiotherapy (or physical therapy) is one modality of returning patients to a satisfactory level of rehabilitation.

It is important in all cases to consider that excessive or premature physiotherapy may cause harm; therefore, guidance from a professional veterinary physiotherapist should be sought to achieve an optimal outcome. Unlike human healthcare, where the term physiotherapist is protected, the same does not presently apply in the veterinary profession. There are recognized veterinary physiotherapy qualifications but, as they are not protected, many people practise physiotherapy without suitable qualifiations. The responsibility of approving physiotherapy centres for their patients remains with the attending veterinary surgeon and care should be taken to identify suitably qualified physiotherapists. The Association of Chartered Physiotherapists in Animal Therapy (ACPAT) is a good starting point (www.acpat.org).

Following orthopaedic surgery it is important to encourage early limb use in order to maximize the beneficial effects of the surgery.

> The advantages of early limb use following orthopaedic surgery are to:
> - Maintain muscle mass/minimize atrophy
> - Maintain muscle tone and proprioception
> - Maintain joint range of movement
> - Minimize fibrosis
> - Minimize limb oedema

Immobilization can lead to atrophy of the muscles, fibrous contracture of the limb and reduced health of the bone and the cartilage in joints, resulting in a further decrease in use of the affected limb. Ideally, physiotherapy should be incorporated into the rehabilitation protocol following orthopaedic surgery and may involve a range of elements to maximize recovery in the individual patient (Saunders, 2007).

The benefits of physiotherapy are well documented in humans but less clear in animals, with little objective evidence currently available to support its use although it is an evolving field. The use of physiotherapy has been shown to be beneficial in dogs undergoing tibial plateau levelling osteotomy and lateral extracapsular stabilization for cranial cruciate disease (Monk *et al.*, 2006; Jerre, 2009). These studies showed that early physiotherapeutic intervention was beneficial and should be considered to maximize recovery and limb function outcomes following surgery.

- **Gentle massage** of the muscles in the affected area should be beneficial to enhance local blood circulation and reduce scar tissue formation and local oedema. There are many reported methods of massage and the techniques used should be modified to suit the individual patient (Saunders, 2007; Shumway, 2007).
- **Hydrotherapy** is another modality that may be incorporated into a rehabilitation process. Walking on an underwater treadmill (Figure 17.9) allows an adjustable degree of weight-bearing in a buoyant environment so a lower load is placed on the affected limb. It is important that qualified physiotherapists (ACPAT or veterinary physiotherapist) are involved at this stage in the process rather than attempting *ad hoc*

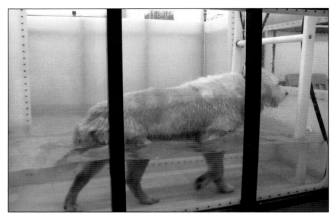

17.9 Use of an underwater treadmill in the rehabilitation of an orthopaedic patient; specifically, and as opposed to a hydrotherapy pool, this allows walking with a variable depth of water that alters the amount of weight-bearing/flotation of the patient.
(Courtesy of Darryl L Millis)

'in-house' solutions. An underwater treadmill is a controlled environment and can be adjusted to each individual patient's requirements.

- **Cold packing** the affected area, starting immediately postoperatively, is often beneficial and can be continued for 2–3 days, or as long as swelling or inflammation is present. Cold packing in the immediate postoperative period may help to reduce inflammation, swelling and improve patient comfort. The application of cold packs for 10–20 minutes immediately following surgery is recommended (Shumway, 2007) (Figure 17.10). A cold pack normally comprises an ice pack that should always be wrapped in a towel or similar, in order to prevent thermal (ice) burns of the skin.

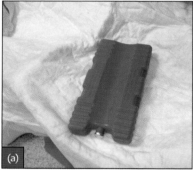

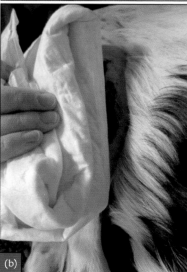

17.10 (a) Preparation of a cold pack by enclosing a frozen ice block within an incontinence sheet or towel. (b) Application of the cold pack to the affected area.

- **Warm packing** can be used after the initial phase of postoperative inflammation has subsided, with the application of warm packs, wrapped in towelling to protect the tissues. This, in combination with gentle range-of-motion exercise and massage, can help to improve blood supply, loosen soft tissues and relax muscles, thus helping to reduce further atrophy or stiffness of the limb (Shumway, 2007). A warm pack could be useful prior to physiotherapy or exercise in order to loosen the tissues.

Even short periods of immobilization can lead to secondary changes in the limb, such as articular degeneration, muscle atrophy and a reduction in the range of motion. These can take several weeks to return to normal and in some cases, the secondary changes of muscle atrophy and restricted range of motion may be irreversible, although this is poorly defined. Early initiation of passive range-of-motion exercises can also reduce the postoperative recovery time.

Some of these techniques are harder or impossible to perform in cats, depending on the nature and temperament of the individual cat. Careful consideration of the individual cat to maximize its care can help to improve outcome.

Too little exercise may be as detrimental as too much, as the joints will tend to stiffen. For controlled exercise programs, walks should be limited to 15–60 minutes (as appropriate to the individual case) on the lead with avoidance of exuberant off-lead activities. Liaison with a qualified physiotherapist could be beneficial

---

Further information is available in the *BSAVA Manual of Canine and Feline Rehabilitation, Supportive and Palliative Care*. The above section is only intended as an overview.

Discharge and re-examination

Most orthopaedic patients are hospitalized until they are able to rise, stand and walk unsupported and all medication can be given orally, and until such time that all other treatments such as physiotherapy exercises and bladder management can be done at home, and the owners are comfortable with performing these tasks. Most orthopaedic patients are discharged home 1–3 days after the surgical procedure.

Factors to consider when deciding when to discharge a patient from hospital include:

- Age of patient
- Nature of injury
- Demeanour of the patient: nervous/depressed/inappetent in the hospital environment
- Mobility of the patient
- Whether any medication can be given orally
- Practicality and capability of the owner(s) to care for the patient
- Whether the patient's condition is stable/there is any likelihood of an imminent complication
- Suitability of the home environment
- Bandage care and location of sutures

Discharge instructions

Comprehensive discharge instructions should be printed that are individualized to the patient, listing treatment performed, prescribed medication, exercise protocols and warning signs to look out for (e.g. wound discharge). This is important as it advises owners what to do and what to expect in the postoperative period (Figure 17.11). Clear instructions are particularly important when casts or bandages have been placed and production of an owner information sheet, detailing daily bandage checks and clinical signs to be aware of, is highly recommended.

Re-examination schedule

Following discharge, the re-check schedule should be designed and advised to allow for adequate assessment of the patient, the progress of healing and appropriate early intervention in the case of complications, without being excessive. The exact timing of re-examinations is somewhat subjective, depends on surgeon preference and is adjusted on a case-by-case basis, but the following is an example schedule:

- 7 days postoperatively: check/replace bandage if present; if not present, optional to check clinical progress
- 10–14 days postoperatively: remove sutures/staples if present; check clinical progress; check/replace bandage if present
- Thereafter, if bandage present, check/replace bandage at least every 7 days until bandage removed
- Every 4–8 weeks: check clinical progress and radiograph the surgical site if bone/fracture healing is to be monitored. Repeat until the patient is signed off.

Factors to consider when assessing clinical progress:
- Wound swelling, bruising, discharge
- Soft tissue/surgical site thickening
- Joint range of movement and crepitus
- Joint/bone pain
- Muscle atrophy
- Limb use; degree of weight-bearing when standing and grade of lameness
- General demeanour of patient

Small Animal Teaching Hospital, University of Liverpool, Leahurst, Chester High Road, Neston, Wirral, CH64 7TE Tel: +44 151 7956100 or 794 4290 Fax: +44 151 7956101 Web: http://www.liv.ac.uk/sath email: sath@liv.ac.uk	Animal name: .... Owner: .... Referring vet/practice: ....
Orthopaedics	Clinician : .... Admittance date: .... Discharge date : ....

Diagnostic findings

Treatment ....

Medication ....

Aftercare

There are staples in the skin which have been covered with a light dressing to protect them. This dressing can be removed in **TWO** days' time. Please check the wound **daily** for signs of swelling, redness or discharge.

It is important to restrict.................. exercise for the first few weeks to allow healing to take place.

- For the first two weeks **strict** rest is required. Only allow.................. to go into the garden on a lead to toilet, and prevent him/her from going up and down stairs, and jumping on and off the furniture. Ensure.................. is kept in a room with non-slip flooring.
- After two weeks.................. can begin **FIVE** minute walks, **three** times daily.
- If there are no problems, then gradually increase the length of each walk by **FIVE** minutes per week.
- It is important that.................. remains on controlled, lead exercise only, as instructed, and is not allowed to run free until we reassess his/her progress when you return for your post-op check in **EIGHT** weeks' time. We will then advise you on how you can begin to gradually increase the level of activity.

Follow-up

Please visit your own veterinary surgeon in **TEN** days' time to have the staples removed.
Make an appointment to bring.................. back to see us in **eight** weeks' time.
It may be necessary to take X-rays at that time, so please ensure your dog has been fasted from **10 pm** the previous evening.
Please complete the course of medication prescribed, and do not hesitate to contact us or your own veterinary surgeon if you have any queries or concerns.

17.11 An example of a discharge instruction template that is given to owners following surgical procedures at the authors' practice.

For most patients undergoing routine orthopaedic surgery, an initial revisit appointment can be scheduled at 10–14 days (the time of suture removal) either with the referring veterinary surgeon or at the referral centre, unless a bandage is in place, in which case a bandage check should be made sooner, typically no more than 7 days after its application. At the same time, clinical progress can also be assessed. Some degree of swelling and bruising is to be expected but excessive levels should be immediately addressed or monitored closely as appropriate (Dymond *et al.*, 2010). For the vast majority of orthopaedic patients and procedures, the patient should be toe touching to weight-bearing within a few days of surgery, and certainly by the time of the first re-check.

Further follow-up appointments can be scheduled as appropriate. If follow-up radiographs are required to assess osseous healing then these should be scheduled at about 4–8 weeks postoperatively dependent upon the age of the animal. At the same time as radiographic assessment (and immediately prior to it) clinical progress should be reviewed. Depending on progress, follow-up appointments can be rescheduled as required. For the most common surgeries, a follow-up appointment is usually performed at 6–8 weeks postoperatively at the authors' practice, when radiographs are taken for fracture/osteotomy/joint replacement patients. Further patient checks are usually limited to telephone updates thereafter unless complications are reported.

In general, juvenile animals should be seen earlier and more frequently than skeletally mature animals. Healing is more rapid (bone should heal quicker) in juvenile animals, as is the production of potentially deleterious periarticular fibrosis; therefore, early intervention is preferable to prevent permanent loss of motion. Implant loosening may be more likely in younger animals as the bone is softer due to the relative lack of mineralization.

Radiographic checks with respect to patient age (approximate guideline):

- Patients less than 4 months of age, particularly those with articular fractures, should be checked every 10–14 days
- Patients 4–6 months of age should be checked every 2–4 weeks
- Patients 6–10 months of age should be checked every 4–6 weeks
- Patients over 10 months of age should be checked every 6–8 weeks.

Radiographs are taken to be certain that healing is progressing as expected, the implants are stable and that bone alignment is maintained

---

Exercise management

Exercise management/restriction is very important because excessive activity at too early a stage postoperatively may predispose to implant failure, which is a major complication with potentially disastrous results. Precise exercise management at home is somewhat case-dependent but some general rules apply. For dogs, exercise should initially be restricted to short lead walks. The duration of these can be gradually increased depending on clinical progress, but unrestricted activity should be avoided. Between walks, the precise management is dependent upon the nature of the patient. If the animal will tolerate cage rest then it is prudent to use one, in order to prevent any sudden movement or excessive loading of the limb/implant. If the patient will not tolerate being restricted to a cage, then it should be kept in as small an area as is practical and prevented from vigorous activities, including jumping. Feline patients are best managed in a cage, but it is important to interact with the patient to provide stimulation and ensure some controlled gentle movement. The cage should be big enough to contain a bed, litter tray and food, but prevent vigorous activities.

References and further reading

Arnold M and Barbul A (2006) Nutrition and wound healing. *Plastic and Reconstructive Surgery* **117**, 42S–58S

Bhende S, Rothenburger S, Spangler DJ and Dito M (2002) Surgical Infections. *Surgical Infections (Larchmont)* **3**, 251–257

Duke-Novakovsky, de Vries M and Seymour C (2016) *BSAVA Manual of Canine and Feline Anaesthesia and Analgesia, 3rd edn.* BSAVA Publications, Gloucester

Dymond NL, Goldsmid SE and Simpson DJ (2010) Tibial tuberosity advancement in 92 canine stifles: initial results, clinical outcome and owner evaluation. *Australian Veterinary Journal* **88**, 381–385

Innes JF, Clayton J and Lascelles BDX (2010) Review of the safety and efficacy of long-term NSAID use in the treatment of canine osteoarthritis. *Veterinary Record* **166**, 226–230

Jerre S (2009) Rehabilitation after extra-articular stabilization of cranial cruciate ligament rupture in dogs. *Veterinary and Comparative Orthopaedics and Traumatology* **22**, 148–152

Lindley S and Watson P (2010) *BSAVA Manual of Canine and Feline Rehabilitation, Supportive and Palliative Care.* BSAVA Publications, Gloucester

Meeson RL, Davidson C and Arthurs GI (2011) Soft-tissue injuries associated with cast application for distal limb orthopaedic conditions. A retrospective study of sixty dogs and cats. *Veterinary and Comparative Orthopaedics and Traumatology* **24(2)**, 126–131

Monk ML, Preston CA and McGowan CM (2006) Effects of early intensive postoperative physiotherapy on limb function after tibial plateau leveling osteotomy in dogs with deficiency of the cranial cruciate ligament. *American Journal of Veterinary Research* **67**, 529–536

Saunders DG (2007) Physical therapy in small animals: therapeutic exercise. *Clinical Techniques in Small Animal Practice* **22**, 155–159

Shumway R (2007) Physical therapy in small animals: rehabilitation in the first 48 hours after surgery. *Clinical Techniques in Small Animal Practice* **22**, 166–170

Unis MD, Roush JK, Bilicki KL and Baker SG (2010) Effect of bandaging on postoperative swelling after tibial plateau levelling osteotomy. *Veterinary and Comparative Orthopaedics and Traumatology* **23(4)**, 240–244

OPERATIVE TECHNIQUE 17.1

Application of a soft padded dressing

POSITIONING

The dog or cat is placed in lateral recumbency with the affected limb uppermost. The joints are positioned to mimic a functional standing position.

ASSISTANT

In most cases it is necessary to sedate the patient in order to keep the limb in the correct position and aid correct placement of the bandage. Some patients will allow conscious dressing changes, in which case an assistant is essential.

EQUIPMENT EXTRAS

Adhesive tape; cast padding or cotton wool; conforming bandage; a suitable outer self-adherent or adhesive wrap.

APPLICATION

With the patient in lateral recumbency and the affected limb uppermost, the joints of the limb are placed in a functional weight-bearing position.

To prevent slippage of the bandage, 'stirrups' are placed: two strips of adhesive tape are placed on the distal limb on the dorsal and palmar (plantar) or medial and lateral surfaces to the level of the carpus or tarsus (Figure 17.12a). It is important that these do not contact or stick to the surgical wound. A dressing may be placed directly over the incision or wound, if present. Cotton wool is placed between the digits to prevent rubbing and associated skin wounds (Figure 17.12b).

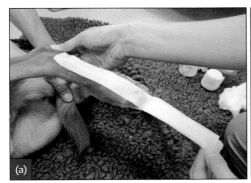
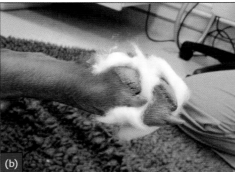

17.12 (a) Two strips of adhesive tape are placed on the distal limb on the medial and lateral surfaces (or dorsal and palmar/plantar surfaces) to the level of the carpus/tarsus. (b) Cotton wool is placed between the digits to prevent rubbing.

Starting distally, the cast padding or cotton roll is wrapped spirally up the limb, overlapping layers by 50% on each rotation (Figure 17.13a). The bottom of the bandage should be at the level of the nail beds of the middle digits. The proximal portion of the bandage should extend at least to the joint above the pathology, and often to above the elbow/stifle joint (Figure 17.13b), ensuring all bony prominences are well padded to prevent any pressure sores from developing as a result of the bandage.

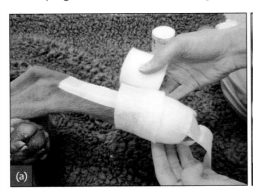
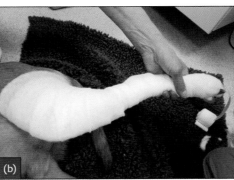

17.13 (a) Starting distally, the cast padding or cotton wool roll is wrapped spirally up the limb, overlapping layers by 50% on each rotation. (b) The dressing is continued proximal to the pathology/wound, or proximal to the elbow/stifle.

→ OPERATIVE TECHNIQUE 17.1 CONTINUED

If necessary, extra padding should be added to those areas with poor soft tissue coverage and covered with a further layer of cast padding/cotton wool (Figure 17.14). Padding support should be gently applied circumferentially around the limb with care taken that it is applied evenly and does not bunch up, as this can potentially cause focal areas of increased pressure and sores.

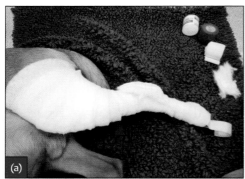
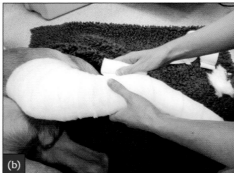

17.14 (a) Extra padding should be added to those areas with poor soft tissue coverage. This should be applied evenly and care should be taken that the extra padding does not bunch or cause uneven pressure on the underlying skin. (b) Any extra padding can be covered with a further even layer of cast padding/cotton wool.

The optimum amount of padding is unknown. Too little padding and the dressing may be too tight and cause distal limb swelling and/or ischaemic necrosis; too much padding and the dressing may be too loose and slip.

The conforming bandage should be applied next, following the same placement technique used for the cotton wool/cast padding (Figure 17.15a). The conforming bandage should be placed with a small amount of tension, but not so tight as to result in venous stasis and swelling of the digits (Figure 17.15b). The conforming bandage should not extend beyond the level of the padding/cotton wool otherwise a constrictive effect directly on the skin might result.

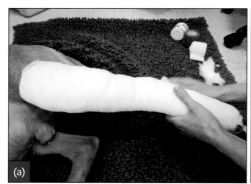
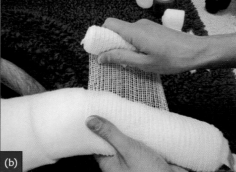

17.15 (a) The conforming bandage is applied next, following the same placement used for the cotton wool/cast padding. (b) This should be placed with a small amount of tension, but not so tight as to result in venous stasis and swelling of the digits.

The tape stirrups are separated from each other, rotated 180 degrees, and stuck proximally to the conforming bandage material to prevent the entire bandage from slipping (Figure 17.16).

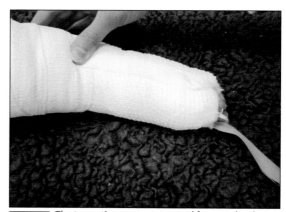

17.16 The tape stirrups are separated from each other, rotated 180 degrees and placed proximally on the bandage material to prevent it from slipping.

→ **OPERATIVE TECHNIQUE 17.1 CONTINUED**

The outer tertiary layer is then applied using a dressing material such as Vetrap (3M), ensuring adequate coverage of the underlying layers (Figure 17.17a). The outer tertiary layer should not be pulled tightly at the ends of the bandage; rather the covering should be pulled free from the roll, the tension released and the material simply placed over the cotton wool/cast padding (Figure 17.17b).

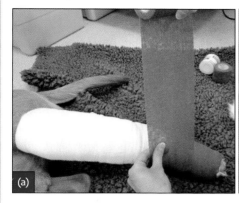 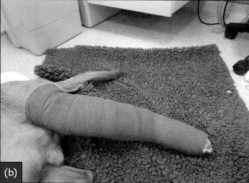

17.17 (a) The outer layer is applied, ensuring adequate coverage of the underlying layers. (b) This layer should be pulled free from the roll, the tension released and the material simply placed over the underlying bandage.

A date can be marked on the outer dressing surface to show when the dressing was last changed. This should also be recorded on the hospital sheet.

AFTERCARE

The bandage should be monitored throughout the day for swollen toes, warmth, wetness, soiling or slippage and changed if necessary. It must be kept clean and dry, and the patient restricted from access to outside as much as possible; before the patient is taken outside, the bandage should be covered with a thick durable plastic bag. This plastic bag must be removed when the animal is indoors.

If no open wounds are present under the bandage and it remains in place, clean and dry and without any concerns about compromised circulation, then it could be changed once a week. If open wounds are present then the bandage needs to be replaced and the wound checked (with minimal interference) as often as is deemed essential, usually at least once daily.

WARNING

Take great care with dressings. A dressing that is excessively tight, has insufficient padding or is not monitored sufficiently frequently and carefully can result in serious complications including distal limb ischaemic necrosis, which may necessitate amputation in the worst case scenario.

Bandage-related skin wounds and complications are not necessarily obvious from the outside. The only way to be sure is to remove the dressing, inspect the skin, and then reapply the dressing if appropriate

Chapter 18

The shoulder

Steve Butterworth and Rob Pettitt

Introduction

Diseases and disorders of the shoulder are a frequent cause of lameness in dogs and can also be seen in cats. In adult dogs, definitive diagnosis of shoulder-related lameness can be challenging. It is vital for the practitioner to have a comprehensive understanding of shoulder problems in order to identify and distinguish them from other causes of thoracic limb lameness and ensure optimal treatment.

Fractures of the scapula and proximal humerus may be responsible for shoulder lameness; these are covered in the BSAVA Manual of Canine and Feline Fracture Repair and Management.

Causes of shoulder lameness which are discussed in this chapter include:

- Congenital/developmental:
  - Scapulohumeral luxation
  - Scapulohumeral dysplasia
  - Osteochondrosis – osteochondritis dissecans (OCD) of the humeral head, ununited caudal glenoid.
- Acquired:
  - Luxations – scapulohumeral luxation, dorsal luxation of the scapula
  - Muscle-related – contracture of the spinatus muscles, teres minor myopathy
  - Tendon or ligament-related – biceps brachii tendinitis/tenosynovitis, rupture of the biceps brachii tendon sheath, medial luxation of the biceps brachii tendon, biceps brachii tendon rupture/avulsion, subscapularis tears, supraspinatus mineralizing tendinopathy, infraspinatus bursal ossification, medial or lateral collateral instability
  - Osteoarthritis (see also Chapter 6)
  - Inflammatory arthritis – infective, immune-mediated (see also Chapter 6)
  - Neoplasia – osteosarcoma, synovial sarcoma, other sarcomas (chondrosarcoma, fibrosarcoma, haemangiosarcoma) (see also Chapter 11).

Functional anatomy

The scapulohumeral joint is an enarthrodial joint formed by the articulation of the scapular glenoid with the humeral head (Figure 18.1ab). The scapula is made up of a flat blade, lying in the sagittal plane. The scapular spine arises on the blade's lateral aspect, projecting almost perpendicularly from it and ending distally as the acromion process. Distally, the scapular blade becomes narrower, creating the scapular neck, before expanding to form the glenoid with its cranial prominence, the scapular tuberosity (comprising the supraglenoid tuberosity and coracoid process) and its concave articular surface. The surface area of the glenoid is extended in some dogs by a cartilaginous labrum. The concave glenoid and labrum articulate with the convex surface of the humeral head. Cranially, the proximal humerus possesses two tubercles, the greater and lesser tubercles, which are respectively positioned laterally and medially and separated by the intertubercular groove.

The joint capsule is attached to the rim of the glenoid and to the humeral head and has several outpouchings. The most significant of these are the caudal pouch and the cranial extension, which forms a tendon sheath around the tendon of origin of the biceps brachii muscle as it passes through the intertubercular groove. Within the joint capsule are the lateral and medial glenohumeral ligaments.

The glenohumeral joint is stabilized by active and passive mechanisms. Active (dynamic) stabilization comes from the coordinated or selective contraction of adjacent ('cuff') muscles. The supraspinatus and infraspinatus muscles arise from the scapular blade, cranial and caudal to the scapular spine, respectively, and insert on the cranial and lateral aspects of the greater tubercle (Figure 18.1f). Medially, the subscapularis muscle arises from the scapular blade and inserts on the lesser tubercle; cranially, the biceps brachii muscle arises from the supraglenoid tuberosity and passes through the intertubercular groove where it is constrained cranially by the intertubercular ligament (Figure 18.1d). The tendons of all these muscles have very close associations with the joint capsule. In addition, there are several other muscles, such as the deltoid, teres minor and major and coracobrachialis, which lend some support to the joint without such intimate contact with the capsule (Figure 18.1ef).

Passive joint stability is dependent on the concavity compression mechanism of the joint, its limited joint volume, the fibrous joint capsule and the glenohumeral ligaments (Figure 18.1cd). An in vitro analysis of shoulder stability showed that removal of all the 'cuff' muscles had little effect on the passive stability of the joint and that it was necessary to damage the capsule itself before increased laxity could be detected (Vasseur et al., 1982). Another in vitro study reported that the biceps brachii tendon contributes to passive shoulder joint stability and that the medial glenohumeral ligament is important for medial stability in dogs (Sidaway et al., 2004).

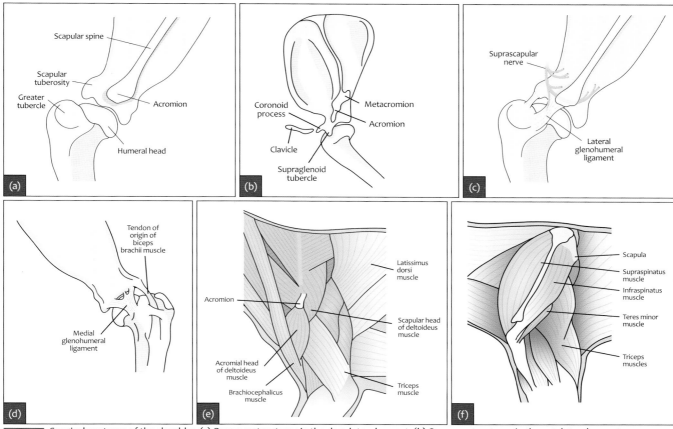

18.1 Surgical anatomy of the shoulder. (a) Osseous structures in the dog, lateral aspect. (b) Osseous structures in the cat, lateral aspect. (c) Ligaments and nerves of the shoulder joint, lateral aspect in the dog. (d) Ligaments of the shoulder joint, medial aspect in the dog. (e) Superficial muscles over the lateral aspect of the shoulder in the dog. (f) Deep muscles over the lateral aspect of the shoulder in the dog.

Neurovascular structures that are important with respect to surgery (see relevant Operative Techniques) include:

- The omobrachial vein (a branch of the cephalic vein), which passes across the craniolateral aspect of the joint
- The caudal circumflex artery and vein and the axillary nerve, which cross the caudal aspect of the joint capsule
- The suprascapular nerve (Figure 18.1c), which courses from cranial to caudal under the tendons of insertion of the suprascapular muscles and the acromion of the scapula.

Clinical examination

As with other joints, patients with lameness relating to the shoulder will show particular features on clinical examination:

- Gait is usually affected in a non-specific way such that the only abnormality visible is reduced weight-bearing. Reluctance to extend the joint fully may cause a shortened cranial phase to the stride but this can be difficult to appreciate. Some specific conditions (e.g. infraspinatus contracture) may cause a characteristic change in gait pattern
- Palpation may reveal atrophy of the spinatus muscles; this can be seen as part of a generalized proximal limb muscle atrophy associated with any chronic thoracic limb lameness, but it is often seen sooner and more prominently in cases with shoulder pain

- There may be an abnormal relationship of anatomical landmarks, for example the relative positions of the acromion and the greater tubercle in a case of luxation
- The finding of 'point pain' on palpation of specific structures, such as the biceps tendon of origin, can be important, but care should be taken in overinterpreting such findings.

Manipulation of the joint should include extension, flexion, abduction and adduction. In the dog (and cat) normal limits of flexion and extension are 57 (32) degrees and 165 (164) degrees, respectively. It is difficult to extend the shoulder without simultaneously extending the elbow and so pain on such manipulation could emanate from either joint. However, the elbow can be extended without extending the shoulder and this can help to show the elbow is not the source. Some care needs to be taken with this interpretation as extending the elbow does place tensile stress on the biceps tendon of origin, pathology of which can be responsible for shoulder lameness. Flexion of the shoulder should be carried out with the elbow in flexion and then in extension. This may provide useful information since flexion of the shoulder with the elbow extended creates more tension in the biceps tendon of origin and so pain from this structure should be exacerbated. Furthermore, digital pressure over the biceps tendon might produce evidence of 'point pain' at this site. Palpation should also be undertaken during manipulation so that any changes in anatomy can be appreciated, e.g. scapulohumeral luxation or displacement of the biceps tendon of origin. Manipulation should test joint stability to reveal such problems as luxation. The scapulohumeral joint has one of the largest ranges of motion of all the synovial joints in the body. Care should be taken not to mistake joint laxity for instability; if doubt exists, a comparison should always be made with the non-lame limb. Joint subluxation has been proposed as a cause of lameness resulting from instability (Bardet, 1998; Cook, 2003) and, although the clinical tests used to detect instability are not universally accepted as reliable, the evidence for this and the condition as an entity is growing (Cook *et al.*, 2005ab; Devitt *et al.*, 2007).

It should be remembered that developmental elbow disease in medium to large-breed dogs is common. As a result coexistent pathology may be identifiable both clinically and radiographically in the elbow joints of dogs with shoulder lameness. As always, the interpretation of such findings is based on careful clinical assessment. Differentiating between the shoulder and elbow as the source of lameness can be very challenging and the shoulder is often suspected once significant pathology in the distal limb has been ruled out. It is important to resist any temptation to label this as shoulder lameness unless lameness can be definitively localized to the joint.

A brief neurological evaluation is undertaken as routine when evaluating suspected shoulder lameness particularly in skeletally mature dogs. Brachial plexus and lower cervical spinal disease can both produce a thoracic limb lameness seemingly associated with pain on shoulder manipulation. In such cases, axillary or neck pain may be evident and the presence of any neurological deficits, such as a reduced or absent withdrawal reflex, ipsilateral absence of the panniculus reflex or presence of Horner's syndrome indicates a neurological rather than an orthopaedic problem (see the *BSAVA Manual of Canine and Feline Neurology*).

Diagnostic imaging

Specific details on appropriate imaging techniques for the shoulder are provided in the imaging section at the end of this chapter. For more general information on imaging techniques and their application, see Chapter 3.

Congenital/developmental conditions

Scapulohumeral luxation

This condition is rare and there appears to be a breed predisposition, with Toy Poodles and Shetland Sheepdogs being over-represented alongside some other toy breeds.

Affected dogs are usually presented for recurrent lameness, which develops at 3 to 10 months of age. Occasionally they will be presented after reaching skeletal maturity, following minor trauma. Patients characteristically adopt a begging posture, with the joint held partially flexed. In some cases the problem is bilateral and such dogs may be found to have much better developed hindquarters or even a tendency to try to walk upright on their pelvic limbs. The direction of luxation is invariably medial. This can easily be appreciated; the acromion is much more prominent as a result of medial displacement of the humerus.

Medial luxation is confirmed on caudocranial radiographs and mediolateral views will demonstrate a flattened or convex glenoid and a relatively large and flattened humeral head (Figure 18.2). If the humeral head

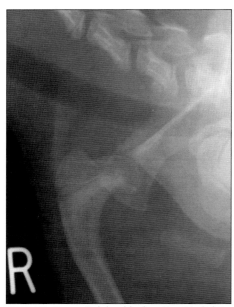

18.2 Congenital shoulder luxation. Mediolateral radiograph of the shoulder of a 3-month-old Jack Russell Terrier with medial luxation. There is deformity of the articular surfaces, making the joint inherently unstable. Orthogonal views are advised but the direction of luxation – medial or lateral – is usually evident on examination.

and glenoid are not in proper contact during the period of skeletal growth and development, the articular surfaces do not develop a normal shape and gross malformation develops very rapidly. In a patient of this age reduction becomes impossible within a very short space of time. If, however, the problem is diagnosed early, reduction may be possible and successful treatment by application of a closed transarticular pinning technique has been described (Read, 1994). In cases where reduction cannot be achieved, conservative measures are advisable in the first instance. The joint tends to stabilize and the degree of lameness/incapacity improves as the dog matures. In general it may be anticipated that, by 1 year of age, these dogs will be somewhat disabled but pain-free and able to lead relatively normal lives. If lameness persists, salvage procedures, such as excision arthroplasty or arthrodesis, should be considered.

Shoulder dysplasia

Shoulder dysplasia is defined as abnormal development of the joint. Shoulder dysplasia resulting in excessive joint laxity has been documented as a cause of lameness in only two single case reports, one involving a 3.5-year-old Collie and the other a 10-month-old Labrador Retriever. However, one of the authors has seen several dogs of chondrodystrophic breeds, most notably Bassett Hounds, presented for non-specific thoracic limb lameness with mild discomfort on shoulder extension. Radiographically they were found to have a shallow glenoid and flattened humeral head, as expected for the breed (Figure 18.3). No other abnormality could be found clinically or radiographically. The lameness was successfully managed by conservative means and, in the case of immature dogs, improvement seemed to occur as they reached skeletal maturity. There are no established criteria by which shoulder dysplasia can be specifically diagnosed and its relevance to the presenting signs are evaluated clinically and by exclusion of other differential diagnoses.

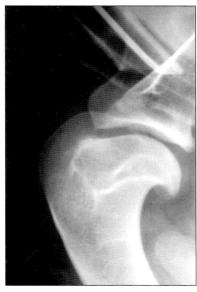

18.3 Shoulder dysplasia. Mediolateral radiograph of the left shoulder of a 3-year-old Bassett Hound that showed intermittent lameness associated with shoulder pain. The glenoid appears shallow and the humeral head flattened.

Osteochondrosis

Osteochondrosis usually involves the articular cartilage of the medial aspect of the caudal third of the humeral head but, uncommonly, the caudal rim of the glenoid may also be involved. The under-run cartilage of the humeral head may split vertically, causing flap formation, whereupon the term osteochondritis dissecans (OCD) is used to indicate separation of the flap. This may become mineralized and thus visible radiographically. In addition, it may break free and form a 'joint mouse', which can absorb nutrients from the synovial fluid, grow and possibly become mineralized. Occasionally such osteochondral fragments will migrate later in life into the biceps tendon sheath and cause lameness, necessitating their late removal. Once the flap has become detached the defect may fill in with granulation tissue that is then converted into fibrocartilage.

Signalment and history

The condition is associated with a number of breeds, including giant breeds such as the Great Dane, Pyrenean Mountain Dog and Irish Wolfhound. Other associated breeds include the Labrador Retriever, Golden Retriever, Bernese Mountain Dog, Border Collie, Cocker Spaniel and Pug (Bruggeman *et al.*, 2010). Although the ratio of males to females varies between reports, there is general consensus that more males are affected clinically. One large retrospective study (Rudd *et al.*, 1990) gave a male:female ratio of 2.24:1. The condition is radiographically bilateral in just over 50% of clinical cases, although few are bilaterally lame.

The lameness usually begins when the dog is between 4 and 7 months of age, although the owners may delay presentation because the onset is somewhat insidious. This age of onset might be expected since it is the period of most rapid growth. However, in one study, 36% of dogs were over 1 year of age at the time of diagnosis (Rudd *et al.*, 1990). Thus, the condition should not be excluded as a cause of shoulder lameness simply because a dog is older than 12 months. The degree of lameness varies but is usually mild to moderate and may be intermittent. The owner will usually report that the lameness deteriorates with exercise and that there is stiffness after rest, particularly following exercise. Restriction of exercise tends to improve the lameness.

Clinical findings

Lameness is usually evident, although if both shoulders are affected clinically, the dog might show more of a stiff shuffling thoracic limb gait rather than overt lameness. Disuse atrophy, especially of the spinatus muscles, may be present, which makes the scapular spine more prominent. Pain is usually elicited on extension of the joint.

Diagnosis

Diagnosis can generally be confirmed by radiography/arthrography (Figure 18.4) but, in some cases, computed tomography (CT), ultrasonography, magnetic resonance imaging (MRI) or arthroscopy may be required to confirm it (Wall *et al.*, 2015). A mediolateral view of the extended shoulder will usually suffice but occasionally inwardly and/or outwardly rotated views may prove necessary to skyline the lesion (see Imaging Techniques). Changes that may be observed on plain radiographs in cases involving the humeral head include:

- A subchondral defect with flattening of the caudal humeral head
- A sclerotic margin to any such defect
- The presence of a cartilage flap (only visible if mineralized)
- The presence of 'joint mice' (only visible if mineralized), most commonly found in the caudal recess of the joint
- Vacuum phenomenon (van Bree, 1992) – gas opacity in the articular space creating an image resembling a negative arthrogram (seen in 20 of 100 radiographs of shoulders affected by osteochondrosis and none of 30 normal shoulders)
- Secondary osteoarthritis, most often seen as osteophyte formation on the caudal borders of the glenoid and/or the humeral head.

Both shoulders should be imaged as changes are often bilateral. This may be helpful in cases that have suffered subclinical osteochondrosis in one shoulder and then developed a clinical lameness due to the same problem in the second limb. The changes in the latter may have not yet developed or be quite subtle, and the finding of changes in the 'normal' limb helps to reinforce the clinical picture with respect to diagnosis of osteochondrosis in the lame limb.

Positive contrast arthrography (Figure 18.5) may help to assess whether a non-mineralized cartilage flap or 'joint mouse' is present. However, with the rapidly expanding use and availability of CT, contrast CT and arthroscopy, there are more accurate and less equivocal diagnostic tools available. Arthroscopy may be used diagnostically to examine the articular surface and determine the extent and severity of articular cartilage damage if radiography is equivocal (Figure 18.6).

Conservative treatment

In some cases lameness may resolve with 6–8 weeks of controlled (lead) exercise. Whether such resolution is a result of failure of osteochondral flap formation and resolution of osteochondrosis or because of dislodgement of an osteochondral flap and subsequent healing by fibrocartilage formation is a point of conjecture. If such measures are continued then the majority of cases will eventually become sound, but this may take several months. While these dogs are being rested the use of non-steroidal anti-inflammatory drugs (NSAIDs) should be considered to limit pain and lameness. Some authors advocate a regime of vigorous

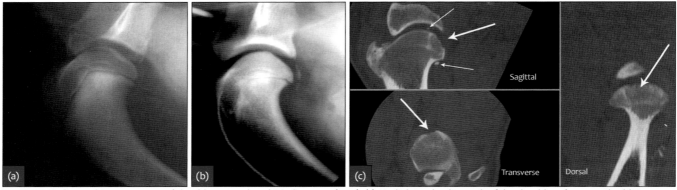

18.4 Radiographic appearance of shoulder osteochondritis dissecans (OCD). (a) Mediolateral radiograph of the shoulder of a 5-month-old Bernese Mountain Dog. A subchondral defect is clearly present in the caudal humeral head, with a sclerotic margin. (b) Mediolateral radiograph of the shoulder of an 11-month-old Border Collie. The caudal humeral head appears flattened and a mineralized flap is evident in the caudal joint space. (c) Multiplanar CT reconstructions of an 11-month-old crossbreed dog with shoulder OCD. A large subchondral defect (thick arrows) in the humeral head and mineralized intra-articular detached flap fragments (thin arrows) are visible.
(Courtesy of Gordon Brown)

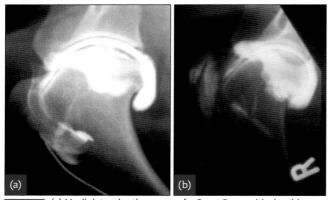

18.5 (a) Mediolateral arthrogram of a Great Dane with shoulder osteochondritis dissecans (OCD). A low dose of contrast medium is required, otherwise the articular surface of interest becomes obliterated; with such a low dose the tendon sheath of the biceps brachii is often poorly filled. (b) A low-dose normal arthrogram for comparison. Note the intact cartilage line over the humeral head.

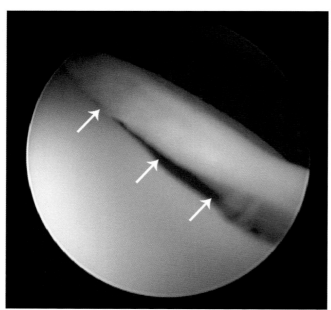

18.6 Arthroscopic view of an osteochondritis dissecans (OCD) lesion of the humeral head. (Arrows indicate the OCD cleavage site.)

exercise for these dogs, with the aim of promoting detachment of the cartilage flap and resolution of the lameness once the subchondral defect has filled in with fibrocartilage. The results following conservative measures are poorly documented but suggest a slower and less optimal outcome than that associated with surgical management. The use of polysulphated glycosaminoglycan preparations, such as sodium pentosan polysulphate, has been advocated, but there has been no documented evidence that it produces an improvement beyond that expected with restricted exercise alone.

Surgical treatment

Surgery is preferred to conservative management because the success rate is high and the period of convalescence relatively short. Early diagnosis and treatment is associated with optimal results and the majority of patients will be sound by 6–8 weeks after surgery. The aim of surgery is to remove the (partially) detached articular cartilage (free body or flap). Curettage or micropicking of the exposed subchondral bone to produce a bleeding bed and facilitate its repair through the formation of fibrocartilage is often advocated, but without sound evidence of its benefit. The cells responsible for producing this fibrocartilage are pluripotential mesenchymal cells that migrate in from subchondral bone. Such surgery can be undertaken at arthrotomy or arthroscopically. A caudal or caudolateral approach (see Operative Technique 18.3) to the joint provides good exposure of the affected portion of the humeral head. Arthroscopic removal of shoulder OCD lesions was first described by Van Ryssen *et al.* (1993). Arthroscopy reduces the morbidity of the procedure and hence aids recovery (Olivieri *et al.*, 2007). In addition, arthroscopy allows for a greater inspection of the joint and may be useful for retrieval of joint mice from unusual positions (e.g. medial to glenoid or caudal joint recess). It has been advocated in some reports as being less invasive than arthrotomy, having a lower incidence of postoperative seroma formation and producing a more cosmetic result, while achieving the same long-term results (Meyer-Lindenberg *et al.*, 2002).

Osteochondral autograft transfer is technically feasible (Fitzpatrick *et al.*, 2010) and is able to achieve better articular contour reconstruction and resurfacing of osteochondral defects than can be expected following simple cartilage flap removal and curettage. While technically possible, the benefit to the patient is unproven.

Arthrotomy: A caudolateral approach (see Operative Technique 18.4) is used. If 'joint mice' have been identified elsewhere in the joint, additional approaches may be required but such a situation is rare. Bilateral arthrotomies can be performed under the same general anaesthetic, if required, but this is not commonly indicated.

Arthroscopy: A lateral arthroscopy portal is used with a caudolateral instrument portal and craniolateral egress portal (see Operative Technique 18.5). Bilateral arthroscopies can be performed under the same general anaesthetic, if required, but this is not commonly indicated.

Postoperative care

Following arthrotomy or arthroscopy, the dog should be restricted to lead exercise and room rest for 6–8 weeks while healing of the cartilage defect takes place. The distance walked is governed only by what does not make the patient significantly worse (in terms of degree of lameness or stiffness after rest). After that period, most patients will be sound and can be returned to normal exercise over the following month.

Prognosis

Following removal of an OCD flap and any resulting 'joint mice', Clayton Jones and Vaughan (1970) reported that 28 of 29 cases recovered full use of their operated limb with no lameness, while Rudd *et al.* (1990) found that 30 of 40 dogs treated surgically became sound.

Ununited caudal glenoid (or incomplete fusion of the accessory caudal glenoid ossification centre)

In young dogs a separate centre of ossification of the caudal glenoid may be noted on mediolateral plain radiographs; the normal variant has a smooth non-displaced appearance and should not be interpreted as a pathological lesion. If any doubt exists it is worth repeating the radiographs 6 weeks later. In some clinical cases with compatible signalment and features for osteochondrosis, radiography will show lack of fusion of the centre of ossification relating to the caudal rim of the glenoid (Olivieri *et al.*, 1999; Monaco and Schwartz, 2011). Arthroscopy with gentle probing of the lesion may be used to confirm the presence of a separate mobile part of the glenoid (Figure 18.7). If this is the cause of lameness, surgical removal

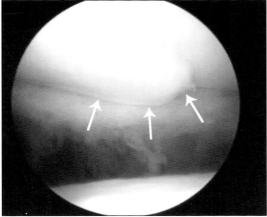

18.7 Arthroscopic view of a mildly displaced incomplete ossification of the caudal glenoid (arrowed).

may be successful where conservative management has failed (Olivieri *et al.*, 2004). A similar lesion affecting the cranial glenoid has also been reported in an 8-month-old English Setter (DeSimone *et al.*, 2013).

Acquired luxations
Scapulohumeral luxation

Luxation of the shoulder is an uncommon condition. Scapulohumeral luxation results in loss of joint function, a decreased range of joint movement and pain on manipulation, which decreases as the condition becomes chronic.

Acquired luxations are usually associated with a fall or knock, particularly when a dog turns at speed. The direction of luxation is generally either lateral or medial. It has been said that smaller breeds tend to suffer medial luxation while lateral luxations are seen more in larger breeds. However, review of the literature suggests there is no correlation and each case should be judged on its own merit. Cranial and caudal luxations are rarely encountered. The author has seen cranial luxation associated with rupture of the transverse humeral ligament allowing displacement of the biceps brachii tendon and loss of cranial support (see Medial luxation of the biceps brachii tendon).

Clinical findings

Affected dogs will be presented with a history of acute onset severe (usually non-weight-bearing) thoracic limb lameness as a consequence of moderate to severe trauma. The elbow is held flexed and adducted, with the distal limb held abducted in cases of medial luxation, and adducted if the luxation is lateral. There may be palpable asymmetry between the acromion and greater tubercle when compared to the unaffected shoulder. In more long-standing cases, especially those with recurrent luxation that reduce spontaneously and cause an intermittent lameness, muscle atrophy may be noted. Manipulation will reveal a reduced range of movement and pain on extension or flexion. In some cases the luxation will reduce spontaneously on manipulation of the joint, particularly when the patient is positioned for radiography. It is therefore important not to rely on radiography for a definitive diagnosis, rather to clinically evaluate joint stability. This is done by holding the scapula in a fixed position while the shoulder joint is flexed, extended, rotated, abducted and adducted. It is imperative that any suspected abnormality is evaluated by comparison with the contralateral limb as instability can easily be misdiagnosed, particularly when the dog is sedated or anaesthetized for radiography.

The possibility of concurrent injuries should be considered. Crepitation might suggest a fracture or indicate articular cartilage loss, while neurological deficits might indicate brachial plexus involvement (particularly in lateral luxations).

Diagnosis

Standard mediolateral and caudocranial radiographic views (Figure 18.8) are used to assess the direction of luxation, the contour of the joint surfaces, osteophyte formation and the existence of concurrent fractures. Since shoulder luxations have a tendency to reduce spontaneously during positioning for radiography, plain radiographs may show no abnormality. If the instability is clearly evident clinically, radiography might be used simply to screen the joint for complicating factors. If, however, radiographs are required

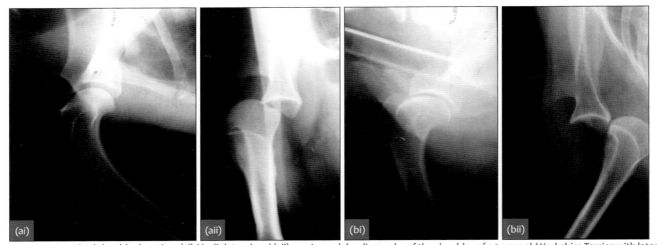

18.8 Acquired shoulder luxation. (ai) Mediolateral and (aii) craniocaudal radiographs of the shoulder of a 2-year-old Yorkshire Terrier with lateral luxation as a result of being attacked by another dog. Note the apparently normal appearance of the joint in the mediolateral view. (bi) Mediolateral and (bii) craniocaudal radiographs of the shoulder of a 12-year-old Shetland Sheepdog, showing medial luxation resulting from the dog being 'extracted' from under an armchair.
(a, Courtesy of ARS Barr)

to demonstrate the instability, then stressed views may be necessary, but can be difficult to obtain and interpret. Views of both limbs must be taken for comparison, as the range of 'normal' appearance is great. It must be stressed that the most reliable test for instability is clinical manipulation.

The direction of luxation is important in determining the method of stabilization (see below). If the luxation is long-standing then the joint surfaces may show remodelling, in which case stability may be more difficult to establish, or osteophytes may be present indicating secondary osteo-arthritis. Both these will tend to make the prognosis worse. If concurrent fractures are present they may interfere with reduction or inherent stability and indicate the need for open reduction and fixation.

Conservative treatment

This is generally successful where luxation has not previously occurred and there are no concurrent fractures. Closed reduction is generally possible, followed by external support. A Velpeau sling (Figure 18.9) should be employed to bandage the affected limb to the body wall in medial luxations, as this creates lateral pressure on the humeral head, thus maintaining the reduction. A non-weight-bearing sling (Figure 18.10) is used for lateral luxations or in cases where the direction is uncertain. Alternatively a body cast may be used. This is best fitted in

the conscious dog with the limb in a weight-bearing position so that the cast can be closely applied; otherwise it may not serve its purpose and/or be uncomfortable for the dog. Whichever method is used, the joint should always be re-radiographed following application of the sling or cast to ensure that reduction has been achieved and maintained. The external support is maintained for 2–6 weeks to allow the soft tissues to heal, and exercise is restricted for a further 2–4 weeks after removal of the support.

Surgical treatment

Surgical treatment is required if the luxation is recurrent or a fracture fragment has to be re-attached or removed. There are several techniques described in the literature, all of which aim to re-establish collateral support by placement of non-absorbable material (e.g. LigaFiba) between tunnels or implants placed near the origin and insertion of the respective ligament (see Operative Techniques 18.6 and 18.7B).

For simultaneous restoration of lateral and medial support, a combination of lateral and medial shoulder stabilization may be used by combining techniques; alternatively, it is possible for one prosthesis to serve both functions. Transverse tunnels are created in a lateral to medial direction through the scapular neck (cranial to the scapular spine and avoiding the suprascapular nerve) and through the greater tubercle (starting at a point close to

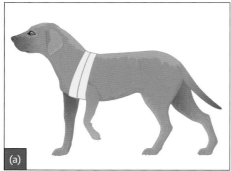
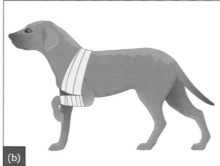
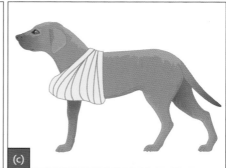

18.9 Application of a Velpeau sling for the treatment of medial shoulder luxation. (a) The bandage is used to hold the distal humerus adducted against the chest wall. (b) Cotton wool is placed around the antebrachium for padding. (c) The entire limb is enclosed in the bandage, including the cranial aspect, so that the dog does not step out of the sling.
(Redrawn after the *BSAVA Manual of Small Animal Arthrology*)

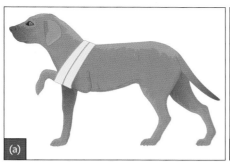 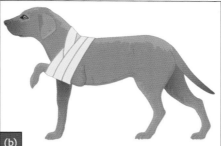 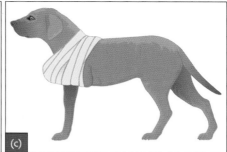

18.10 Application of a non-weight-bearing sling for the treatment of lateral shoulder luxation. (a–b) The distal limb is flexed and the antebrachium bandaged to the body. (c) The entire limb is enclosed in the bandage, including the cranial aspect, so that the dog does not step out of the sling.
(Redrawn after the *BSAVA Manual of Small Animal Arthrology*)

the insertion of the teres minor tendon). Non-absorbable material (e.g. LigaFiba) is then placed through these tunnels and secured laterally, thereby creating both lateral and medial support for the joint.

Although it is often considered appropriate to restore the lateral support in medial luxations and medial support in lateral luxations (or both in either), one of the authors [SB] routinely replaces only the lateral support for luxations in either direction unless the joint is grossly unstable on reduction.

Following surgery, the dog should be restricted to lead exercise and room rest for 6–8 weeks while fibrosis around the prosthesis becomes established. The distance walked is governed only by what does not make the patient significantly worse in terms of degree of lameness or stiffness after rest. After that period most dogs can be returned to normal exercise over the following month.

In order to create collateral support after surgery and to reduce the risk of reluxation, a temporary transarticular pin may be placed across the joint from distal to proximal for a period of 4–6 weeks (Figure 18.11).

An alternative approach has been described for the management of a traumatic shoulder luxation, through application of a temporary transarticular locking plate while the damaged shoulder soft tissues heal (Post *et al.*, 2008).

Prognosis

Maintaining reduction of an acquired shoulder luxation may be problematical. If conservative measures fail, surgery should be undertaken but the prognosis remains only fair to good for a return to complete normality, particularly in cases with medial luxation. In the authors' experience, if surgery has failed to maintain reduction then revision surgery is also prone to failure, unless a definite reason for failure has been identified. In these cases, it may be more appropriate to consider a salvage procedure, such as arthrodesis or excision arthroplasty.

Dorsal luxation of the scapula

This is an uncommon condition seen more frequently in the cat. It is invariably a result of trauma (a jump or fall from height or a road accident) which causes rupture of the serratus ventralis muscle near its insertions on the scapula and possibly additional tearing of the trapezius, rhomboideus, teres major and latissimus dorsi muscles. Diagnosis is based on the clinical appearance of dorsal displacement of the scapula that is clearly evident on weight bearing. Conservative management in cats will usually ultimately result in pain-free limb function but the abnormal gait characterized by dorsal displacement persists. Surgical treatment requires a caudolateral approach to allow re-apposition of the torn muscles and reattachment of any avulsed muscles to the scapula using sutures of stainless steel wire or nylon by way of bone tunnels (Perry *et al.*, 2012). Further support is usually required and the caudal edge of the scapula may be attached to one or more of the underlying ribs using stainless steel wire. Postoperatively, the limb is supported in flexion for 2–3 weeks and exercise is restricted for 6 weeks. The prognosis appears to be reasonably good.

Conditions affecting the soft tissues of the shoulder

Muscle disorders

Infraspinatus (or supraspinatus) contracture

This uncommon condition may involve dogs of any breed or age, but most cases are in medium-sized working dogs or particularly active pets (Bennett, 1986). The infraspinatus is affected much more frequently than the supraspinatus (Vaughan, 1979) and the condition can be bilateral (Franch *et al.*, 2009). A traumatic aetiology is suspected, since histological examination shows evidence of haemorrhage, degeneration, atrophy and fibrosis. There will often be a history of previous acute onset lameness, usually starting at or soon after exercise, which improved over the following few days. The progressive lameness then develops a few weeks later.

18.11 Mediolateral postoperative radiograph of a 9-year-old Toy Poodle following placement of a transarticular pin to stabilize a medial subluxation after revision surgery to replace a collateral prosthesis. The first prosthesis had failed after 2 weeks. The pin was left *in situ* for 4 weeks and the shoulder remained stable.

Clinical findings: Dogs do not show discomfort and are still keen to exercise. When they are standing, the limb can be positioned normally, though in chronic cases it may be held slightly adducted at the elbow with external rotation of the antebrachium creating lateralization of the distal limb (Figure 18.12), an appearance that is pathognomonic for the condition. At a walk and trot there is obvious circumduction of the limb on protraction and a flip-like extension of the paw as the limb moves forwards. Manipulation of the joint causes no pain but flexion is reduced. If the whole limb is flexed, the antebrachium tends to deviate laterally from the body instead of remaining in a straight line. Palpation will normally reveal atrophy of the suprascapular muscles and possibly similar changes in other shoulder muscles. The condition may be bilateral.

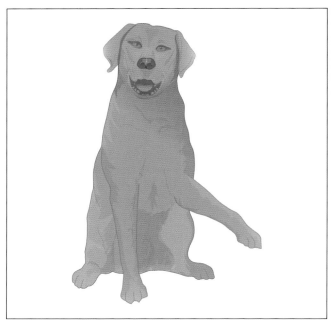

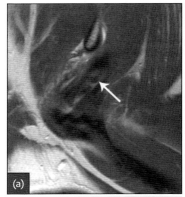 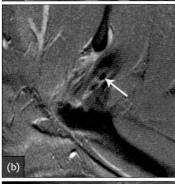 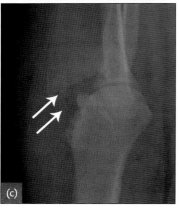

18.13 (a) Sagittal plane PD-weighted and (b) T2*GRE MR images and (c) caudocranial radiograph of a 4-year-old Labrador Retriever with lameness due to infraspinatus tendonopathy. There is dystrophic mineralization present within the tendon (arrowed). Identifying small areas of soft tissue mineralization may be difficult on MRI and it is easier to identify on the radiograph. (Courtesy of Torrington Orthopaedics)

18.12 Patients with contracture of the infraspinatus muscle may adopt this typical posture when sitting. The elbow is held adducted with the distal limb externally rotated.
(Redrawn after the *BSAVA Manual of Small Animal Arthrology*)

Diagnostic imaging: A mediolateral radiographic view may show a relative reduction in the width of the caudal joint space. In the caudocranial view there may be a reduction in the distance between the acromion or the rim of the glenoid and the greater tubercle of the humerus. It is useful to take similar views of the contralateral shoulder for comparison. However, these radiographic features are secondary to the characteristic clinical features when reaching a diagnosis. Ultrasonography can be used to demonstrate muscle pathology and its replacement with fibrous tissue and MRI can be expected to show an abnormal heterogeneous hypointensity within the affected muscle (Figure 18.13) (Orellana-James *et al.*, 2013).

Treatment: Treatment involves tenotomy of the affected tendon to restore normal thoracic limb function and carriage. A lateral approach to the greater tubercle provides good exposure of the tendon, which appears scarred and fibrotic. The tendon is sectioned at its insertion; this may involve elevation from the joint capsule and the breakdown of adhesions. Following this, normal movement of the joint should be restored immediately. The dog should be rested until the skin sutures are removed and then rapidly returned to a normal exercise regime to prevent the formation of adhesions. Following surgery the prognosis is favourable for a return to normal function. No recurrences have been recorded.

Teres minor myopathy

Lameness associated with shoulder pain was reported in a 5-year-old working Labrador Retriever in which ultrasonography suggested pathology in the teres minor muscle (Bruce *et al.*, 1997). After conservative management failed to improve the lameness, surgical excision of the muscle led to complete recovery. Histopathology confirmed a diagnosis of teres minor myopathy.

Tendon and ligament disorders

The aetiology of many conditions affecting the ligamentous restraints and cuff muscles of the shoulder is poorly understood but is thought to be related to trauma, often of a chronic repetitive nature. These conditions are generally seen in older, medium to large-breed dogs although smaller breeds may sometimes be affected. The onset of lameness may be acute (following a particularly active period of exercise) or more chronic and insidious. Affected dogs often lead active or working lives and owners will frequently report a lameness that deteriorates with excessive exercise but improves with rest; there may be some stiffness for a few minutes on rising. The degree of lameness may range from mild to severe and pain will be evident on manipulation of the shoulder. Determination of a precise diagnosis can be challenging but thorough, methodical clinical examination can be helpful in localizing the structures involved. Flexion of the shoulder stresses the biceps tendon, especially if the elbow is kept extended, and may exacerbate the pain. Full extension of the joint also seems to cause discomfort, but this may be because of the pressure applied to the cranial aspect of the proximal humerus when such a manipulation is performed. Direct pressure applied over a particular tendon or ligament may produce evidence of 'point pain' that can help to determine the likely structure involved. Evaluation of joint instability in cases suspected of having collateral insufficiency is probably best reserved for the anaesthetized patient. Patients vary in their 'normal' reactions to such manipulations and a comparison of both thoracic limbs should always be made.

In very general terms, conservative treatment, with strict rest for 4 to 6 weeks, may improve the clinical signs and NSAID administration may help during this period. If such measures fail, the injection of 20–60 mg of methylprednisolone (40 mg for a dog of about 30 kg) either around the affected tendon or into the joint under strict asepsis, followed by 4 weeks of strict rest and then a gradual return to normal exercise, may alleviate the signs. The response to such an injection is usually quite rapid, although the patient may be more uncomfortable for a few days following investigation and injection. In one study, about 50% of cases treated for non-specific shoulder lameness (where the clinical and radiographic features were consistent with those described above but a definitive diagnosis was never made) showed long-term improvement (Butterworth, 2003). In other cases there may be temporary improvement, which still helps confirm the shoulder as the source of lameness. When a specific tendon is implicated on clinical examination, personal observation suggests that some dogs respond better to peritendinous injection of methylprednisolone while others respond more favourably when it is administered intra-articularly. Where such conservative measures have failed to improve a patient, then the option of physiotherapy should be considered as this will often lead to improvement and avoid the need for more advanced imaging techniques and surgical intervention.

Disorders affecting the biceps tendon

Bicipital tenosynovitis: The clinical diagnosis of bicipital tenosynovitis can be difficult (Lincoln and Potter, 1984), particularly with respect to differentiation of this from such conditions as glenohumeral ligament pathology and mineralizing supraspinatus tendinopathy (see below). It is a relatively uncommon condition (Bardet, 1999; Devitt *et al.*, 2007).

Plain radiographs may demonstrate new bone deposition superimposed on the greater tubercle that may be located within the intertubercular groove (Figure 18.14ab). In some instances minor lucencies may be observed superimposed on the greater tubercle. The significance of these changes has been brought into question by the fact that many normal dogs, without clinical lameness, show similar changes.

Arthrography may demonstrate poor filling of the tendon sheath due to adhesions and confirm the diagnosis (Figure 18.14cd). Unfortunately, as in human patients, radiographs (including arthrograms) may appear normal. This is not surprising when one considers that it is secondary changes that are being observed, rather than the primary problem.

Ultrasonography (Figure 18.14e) has been investigated as a diagnostic technique; although studies in the past suggested it was less sensitive than arthrography (Rivers

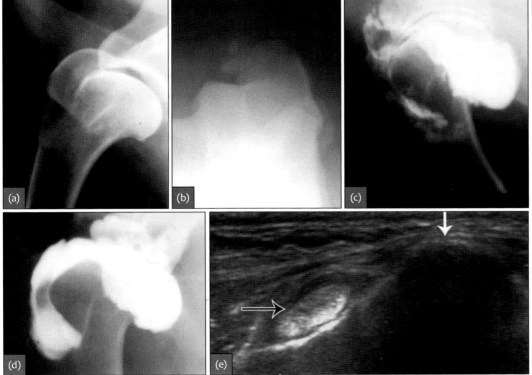

18.14 Bicipital tenosynovitis.
(a) Mediolateral radiograph of a 12-year-old Border Collie with thoracic limb lameness associated with pain on shoulder extension or direct pressure applied over the biceps tendon. There is new bone deposition superimposed on the greater tubercle.
(b) A tangential view shows osteophytes medial to the greater tubercle.
(c) Mediolateral arthrogram (post injection of 6 ml of contrast medium) of a shoulder of a 7-year-old Airedale that was showing similar signs to the dog in (a). There is poor filling of the bicipital tendon sheath.
(d) A normal arthrogram for comparison. (e) Ultrasound image showing a thickened biceps tendon of mixed heterogenous echogenicity (black arrow) surrounded by increased fluid (the black surrounding ring). The white arrow indicates the cranial aspect of the greater tubercle.
(e, Courtesy of Gareth Arthurs and Marie-Aude Genain)

et al., 1992), a more recent study suggested it could be used reliably to detect pathology of the biceps tendon (Kramer *et al.*, 2001). MRI has been shown to be a reliable and sensitive method of assessing biceps pathology although it requires the correct sequences to be read by an experienced reviewer and remains relatively expensive (Murphy *et al.*, 2008).

Arthroscopy was first suggested as a means of evaluating the biceps tendon by Person (1986). Since then it has become the 'gold standard' for diagnosing bicipital pathology as well as other conditions of the shoulder joint (Bardet, 1999). The normal tendon appears as a smooth white structure with variable amounts of vasculature and some fat and synovial folds proximally. Changes that occur with bicipital tenosynovitis include thickening and/or discoloration of the tendon, synovitis and adhesions of the tendon sheath. In chronic cases the tendon may actually rupture. Care must be taken in interpreting pathology as primary bicipital tenosynovitis because synovial hyperplasia may occur secondary to other pathological processes in the shoulder (Figure 18.15), such as OCD and medial shoulder instability, or simply reflect more global joint pathology. Treatment of the primary cause will often resolve these changes seen on the tendon and in the authors' opinion, synovitis of the tendon sheath is merely an extension of generalized synovitis of the shoulder and is rarely a primary synovitis of the biceps tendon.

Treatment: Surgical management should be considered if conservative measures (detailed above) fail. Tenotomy and/or tenodesis of the biceps brachii tendon of origin may be considered and can be performed arthroscopically or via arthrotomy.

Arthroscopy, if available, is the preferred method of diagnosis and treatment due to the relatively low invasiveness and, in experienced hands, the speed of the procedure. Tenotomy can be achieved with standard camera and instrument portals at the time of the initial examination (Holsworth *et al.*, 2002) and this has been reported to produce results comparable to tenodesis. The instrument portal is created craniolaterally, with a lateral arthroscope portal. The biceps tendon is transected using an arthroscopic blade (or a No. 11 blade) or a radiofrequency probe. Arthroscopic tenotomy and tenodesis have also been described by Cook *et al.*, 2004.

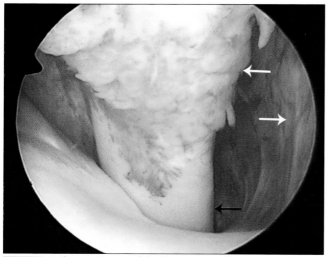

18.15 Arthroscopic view of the biceps tendon (black arrow) showing severe synovial hyperaemia at the proximal end of the tendon and of the craniomedial joint capsule (white arrows).

If arthroscopy is not available then arthrotomy is a viable alternative. The tendon is exposed using a craniomedial approach. Several methods exist (see Operative Technique 18.8), but there are insufficient numbers of cases recorded to establish which of the techniques, if any, is most appropriate. Advocates of tenodesis suggest that securing the biceps tendon proximally is likely to result in a more rapid and predictable return to function. It has also been reported that some dogs remain lame after tenotomy but improve after subsequent tenodesis. Stobie *et al.* (1995) reported excellent or good outcomes for all 14 dogs treated for this condition by tenodesis after medical treatment had failed. The dog should be rested for between 4 and 6 weeks after surgery.

Rupture/avulsion of the biceps brachii tendon of origin: This is an uncommon injury but has been recorded in cases with shoulder luxation (in combination with glenohumeral ligament rupture) particularly those occurring in a craniomedial direction (Bennett and Campbell, 1979). The possibility of biceps tendon injury in these cases should be investigated at surgery. Clinically, there is swelling and pain over the cranial aspect of the shoulder. Plain radiography is of limited use unless part of the scapular tuberosity has been avulsed (Figure 18.16a). Arthrography may demonstrate disruption of the tendon sheath at the site of rupture and arthroscopy can be used to view the damage (Figure 18.16bc).

If the shoulder is stable, conservative measures may be employed (see above). Should these fail then tenodesis should be considered (see Operative Technique 18.8). If joint instability is present then surgery to reconstruct collateral support (see under Luxation), together with tendon repair or tenodesis of the biceps tendon, is indicated.

Partial tears of the biceps tendon are common, especially in agility and working dogs (Figure 18.16c). Conservative management improves the lameness but this usually recurs on recommencement of exercise. Cases with partial rupture of the biceps tendon usually respond well to arthroscopic tenotomy, which yields favourable results in both the short and long term (Bergenhuyzen *et al.*, 2010).

Rupture of the biceps tendon sheath: In two dogs with clinical signs as described above, arthrography showed leakage of contrast agent from the distal portion of the tendon sheath (Figure 18.17). Conservative management (as described above) failed to improve the lameness and surgery to promote biceps tenodesis was reported to improve matters (see Operative Technique 18.8) (Innes and Brown, 2004). No other pathology was recognized arthroscopically in either of the two cases but in one, the resected tendon was submitted for histopathology and revealed concomitant bicipital tendinopathy. Given that tenodesis could improve lameness resulting from tendinopathy, the significance of the sheath rupture may be brought into question in terms of its association with lameness.

Medial luxation of the biceps brachii tendon: This is an uncommon cause of lameness that has been reported in racing Greyhounds, a German Shepherd Dog, an Afghan Hound and a Border Collie (Bennett and Campbell, 1979; Goring *et al.*, 1984; Fox and Bray, 1992; Boemo and Eaton-Wells, 1995). Lameness is gradual in onset and worsens with exercise. There may be evidence of pain and/or crepitus on shoulder manipulation. As the shoulder is flexed the tendon may be felt to 'pop' out of the intertubercular groove in a medial direction and then return to its normal position on extension of the joint. There may be associated

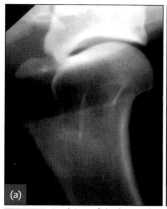
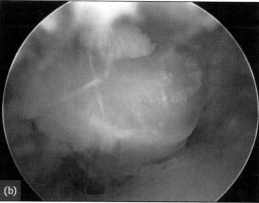
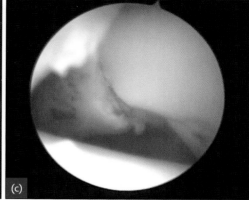

18.16 Avulsion of the biceps brachii tendon. (a) Mediolateral radiograph of the shoulder of a 4-year-old Irish Setter that developed acute onset thoracic limb lameness. The biceps brachii tendon had avulsed from the scapular tuberosity, from which a small fragment of bone has also been avulsed. (b) Arthroscopic view of an avulsed biceps tendon. (c) Arthroscopic view of a partial biceps tendon avulsion in a 7-year-old Bernese Mountain Dog.
(c, Courtesy of Simon Gilbert)

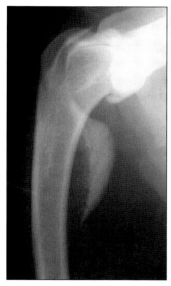

18.17 Mediolateral arthrogram of a 4-year-old Border Collie, showing leakage of contrast agent from the distal margin of the biceps tendon sheath, possibly indicating rupture.

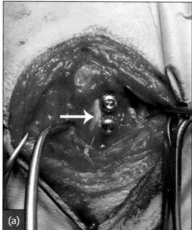

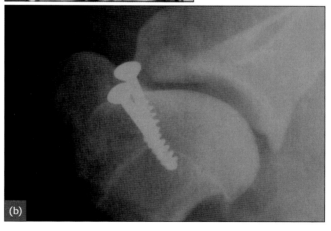

18.18 Medial displacement of the biceps brachii tendon of origin. (a) Intraoperative image after medial placement of two stabilizing screws. The biceps tendon is indicated by the arrow and is positioned lateral to the screws. (b) Postoperative radiograph following relocation of the tendon in the intertubercular groove and stabilization with two 4.0 mm partially threaded cancellous screws.
(Courtesy of Malcolm McKee)

luxation of the shoulder joint due to loss of cranial support, though this also requires damage to additional structures.

Displacement of the biceps tendon follows rupture of the transverse humeral ligament. Treatment involves relocation and retention of the tendon in the intertubercular groove using a cranial approach. The function of the ruptured intertubercular retinaculum can be replaced by placement of orthopaedic wire or polypropylene mesh with a favourable prognosis (Barnes, 2013). An alternative technique involves placement of a partially threaded bone screw in the lesser tubercle, medial to the tendon (Figure 18.18a) (McKee and Macias, 2004). The shank of the screw and the ensuing fibrous reaction prevent re-luxation of the tendon (Figure 18.18b).

Supraspinatus tendinopathy

Dystrophic mineralization within the soft tissues superimposed on the greater tubercle, in particular the supraspinatus tendon of insertion, seen as multi-focal areas of increased radiopacity, is a common incidental radiographic finding (Figure 18.19a). Accurate localization of such pathology with respect to the tendon involved can be challenging and requires CT, MRI or ultrasound examination.

Although such changes may be seen in many clinically normal dogs, supraspinatus tendinopathy (which may be mineralized or non-mineralized) has been reported as a cause of thoracic limb lameness (Muir and Johnson, 1994; Kriegleder, 1995; Lafuente *et al.*, 2009). Conversely, a CT study of lame dogs found that periarticular mineralization, especially of the supraspinatus tendon, was not a significant cause of lameness in the majority of dogs (Figure 18.19b) (Maddox *et al.*, 2013). It is possible that when this condition is associated with lameness it is because of encroachment of the mineralized tissue on the biceps tendon or its sheath; however, this may be a positional

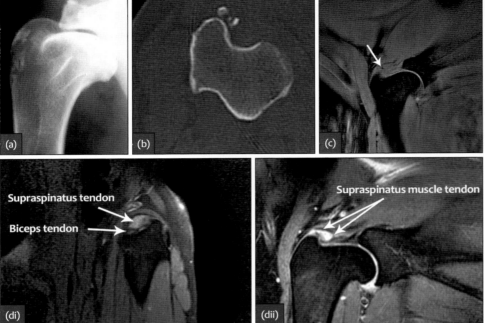

18.19 (a) Mediolateral radiograph of a 9-year-old German Shepherd Dog showing mineralization over the cranial aspect of the greater tubercle in the vicinity of the supraspinatus tendon of insertion. There is also mineralization further caudally, which could involve the intertubercular groove. (b) Transverse CT image at the level of the greater tubercle showing mineralization craniomedial to the greater tubercle, consistent with supraspinatus tendon mineralization. (c) Fat-saturated three-dimensional fast spoiled gradient-echo sequence (3D-WATSC) MR image of supraspinatus mineralization (arrowed) in a dog. (di–ii) PD-weighted fat-saturated MR images of non-mineralized supraspinatus tendinopathy showing increased signal in the supraspinatus muscle tendon on the medial aspect of the greater tubercle insertion and slight medial displacement of the biceps tendon with some flattening.
(Courtesy of Gordon Brown)

artefact and not a true cause of lameness. Ultrasound examination of the region is aimed at assessing the associated tendon and surrounding structures. The relevant findings are a large area of hypoechoic shadowing adjacent to the lesion with associated changes within the tendon. Of those cases that fail to improve with conservative management (as described above), some will improve after surgical removal of the mineralized tissue (Flo and Middleton, 1990; Muir *et al.*, 1996; Laitinen and Flo, 2000; Lafuente *et al.*, 2009). Extracorporeal shock wave therapy has been suggested to have a role in treatment but has yet to be fully evaluated (Danova and Muir, 2003).

Infraspinatus bursal ossification

Radiographs may show evidence of ossification within the infraspinatus bursa. In the mediolateral view the opacity is superimposed on the greater tubercle, but in the caudocranial view the opacity lies lateral to the proximal humerus (McKee *et al.*, 2007) (Figure 18.20). These changes have been associated with clinical lameness in some Labrador Retrievers, although in most of those where arthroscopy

was performed (six out of seven) other pathology was also recognized, which brings into question how significant the bursal ossification was in relation to the lameness. Surgical resection of the ossified masses and release of the associated infraspinatus tendon has been advocated where conservative measures (as described above) fail although some residual lameness is common.

Shoulder joint instability/subluxation

Shoulder instability is defined as an abnormally increased range of motion between the humeral head and the glenoid fossa resulting in discomfort and dysfunction of the shoulder due to the incompetence or disruption of the joint stability mechanisms. Shoulder instability in adult dogs may occur in two forms:

- Traumatic luxations (see Luxations, above)
- Acquired chronic shoulder laxity associated with loss of integrity of the soft tissue supporting structures of the shoulder. This has been recognized in recent years aided by the increasingly widespread use of arthroscopy. While there is still a poor understanding of shoulder instability, it appears that the structures most commonly affected are the medial glenohumeral ligament and the subscapularis tendon (Bardet, 1998) (Figure 18.21) and less commonly, the lateral glenohumeral ligament (Mitchell and Innes, 2000; Pettitt and Innes, 2008) (Figure 18.22).

It has been suggested that insufficiency in the medial support (provided by the medial glenohumeral ligament and subscapularis muscle tendon of insertion) can be evaluated by assessing the angle of abduction through the shoulder when compared with the normal limb or what has been described as 'normal' (Cook *et al.*, 2005a). When measured with a goniometer, the angle of abduction in normal shoulders was reported to be about 33 degrees compared to 54 degrees in shoulders diagnosed as having medial shoulder instability. However, this measurement is subjective and difficult to standardize. It is important when

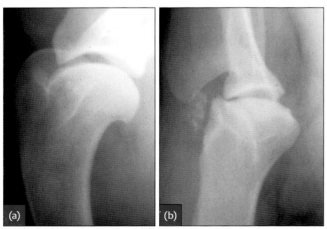

18.20 (a) Mediolateral and (b) craniocaudal radiographs, showing mineralization within the infraspinatus bursa.
(Courtesy of WM McKee)

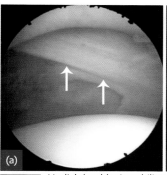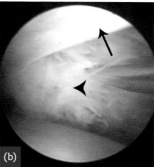

18.21 Medial shoulder instability: arthroscopic views. (a) Normal medial glenohumeral ligament (arrowed). (b) Normal medial glenohumeral ligament (arrowed) and subscapularis tendon with partial tearing (arrowhead).

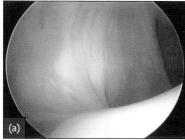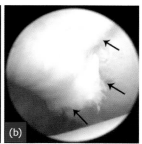

18.22 Lateral shoulder instability: arthroscopic views. (a) Normal lateral glenohumeral ligament. (b) Ruptured lateral glenohumeral ligament (arrowed).

performing this test to have the shoulder and elbow in full extension to prevent inadvertent rotation of the limb as it is abducted.

There are no specific radiographic findings and the definitive diagnosis is based on the arthroscopic examination of the glenohumeral ligaments and subscapularis tendon. Separation of the glenohumeral ligaments from the rim of the glenoid and mid-substance tears (in the ligaments or the subscapularis tendon) have been recognized (Cook *et al.*, 2005a) (see Figures 18.21b and 18.22b). Unfortunately, the significance of these findings alone is somewhat unreliable since they are sometimes seen in combination with other shoulder pathology, and when the latter is treated the lameness may improve. In a study by Devitt *et al.* (2007), shoulder abduction and mediolateral instability tests were shown to have only a minimal to small effect on the probability of detecting changes to the medial compartment structures. They concluded that while an increased angle of abduction greater than 50 degrees is a consistent feature of medial shoulder instability, it is also a consistent finding in dogs with thoracic limb pathology leading to a loss of muscle strength or mass. This means that by itself, an increased abduction angle is not pathognomonic for medial shoulder instability.

Surgical treatment

Surgery is considered where conservative measures (as described above) have failed to improve the lameness associated with suspected medial or lateral shoulder instability. In general, it would appear that there is a higher chance of achieving a successful outcome with surgical treatment compared with conservative management (Franklin *et al.*, 2013).

Surgical options for medial glenohumeral ligament insufficiency include:

- Subscapular imbrication (Pettitt *et al.*, 2007) (see Operative Technique 18.7A)
- Medial prosthesis placement (Fitch *et al.*, 2001; Ringwood *et al.*, 2001) (see Operative Technique 18.7B)
- Thermal modification ('shrinkage') of the joint capsule (O'Neill and Innes, 2004; Cook *et al.*, 2005a; Cook *et al.*, 2005b).

Surgical options for lateral glenohumeral ligament insufficiency include:

- Lateral capsulorrhaphy (Mitchell and Innes, 2000)
- Arthroscopic suturing of the lateral glenohumeral ligament (Pettitt and Innes, 2008).

Neoplasia

Lameness relating to pain on shoulder manipulation caused by neoplasia is uncommon in dogs. The types of neoplasia responsible for this condition include:

- Sarcoma of the proximal humerus and occasionally the scapula (see Chapter 11 and also the *BSAVA Manual of Canine and Feline Oncology*
- Brachial plexus neoplasia (see Chapter 12 and also the *BSAVA Manual of Canine and Feline Neurology*
- Sarcomas of the scapulohumeral joint.

Neoplasms of the scapulohumeral joint itself are rare but if they occur they are likely to be, in order of incidence, histiocytic sarcoma (HS), synovial sarcoma (SCS), or synovial myxomas (SM) (Craig *et al.*, 2002). Such neoplastic lesions cause shoulder lameness in middle-aged to old dogs and are associated with chronic progressive clinical signs. Pain is evident on shoulder manipulation and soft tissue swelling may be palpable. Enlargement of the axillary lymph node may be present, possibly indicating lymphatic metastasis. Treatment involves forequarter amputation, with or without chemotherapy. Metastatic rates vary from 90% for HS to 25% for SCS and reduced the time of survival to 5 months for HS and 30 months for SCS and SM. SM was not reported to metastasize. Readers are referred to Chapter 11 and also the *BSAVA Manual of Canine and Feline Oncology* for further information.

Salvage procedures for the scapulohumeral joint

As for all joints, salvage procedures for the scapulohumeral joint should only be undertaken when all other management options have failed or would be inappropriate. Such situations include:

- Irreparable fractures of the glenoid or humeral head
- Recurrent luxation with erosive deformation of the glenoid, rendering surgical stabilization impossible
- Severe, clinically significant shoulder dysplasia
- Chronic pain associated with severe osteoarthritis
- Chronic sepsis of the scapulohumeral joint (only once the infection has been eliminated or following an extended course of antibiotics).

The options available for salvage surgery for this joint include excision arthroplasty, arthrodesis and total joint replacement. The decision to undertake any such surgery should not be taken lightly; the clinical signs of shoulder disease should be severe enough to warrant such intervention. Following salvage, some degree of mechanical alteration of gait is inevitable and client counselling prior to the surgery is important so that there is a clear understanding of the goals of this surgery.

Excision arthroplasty for the scapulohumeral joint

This is the simplest form of salvage procedure for this joint and the technique was first described by Bruecker and Piermattei (1988). In their series of three cases (ranging from terrier-sized to Labrador Retriever) the results were considered satisfactory, though optimal function took several months to be achieved. A modified technique involving only excision of the glenoid was described by Franczuszki and Parkes (1988). Their series comprised 10 dogs ranging in size from Yorkshire Terriers to a German Shepherd Dog and outcomes at follow-up ranging from 4 months to 6 years were all either excellent or good.

Arthrodesis of the scapulohumeral joint

This is the most commonly used salvage procedure to regain forelimb function in the presence of debilitating scapulohumeral pain.

A craniolateral approach is used followed by preparation for arthrodesis, bone grafting and internal fixation (Figure 18.23a). Plate and screws are generally used for fixation; in theory, locking plates may be advantageous because of limited screw-holding strength in the scapula, but this has not been shown clinically. Dynamic compression plates facilitate compression across the osteotomized sections, which increases stability of the repair and locking compression plates offer both advantages.

Following successful arthrodesis at a functional angle (105–110 degrees), limb function can be good. Lost mobility from the arthrodesed shoulder is compensated by extra movement of the scapula across the thoracic wall and increased movement of the elbow and carpal joints. The additional movement in the omothoracic junction may cause soft tissue problems following scapulohumeral arthrodesis (Figure 18.23bc). Physiotherapy in the months following surgery can be helpful in overcoming these problems. One study of 14 dogs receiving shoulder arthrodesis

(Fitzpatrick *et al.*, 2012) concluded that acceptable limb function can be achieved in the majority of cases despite a high incidence of complications.

Total joint replacement

Recently the technique of scapulohumeral joint replacement has been introduced in small animal orthopaedics. No case series have yet been published but it may be anticipated that this surgical technique will take its place amongst the total joint replacements used in small animals.

References and further reading

Agnello KA, Puchalski SM, Wisner ER *et al.* (2008) Effect of positioning, scan plane, and arthrography on visibility of periarticular canine shoulder soft tissue structures on magnetic resonance images. *Veterinary Radiology and Ultrasound* **49**, 529–539

Bardet JF (1998) Diagnosis of shoulder instability in dogs and cats: a retrospective study. *Journal of the American Animal Hospital Association* **34**, 42–54

Bardet JF (1999) Lesions of the biceps tendon; diagnosis and classification. *Veterinary and Comparative Orthopaedics and Traumatology* **12**, 188–195

Barnes DM. (2013) Bilateral medial displacement of the biceps tendon of origin: repair using polypropylene mesh and staples. *Journal of Small Animal Practice* **54**, 499–501

Bennett RA (1986) Contracture of the infraspinatus muscle in dogs: a review of 12 cases. *Journal of the American Animal Hospital Association* **22**, 481–487

Bennett D and Campbell JR (1979) Unusual soft tissue orthopaedic problems in the dog. *Journal of Small Animal Practice* **20**, 27–39

Bergenhuyzen A, Vermote K, van Bree H and Van Ryssen B (2010) Long-term follow-up after arthroscopic tenotomy for partial rupture of the biceps brachii tendon. *Veterinary and Comparative Orthopaedics and Traumatology* **23**, 51–55

Boemo CM and Eaton-Wells RD (1995) Medial displacement of the tendon of origin of the biceps brachii muscle in 10 greyhounds. *Journal of Small Animal Practice* **36**, 69–73

Bruce WJ, Spence S and Miller A (1997) Teres minor myopathy as a cause of lameness in a dog. *Journal of Small Animal Practice* **38**, 74–77

Bruecker KA. and Piermattei DL. (1988) Excision arthroplasty of the canine scapulohumeral joint: Report of three cases. *Veterinary and Comparative Orthopaedics and Traumatology* **3**, 134–140

Bruggeman M, Van Vynckt D, Van Ryssen B *et al.* (2010) Osteochondritis dissecans of the humeral head in two small-breed dogs. *Veterinary Record* **166**, 139–142

Butterworth SJ (2003) The use of methylprednisolone in the management of shoulder lameness in the dog. Abstract from BSAVA Congress 2003. *Journal of Small Animal Practice* **44**, 336

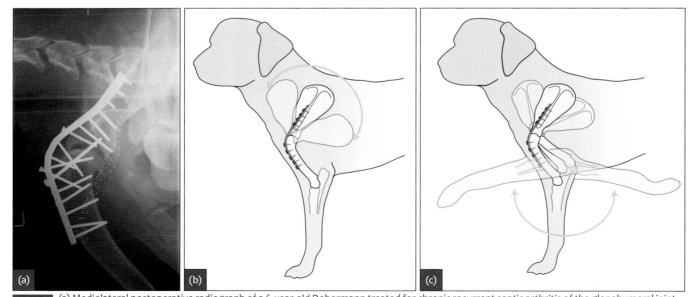

18.23 (a) Mediolateral postoperative radiograph of a 6-year-old Dobermann treated for chronic recurrent septic arthritis of the glenohumeral joint by arthrodesis. (b–c) Following arthrodesis, mobility through the omothoracic junction allows a good range of motion through the distal limb to compensate for loss of movement in the scapulohumeral joint.

Clayton Jones DG and Vaughan LC (1970) The surgical treatment of osteochondritis dissecans of the humeral head in dogs. *Journal of Small Animal Practice* **11**, 803–812

Cook JL (2003) Diagnosis and treatment of shoulder instability in dogs. *Proceedings of the 13th Annual Symposium of the American College of Veterinary Surgeons,* Washington DC

Cook JL, Kenter K and Fox DB (2004) Arthroscopic biceps tenodesis in dogs: technique and results in 6 cases. *Journal of the American Animal Hospital Association* **41**, 121–127

Cook JL, Renfro DC, Tomlinson JL and Sorensen JE (2005a) Measurement of angles of abduction for diagnosis of shoulder instability in dogs using goniometry and digital image analysis. *Veterinary Surgery* **34**, 463–468

Cook JL, Tomlinson JL, Fox DB, Kenter K and Cook CR (2005b) Treatment of dogs diagnosed with medial shoulder instability using radiofrequency-induced thermal capsulorrhaphy. *Veterinary Surgery* **34**, 469–475

Craig LE, Julian ME and Ferracone JD (2002) The diagnosis and prognosis of synovial tumors in dogs: 35 cases. *Veterinary Pathology* **39**, 66–73

Danova NA and Muir P (2003) Extracorporeal shock wave therapy for supraspinatus calcifying tendinopathy in two dogs. *Veterinary Record* **152**, 208–209

DeSimone A, Gernone F and Ricciardi M (2013) Imaging diagnosis – bilateral abnormal ossification of the supraglenoid tubercle and cranial glenoid cavity in an English Setter. *Veterinary Radiology and Ultrasound* **54**, 159–163

Devitt CM, Neely MR and Vanvechten BJ (2007) Relationship of physical examination test of shoulder instability to arthroscopic findings in dogs. *Veterinary Surgery* **36**, 661–668

Dobson J and Lascelles D (2014) *BSAVA Manual of Canine and Feline Oncology, 3rd edn.* BSAVA Publications, Gloucester

Erdem V and Pead MJ (2000) Haemangiosarcoma of the scapula in three dogs. *Journal of Small Animal Practice* **41**, 461–464

Fitch RB, Breshears L, Staatz A and Kudnig S (2001) Clinical evaluation of prosthetic medial glenohumeral ligament repair in the dog (ten cases). *Veterinary and Comparative Orthopaedics and Traumatology* **14**, 222–228

Fitzpatrick N, van Terheijden C, Yeadon R and Smith TJ (2010) Osteochondral autograft transfer for treatment of osteochondritis dissecans of the caudocentral humeral head in dogs. *Veterinary Surgery* **39**, 925–935

Fitzpatrick N, Yeadon R, Smith TJ et al. (2012) Shoulder arthrodesis in 14 dogs. *Veterinary Surgery* **41**, 745–754

Flo GL and Middleton D (1990) Mineralization of the supraspinatus tendon in dogs. *Journal of the American Veterinary Medical Association* **197**, 95–97

Fowler JD, Presnell KR and Holmberg DL (1988) Scapulohumeral arthrodesis: results in seven dogs. *Journal of the American Animal Hospital Association* **24**, 667–672

Fox SM and Bray JP (1992) Surgical correction for rupture of the transverse humeral ligament in a racing greyhound. *Australian Veterinary Practitioner* **22**, 2–5

Franch J, Bertran J, Remolins G et al. (2009) Simultaneous bilateral contracture of the infraspinatus muscle. *Veterinary and Comparative Orthopaedics and Traumatology* **22**, 249–252

Franczuszki D and Parkes LJ (1988) Glenoid excision as a treatment in chronic shoulder disabilities: Surgical technique and clinical results. *Journal of the American Animal Hospital Association* **24**, 637–643

Franklin SP, Devitt CM, Ogawa J, Ridge P and Cook JL (2013) Outcomes associated with treatments for medial, lateral, and multidirectional shoulder instability in dogs. *Veterinary Surgery* **42**, 361–364

Gahring DR (1985) A modified caudal approach to the canine shoulder joint. *Journal of the American Animal Hospital Association* **21**, 613–618

Gemmill T and Clements D (2016) *BSAVA Manual of Canine and Feline Fracture Repair and Management, 2nd edn.* BSAVA Publications, Gloucester

Gibbs C, Denny HR and Kelly DF (1984) The radiological features of osteosarcoma of the appendicular skeleton in dogs: a review of 74 cases. *Journal of Small Animal Practice* **25**, 177–192

Goring RL, Parker RB, Dee L and Eaton-Wells RD (1984) Medial displacement of the tendon of origin of the biceps brachii muscle in the racing greyhound. *Journal of the American Animal Hospital Association* **20**, 933–938

Holsworth IG, Schulz KS and Ingel K (2002) Cadaveric evaluation of canine arthroscopic bicipital tenotomy. *Veterinary and Comparative Orthopaedics and Traumatology* **15**, 215–222

Houlton J and Collinson RW (1994) *BSAVA Manual of Small Animal Arthrology.* BSAVA Publications, Cheltenham

Innes JF and Brown G (2004) Rupture of the biceps brachii tendon sheath in two dogs. *Journal of Small Animal Practice* **45**, 25–28

Kramer M, Gerwing M, Sheppard C and Schimke E (2001) Ultrasonography for the diagnosis of diseases of the tendon and tendon sheath of the biceps brachii muscle. *Veterinary Surgery* **30**, 64–71

Kriegleder H (1995) Mineralization of the supraspinatus tendon: clinical observations in seven dogs. *Veterinary and Comparative Orthopaedics and Traumatology* **8**, 91–97

Lafuente MP, Fransson BA, Lincoln JD et al. (2009) Surgical treatment of mineralized and nonmineralized supraspinatus tendinopathy in twenty-four dogs. *Veterinary Surgery* **38**, 380–387

Laitinen OM and Flo GL (2000) Mineralization of the supraspinatus tendon in dogs: long-term follow-up. *Journal of the American Animal Hospital Association* **36**, 262–267

Llhermette P and Sobel D (2008) *BSAVA Manual of Canine and Feline Endoscopy.* BSAVA Publications, Gloucester

Lincoln JD and Potter K (1984) Tenosynovitis of the biceps brachii tendon in dogs. *Journal of the American Animal Hospital Association* **20**, 385–392

Maddox TW, May C, Keeley BJ and McConnell JF (2013) Comparison between shoulder computed tomography and clinical findings in 89 dogs presented for thoracic limb lameness. *Veterinary Radiologyy and Ultrasound* **54**, 358–364

McKee WM and Macias C (2004) Orthopaedic conditions of the shoulder in the dog. *In Practice* **26**, 118–129

McKee WM, May C, Macias C and Scurrell EJ (2007) Ossification of the infraspinatus tendon-bursa in 13 dogs. *Veterinary Record* **161**, 846–852

Meyer-Lindenberg A, Koppler M and Fehr M (2002) Treatment of osteochondrosis dissecans of the shoulder joint in dogs: arthroscopic *versus* conventional removal. Abstract from BSAVA Congress 2002. *Journal of Small Animal Practice* **43**, 302a

Mitchell RAS and Innes JF (2000) Lateral glenohumeral ligament rupture in three dogs. *Journal of Small Animal Practice* **41**, 511–514

Monaco T and Schwartz P (2011) What is your diagnosis? Incomplete fusion of the caudal glenoid ossification centre. *Journal of the American Veterinary Medical Association* **239**, 1545–1546

Muir P and Johnson KA (1994) Supraspinatus and biceps brachii tendinopathy in dogs. *Journal of Small Animal Practice* **35**, 239–243

Muir P, Johnson KA and Manley PA (1996) Force-plate analysis of gait before and after surgical excision of calcified lesions of the supraspinatus tendon in two dogs. *Veterinary Record* **139**, 137–139

Murphy SE, Ballegeer EA, Forrest LJ and Schaefer SL (2008) Magnetic resonance imaging findings in dogs with confirmed shoulder pathology. *Veterinary Surgery* **37**, 631–638

Olivieri M, Ciliberto E, Hulse DA et al. (2007) Arthroscopic treatment of osteochondritis dissecans of the shoulder in 126 dogs. *Veterinary and Comparative Orthopaedics and Traumatology* **20**, 65–69

Olivieri M, Piras A, Marcellin-Little et al. (2004) Accessory caudal glenoid ossification centre as possible cause of lameness in nine dogs. *Veterinary and Comparative Orthopaedics and Traumatology* **17**, 131–135

Olivieri M, Piras A and Vezzoni A (1999) Ununited caudal glenoid ossification centre in 5 dogs: arthroscopic diagnosis and treatment (Abstract ECVS). *Veterinary Surgery* **28**, 213–214

O'Neill T and Innes JF (2004) Use of thermal capsulorrhaphy to treat instability of the shoulder joint in a dog. *Journal of Small Animal Practice* **45**, 521–524

Orellana-James NG, Ginja MM, Regueiro M et al. (2013) Sub-acute and chronic MRI findings in bilateral canine fibrotic contracture of the infraspinatus muscle. *Journal of Small Animal Practice* **54**, 428–431

Perry KL, Lam R, Rutherford L and Arthurs GI (2012) A case of scapular avulsion with concomitant scapular fracture in a cat. *Journal of Feline Medicine and Surgery* **14**, 946–951

Person MW (1986) Arthroscopy of the canine shoulder joint. *Compendium on Continuing Education for the Practicing Veterinarian* **8**, 537–547

Pettitt RA, Clements DN and Guilliard MJ (2007) Stabilization of medial shoulder instability by imbrication of the subscapularis muscle tendon of insertion. *Journal of Small Animal Practice* **48**, 626–631

Pettitt RA and Innes JF (2008) Arthroscopic management of a lateral glenohumeral rupture in two dogs. *Veterinary and Comparative Orthopaedics and Traumatology* **21**, 302–306

Platt S and Olby N (2013) *BSAVA Manual of Canine and Feline Neurology, 4th edn.* BSAVA Publications, Gloucester

Post C, Guerrero T, Voss K and Montavon PM (2008) Temporary transarticular stabilization with a locking plate for medial shoulder luxation in a dog. *Veterinary and Comparative Orthopaedics and Traumatology* **21**, 166–170

Read RA (1994) Successful treatment of congenital shoulder luxation in a dog by closed pinning. *Veterinary and Comparative Orthopaedics and Traumatology* **7**, 170–172

Ringwood PB, Kerwin SC, Hosgood G and Williams J (2001) Medial glenohumeral ligament reconstruction for ex-vivo medial glenohumeral luxation in the dog. *Veterinary and Comparative Orthopaedics and Traumatology* **14**, 196–200

Rivers B, Wallace L and Johnstone GR (1992) Biceps tenosynovitis in the dog: radiographic and sonographic findings. *Veterinary and Comparative Orthopaedics and Traumatology* **5**, 51–57

Rudd RG, Whitehair JG and Margolis JH (1990) Results of management of osteochondritis dissecans of the humeral head in dogs: 44 cases (1982–1987). *Journal of the American Animal Hospital Association* **26**, 173–178

Schaefer SL, Baumel CA, Gerbig JR et al. (2010) Direct magnetic resonance arthrography of the canine shoulder. *Veterinary Radiology and Ultrasound* **51**, 391–396

Sharp NJ (1988) Craniolateral approach to the brachial plexus. *Veterinary Surgery* **17**, 18–21

Sharp NJ (1995) Neoplasia of the brachial plexus and associated nerve roots. In: *Manual of Small Animal Neurology, 2nd edn*, ed. SJ Wheeler, pp. 164–166. BSAVA Publications, Cheltenham

Sidaway BK, McLaughlin RM, Elder SH, Boyle CR and Silverman EB (2004) Role of the tendons of the biceps brachii and infraspinatus muscles and the medial glenohumeral ligament in the maintenance of passive shoulder stability in dogs. *American Journal of Veterinary Research* **65**, 1216–1222

Silva HR, Uosyte R, Clements DN *et al.* (2013) Computed tomography and positive contrast computed tomographic arthrography of the canine shoulder: Normal anatomy and effects of limb position on visibility of soft tissue structures. *Veterinary Radiology and Ultrasound* **54**, 470–477

Stobie D, Wallace LJ, Lipowitz AJ, King V and Lund EM (1995) Chronic bicipital tenosynovitis in dogs: 29 cases (1985–1992). *Journal of the American Veterinary Medical Association* **207**, 201–207

Targett MP, Dyce J and Houlton JEF (1993) Tumours involving the nerve sheaths of the forelimb in dogs. *Journal of Small Animal Practice* **34**, 221–225

van Bree HJJ (1992) *Positive Shoulder Arthrography in the Dog: the Application in Osteochondrosis Lesions Compared with other Diagnostic Imaging Techniques* [thesis]. Utrecht University Press, Utrecht

Van Ryssen B, van Bree H and Missinne S (1993) Successful arthroscopic treatment of shoulder osteochondrosis in the dog. *Journal of Small Animal Practice* **34**, 521–528

Vasseur PB, Moore D, Brown SA and Eng D (1982) Stability of the canine shoulder joint: an in vitro analysis. *American Journal of Veterinary Research* **43**, 352–355

Vaughan LC (1979) Muscle and tendon injuries in dogs. *Journal of Small Animal Practice* **20**, 711–736

Vaughan LC and Jones DGC (1968) Osteochondritis dissecans of the head of the humerus in dogs. *Journal of Small Animal Practice* **9**, 283–294

Wall CR, Cook CR and Cook JL (2015) Diagnostic sensitivity of radiography, ultrasonography, and magnetic resonance imaging for detecting shoulder osteochondrosis/osteochondritis dissecans in dogs. *Veterinary Radiology and Ultrasound* **56**, 3–11

IMAGING TECHNIQUES

Thomas W. Maddox

Radiography is the imaging modality most commonly employed in investigating shoulder disease but it is poor for assessment of anything other than the osseous structures. The surrounding soft tissues are poorly delineated and even a significant joint effusion will not be apparent. The use of contrast media in the form of shoulder arthrography can overcome some of the limitations of plain radiography and allows some outline visualization of intra-articular soft tissue structures, but the information gained is still limited and can be difficult to interpret. Given that much shoulder lameness in skeletally mature dogs is the result of injury to the associated soft tissues, there is increasing use of other modalities (particularly MRI and ultrasonography) that can provide much more detailed and useful information on these cases.

RADIOGRAPHY

Standard views

The standard orthogonal views obtained are the mediolateral and caudocranial views. The use of a grid is advised for any patients other than small dogs.

Mediolateral view

This view allows good visualization of the humeral head, glenoid and supraglenoid tubercle.

- The animal is placed in lateral recumbency with the target limb protracted cranially and dependent against the cassette/plate, with the contralateral limb retracted caudally (Figure 18.24). It is important that the limb is sufficiently cranial so that the thorax is not superimposed over the shoulder.
- Slight dorsal extension of the neck can alleviate superimposition of the trachea and neck muscles. The sternum is slightly rotated away from the target limb.
- The primary beam is centred just distal to the acromion.
- Collimate proximally and distally to include approximately one-third of the scapula and humerus.
- The shoulder can be slightly pronated or supinated to highlight the caudomedial/caudolateral aspect of the humeral head, which sometimes allows better depiction of osteochondrosis lesions (Figure 18.25).

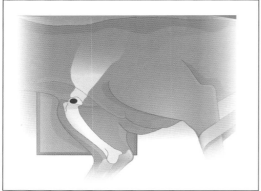

18.24 Patient positioning for a mediolateral view of the shoulder.

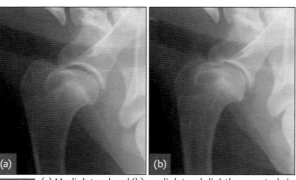

18.25 (a) Mediolateral and (b) mediolateral slightly pronated views of the shoulder. The flattening and adjacent fine mineralized flap on the caudal aspect of the humeral head are not apparent on the original image, but mild pronation skylines the lesion more effectively.

→ IMAGING TECHNIQUES CONTINUED

Caudocranial view

- The animal is placed in dorsal recumbency with the target limb extended cranially and the scapular spine approximately parallel to the cassette/plate (Figure 18.26).
- The primary beam is centred just medial to the acromion.
- Collimate to include the skin margins medial to lateral and approximately one-third of the scapula and humerus proximal to distal.

Speical views

Cranioproximal–craniodistal view

This view provides a skyline view of the intertubercular or bicipital groove, for assessment of new bone formation and mineralization of the supraspinatus and biceps tendon.

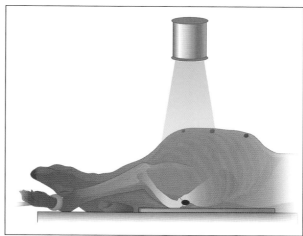

18.26 Patient positioning for a caudocranial view of the shoulder.

- The animal is placed in sternal recumbency with the shoulder and elbow of the target limb flexed and prevented from abduction by laterally placed sandbags (Figure 18.27).
- The head and neck are laterally flexed to the contralateral side.
- The cassette is placed into the crook of the elbow on the cranial surface of the antebrachium.
- The primary beam is centred on the greater tubercle.
- Collimate tightly on the proximal humerus.

ARTHROGRAPHY

The shoulder joint was previously the most common joint in which positive contrast arthrograms were performed. This technique has largely been superseded by the use of CT, MRI and ultrasonography. It can, however, be used to delineate osteochondrosis lesions of the caudal humeral head and although these can often be identified on plain radiographs, contrast may under-run and outline a cartilage flap of osteochondritis dissecans. Potentially more valuable is the ability to visualize the biceps tendon and associated synovial tendon sheath.

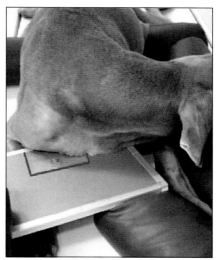

18.27 Patient positioning for a cranioproximal–craniodistal view of the shoulder.

- A small volume (1–5 ml) of non-ionic, low osmolar contrast medium (e.g. iohexol, iopromide) is diluted to approximately 100 mg iodine/ml. Too high a concentration of iodine can result in subtle lesions being masked and care must be taken not to introduce gas bubbles.
- The diluted contrast is injected into the shoulder joint after aseptic preparation.
- Mediolateral and caudocranial radiographs are obtained within 5 minutes of injection.

COMPUTED TOMOGRAPHY

CT has increased soft tissue contrast compared with radiography, but only mineralizing pathology of tendons and muscles is likely to be detected on plain images. Osseous lesions are seen well with CT; however, unlike some other joints, the commonly encountered lesions are also likely to be readily apparent on good quality radiographs. CT does offer some advantages: individual muscles and tendons can be identified and so the origin of periarticular mineralization can be determined (Maddox et al., 2013). Furthermore, images can be acquired concurrently with those of other parts of the thoracic limb, with only a small increase in scan times.

Standard technique

- Scan times are short with multidetector (more than 4-slice) CT units and so images can normally be acquired under sedation.
- The animal should be placed in sternal recumbency with the thoracic limbs fully extended (Figure 18.28).
- The scan margins should extend from slightly proximal to the acromion to include the proximal quarter of the humerus.

→

→ IMAGING TECHNIQUES CONTINUED

- Once acquired, separate images of both shoulders should be reconstructed with as small a field of view as feasible.
- Image reconstruction using both bone and soft tissue algorithms is advisable.

CT arthrography

Like conventional radiographs, intra-articular iodinated media can be used to allow better visualization of soft tissue structures (Silva *et al.*, 2013). A diagnostic quality CT arthrogram allows the medial and lateral glenohumeral ligaments and joint capsule to be identified (Figure 18.29).

The technique is similar to that used for radiographic arthography, with approximately the same volume but a lower concentration of contrast medium generally required (30–80 mg iodine/ml).

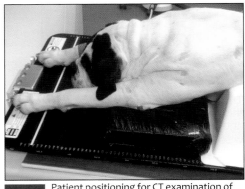

18.28 Patient positioning for CT examination of the shoulder.

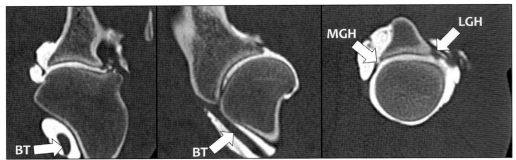

18.29 CT arthrograms of the shoulder of a dog. The biceps tendon (BT) can be seen within the tendon sheath, as well as the medial glenohumeral (MGH) and lateral glenohumeral (LGH) ligaments.

ULTRASONOGRAPHY

Diagnostic ultrasonography is well suited to the imaging of the soft tissue structures of the shoulder. Lesions of the biceps, supraspinatus and infraspinatus tendons can be well characterized and the caudal humeral head and its articular cartilage can be visualized. However, complete evaluation of the medial soft tissue structures of the shoulder, such as the subscapularis, is not generally possible.

The examination is performed with a high frequency linear ultrasonography probe. Abduction and external rotation of the limb is beneficial, especially for the biceps tendon, as this allows a cross-sectional image of the intertubercular groove to be obtained (Figure 18.30).

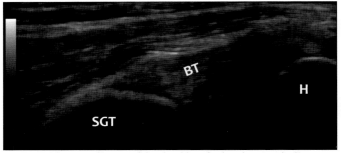

18.30 Ultrasound image of the shoulder of a dog showing the linear fibres of the biceps tendon (BT) originating from the supraglenoid tubercle (SGT) and passing over the proximal humerus (H).

MAGNETIC RESONANCE IMAGING

Magnetic resonance imaging (MRI) offers moderately superior soft tissue contrast to ultrasonography and has the added advantage that the medial structures of the shoulder can be well evaluated. These benefits can justify the increased cost and necessity for general anaesthesia and mean that it is increasingly used more frequently than CT for advanced imaging of the shoulder.

Most of the principal soft tissue structures of the shoulder can be readily evaluated, particularly if intra-articular contrast media are used (Figure 18.31).

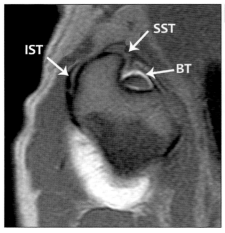

18.31 Transverse T1-weighted MR image (postarthrogram) of the shoulder of a dog, showing the biceps tendon (BT), infraspinatus tendon (IST) and supraspinatus tendon (SST).

→ **IMAGING TECHNIQUES CONTINUED**

Animals are generally scanned in lateral recumbency with the target limb dependent and mildly flexed (Agnello *et al.*, 2008). T1-weighted and T2-weighted sequences are routinely acquired in all three conventional planes (dorsal, sagittal and transverse), with further sequences such as STIR acquired dependent on machine capabilities and suspected pathology.

MRI arthrography

The intra-articular injection of diluted, gadolinium-based contrast medium can further enhance the visibility of the soft tissues, particularly intra-articular structures such as the medial glenohumeral ligament (Schaefer *et al.*, 2010). Volumes and concentrations of gadolinium contrast used have varied, but are generally 4–6 ml of 0.5 mol/l gadolinium diluted with sterile saline to a concentration of between 1:800 and 1:1200.

OPERATIVE TECHNIQUE 18.1

Craniomedial approach to the shoulder

INDICATIONS

This approach is used relatively infrequently but is indicated for the following procedures:

- Exposure of the biceps brachii tendon of origin for investigation and treatment of:
    - Tendon rupture (partial or complete)
    - Medial displacement due to rupture of the transverse humeral ligament
    - Bicipital tenosynovitis
    - Traumatic shoulder luxation by means of bicipital tendon transposition
- Exposure of the scapular tuberosity for treatment of avulsion fractures.

POSITIONING

Dorsal recumbency with the operative limb drawn caudally with a tie; the incision is made over the craniomedial aspect of the joint. Placement of a sterile foam wedge between the limb and thoracic wall can aid access to the craniomedial aspect of the shoulder.

ASSISTANT

Preferable.

EQUIPMENT EXTRAS

Treves self-retaining retractors; Weitlander self-retaining retractors; Gelpi retractors (large and/or small); instruments for placement of any implants required for fixation of a planned greater tubercle osteotomy (Kirschner wires, orthopaedic wire).

SURGICAL TECHNIQUE

A skin incision is made from a point just medial and caudal to the acromion, passing distally over the craniomedial aspect of the humerus (Figure 18.32a). The fascia along the lateral border of the brachiocephalicus muscle is incised (with or without ligation of the omobrachial vein) to allow retraction of the muscle (Figure 18.32b) and exposure of the superficial pectoral muscle (Figure 18.32c), which is elevated and retracted. This is followed in a similar manner by the deep pectoral muscle. The biceps brachii muscle and tendon of origin will be exposed (Figure 18.32d) and can be followed proximally to the transverse humeral ligament and then to the scapular tuberosity.

> **PRACTICAL TIP**
>
> Exposure of the tuberosity can be improved by osteotomy of the greater tubercle (Figure 18.32e), which allows reflection of the supraspinatus muscle, followed by incision of the joint capsule

→ **OPERATIVE TECHNIQUE 18.1 CONTINUED**

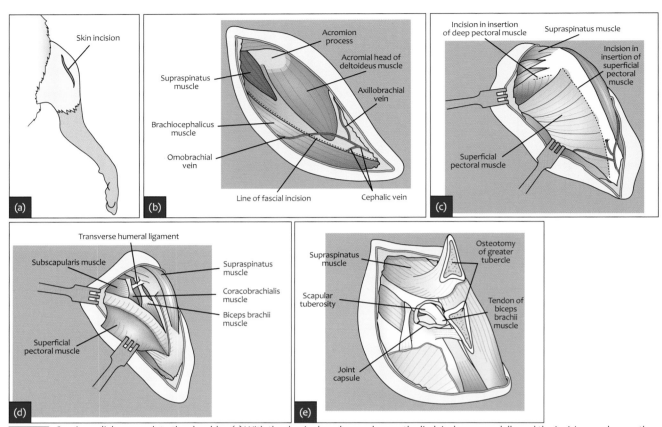

18.32 Craniomedial approach to the shoulder. (a) With the dog in dorsal recumbency, the limb is drawn caudally and the incision made over the craniomedial aspect of the joint. (b) The fascia is incised to allow retraction of the brachiocephalicus muscle. (c) The superficial and deep pectoral muscles are released from their insertion on the humerus. (d) Retraction of the pectoral muscles exposes the biceps brachii tendon of origin. (e) Exposure of the more proximal part of the tendon can be improved by osteotomy of the greater tubercle.

Closure

The greater tubercle must be reattached during closure using crossed Kirschner wires, a lagged bone screw, or pins and a tension-band wire. The placement of the implants is easier if the holes are pre-drilled or the implants placed and removed before the osteotomy is made. The remaining closure involves reattachment of the deep and then superficial pectoral muscles to the deltoideus/superficial fascia using absorbable simple continuous or interrupted cruciate sutures.

POSTOPERATIVE CARE

See individual procedures. Generally, 4 weeks of rest if no osteotomy has been performed; if osteotomy has been performed, rest for 8 weeks and confirm osteotomy healing radiographically.

COMPLICATIONS

See individual procedures.

OPERATIVE TECHNIQUE 18.2

Craniolateral approach to the shoulder

INDICATIONS

Indications for a craniolateral approach are limited but include:

- Exposure of the proximal humerus and scapular neck for treatment of scapulohumeral luxations
- Exposure of the spinatus muscle tendons of insertion for treatment of:
  - Infraspinatus contracture
  - Infraspinatus bursal ossification
  - Mineralization of the supraspinatus tendon.

POSITIONING

Lateral recumbency with operative limb uppermost and drawn caudal to the contralateral limb. Placement of a foam wedge between the legs but under the drapes helps support the affected limb.

ASSISTANT

Desirable but not essential. Of the indications listed, an assistant is possibly most useful for treatment of shoulder luxation.

EQUIPMENT EXTRAS

Treves self-retaining retractors; Weitlander self-retaining retractors; Gelpi retractors (large and/or small).

SURGICAL TECHNIQUE

A skin incision is made from about one-third to halfway up the scapular spine to the distal end of the deltoid tuberosity, passing cranial to the acromion process. (Figure 18.33a). The deep fascia is incised over the scapular spine (Figure 18.33b), which releases the insertions of the omotransversarius and trapezius muscles cranially and the origin of the scapular head of the deltoid muscle caudally. This incision is extended distally towards the omobrachial vein to expose the acromial head of the deltoid muscle which, when reflected caudally, exposes the supraspinatus, infraspinatus and teres minor muscles (Figure 18.33c). Tenotomy of the infraspinatus muscle tendon of insertion improves exposure of the lateral joint capsule (Figure 18.33d). The scapular neck can now be exposed by elevation of the spinatus muscles.

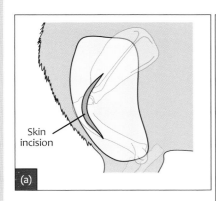

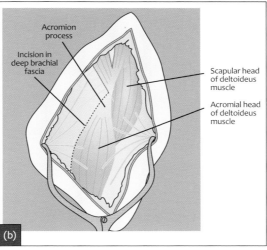

18.33 Craniolateral approach to the shoulder. (a) With the dog in lateral recumbency a skin incision is made from about a third to halfway up the scapular spine to the distal limit of the deltoid tuberosity, passing cranial to the acromion process. (b) An incision is made in the deep brachial fascia. The length of the incision is dictated by which structures are required to be exposed. (continues) ▶

→ **OPERATIVE TECHNIQUE 18.2 CONTINUED**

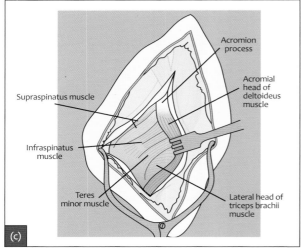
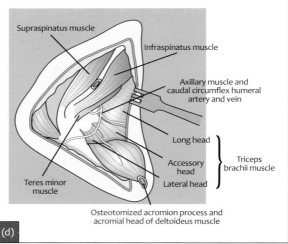

18.33 (continued) Craniolateral approach to the shoulder. (c) Retraction of the acromial head of the deltoid muscle caudally exposes the insertions of the supraspinatus, infraspinatus and teres minor muscles, which can be incised and reflected to expose the lateral glenohumeral ligament and capsule. (d) Tenotomy of the acromial head of the deltoid muscle or osteotomy of the acromion process allows reflection of the deltoid muscle for improved exposure of the lateral aspect of the joint.

PRACTICAL TIP

Improved exposure of the scapular neck can be achieved by reflection of the acromial head of the deltoid muscle, either by tenotomy or osteotomy of the acromial process (see Figure 18.33d). However, for the indications listed, exposure of the scapular neck can usually be achieved without the need for these additional steps

Closure

If tenotomy has been performed, repair requires tendon sutures in the acromial head of the deltoid, infraspinatus muscles or teres minor muscles, and if acromial osteotomy has been performed, reattachment of the acromion is needed, using either Kirschner wires and a tension band or wire sutures (Figure 18.34). The remaining closure involves reattachment of fascia, including insertions of the omotransversarius and trapezius muscles, with simple continuous or interrupted cruciate sutures using an absorbable suture material (e.g. polydioxanone).

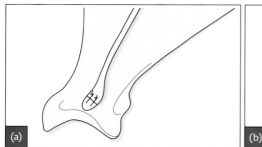
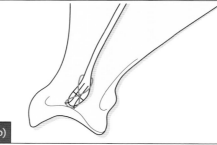

18.34 If an acromion osteotomy has been performed, closure will include reattachment of the process with (a) wire sutures or (b) a pin and tension-band technique.

POSTOPERATIVE CARE

See individual procedures. Generally, 4 weeks of rest if no osteotomy has been performed; if osteotomy has been performed, rest for 8 weeks and confirm osteotomy healing radiographically.

COMPLICATIONS

See individual procedures.

OPERATIVE TECHNIQUE 18.3

Caudolateral approach to the shoulder

INDICATIONS

This is the most frequently used open approach to the shoulder joint. Indications include:

- Exposure of the caudal humeral head for treatment of OCD
- Exposure of the caudal rim of the glenoid for treatment of osteochondrosis (osteochondral fragmentation) or fragmented osteophytes (see Osteophyte removal in Chapter 13).

POSITIONING

Lateral recumbency with operative limb uppermost and drawn cranial to the contralateral limb. Placement of a foam wedge between the legs but under the drapes helps support the affected limb.

ASSISTANT

An assistant is essential in aiding exposure of the caudal humeral head, in particular, since this requires marked internal rotation of the limb.

EQUIPMENT EXTRAS

Treves self-retaining retractors; Weitlander self-retaining retractors; Gelpi retractors (large and/or small).

SURGICAL TECHNIQUE

There are three variations of this surgical approach. The first two give satisfactory exposure but the second is slightly more limited, and the third creates a 'deeper' approach requiring retraction of larger muscle masses (if no assistant is available, it is often easier to expose an OCD lesion using this approach with the aid of self-retaining retractors alone).

A skin incision is made from halfway along the scapular spine, passing caudal to the acromion and curving distally to and about one-third of the way down the humerus (approximately at the distal end of the deltoid tuberosity) (Figure 18.35a). The subcutaneous tissues and fascia are dissected to allow identification of the two heads of the deltoid muscle (Figure 18.35b). These are then separated by blunt dissection and retracted (Figure 18.35c).

Variation 1

The teres minor muscle is identified along with a neurovascular bundle just caudal to it (made up of the cephalic vein, muscular branch of the axillary nerve and the caudal circumflex humeral vessels). The muscle is retracted cranially and the nerves and vessels carefully dissected off the joint capsule and then pushed, or retracted, caudally (Figure 18.35d). An incision is made through the joint capsule to expose the caudal humeral head (Figure 18.35e).

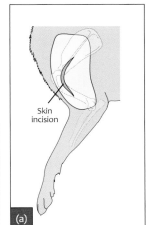
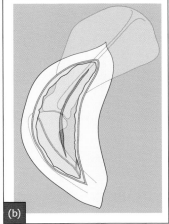
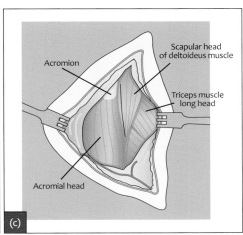

18.35 Caudolateral approach to the shoulder. (a) With the dog in lateral recumbency a skin incision is made from midway down the scapular spine to the distal limit of the deltoid tuberosity, passing caudal to the acromion process. (b) The fascia overlying the deltoid muscle is incised over the division between the scapular and acromial heads of the muscle, which can be seen or palpated; the omobrachial vein normally forms the distal limit of this incision, and where the division meets the scapular spine forms the proximal limit. (c) Using blunt dissection the two heads of the deltoid muscle are then separated to the same limits as in (b). (continues)

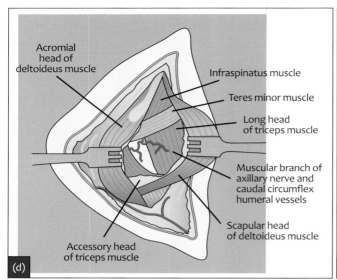

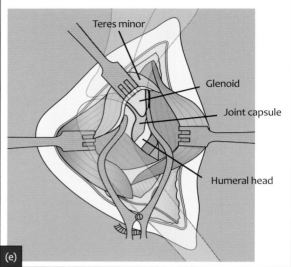

18.35 (continued) Caudolateral approach to the shoulder. (d) Cranial retraction of the acromial head and caudal retraction of the scapular head of the deltoid muscle exposes the teres minor muscle and the neurovascular bundle over the caudal joint capsule. (e) Undermining the neurovascular bundle with blunt dissection will allow it to move caudally, providing ready access to the caudal joint capsule, which is then incised to expose the caudal humeral head.

Variation 2

Having separated the heads of the deltoid muscle, it is possible to gain access to the joint by blunt dissection between the teres minor and infraspinatus muscles (and thus avoid being close to the nerves and vessels mentioned above).

Variation 3

With this approach it is better to make a straight incision between the proximal and distal landmarks described above, rather than the curved incision used for the standard approach. Exposure of the joint capsule may be achieved by separating the scapular head of the deltoid muscle and the lateral head of the triceps muscle (Gahring, 1985) (Figure 18.36).

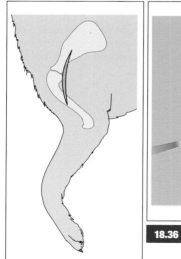

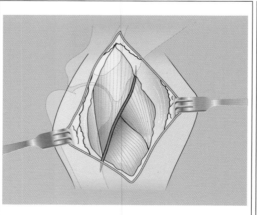

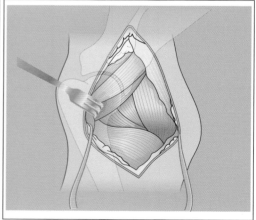

18.36 Caudolateral approach to the shoulder achieved by separating between the scapular head of the deltoid muscle and lateral head of the triceps muscle.

Closure

During closure of variation 1, it is generally possible to suture the joint capsule, or at least suture the caudal margin of the capsule, to the teres minor muscle. The deltoid muscle bellies are then apposed and the overlying fascia sutured. For variation 2, the joint is closed by appositional suturing of the teres minor muscle to the infraspinatus muscle. For variation 3, it may be possible to suture the joint capsule. The bellies of the deltoid muscle and triceps muscle are then apposed.

→ **OPERATIVE TECHNIQUE 18.3 CONTINUED**

PRACTICAL TIP

During routine closure of the subcutaneous fat, picking up the underlying fascia with every other throw helps to close dead space and significantly reduces the likelihood of postoperative seroma formation. If a subcuticular suture is placed then it is again best to pick up the subcutaneous tissue with every other throw for the same reason

POSTOPERATIVE CARE

See individual procedures. Generally, 4 weeks of rest.

COMPLICATIONS

Seroma formation can occur but is very uncommon if the practical tip relating to closure is observed. If seen, it is best treated conservatively and will generally resolve slowly; drainage is not recommended because of the risk of introducing infection.

OPERATIVE TECHNIQUE 18.4

Caudolateral arthrotomy for osteochondritis dissecans of the humeral head

POSITIONING

Lateral recumbency with operative limb uppermost and drawn cranial to the contralateral limb. Placement of a foam wedge between the legs but under the drapes helps support the affected limb.

ASSISTANT

Essential in aiding exposure of the caudal humeral head in particular, since this requires marked internal rotation of the limb facilitating outward rotation of the caudal humeral head to expose the remaining attachment of the OCD flap, which is invariably medial.

EQUIPMENT EXTRAS

Treves self-retaining retractors; Weitlander self-retaining retractors; Gelpi retractors (large and/or small); Hohmann retractors (of appropriate size and including blunt-ended variants); OCD curette(s); Kirschner wires or small drill bits for forage of any eburnated subchondral bone; forceps designed for arthroscopic surgery (useful because of their size).

SURGICAL TECHNIQUE

Follow Operative Technique 18.3. Once the OCD lesion has been identified, the aim is to remove all the loose and under-run articular cartilage from the humeral head, and any 'joint mice' from the caudal joint pouch (Figure 18.37). The latter can generally be retrieved by probing the caudal joint pouch with a pair of haemostats. It is advisable to refrain from placing a Hohmann retractor into the joint space until the majority of the flap has been removed, otherwise there is a chance that the retractor will push the flap off the humeral head and into the medial or cranial joint space, from which retrieval can be difficult. It is useful to grasp the flap with forceps, place a curette under it to the point where it is attached and then lever the flap from the surrounding cartilage. The margins of the defect are then inspected to ensure the entire area of under-run cartilage has been removed, leaving sharp edges all around. Granulation tissue within the defect is left in place but any areas of eburnated bone may be foraged with a Kirschner wire or small drill bit to encourage granulation.

Closure

After thorough flushing of the joint with sterile normal saline, closure is achieved as described in Operative Technique 18.3.

→ OPERATIVE TECHNIQUE 18.4 CONTINUED

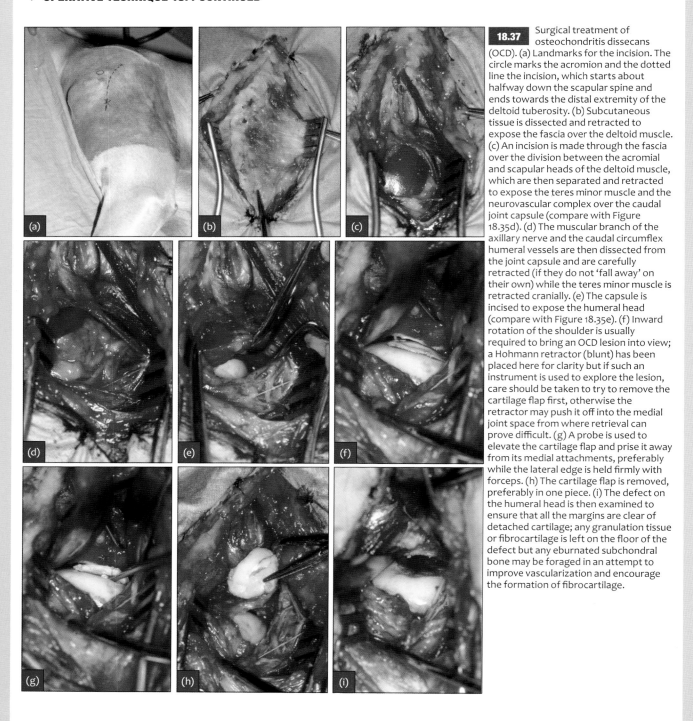

18.37 Surgical treatment of osteochondritis dissecans (OCD). (a) Landmarks for the incision. The circle marks the acromion and the dotted line the incision, which starts about halfway down the scapular spine and ends towards the distal extremity of the deltoid tuberosity. (b) Subcutaneous tissue is dissected and retracted to expose the fascia over the deltoid muscle. (c) An incision is made through the fascia over the division between the acromial and scapular heads of the deltoid muscle, which are then separated and retracted to expose the teres minor muscle and the neurovascular complex over the caudal joint capsule (compare with Figure 18.35d). (d) The muscular branch of the axillary nerve and the caudal circumflex humeral vessels are then dissected from the joint capsule and are carefully retracted (if they do not 'fall away' on their own) while the teres minor muscle is retracted cranially. (e) The capsule is incised to expose the humeral head (compare with Figure 18.35e). (f) Inward rotation of the shoulder is usually required to bring an OCD lesion into view; a Hohmann retractor (blunt) has been placed here for clarity but if such an instrument is used to explore the lesion, care should be taken to try to remove the cartilage flap first, otherwise the retractor may push it off into the medial joint space from where retrieval can prove difficult. (g) A probe is used to elevate the cartilage flap and prise it away from its medial attachments, preferably while the lateral edge is held firmly with forceps. (h) The cartilage flap is removed, preferably in one piece. (i) The defect on the humeral head is then examined to ensure that all the margins are clear of detached cartilage; any granulation tissue or fibrocartilage is left on the floor of the defect but any eburnated subchondral bone may be foraged in an attempt to improve vascularization and encourage the formation of fibrocartilage.

POSTOPERATIVE CARE

The dog should be restricted to lead exercise and room rest for 6–8 weeks while the cartilage defect heals. The distance walked is governed only by what does not make the patient significantly worse (in terms of degree of lameness or stiffness after rest). After that period most cases should be sound and can be returned to normal exercise over the following month.

COMPLICATIONS

- Seroma formation (see Operative Technique 18.3).
- If there is failure to remove completely all the under-run cartilage, lameness may persist and repeat surgery is indicated.

OPERATIVE TECHNIQUE 18.5

Arthroscopy of the shoulder joint

INDICATIONS

Arthroscopy allows magnification of intra-articular structures so is a useful diagnostic tool for occult lameness localized to the shoulder. Other indications include:

* Management of humeral head OCD
* Diagnosis and management of biceps brachii pathology
* Diagnosis and management of glenohumeral ligament pathology.

POSITIONING

Lateral recumbency with operative limb uppermost. Placement of a foam wedge between the legs but under the drapes helps support the affected limb and prevent the shoulder joint space from closing.

ASSISTANT

Not necessary for diagnostic arthroscopy. Desirable for operative arthroscopy, particularly for right shoulder for the right-handed surgeon (and left shoulder for left-handed surgeon).

EQUIPMENT EXTRAS

Arthroscopy tower with light source, camera unit, monitor; 2.7 mm 30-degree arthroscope with sleeve and blunt obturator (2.4 mm arthroscope in small dogs and cats and 4 mm arthroscope in giant breeds); two 50 mm (2 inch) 20 G needles; two 10 ml hypodermic syringes; fluid giving set either in an infusion pressure jacket or a dedicated fluid pump; sufficient quantity of Hartmann's solution (usually 1 litre); for operative arthroscopy appropriate operative instruments will be needed, e.g. appropriately sized cannulas, switching stick, range of arthroscopic grasping forceps, arthroscopic probe.

SURGICAL TECHNIQUE

Lateral portals

A hypodermic needle is placed into the craniolateral aspect of the shoulder joint between the acromion process and the greater tubercle to create an egress portal. Synovial fluid is aspirated and 5–10 ml of Hartmann's solution injected into the joint space. A second hypodermic needle is placed into the joint approximately 1 cm distal to the acromion process (or slightly caudal to this). The needle should pass easily into the joint and move freely (Figure 18.38).

An alternative approach, as used by the authors, is to place the lateral needle first and use this portal to inject the saline. Identification of the craniolateral portal position is more straightforward in this way. A stab incision is made with a No. 11 blade along the path of the lateral needle to enter the joint space. The arthroscope sleeve and blunt obturator are then passed along this tissue track after which the needle is removed. The joint is entered, the obturator is removed and the arthroscope inserted. The light source, camera and giving set are attached and the fluid flow commenced.

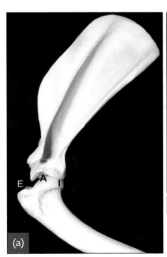
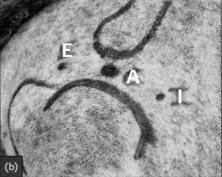
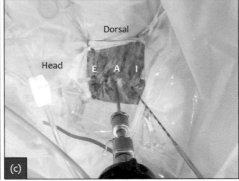

18.38 Arthroscopy of the shoulder joint. (a) Skeleton model demonstrating the portals for a lateral shoulder arthroscopy. (b) Cadaver with lateral shoulder arthroscopy portals marked. (c) Arthroscope *in situ*. A = arthroscope/camera portal; E = egress portal; I = instrument portal.
(a, Reproduced from the *BSAVA Manual of Canine and Feline Endoscopy and Endosurgery*)

→ **OPERATIVE TECHNIQUE 18.5 CONTINUED**

The joint should be inspected in an orderly fashion, starting cranially and medially and passing caudally. After the medial aspect of the joint has been inspected, the articular surfaces are observed, followed by the craniolateral and caudolateral aspects.

An instrument portal is usually established caudolaterally or craniolaterally, initially by placement of a hypodermic needle under arthroscopic guidance. A stab incision along the line of this needle then allows placement of a switching stick over which the instrument cannula is placed. Removal of the switching stick allows placement of operative instruments.

Craniomedial portal (push-through technique)

If a craniomedial portal is required, this can be established using a push-through technique. Using the lateral portal, the arthroscope is pushed against the joint capsule between the subscapularis tendon and the biceps brachii tendon. The sleeve is held in this position as the arthroscope is removed and a switching stick inserted and used to puncture the capsule and push through the soft tissues to exit under the skin craniomedially. An incision over the protruding switching stick allows the stick to be pushed further and the arthroscope sleeve is moved from the lateral position over the stick and guided into the joint craniomedially. This portal allows inspection of the medial gutter and the lateral aspect of the joint.

> **Note:** A larger clip and draping area is required for this portal and the head and neck may inhibit access to this region. If so, a hanging limb technique is preferable

PRACTICAL TIP

All portals are interchangeable as necessary

See *BSAVA Manual of Canine and Feline Endoscopy and Endosurgery* for more details on surgical technique.

Closure

Single skin sutures are placed in the portal sites.

POSTOPERATIVE CARE

Generally, 48 hours rest following diagnostic arthroscopy. If arthroscopic surgery is performed, the period of rest is extended as appropriate for each individual procedure.

COMPLICATIONS

Accumulation of extravasated subcutaneous fluid can occur during the procedure. This can cause some joint space collapse; it resolves within 48–72 hours.

OPERATIVE TECHNIQUE 18.6

Lateral shoulder stabilization

POSITIONING

See Operative Technique 18.2.

ASSISTANT

Desirable but not essential.

EQUIPMENT EXTRAS

Periosteal elevator; drill bits and sleeves of appropriate sizes to create bone tunnels; wire to create loops to facilitate placement of prosthesis through tunnels:

- Bone screws and spiked washers, together with appropriate drill bit, depth gauge, (tap) and screwdriver; or
- Suture screws, together with appropriate drill bit, depth gauge and screwdriver; or
- Tissue anchors, together with the appropriate 'driving' instrumentation.

Material for the prosthesis, generally non-absorbable and either coated braided polyester or monofilament nylon (leader line); crimps and crimping pliers if these are to be used to secure the material and Ligafiba.
See Operative Technique 18.2.

SURGICAL TECHNIQUE

Follow Operative Technique 18.2. In order to expose the distal aspect of the scapular spine for anchorage of a lateral prosthesis, osteotomy of the acromion can be performed (Figure 18.39a). However, by separating the two heads of the deltoid muscle it is quite possible to retrieve suture material placed through a tunnel in the scapular spine and then pass it back under the acromial head of the deltoid muscle. A cranial to caudal tunnel is drilled through the scapular spine as far distally as possible while avoiding penetration of the concave articular surface, and the prosthesis anchored proximally by passage through this and back under the acromial head of the deltoid muscle (Figure 18.39b). Alternatively, a suture screw or tissue anchor can be used to secure the origin of the prosthesis. This is placed in the scapular neck cranial to the scapular spine, with care taken to avoid the suprascapular nerve (Figure 18.39c).

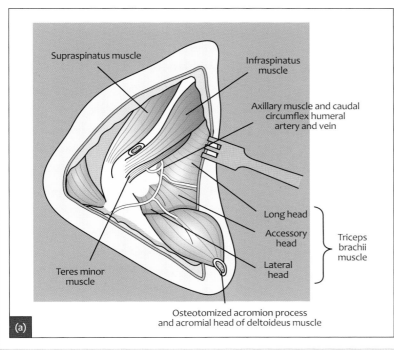

18.39 Lateral stabilization of the shoulder joint. (a) The caudal aspect of the scapular spine can be accessed by osteotomy of the acromion process, but separation of the two heads of the deltoid muscle will usually suffice; osteotomy is shown here for clarity. (continues) ▶

→ **OPERATIVE TECHNIQUE 18.6 CONTINUED**

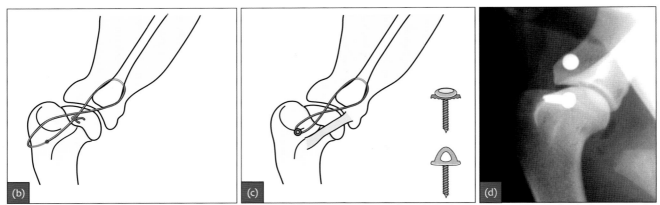

18.39 (continued) Lateral stabilization of the shoulder joint. (b) A lateral prosthesis of braided polyester or monofilament leader line is passed through a tunnel created in the distal scapular spine and a second tunnel drilled in the greater tubercle or (c) is anchored around or through an implant (bone screw with spiked washer, suture screw, tissue anchor) placed in the greater tubercle close to the insertion of the teres minor muscle. (d) Postoperative mediolateral radiograph of the shoulder of 3-year-old Border Collie treated for lateral luxation.

The distal attachment point for the prosthesis is on the lateral aspect of the greater tubercle, either where the ligament insertion can be seen or close to the insertion of the infraspinatus muscle if the remnants of the ligament cannot be identified. Fixation of the prosthesis can be achieved by creation of a caudocranial tunnel (Figure 18.39b) in the greater tubercle (which can be difficult to execute). Alternatives to this include fixation under a bone screw and spiked washer, through a suture screw or a tissue anchor (Figure 18.39cd). When tying or crimping the prosthesis it is important not to over-tighten, since this will create abduction of the limb and encourage early failure of the prosthetic material.

PRACTICAL TIP

Placement of a combined lateral and medial prosthesis (Figure 18.40a–d) requires access to the medial aspect of the joint. This can be achieved by retraction of the supraspinatus muscle

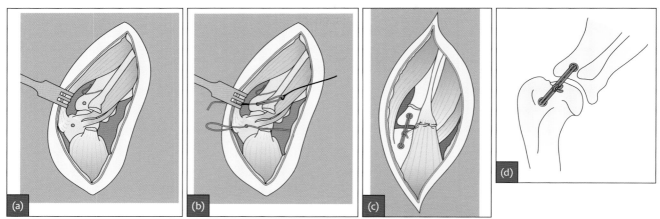

18.40 Lateral shoulder stabilization including modification to combine lateral and medial stabilization. (a) The scapular neck and proximal humerus are exposed as shown in Figure 18.33. (b) Transverse tunnels are created in the scapular neck and humerus close to the insertion of the teres minor muscle. A prosthesis of braided nylon or leader line is passed through these tunnels. (c) After repair of any available joint capsule, the prosthesis is tightened so the joint is stable but not restricted in range of motion, and tied (or crimped). (d) Position of the prosthesis.

Closure

See Operative Technique 18.2.

POSTOPERATIVE CARE

Following surgery the dog should be restricted to gradually increasing lead exercise and room rest for 6–8 weeks while fibrosis becomes established. After that period most cases should be sound and can be returned to normal exercise over the following month.

COMPLICATIONS

Implant failure is an uncommon complication.

OPERATIVE TECHNIQUE 18.7A

Medial shoulder stabilization – imbrication of the subscapularis muscle

POSITIONING

See Operative Technique 18.1.

ASSISTANT

Essential, as limb needs to be externally rotated.

EQUIPMENT EXTRAS

Treves self-retaining retractors; Weitlander self-retaining retractors; Gelpi retractors (large and/or small); periosteal elevator; 3.5 metric (0 USP) or 4 metric (10 USP) polydioxanone or monofilament nylon.

SURGICAL TECHNIQUE

Follow Operative Technique 18.1. After identification of the biceps tendon, the coracobrachialis and subscapularis tendons are found immediately caudal to it. The tendon of the subscapularis muscle can be isolated using Mayo or Metzenbaum scissors (Figure 18.41a). One or two horizontal mattress sutures are placed in the proximal to distal extremities of the tendon and tightened in order to imbricate the tendon (Figure 18.41b).

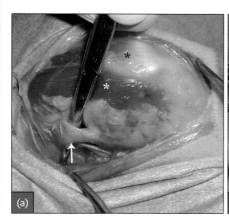
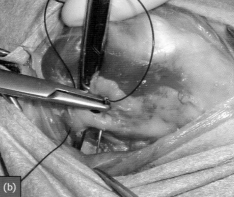

18.41 (a) Identification of the subscapularis muscle tendon of insertion (arrowed), supraspinatus muscle (white asterisk) and greater tubercle (black asterisk). (b) Placement of the horizontal mattress suture through the tendon of the subscapularis muscle.

Note: It is important to isolate the tendon when placing the sutures in order that inadvertent entrapment of other local structures is avoided. Place the proximal arm of the suture superficially and the distal arm through the main body of the tendon

---

Closure

See Operative Technique 18.1.

POSTOPERATIVE CARE

Following surgery the dog should be restricted to lead exercise and room rest for 6–8 weeks while fibrosis becomes established.

COMPLICATIONS

* Seroma formation.
* Wound dehiscence.

OPERATIVE TECHNIQUE 18.7B

Medial shoulder stabilization – placement of a medial collateral prosthesis

POSITIONING

See Operative Technique 18.1.

ASSISTANT

Essential, as the limb needs to be held externally rotated.

EQUIPMENT EXTRAS

See Operative Technique 18.1; suture screws or tissue anchors, with instrumentation to apply them; crimps and pliers for crimping if these are to be used to secure the sutures; small Hohmann retractors.

SURGICAL TECHNIQUE

Follow Operative Technique 18.1. The subscapularis muscle is incised and elevated to reveal the medial joint capsule and remnants of the medial glenohumeral ligament. This exposure is aided by placement of Gelpi retractors or by using small Hohmann retractors behind the scapula and cranially under the supraspinatus muscle (Figure 18.42a). Suture screws or tissue anchors are then placed at the points of origin (two) and insertion (one) of the ligament. Sutures of braided polyester or monofilament nylon are then placed to recreate both components of the ligament (Figure 18.42b). When tying or crimping the prosthesis, it is important not to over-tighten since this will result in adduction of the limb and encourage early failure of the material.

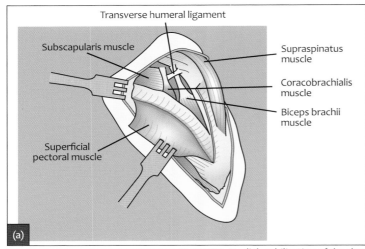

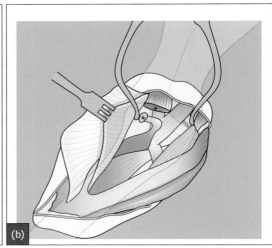

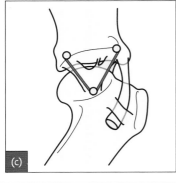

18.42 Medial stabilization of the shoulder joint. (a) Retraction of the pectoral muscle exposes the biceps brachii tendon of origin. (Note this is an extension of the technique shown in Figure 18.32d.) (b) Incisions are made in the coracobrachialis (∗) and subscapularis (+) tendons to expose the joint capsule and glenohumeral ligament. Exposure can be helped by placement of Gelpi retractors or using a small Hohmann retractor caudal to the scapula and a second one under the supraspinatus muscle, passing cranial to the scapula. (c) Suture screws or tissue anchors are then introduced at the points of origin and insertion of the medial glenohumeral ligament, and two separate sutures of braided polyester or monofilament leader line are used to replace both the cranial and caudal components of the ligament. (Note that these are simplified drawings showing schematic examples of the surgical procedure. Certain anatomical features have been omitted for clarity.)

→ **OPERATIVE TECHNIQUE 18.7B CONTINUED**

Closure

See Operative Technique 18.1.

Following surgery the dog should be restricted to room rest for 6–8 weeks. After that, a gradual return to lead exercise is recommended; the distance walked is governed only by what does not make the patient significantly worse (in terms of degree of lameness or stiffness after rest).

COMPLICATIONS

Implant failure is an uncommon complication.

OPERATIVE TECHNIQUE 18.8

Tenotomy or tenodesis of the biceps brachii tendon of origin

POSITIONING

See Operative Technique 18.1.

ASSISTANT

Desirable but not essential.

EQUIPMENT EXTRAS

See Operative Technique 18.1.

- Tenotomy: No. 11 scalpel blade.
- Tenodesis – there are two methods to fixate the tendon origin:
  - Method 1 – ligament staple of appropriate size (usually 8 or 11 mm) and a means of driving it home (mallet ± staple guide)
  - Method 2 – bone screw and spiked washer; appropriate drill bit; sleeve; depth gauge; (tap if non-self-tapping screw); screw driver.

SURGICAL TECHNIQUE

Follow Operative Technique 18.1 to expose the biceps tendon (Figure 18.43). In the case of tenotomy, the tendon can be followed proximally to its point of origin on the supraglenoid tubercle and released using a scalpel blade. Note that tenotomy may also be undertaken arthroscopically (see Operative Technique 18.5).

Tenodesis can be achieved by two different methods.

Method 1

The simplest technique is to place a ligament staple over the tendon and drive it into the humerus (Figure 18.44a). A tenotomy can then be performed, the tendon folded over the staple and sutured to itself with 3 or 3.5 metric (2/0 or 0 USP) polydioxanone.

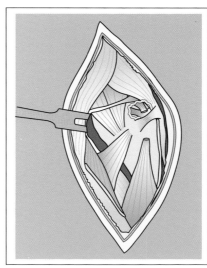

18.43 The biceps brachii tendon of origin is exposed by way of a craniomedial approach.

→ **OPERATIVE TECHNIQUE 18.8 CONTINUED**

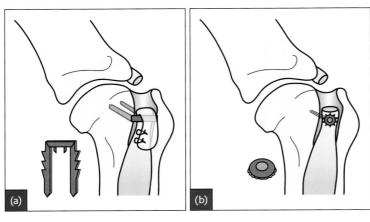

18.44 Methods of achieving biceps tenodesis. (a) A ligament staple is used to secure the tendon to the proximal humerus; the tendon is then incised from the scapular tuberosity, folded over the staple and sutured to itself. (b) A bone screw and spiked washer are used to secure the tendon to the proximal humerus before or after it is incised from the scapular tuberosity.

Method 2

Alternatively, the biceps tendon can be secured to the humerus with a bone screw and spiked washer (Figure 18.44b).

> **WARNING**
>
> In all cases, it is important that the elbow is held in extension when the tendon is fixed to the humerus, otherwise the joint will have a reduced range of motion postoperatively

Closure

See Operative Technique 18.1.

POSTOPERATIVE CARE

Following surgery the dog should be restricted to lead exercise and room rest for 6–8 weeks while the tendon heals or the tenodesis becomes established. The distance walked is governed only by what does not make the patient significantly worse (in terms of degree of lameness or stiffness after rest). After that period most cases should be sound and can be returned to normal exercise over the following month.

COMPLICATIONS

Implant failure is an uncommon complication.

Chapter 19

The elbow

Neil Burton

Elbow disease is the most common cause of thoracic limb lameness in medium to large-breed dogs due in large part to the prevalence and consequences of developmental disease affecting this joint. The elbow has a complex articular topography and this, coupled with small joint spaces, renders a low tolerance to disturbances of growth and articulation that may occur during development. Recent advances in dynamic elbow imaging, such as fluoroscopic kinematography (comprising bi-planar high-speed fluoroscopy), are permitting objective mapping of elbow articulation during gait for the first time. This is revealing that complex axial, translatory and rotatory relationships exist between the humeral, radial and ulnar articulations. Additionally, the increased use and accessibility of arthroscopy, advanced imaging and gait analysis in veterinary surgery are giving a wider appreciation of articular lesions, as well as providing data that have challenged the efficacy of previously well established treatments for elbow disease.

Clinical anatomy

The elbow joint is a compound ginglymus or hinge joint. Normal passive range of motion has been previously defined as approximately 130 degrees in the Labrador Retriever (166 degrees extension to 36 degrees flexion) and 141 degrees in the cat (163 degrees extension to 22 degrees flexion), with approximately 70 degrees of rotation (Jaeger et al., 2002; Jaeger et al., 2007). In the dog, both breed and conformational differences probably exist but have not been defined.

Bony anatomy

Three articulations, humeroradial, humeroulnar and radioulnar, are present within a common joint cavity (Figure 19.1). The articular surface of the distal humerus, the humeral condyle, is helical in morphology and offset cranially from the long axis of the humerus. It comprises a smaller lateral capitulum articulating with the radial head and a more prominent medial trochlea articulating with the trochlear notch of the ulna. The humeral condyle develops as separate lateral and medial ossification centres that fuse by 12 weeks to become a single condyle. The lateral and medial epicondyles are readily palpable surgical landmarks and are located both caudal and proximal to the centre of the humeral condyle, an important consideration when placing transcondylar implants.

The proximal ulna has three processes on the cranial surface, the anconeal process and two smaller unnamed processes that lie laterally and medially near the proximo-

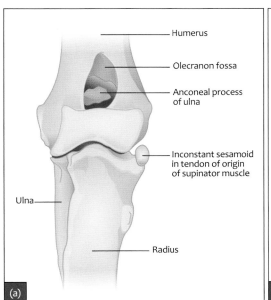

Humerus

Olecranon fossa

Anconeal process of ulna

Inconstant sesamoid in tendon of origin of supinator muscle

Ulna

Radius

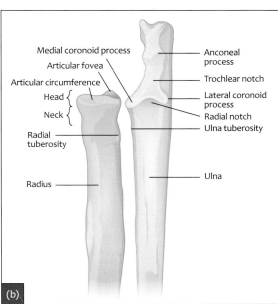

Medial coronoid process

Articular fovea

Articular circumference

Head

Neck

Radial tuberosity

Radius

Anconeal process

Trochlear notch

Lateral coronoid process

Radial notch

Ulna tuberosity

Ulna

19.1 Bony anatomy of the elbow joint. (a) Cranial view of the elbow. (b) Cranial view of the radius and ulna disarticulated.

caudal extremity of the olecranon, these functioning as a groove for the common triceps tendon which attaches near this site. The anconeal process articulates with the caudoproximal intracondylar surface of the humerus and fits into the supratrochlear foramen when the joint is maximally extended. A fossa rather than a foramen is present in the cat. The proximal ulna has a lateral to medial inclination from proximal to distal in the dorsal plane and this should be considered when placing intramedullary fixation. The trochlear notch of the ulna articulates with the trochlea of the humerus and ends distally in two prominences, the medial and lateral coronoid processes. The medial coronoid process is significantly larger and more distally oriented. The radial head articulates with a curved depression called the radial notch which is located between the two coronoid processes, with the medial, axial concave aspect of the notch termed the radial incisure. The radius is held in place by the annular ligament. Static load distribution studies reveal load through the humeroradial and humeroulnar joints to be 51% and 49% respectively (Mason *et al.*, 2005).

Ligaments

The lateral and medial collateral ligaments have their origins on the lateral and medial epicondyles, respectively, and insert as double radial and ulnar branches (Figure 19.2). The lateral collateral ligament blends with the annular ligament before dividing distally into two crura, the larger of these inserting on the radial head, the lesser on the ulna. A sesamoid bone is occasionally found between the lateral collateral ligament and the radial head in the tendon of origin of the supinator muscle. The medial collateral ligament similarly divides into two crura, a lesser branch inserting on the radial head while the larger branch passes deeply into the interosseous space before inserting mainly on the ulna but also on the radius. The annular ligament forms a circumferential loop around the cranial aspect of the radius, with lateral and medial attachments abaxial and distal to the respective coronoid processes of the ulna.

Muscles and tendons

The periarticular muscle groups of the elbow comprise the insertions of the triceps brachii and anconeus caudally (elbow extension) and the insertions of the brachialis and biceps brachii cranially (elbow flexion). The carpal and digital extensor muscles originate directly or indirectly from the lateral epicondyle; from cranially to caudally these are:

- Extensor carpi radialis
- Common digital extensor
- Lateral digital extensor
- Extensor carpi ulnaris.

The supinator muscle originates on the lateral humeral epicondyle and lateral ligament and lies under the extensor carpi radialis; the lateral collateral ligament lies between the lateral digital extensor and extensor carpi ulnaris.

The majority of the carpal and digital flexor muscles originate around the medial epicondyle. From cranially to caudally these are:

- Flexor carpi radialis (humeral head)
- Deep digital flexor (humeral, radial and ulnar heads)
- Superficial digital flexor (humeral head)
- Flexor carpi ulnaris (humeral and ulnar heads).

The pronator teres originates on the medial humeral epicondyle cranial to the flexor carpi radialis and the medial collateral ligament lies between these two muscles.

Neurovascular structures

The radial nerve traverses from proximocaudal to craniodistal across the distal third of the lateral aspect of the humerus with branches supplying the triceps group, responsible for elbow extension (Figure 19.3). The musculocutaneous nerve lies in close proximity to, and innervates, the biceps brachii, responsible for elbow flexion. On the medial aspect of the joint, the ulnar nerve passes caudally and the median nerve cranially relative to the medial

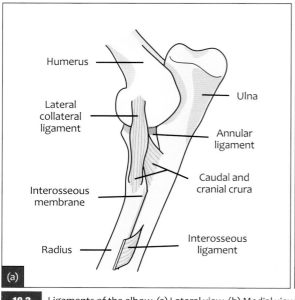

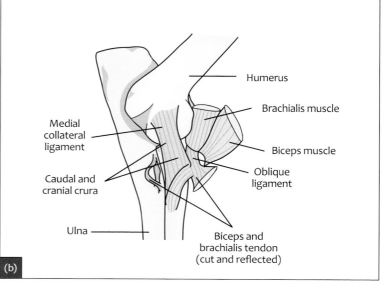

19.2 Ligaments of the elbow. (a) Lateral view. (b) Medial view.

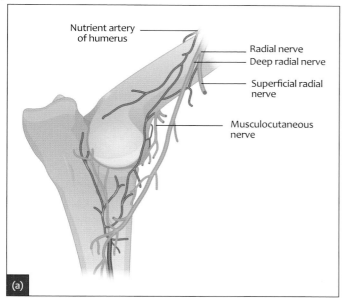

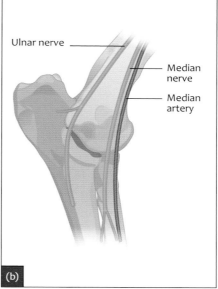

19.3 Neurovascular structures of the elbow. (a) Lateral view. (b) Medial view.

epicondylar ridge. The median nerve gives branches to the pronator teres which inserts on the proximal dorsal radius and both median and ulnar nerves give branches to the carpal flexor muscle groups. A branch of the brachial artery passes distal to the medial aspect of the elbow close to the pronator teres muscle. In the cat, the medial epicondyle contains a supracondylar foramen through which the median nerve, artery and vein pass.

Clinical examination

This should begin with assessment of the conformation of the dog while standing (Figure 19.4) followed by observation of the dog walking and trotting on a lead away and toward the clinician, as well as in front of the clinician to

the left and right, allowing information on stance, swing phases of the gait and angular excursion of the elbow to be subjectively assessed. Should unilateral lameness be present, this will be characterized by a downward nod of the head as the sound limb enters stance. However, the clinician should be mindful that bilateral developmental elbow disease is common and in such cases lameness can erroneously appear unilateral should one elbow be more painful than the other. Equally, if lameness is of similar magnitude bilaterally, no head nod may be present. However, abduction of the elbows, reduced angular excursion during stance and 'flicking' or accelerated carpal extension during the swing phase of gait are adaptive responses that may be appreciable.

Manipulation of the elbow should include assessment of range of motion; a goniometer allows objective assessment. The joint should be assessed for the presence or

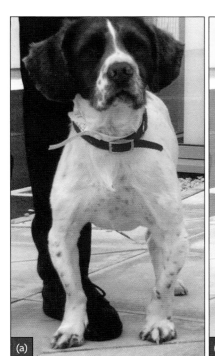

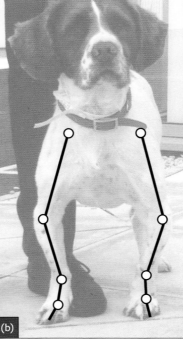

19.4 Clinical examination should begin with assessment of conformation of the dog when standing. (a) A 3-year-old neutered male Springer Spaniel presented with bilateral thoracic limb lameness and was subsequently diagnosed with both bilateral medial coronoid process disease and incomplete ossification/intracondylar fissure-fracture of the humeral condyle (IOHC/ICFF). (b) Overlay illustrating the cranial long axes of the brachii, antibrachii and manus. Even allowing for breed conformation, the dog is standing with marked abduction of both elbows and external rotation of the manus, an adaptive posture suggestive of bilateral elbow medial compartment pain.

absence of crepitus, thickening due to fibrosis and for effusion, the latter being most readily palpable on the caudolateral aspect of the joint. Observation of the patient for a pain response during both full extension and full flexion of the elbow, each with concurrent supination of the antebrachium (which selectively compresses the medial joint compartment) are useful tests (Figure 19.5). Reassessment of gait for any exacerbation of lameness immediately following these manoeuvres can be helpful. Palpation of the lateral epicondylar crest and compressive deep palpation applied transversely across the condyle may evoke a pain response in cases of incomplete ossification/intracondylar fissure-fracture of the humeral condyle (IOHC/ICFF).

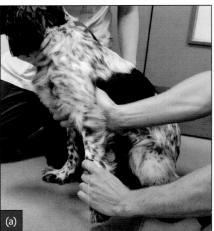

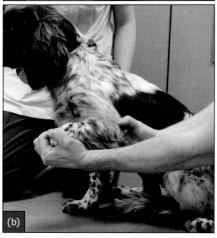

19.5 Examination for evidence of elbow pain. (a) Full extension of the elbow; a hand is placed behind the olecranon and the antebrachium is pushed caudally and firmly held in this position for a few seconds. (b) Flexion of the elbow with concurrent supination (external rotation) of the antebrachium compresses the medial joint compartment.

Diagnostic imaging

Specific details on appropriate imaging techniques for the elbow are provided in the imaging section at the end of this chapter. For more general information on imaging techniques and their application, see Chapter 3.

Arthroscopy

Arthroscopic examination of the elbow provides detailed information on the morphology of articular cartilage. Its use in the quantification of joint congruity has also been described (Wagner *et al.*, 2007); however, a recent study has revealed that congruence may be altered significantly

as a function of arthroscope placement (Skinner *et al.*, 2015). In both dogs and cats, the arthroscope, instrument portal and egress needle are usually placed medially (Van Ryssen *et al.*, 1993; Staiger and Beale, 2005) (see Operative Technique 19.1).

From a medial portal the following structures can be assessed (Figure 19.6):

- Cranial and medial aspects of the anconeal process
- Medial trochlear notch of the ulna
- The humeral trochlea and axial capitulum of the humerus
- Medial and lateral coronoid processes
- Medial, cranial and caudal aspects of the radial head
- Synovium and annular ligament.

More details on arthroscopy can be found in Chapter 15.

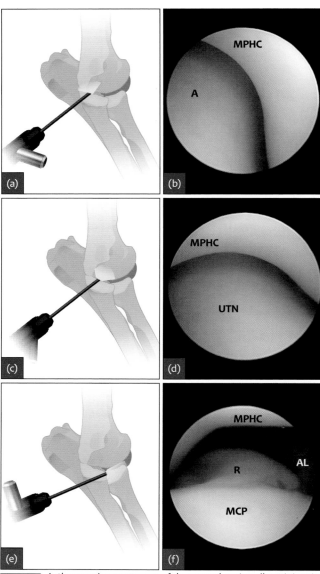

19.6 Arthroscopic appearance of the normal canine elbow joint via a medial portal. (a) The light post is positioned to view the caudomedial joint. (b) View of the caudomedial joint showing the anconeal process (A) and medial portion of the humeral condyle (MPHC). (c) The light post is positioned to view the centromedial joint. (d) The centromedial joint showing the MPHC and ulnar trochlear notch (UTN). (e) The light post is positioned to view the craniomedial joint. (f) The craniomedial joint showing the MPHC, medial coronoid process (MCP), radial head (R) and annular ligament (AL).

Surgical approaches to the elbow

Caudolateral approach

This approach (see Operative Technique 19.2) is indicated for excision or internal fixation of an ununited anconeal process, surgical reduction of lateral elbow luxation or fracture fixation of the lateral portion of the humeral condyle.

Medial approach

The medial approach (see Operative Technique 19.3) is indicated for exploration of the medial compartment of the elbow, subtotal coronoidectomy (see Operative Technique 19.4), removal of large medial coronoid process fragments that cannot be retrieved arthroscopically and for debridement of large osteochondritis dissecans (OCD) lesions (see Operative Technique 19.5). The approach can also be extended proximally for fracture fixation of the medial portion of the humeral condyle.

Elbow luxation

Luxation of the elbow can be classified as traumatic, developmental (attributable to asynchronous radial and ulnar growth) or congenital (Langley-Hobbs and Carmichael, 1996).

Traumatic luxation

The incidence of traumatic elbow luxation is low when compared to that of hip luxation (Billings et al., 1992) as trauma to the elbow joint more often results in fracture rather than luxation (Walker and Hickman, 1958). Luxation most commonly occurs as a result of vehicular trauma with around 90% of cases resulting in lateral displacement of the radius and ulna relative to the humerus (O'Brien et al., 1992). Lateral luxation appears predisposed due to a substantially larger medial condyle precluding medial ulnar displacement. Conversely the smaller, rounded topography of the lateral condyle allows the anconeal process to clear the lateral epicondylar crest when the elbow is in greater than 90 degrees of flexion. Partial luxation (with retention of the anconeus in the olecranon fossa) as well as complete medial (Bongartz et al., 2008) and caudal luxations have also been reported (Figure 19.7). In the cat, lateral, medial and cranial luxations are described. In each case, the mechanism of luxation is thought to be via internally induced musculotendinous torsional moments across the joint experienced at the time of trauma (Campbell, 1971).

Diagnosis

As a high proportion of cases follow vehicular trauma, it is important that initial assessment of the patient should investigate the presence of concurrent cervicothoracic or abdominal trauma. A neurological examination of the limb should also be performed, at least to check cutaneous and deep pain sensation in the distal limb, although the incidence of concurrent brachial plexus/peripheral nerve injury is rare. In the case of lateral luxation, affected animals adopt a characteristic posture with semi-flexion of the elbow combined with abduction and supination of the antebrachium and manus. There is marked soft tissue swelling around the elbow joint with crepitus, pain and a reduced range of motion on manipulation. The laterally displaced trochlear notch and radial head are readily palpable with the lateral epicondyle of the humerus being more difficult to identify. Orthogonal radiographs or computed tomography (CT) of the elbow should be performed and evaluated for evidence of concurrent articular fracture and avulsion fracture of the origin/insertion of the collateral ligament(s).

Treatment

Closed reduction is performed under general anaesthesia and is usually successful (see Operative Technique 19.6). It should be attempted as soon as the patient is stable and

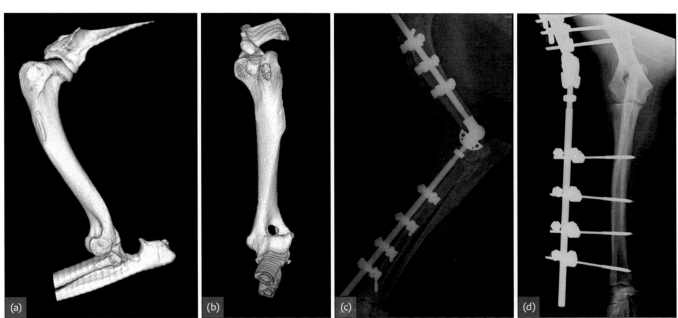

19.7 (a–b) Volume rendered CT images of a rare, traumatic caudal elbow luxation in a 5-year-old neutered male Labrador Retriever. (c–d) The joint was reduced closed and a transarticular external skeletal fixator applied to the humerus and radius for 3 weeks.
(© Dr Kevin Parsons)

before organization of the intra-articular haematoma and muscle contracture make reduction difficult. Following closed reduction of the elbow, orthogonal radiographs should be repeated to confirm reduction. If the elbow is deemed to be palpably stable, a Spica splinted dressing is applied to the limb for 10–14 days followed by a further 2 weeks of room rest and strictly controlled lead exercise, with a subsequent incremental return to normal exercise over the ensuing 4–6 week period.

Surgical intervention is indicated where closed reduction has failed and to repair/replace collateral support when indicated. Additionally it allows inspection of the articular surfaces and removal of any chip fractures. Open reduction is undertaken via a caudolateral approach and the joint is cleared of haematoma/granulation tissue prior to careful reduction.

Following either closed or open reduction, quantification of adjunctive collateral ligament damage is imperative for successful management. In dogs, opinion between studies is split as to whether collateral ligament damage occurs in only a proportion of cases (18–50%) or whether damage, particularly to the lateral collateral in the case of lateral luxation, may be a prerequisite for luxation to occur (Billings *et al.*, 1992; Farrell *et al.*, 2007). It has been suggested that collateral ligament integrity can reliably be evaluated following closed reduction by measurement of the amount of supination and pronation of the manus achievable with both the carpus and elbow held at 90 degrees of flexion (Campbell, 1969). In cadaver limbs with intact collateral ligaments, supination of 60–70 degrees and pronation of 40–50 degrees was possible, increasing to 120–140 degrees of supination with lateral collateral ligament (LCL) transection and 100 degrees of pronation with medial collateral ligament (MCL) transection (Figure 19.8) (Campbell, 1969). A recent *in vitro* study has validated this test as reliable but highlighted that significant inter-animal variability may exist with a strong correlation between increased size and smaller angle of rotation (Farrell *et al.*, 2007); thus the contralateral elbow should always be used as a control. This study also defined normal feline supination as 108–151 degrees, increasing to 167 degrees (± 13.1 degrees) with LCL sectioning, and normal pronation as 79–112 degrees, increasing to 99 degrees (± 17.6 degrees) with MCL sectioning. Elbow luxation was not possible in the cat unless both lateral and medial collateral ligaments were sectioned.

Should the joint be deemed unstable then surgical stabilization of the collateral ligament(s) is indicated (see Operative Technique 19.7). Avulsion fracture of the origin of the collateral ligament can be repaired with a suture placed through bone tunnels or with screws and washers, while insertional avulsions are either similarly repaired or sutured to the annular ligament. Mid-body tears can be sutured primarily, with or without augmentation with suture or autogenous graft (Campbell, 1971). Regardless of the repair technique, the limb is coapted with a Spica splint for 2 weeks and exercise controlled as for closed reduction.

Where primary repair is not possible, a collateral ligament prosthesis may be placed through bone tunnels in the humerus, radius and ulna and secured with a self-locking knot with the elbow in 135 degrees of extension (Figure 19.9) (Farrell *et al.*, 2009). In dogs, a non-absorbable encircling suture (e.g. 7 metric FiberWire®, Arthrex) is used (Farrell *et al.*, 2007) and in cats, a 4 metric (1 USP) polydioxanone suture is placed. Alternatively, transarticular external skeletal fixation can be applied for 4–6 weeks, either as a primary stabilization technique, or to protect the primary repair (see Figure 19.7).

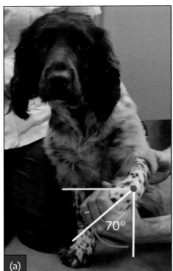

(a)

70°

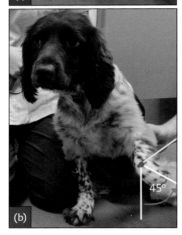

(b)

45°

19.8 Testing for collateral ligament integrity following closed reduction of the joint. The carpus and elbow are both flexed to 90 degrees and the elbow supported.
(a) Lateral collateral integrity testing: supination is limited to about 70 degrees by the lateral collateral ligament (white lines) but rupture may allow this to increase to more than 140 degrees (yellow line).
(b) Medial collateral integrity testing: pronation is limited to about 45 degrees by the medial collateral ligament (white lines) but rupture may allow this to increase to more than 90 degrees (yellow line).

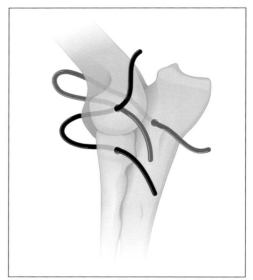

19.9 Lateral view of the elbow with placement of a Farrell suture for traumatic elbow luxation. Transverse bone tunnels are drilled in the humeral condyle at the level of the lateral and medial collateral ligament origins craniodistal to the epicondyles, through the radial head at the level of the insertion of the collateral ligament and through the ulna at the mid-portion of the ulnar trochlear notch equidistant between the articular surface and caudal ulnar cortex. Suture material is pre-placed through the humeral and ulnar and the humeral and radial holes prior to tying with the elbow at a mid-stance angle of 135 degrees.
(Redrawn after Farrell *et al.*, (2007) © John Wiley and Sons)

Prognosis

A good prognosis is reported in 87% of cases receiving prompt closed reduction and in 56% of cases requiring open reduction (O'Brien *et al.*, 1992). Osteoarthritis is reported as a sequel in between 50 and 100% of cases (Meyer-Lindenberg *et al.*, 1991; Billings *et al.*, 1992). In one study, re-luxation did not occur in any of the cats following closed reduction (Mitchell, 2011).

Congenital luxation

Congenital elbow luxation is rare, with three clinical manifestations described: humeroradial (Type I), humeroulnar (Type II) and combined humeroradial and humeroulnar luxation (Type III). The precise aetiopathogenesis of luxation is unknown, with a possible hereditary basis having been proposed (Bingel and Riser, 1977). Concurrent abnormalities may include patellar luxation, hydrocephalus and femoral head and neck necrosis. Because the condition is uncommon and published case series are limited, guidelines on the most appropriate treatment strategies are, to a degree, speculative. Diagnosis of congenital elbow luxation is based on early onset of clinical signs and radiographic features. In cases presenting during later stages of growth it should be differentiated from developmental elbow luxation as a result of asynchronous antebrachial growth.

Type I – Humeroradial luxation

Luxation of the radial head is usually caudolateral with the ulna in a relatively normal location with respect to the humeral condyle. There appears to be no sex predisposition. Boxers, Bulldogs and Labrador Retrievers appear in case reports describing the condition. Luxation is frequently bilateral and, while it may be evident from birth, it more often manifests clinically at around 3 months of age (Campbell, 1979). Hypoplasia or aplasia of the anconeal process, medial coronoid process or annular ligament have been suggested as primary contributory factors (Milton and Montgomery, 1987).

Diagnosis: Clinical signs include mild forelimb lameness, elbow varus and carpal valgus with demonstrable elbow pain and a reduced range of motion. A prominent radial head is palpable laterally. Orthogonal radiographs of the elbow demonstrate a caudolaterally (sub)luxated radial head that is often convex (Figure 19.10). Concurrent anomalies may also include agenesis of the anconeal process, hypoplasia of the medial coronoid process, distal humeral and proximal radial angular deformity, caudal bowing of the ulna and medial deviation of the olecranon.

Treatment: Surgical descriptions for management are numerous and include:

- Oblique or wedge osteotomy/ostectomy of the proximal radius or oblique proximal ulnar osteotomy with soft tissue imbrication
- In the skeletally mature dog, proximal ulnar osteotomy with temporary screw placement between proximal radius and ulna
- Oblique radial osteotomy and progressive correction using traction external skeletal fixation
- Radial head ostectomy
- Reconstruction of the annular ligament, radial osteotomy and temporary transarticular pinning
- Radial osteotomy and plate fixation in combination with a temporary transarticular humeroradial pin
- Arthrodesis.

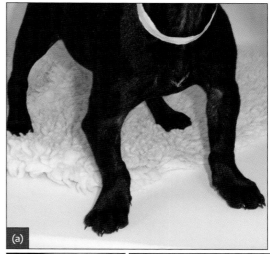

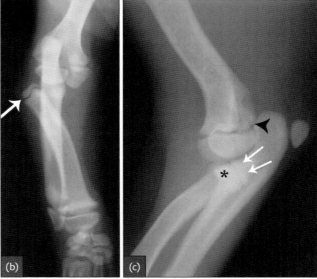

19.10 (a) A 12-week-old entire female Staffordshire Bull Terrier with congenital right humeroradial elbow luxation. Note the prominent radial head laterally. (b) Craniocaudal radiograph showing lateral luxation of the radial head (arrowed). (c) Mediolateral radiograph revealing that the radial head (arrowed) is caudolaterally displaced relative to the humeral condyle, a hypoplastic medial coronoid process and trochlear notch (*), and a hypoplastic anconeal process (arrowhead).

Small case numbers in published series, multiple techniques and short follow-up times make it difficult to formulate precise recommendations for the most appropriate surgical techniques. In practice, failure to maintain radiohumeral reduction is common and conservative management is advised for the majority where both lameness and subluxation are mild (Dassler and Vasseur, 2003).

Type II – Humeroulnar luxation

This condition can be uni- or bilateral and occurs most commonly in small-breed dogs such as the Yorkshire Terrier, Boston Terrier, Pug, Pomeranian, Miniature Poodle and Chihuahua with a higher prevalence in males.

Diagnosis: Severe, early limb deformity and lameness are usually present, allowing identification from birth to 6 weeks of age. There is typically 90 degrees outward rotation of the proximal ulna relative to the humerus with associated marked external rotation of the antebrachium and manus. Palpation reveals a reduced range of motion of the elbow and palpable lateral ulnar displacement relative to the distal humerus. Orthogonal radiographs clearly demonstrate the luxation with a craniocaudal view of the humerus revealing a mediolateral view of the ulna, the ulna being orthogonally rotated relative to the humerus (Figure 19.11). Concurrent changes may include aplasia or hypoplasia of the trochlear notch, anconeal process, medial coronoid process, humeral condyle and olecranon (Kene *et al.*, 1982).

Treatment: Conservative management cannot be advocated, as lameness will predictably worsen with skeletal maturation. Early surgical management, comprising closed reduction of the humeroulnar articulation with placement of a temporary ulnohumeral transarticular pin with the elbow in 140 degrees of extension, is advocated (Rahal *et al.*, 2000). Sometimes closed reduction is not possible, in which case open reduction via an extended caudolateral approach with sectioning of the brachial fascia along the lateral head of the triceps, as well as the anconeus muscle, facilitates reduction. Following placement of the transarticular pin, stabilization should be supported with a padded dressing with pin removal 10–14 days later. In a small case series of eight dogs, six dogs subjectively showed near-normal return to function (Rahal *et al.*, 2000). An alternative surgical approach comprising medial capsulorrhaphy, lateral desmotomy, rotational proximal ulnar osteotomy, olecranon transposition, fixation of the proximal ulna to the radius and anconeal resection has been described (Milton *et al.*, 1979).

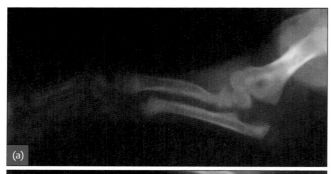
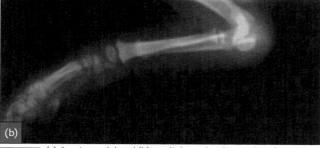

19.11 (a) Craniocaudal and (b) mediolateral radiographs of an 8-week-old entire male Pug with bilateral congenital humeroulnar luxation. Note the humeroulnar joint space is markedly widened and the proximal ulna is rotated approximately 90 degrees relative to the humeral condyle.

Type III – combined humeroradial and humeroulnar luxation

There is no breed predisposition and the condition is frequently associated with a generalized joint laxity (arthrodysplasia) and concurrent multiple developmental anomalies such as ectrodactyly (Montgomery and Tomlinson, 1985). Treatment is rarely undertaken.

Elbow dysplasia

Elbow dysplasia is the collective term for multiple developmental abnormalities of the elbow joint which may coexist, including elbow incongruity, ununited anconeal process (UAP), medial coronoid process disease (MCPD) and osteochondral lesions of the humeral condyle. Elbow dysplasia is a challenging condition to manage; the precise aetiopathogenesis of how these lesions are formed appears multifactorial, most likely comprising both inherited and developmental factors and remains incompletely understood. Equally, the most appropriate treatment strategy for each condition is highly speculative due to a lack of objective comparative studies evaluating different treatment modalities. Osteoarthritic change is an inevitable consequence.

Incongruity

Incongruity is a term describing anatomical malalignment of the articular surfaces. Incongruity was initially proposed as the primary aetiopathogenesis of elbow dysplasia in two seminal papers documenting radiographic and postmortem abnormalities in dogs with elbow dysplasia lesions (Wind, 1986; Wind and Packard, 1986). These studies revealed an axial mismatch in radial length relative to the ulna or an underdevelopment of the ulnar trochlear notch resulting in a bicentric humeroulnar incongruity (Figure 19.12). Axial mismatch in radioulnar length as a primary cause is further supported by cadaveric studies showing increased coronoid loading with artificial radial shortening (Preston *et al.*, 2000) and the coexistence of MCPD in dogs with a short radius secondary to premature closure of the distal radial physis (Macpherson *et al.*, 1992). Bicentric humeroulnar incongruity is similarly supported by studies comparing trochlear notch radius of curvature of breeds predisposed to MCPD, such as the Bernese Mountain Dog and Rottweiler, *versus* controls (Viehmann *et al.*, 1999; Collins *et al.*, 2001). Collectively, these changes in joint congruence have been proposed to result in focal topographical increases in load at the medial coronoid process and anconeus, resulting in damage to the articular surface and/or subchondral bone and, in the case of the latter, failure of fusion. However, in contrast to this body of evidence, some studies reveal a significant proportion of dogs with dysplastic lesions to have no evidence of incongruity at the time of clinical diagnosis (Gemmill *et al.*, 2005; Kramer *et al.*, 2006) as well as incongruity being present but in an opposite form to that expected to explain the articular lesions observed (Meyer-Lindenberg *et al.*, 2006). Recent research has suggested additional incongruities may exist; a primary rotational incongruence of the radius and ulna had been proposed with compression of the coronoid between radial head and humeral condyle, as well as mismatch between the contour arc of the incisures of the medial coronoid process and radial head (Fitzpatrick and Yeadon, 2009). In addition, rotational abutment of the radial head against the medial coronoid process has been demonstrated in *ex vivo* dynamic elbow loading (Burton *et al.*, 2013). Dynamic radiostereometric analysis (an imaging technique accurately determining the three-dimensional (3D) movement of bone) has revealed axial movements of the proximal radius and ulna relative to each other (Guillou *et al.*, 2011) and fluoroscopic kinematography of the dysplastic elbow has revealed craniomedial rotation of the humerus with compression of the humeral trochlea against the craniolateral aspect of the medial coronoid (Schmidt *et*

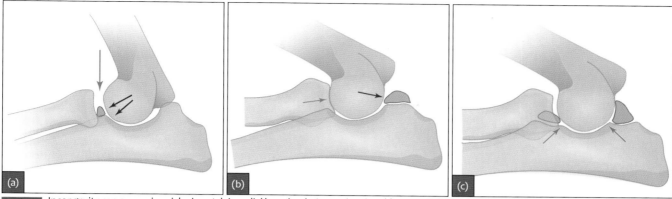

19.12 Incongruity can occur via axial mismatch in radial length relative to the ulna. (a) Relative radial shortening with an increase in humeroradial joint space (red arrow) increasing load on the medial coronoid process (blue arrows). (b) Relative radial overlength (red arrow) increasing load on the anconeal process (blue arrow) and causing humeroulnar and radioulnar incongruity. (c) An underdevelopment of the ulnar trochlear notch may result in a bicentric humeroulnar incongruity with focal overload of the medial coronoid process and anconeal processes concurrently (red arrows).

al., 2012). These recent studies raise the question as to whether, akin to hip dysplasia, soft tissue laxity may be a contributory factor to dynamic incongruity in predisposed breeds. The influence of incongruity over the development of dysplastic lesions is complicated by studies suggesting a degree of physiological incongruity to be endemic within the normal canine elbow joint (Preston et al., 2000; Blond et al., 2005). Furthermore, physiological incongruity may vary as a function of elbow angle as well as with concurrent supination or pronation, as contact mechanics are significantly altered by these movements (Cuddy et al., 2012). Inconsistency in the presence, absence or type of incongruence, which may vary as a function of stage of development, both within individual study cohorts as well as contradictory data between studies, makes interpretation of its precise influence over the development of elbow dysplasia lesions difficult to elucidate.

Ununited anconeal process

Aetiology and pathogenesis

The anconeal process is a primary stabilizer of the elbow in pronation and forms as an ancillary centre of ossification in breeds such as the German Shepherd Dog, Bassett Hound, Newfoundland, Mastiff and Greyhound. Ossification begins around 10–13 weeks of age and fusion to the olecranon is complete by 20 weeks of age. If fusion is not evident by this time then a diagnosis of UAP is supported, for which the German Shepherd Dog has the highest reported incidence (Hayes et al., 1979). Males are affected approximately twice as commonly as females.

UAP was historically thought to be an osteochondrosis lesion (Olsson, 1977) but this has not been supported by histological studies (Trostel et al., 2003). Trauma, metabolic and genetic factors have been proposed but are as of yet of unproven influence. Specific incongruities suggested as alternate mechanisms for the formation of UAP are firstly, an over-long radius relative to the ulna, translating the humeral condyle against the anconeal process and secondly, underdevelopment of the trochlear notch, both resulting in focal overload with subsequent disruption of microcirculation (Trostel et al., 2003) and failure of fusion (Wind et al., 1986; Sjostrum et al., 1995). Certainly in the case of a relatively over-long radius, premature closure of the distal ulnar growth plate in breeds such as the Bassett Hound may predictably result in UAP via the humeroulnar incongruence that is induced.

Diagnosis

Lameness attributed to the primary lesion is seen from 4–5 months of age (Guthrie, 1989) and can vary from intermittent and subtle to severe and continuous. The condition is bilateral in approximately 30% of cases, these dogs often displaying varying degrees of shifting forelimb lameness. Dogs may stand with the elbow in an abducted position, with a varying degree of external rotation of the manus. There may be palpable elbow effusion and thickening, with pain elicited on manipulation, especially extension. However, some dogs may only present with lameness later in life due to secondary osteoarthritis. UAP may occasionally be an incidental finding in mature dogs with no clinical signs of lameness.

Diagnosis can be confirmed on a fully flexed mediolateral radiograph that minimizes superimposition of the medial condyle over the anconeal process. Both elbows should be radiographed. Radiographs may demonstrate partial or complete separation of the anconeal process or, more rarely, it may be fused in an abnormal location (Presnell, 1990). Caution should be used when diagnosing adjunctive elbow incongruence from radiographs as interobserver interpretation can vary markedly unless any step is large – typically more than 4 millimetres (Mason et al., 2002). Alternatively, CT allows accurate, concurrent assessment of the anconeal process, medial joint compartment and elbow congruence. The recent evaluation of this imaging modality for dogs with UAP has revealed 92% and 100% of dogs to have concurrent MCPD and incongruence respectively (Gasch et al., 2012). Arthroscopy has been assessed as a tool with apparent high sensitivity in assessing incongruence (Wagner et al., 2007). However, a recent study has revealed incongruence may be influenced by the volume effect of arthroscope placement (Skinner et al., 2015).

Treatment and prognosis

Controversy persists as to the most appropriate means to manage UAP as there is a lack of robust objective data with suitable follow-up to substantiate one treatment strategy over another. One important consideration is the high presence of adjunctive joint anomalies, namely MCPD and incongruence. Failure to address these conditions may adversely affect function as well as predispose to implant failure or failure of fusion with internal fixation. Regardless of the management strategy employed, osteoarthritis is an inevitable consequence (Guthrie, 1989).

Importantly, the precise correlation between the degree of osteoarthritic change that may develop and clinical function is currently unknown. Conservative or surgical management may be used.

Conservative management: In the mature dog with lameness where osteoarthritic change is advanced, or UAP is an incidental finding, or when economic constraints exist, conservative management may be chosen. Little published information is available to document the natural progression of lameness when conservative management is employed.

Surgical management:

Removal of the UAP: Historically this was the treatment of choice, with some evidence to show little change in clinical function and progression of osteoarthritis reported in only 25% of cases (Sinibaldi and Arnoczky, 1975). Intuitively, however, progression of osteoarthritis in all cases of UAP removal should be anticipated. As the anconeal process contributes significantly to elbow stability in extension, removal of the process, especially in young dogs, cannot be advocated (see Operative Technique 19.9).

Proximal ulnar osteotomy (PUO): PUO (see Operative Technique 19.8) aims to improve humeroulnar incongruity while permitting proximal migration of the ulna, thus mitigating the shear force experienced by the trochlear notch and anconeal process. This has been reported to result in spontaneous fusion. Two studies have evaluated cohorts undergoing this surgery with widely variable fusion rates being reported of 30–71% of cases, and with differing criteria denoting 'fusion' (Sjostrum *et al.*, 1995; Turner *et al.*, 1998). In addition, osteotomies were performed at variable sites with differing planes of obliquity. The propensity for fusion of the UAP has so far not been correlated with lameness or clinical outcome. Fusion of the UAP in malalignment is also reported (Matis, 1992). Owners should be counselled that it is not unusual for significant callus formation to occur following PUO that may be easily palpable under the skin or seen as thickening of the limb at this site. Placement of an intramedullary pin down the ulna does not appear to influence the propensity for UAP fusion (Pettitt *et al.*, 2009).

Internal fixation: Lag screw fixation alone does not address joint incongruence that may be present; this may be the reason why a fusion rate of only 50% is reported (Fox *et al.*, 1996; Pettitt *et al.*, 2009). Long-term correlation between propensity for fusion, limb function and progression of osteoarthritis is lacking.

Lag screw fixation and PUO: The most sizeable case series report fusion rates of 84–94% (Meyer-Lindenberg *et al.*, 2001; Pettitt *et al.*, 2009) (Figure 19.13). Similarly, long-term follow-up of the correlation between propensity for fusion, limb function and progression of osteoarthritis is lacking. In light of this evidence and comparatively favourable outcomes, lag screw fixation, with concurrent PUO if incongruity is evident, appears the treatment option of choice. Where the anconeus can be arthroscopically palpated and determined to be stable then PUO alone may be a valid option.

Medial coronoid process disease
Aetiology and pathogenesis

The precise aetiopathogenesis of this disease remains highly controversial. Historically, MCPD has been called fragmented medial coronoid process but a spectrum of

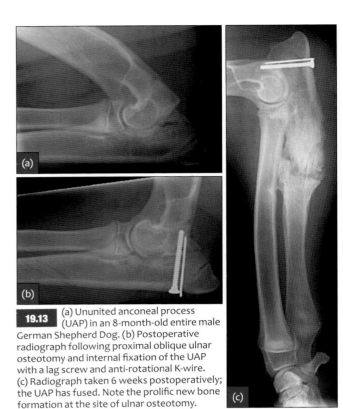

19.13 (a) Ununited anconeal process (UAP) in an 8-month-old entire male German Shepherd Dog. (b) Postoperative radiograph following proximal oblique ulnar osteotomy and internal fixation of the UAP with a lag screw and anti-rotational K-wire. (c) Radiograph taken 6 weeks postoperatively; the UAP has fused. Note the prolific new bone formation at the site of ulnar osteotomy.

pathological changes affecting the medial coronoid process are now recognized, not just fragmentation *per se*. The medial coronoid process develops by appositional ossification with the sequential subperiosteal deposition of bone at its peripheral margin, rather than as a separate ossification centre. The lesion was initially thought to be osteochondrosis (Tirgari, 1980) but much work has refuted this, with alternative theories such as subchondral osteosclerosis (Temwichitr *et al.*, 2010), subchondral microfracture (Danielson *et al.*, 2006), trochlear notch dysplasia and joint incongruity (Wind, 1986) and variant shear stress (Hulse *et al.*, 2010) being proposed. Conflicting studies support primary pathology to be either subchondral, with microcracks and diffuse damage preceding articular fissure formation (Danielson *et al.*, 2006), or articular, with a primary reduction in glycosaminoglycans preceding changes in subchondral density (Lau *et al.*, 2013). In addition, recent micro-CT studies suggest fragmentation can be subdivided topographically into either distinct transverse tip or radial incisure entities (Figure 19.14) with the suggestion that different aberrant loading mechanisms may predispose to each subtype (Fitzpatrick *et al.*, 2011). Changes in bone density in the radial head at the level of abutment with the coronoid may also support the radial head as a distinct entity contributing to coronoid pathology (Philips *et al.*, 2015) (Figure 19.15).

Clinical signs

Clinical signs of lameness classically develop from 5–8 months of age. However, changes are incipient within the joint from 15 weeks of age (Lau *et al.*, 2013). Equally, some dogs present with lameness when mature (Vermote *et al.*, 2010), and in some dogs findings appear incidental. Lameness is often initially subtle and intermittent, later becoming recalcitrant. Dogs often exhibit external rotation of the manus with the elbows either abducted or adducted

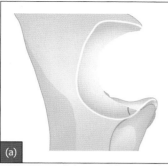
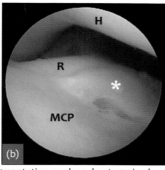
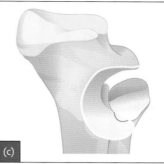
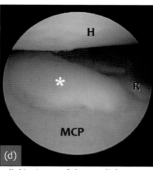

19.14 Medial coronoid process fragmentation can be subcategorized as affecting either (a–b) the tip or (c–d) the radial incisure of the medial coronoid process. H = humeral condyle; MCP = medial coronoid process; R = radial head; * = coronoid fragment.

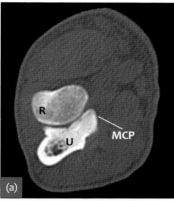

19.15 Transverse CT images of (a) a normal Labrador Retriever elbow and (b) a Labrador Retriever elbow with medial coronoid process disease. Note the sclerotic change in the radial head (arrowed). (c) Arthroscopic image of the dog in (b): there is evidence of cartilage damage on the radial head where it articulates with the medial coronoid process. HC = humeral condyle; MCP = medial coronoid process; R = radial head; U = ulna.

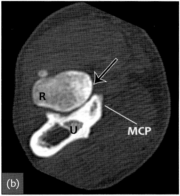

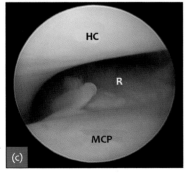

Imaging

Direct observation of the medial coronoid process from plain radiographs is hampered by superimposition of the radial head. Oblique views (distomedial–proximolateral oblique) have been described which increase the sensitivity of detecting fragmentation (Haudiquet *et al.*, 2002). Occasionally, overt fragmentation can be appreciated but this is the exception rather than the rule and diagnosis on plain radiographs usually relies on the assessment of secondary changes of variable incidence, such as trochlear notch sclerosis (87%) and osteophyte production on the anconeus (70%), lateral epicondyle (57%) and radial head (37%) (Fitzpatrick *et al.*, 2009b). However, 3% of cases may not demonstrate any radiological change. Equally, the extent of osteophyte deposition, while supporting a diagnosis of MCPD, is only a poor to moderate predictor of the severity of articular pathology (Fitzpatrick *et al.*, 2009b).

Both MRI and CT have been evaluated for imaging the medial coronoid and both have a sensitivity of around 90% for the detection of overt fragmentation (Figure 19.16). CT has been evaluated in concert with arthroscopy for the detection of coronoid pathology; this study revealed that CT and arthroscopy can provide complementary yet contradictory information in the detection of coronoid pathology (Moores *et al.*, 2008). Arthroscopy provides

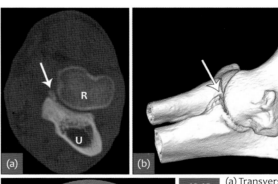

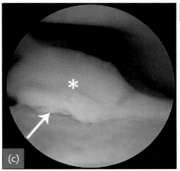

19.16 (a) Transverse and (b) 3D reconstruction CT images of an elbow affected by medial coronoid process disease; a fragment is evident (arrowed). (c) Arthroscopic view of the fragment (*) and fissure line (arrowed) extending along the radial incisure. R = radial head; U = ulna.

(see Figure 19.4) with supination during forward movement and a 'paddling' gait when bilaterally affected. Typical of degenerative joint disease, stiffness and lameness is often at its worst after rest that follows exercise. Examination may reveal pain on full extension or flexion of the joint, each with concurrent supination or pronation of the antebrachium. As the disease progresses and secondary osteoarthritic change is established, reduced range of motion, effusion, joint thickening and crepitus may be palpable.

detailed information on articular cartilage changes but subchondral changes cannot be evaluated. Equally, CT provides detailed information on subchondral changes but no information on cartilage lesions; thus an absence of CT signs does not rule out significant articular pathology.

Arthroscopy

Diagnostic arthroscopy via medial portals (see Operative Technique 19.1) provides exquisite detail of the articular changes affecting the medial compartment. Findings may include synovitis (100%) and fragmentation (64%), fissuring (18%) or a grossly intact medial coronoid process (18%) (Fitzpatrick et al., 2009b). Cartilage damage can be categorized as focal or diffuse, as well as graded in severity from mild fibrillation and chondromalacia through to full-thickness loss (modified Outerbridge scale, Jungius et al., 2006).

Kissing lesions affecting the medial portion of the humeral condyle can be seen with reasonable frequency (49%); this lesion is presumed to occur due to focal overload in direct apposition to the trochlear notch of the ulna subsequent to humeroulnar incongruity during growth. Cartilage loss concurrently affecting the trochlea of the humerus, the axial trochlear notch and medial coronoid is termed medial compartment disease. As well as having a diagnostic role, arthroscopic debridement of the joint can be performed.

Treatment

The most appropriate management strategy for medial coronoid process disease remains highly controversial. Conservative management as well as a plethora of surgical procedures have been proposed. However, in a similar vein to the management of UAP, the vast majority of published studies offer low levels of evidence. They are typically retrospective, employ small case numbers with no control group, use only subjective outcome measures, report only limited follow-up and do not catalogue the exact type of articular pathology present. To complicate decision-making further, recent work suggests that neither owners nor clinicians can reliably assess long-term lameness in dogs with MCPD when compared with quantitative gait analysis, tending to underestimate lameness as a function of time (Burton et al., 2009). Thus studies employing owner and clinician outcome assessment for the treatment of MCPD may overestimate the efficacy of established surgical treatment protocols. It is similarly unclear how the rate of progression of osteoarthritis is influenced, as well as how this correlates with lameness clinically.

Conservative management: Conservative management typically comprises weight restriction, a controlled exercise regime and tactical use of non-steroidal anti-inflammatory medication. Rehabilitation (hydrotherapy/physiotherapy) and complementary therapies such as acupuncture, as well as dietary supplementation with cod liver oil or nutraceuticals, can be employed concurrently but objective data as to their efficacy are currently lacking. Further information on the medical management of degenerative joint disease can be found in Chapter 6. One study suggested inferior results with conservative management compared to fragment removal via arthrotomy; however, outcome measurement was subjective (Read et al., 1990). Two subsequent studies employing gait analysis comparing these treatment modalities failed to find any difference in outcome (Huibregtse et al., 1994; Bouck et al., 1995). Inverse dynamics gait analysis

(see Chapter 1) of juvenile dogs with medically managed MCPD has revealed that lameness improves progressively over the ensuing 6–12 month period following diagnosis (Burton et al., 2011); thus, if a conservative approach is employed, owners should be counselled that improvements, should they occur, will be gradual. To date, only three studies comparing medical and surgical management have used objective outcome measures and a control group (treated medically); all failed to demonstrate superiority of surgery over medical management alone.

Surgical management:

Fragment removal: This can be performed either via arthrotomy or arthroscopically, with or without concurrent debridement of the subchondral bone bed. Convalescence following arthroscopic debridement is purportedly shorter (Meyer-Lindenberg et al., 2003); this study suggested that fewer dogs were lame following arthroscopic debridement. However, subjective outcome assessment was employed and the precise articular changes present were poorly categorized. A recent study using inverse dynamic gait analysis comparing arthroscopic removal of fragments to conservative management failed to demonstrate a therapeutic benefit of fragment removal, but found that surgery exacerbated lameness for between 2 and 6 months postoperatively, although case numbers were limited (Burton et al., 2011). Arthroscopic debridement does not address the subchondral bone abnormalities where fissuring and microfracture appear to be initiated and pain is likely to arise. Debridement of normal cartilage will result in deleterious changes in contact mechanics and accelerate progression of osteoarthritis through the exposure of subchondral bone. In the clinical situation, however, the surgical target articular cartilage that is debrided is abnormal and subchondral bone is frequently already exposed. Finally, arthroscopic debridement does nothing to address wider incongruence within the joint.

Subtotal coronoid ostectomy: This is an osteotomy at the base of the medial coronoid process with removal of the osteochondral fragment (see Operative Technique 19.4). This technique removes a proportion of the subchondral microfractured bone which is likely to contribute to the pain associated with MCPD, but by its very nature it further exposes subchondral bone, which is likely to accelerate osteoarthritis as well as having the potential to deleteriously affect humeroulnar contact mechanics. It is reported that 51% of dogs treated appeared free of lameness postoperatively (Fitzpatrick et al., 2009a) but objective outcome measures were lacking in this study and osteoarthritis progressed in all cases. Recent second-look arthroscopy suggests articular impingement of the trochlea of the humerus on the edge of the osteotomy may occur following this surgery in some cases, leading to rapid full-thickness cartilage wear along the resection line and humeral trochlea and accelerated progression of medial compartment disease (Bräuer and Böttcher, 2015).

Proximal ulnar osteotomy/ostectomy (PUO): PUO (see Operative Technique 19.8) has been described in conjunction with arthrotomy and fragment removal in immature dogs. This surgery attempts to allow migration of the proximal ulna to ameliorate the supraphysiological load on the coronoid process caused by a shortened radius, and this is supported by recent in vivo CT analysis (Böttcher et al., 2013). Subjectively, results have been encouraging with the majority of dogs deemed sound. However, published case numbers are small and subjective assessment of outcome was employed (Ness, 1998). More recently a bi-oblique dynamic PUO has been described which aims to limit morbidity associated with post-osteotomy ulnar instability and appears to allow divergence of the radial incisure of the ulna from the radial head (Fitzpatrick *et al.*, 2013a). PUO does not address incongruence of the trochlear notch, nor abnormalities of the medial coronoid bone, and by its very nature it induces a distolateral rotational incongruence of the joint.

Sliding humeral osteotomy: This procedure comprises a mid-diaphyseal transverse humeral osteotomy, medial translation of the distal humerus and stabilization with a stepped locking plate and screws (Figure 19.17). The surgery is proposed to elicit lateral shifting of the load axis from the medial compartment. A case series of 59 limbs demonstrated resolution of lameness in 65% of cases (Fitzpatrick *et al.*, 2009e) but only subjective outcome assessments were used. Medium term follow-up employing objective outcome measures on a small cohort of dogs revealed significant improvements in forelimb symmetry (Fitzpatrick *et al.*, 2015). The long-term efficacy of this procedure is unknown.

Proximal abducting ulnar osteotomy: The proximal abducting ulnar osteotomy (PAUL) procedure comprises a proximal transverse ulnar osteotomy with medial translation of the distal extent of the proximal ulnar segment; this functionally abducts the proximal aspect of the proximal ulnar segment relative to its preoperative axial alignment. The bone is secured with a stepped locking plate and screws (Figure 19.18). PAUL is purported to have the effect of load transfer to the lateral elbow compartment. Preliminary assessment of outcome in conjunction with medial coronoid process fragment removal suggest 88% of dogs were pain-free (Pfeil *et al.*, 2012) but precise case selection criteria were lacking in this cohort, as were objective outcome measures.

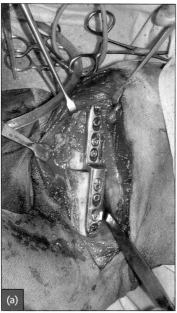
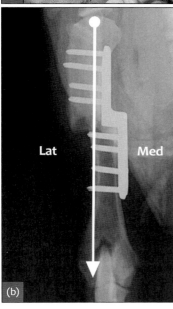

19.17 Sliding humeral osteotomy. (a) A stepped locking plate and screws are applied to the medial aspect of the humerus following transverse osteotomy of the diaphysis. (b) Postoperatively, load is redistributed eccentrically (arrowed) through the lateral joint compartment, hence off-loading the abnormal medial compartment.

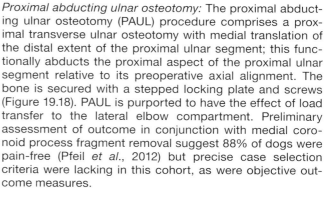
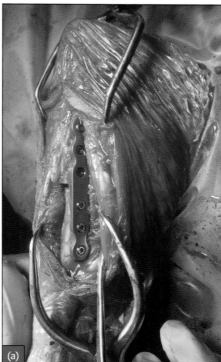
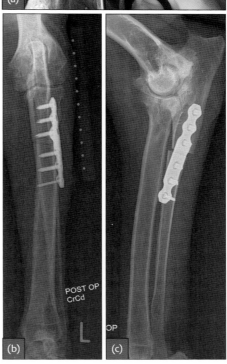

19.18 Proximal abducting ulnar osteotomy (PAUL) procedure. (a) Intraoperative image and (b–c) postoperative radiographs. The surgery involves application of a stepped locking plate to the lateral aspect of the proximal ulna, abducting the ulna and shifting load to the lateral joint compartment.

Bicipital ulnar release: This procedure is hypothesized to remove any torsional–compressive forces that the muscle may exert on the medial joint compartment as a consequence of its attachment to the proximal medial radius and ulna (Hulse *et al.*, 2010). Further work is required to explore any contribution this mechanism may play in MCPD before biceps release can be advocated as a surgical treatment for this disease.

Osteochondral lesions of the humeral trochlea

Aetiology and pathology

Osteochondral lesions of the medial portion of the humeral condyle are reported to account for up to 25% of elbow dysplasia lesions with concurrent MCPD occurring in at least 12% of cases (Denny, 1995). However, with modern imaging techniques such as arthroscopy and CT there is anecdotal evidence that these historic data probably significantly overestimate the incidence of these osteochondral lesions. As with MCPD, a spectrum of severity of lesions from mild fibrillation of the cartilage to overt osteochondral fissuring and flap formation may be evident. There is ongoing debate as to whether these lesions are wholly attributable to osteochondrosis originating in the articular–epiphyseal cartilage complex at this site or due to incongruence during growth overloading the medial humeral joint compartment and causing the osteochondral damage observed. The condition occurs with high frequency in the Labrador and Golden Retriever (Lavrijsen *et al.*, 2012) and is frequently bilateral.

Diagnosis

Clinical signs are very similar to MCPD. Osteochondrosis is most often readily diagnosed on a craniocaudal or mediolateral radiograph as an area of erosion or flattening of the subchondral bone on the medial portion of the humeral condyle. A flap may be visible in cases where there is separation through mineralized subchondral bone. More subtle lesions may require CT and/or arthroscopy for diagnosis (Figure 19.19). Secondary osteoarthritis is often evident concurrently.

Treatment

Osteochondral flaps may be removed either via arthrotomy (see Operative Technique 19.5) or arthroscopically. There is a lack of objective literature documenting outcomes of either conservative or surgical management of this lesion in isolation. Subjectively, there appears to be approximately an 80% chance of 'satisfactory' function with the surgical debridement of concurrent OCD and MCPD lesions. More recently, osteochondral autograft transfer (OATS®) of the medial humeral condyle has been described in a small series of dogs, with 83% of dogs being sound on subjective follow-up assessment (Fitzpatrick *et al.*, 2009c). However, the results of this study are difficult to interpret as concurrent MCPD was present in the majority of dogs and treatment for this was provided in tandem with the OATS® procedure. There is also the important consideration of donor site morbidity with this technique. An alternative novel implant, the SynACART® (Arthrex), can be placed in the osteochondral defect, negating the need to harvest a graft from a donor site. Prospective objective studies are required to establish if these surgical interventions for this condition confer any long-term efficacy beyond flap removal alone.

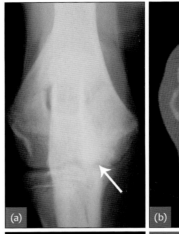
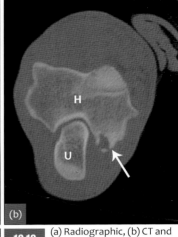
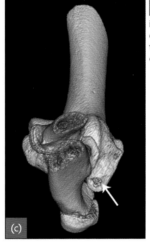

19.19 (a) Radiographic, (b) CT and (c) 3D reconstruction CT images of the appearance of osteochondritis dissecans (arrowed) of the medial portion of the humeral condyle (H). U = ulna.

Elbow incongruity secondary to growth plate disturbance

Distal antebrachial physeal disturbances occur commonly (see Chapter 8). Disturbance may be due to trauma or secondary to conditions affecting the physeal region such as metaphyseal osteopathy and retained cartilage cores, or as a result of a primary osteochondrodysplasia in breeds such as the Dachshund and Bassett Hound. In such breeds, there appears to be a genetic predisposition for premature consolidation of the distal ulnar physis with an absence of trauma; this results in short bowed thoracic limbs with adjunctive humeroulnar subluxation and/or caudolateral subluxation of the radial head. This section will focus on the consequences and treatment for the elbow joint.

Distal ulnar growth plate closure

This is the commonest growth plate to be affected, comprising 75% of all physeal disturbances (Ramadan and Vaughan, 1978) (Figure 19.20). Proximal humeroulnar subluxation may occur as a consequence due to relative axial overgrowth of the radius; therefore this growth deformity may predispose to UAP. Dogs will typically present with elbow pain and a variable degree of adjunctive antebrachial procurvatum, carpal valgus and external rotation of the manus. Correction of elbow incongruity is best achieved via an ulnar osteotomy/ostectomy (see Operative Technique 19.8) with 50% of dogs having a good to excellent outcome 2 years postoperatively (Gilson *et al.*, 1989). It

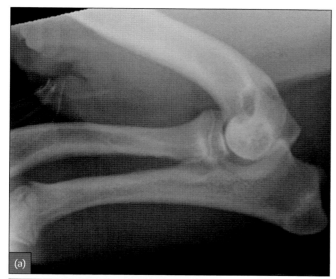

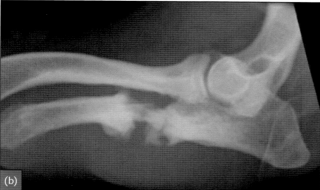

19.20 (a) Humeroulnar and radioulnar subluxation in a 6-month-old Jack Russell Terrier as a result of reduced growth of the distal ulnar physis. Proximal ulnar ostectomy was performed. (b) Radiograph taken 6 weeks following surgery showing improved elbow congruency. Note the prolific new bone formation at the site of ulna ostectomy.

is suggested that ulnar ostectomy alone is an effective treatment in dogs less than 5 months of age with less than 13 degrees of concurrent valgus deformity (DeCamp *et al.*, 1986). In the adult, concomitant correction of distal limb deformity may be required if it is clinically significant.

Distal radial growth plate closure

This occurs much less frequently than distal ulnar physeal closure. Symmetrical or asymmetrical closure can occur, with the latter affecting the lateral side more commonly. The elbow can subsequently be affected by distal humero-ulnar subluxation, and MCPD occurs in 50% of cases as a consequence (Robins, 1987). Clinically, lameness may initially result from elbow incongruity and subsequently, secondary osteoarthritic change. Regardless of the surgical management strategy employed, the elbow should be inspected for concurrent MCPD and treatment of this lesion performed. Surgical correction can comprise either ulnar shortening or radial lengthening (see Operative Technique 19.10) and these are briefly discussed in turn.

Ulnar shortening can be achieved by a proximal segmental ostectomy (Figure 19.21). Ulnar shortening has the benefit of being relatively simple to perform but limb length is lost. Postoperative stabilization of the ulna is unnecessary and while an intramedullary pin may provide adjunctive stability, this may restrict dynamic reduction of the joint and can lead to seroma formation over the olecranon.

Radial lengthening has been described either dynamically, with the use of pins and elastic (Mason and Baker, 1978), statically with a dorsal plate and screws (Vandewater and Olmstead, 1983), or alternatively external skeletal fixation can be used. Radial lengthening has the benefit of preserving limb length, but ensuring that the final position of the radial head achieves good joint congruence can be challenging.

Case series are limited for both techniques but functionally, radial lengthening may confer advantages over ulnar shortening (Barr and Denny, 1985).

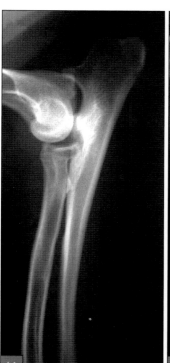
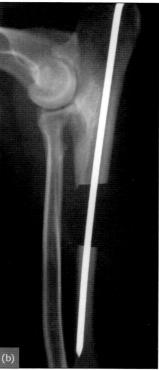
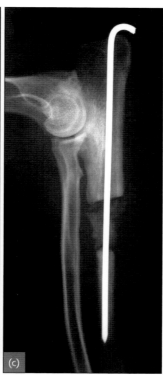

19.21 (a) Preoperative radiograph showing a short radius due to premature closure of the distal radial growth plate, and secondary severe distal humeroulnar subluxation. (b) Postoperative appearance following proximal ulnar ostectomy and placement of an intramedullary pin in the ulna. Note the substantial improvement in humeroulnar and humeroradial congruence. (c) Radiograph taken 4 weeks postoperatively; new bone is present at the site of ulnar ostectomy. (Courtesy of Martin Owen)

Incomplete ossification/ intracondylar fissure-fracture of the humeral condyle

Aetiology and pathogenesis

Morphologically the canine humeral condyle develops from three centres of ossification; the lateral forms the capitulum and lateral portion of the condyle, the medial forms the trochlea and medial portion of the condyle and the third forms the medial epicondyle. During normal development, ossification of the condyle commences at 2 weeks of age and fusion of lateral and medial component parts occurs by 12 weeks of age (Hare, 1961). In certain breeds, most notably spaniels and to a lesser degree, the Labrador Retriever and Rottweiler, failure of ossification may occur (Marcellin-Little et al., 1994). Histologically this is reflected by a band of fibrous tissue between the two halves of the condyle with dense, sclerotic bone presumed to be an adaptive response to instability. The aetiology of IOHC is poorly understood. A recessive mode of inheritance has been proposed (Marcellin-Little et al., 1994) and an increased prevalence in males has led to speculation that low oestrogen levels may lead to the condition due to their stimulatory effect on epiphyseal maturation (Strickland and Sprinz, 1973). Microangiography studies support a decreased vascular density in spaniel breeds (Larsen et al., 1999) but the precise influence of this over the propensity to develop IOHC is ill-defined. More recent evidence suggests that a subset of dogs may develop partial or complete fissuring representing a non-union fracture after ossification is complete (Carrera et al., 2008), in which case use of the term IOHC to describe this lesion is inaccurate. Fissure formation in a previously normal humeral condyle has been documented with CT, supporting this theory (Farrell et al., 2011). Several studies speculate that joint incongruence may predispose to fissure formation due to shear stress across the condyle resulting in stress fracture (Carerra et al., 2008; Charles et al., 2009). However, in a similar vein to MCPD, incongruence is not present in all cases at the time of diagnosis. Fissure propagation appears to originate from the articular surface (Figure 19.22).

IOHC/ICFF has a spectrum of clinical presentations; it may be an incidental finding or it may be associated with recalcitrant lameness, as well as predisposing to fracture of the humeral condyle. Fractures typically occur without a history of significant trauma.

Diagnosis

Clinically, lameness can vary from mild and episodic to severe, with pain often demonstrable on full extension of the elbow, on application of pressure transversely across the condyle or on palpation of the lateral epicondylar crest. A craniocaudal radiograph may reveal IOHC/ICFF as a radiolucent line extending completely or partially from the articular surface to the supratrochlear foramen (Figure 19.23). However, if the primary beam is offset by greater than 5 degrees from the orientation of the fissure it is unlikely to be visible on the radiograph. In 43–80% of dogs, there is evidence of periosteal proliferation and sclerosis affecting the lateral epicondylar crest (Marcellin-Little et al., 1994; Carrera et al., 2008).

MRI and CT are highly sensitive and specific (Carrera et al., 2008; Piola et al., 2012) and allow concurrent assessment of the medial compartment of the joint.

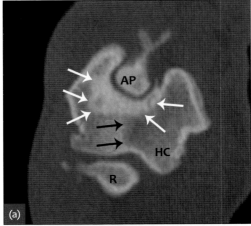

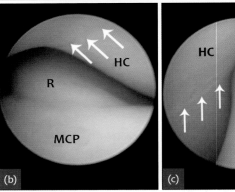

19.22 (a) Computed tomographic and (b–c) arthroscopic appearance of the right elbow of a 3-year-old neutered male Springer Spaniel presenting with elbow pain. (a) Dorsal CT image revealing hypoattenuation of the condylar bone in this region (black arrows). Pronounced regional sclerotic change is present in the proximal portion of the condyle (white arrows). (b) Craniomedial and (c) caudomedial arthroscopic images of the same humeral condyle. A faint line is present in the cartilage (arrowed) at the location that fissure formation would be predicted to occur. AP = anconeal process; HC = humeral condyle; MCP = medial coronoid process; R = radial head.

Variable cavitation and heterogenicity within the condyle are often seen on advanced imaging (Figure 19.23). Both incomplete (52%) and complete fissures (48%) are documented, as well as progression from the former to the latter (Witte et al., 2010). The incidence of bilateral disease is between 42 and 95%.

Management of IOHC pre-fracture

There are numerous management strategies including conservative management, or surgical management to place a transcondylar implant, with or without a bone graft and/or forage, via a lateral or medial approach. There are pros and cons to each of these management strategies and these are discussed in turn.

Conservative management

Conservative management carries a risk of partial and complete fissures progressing to fracture. However, if lameness is mild and readily controlled with tactical use of NSAIDs and reduced exercise, then this approach may be an effective management strategy when financial constraints exist or if owners are uncomfortable with the risk of complications associated with surgery and aware of the risk of condylar fracture occurring at any time.

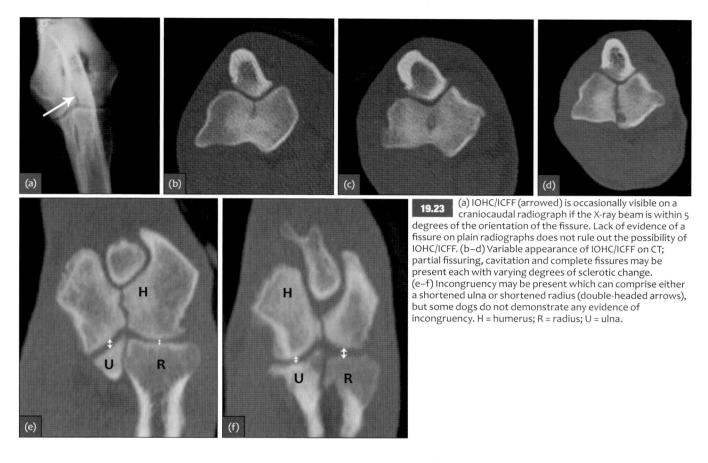

19.23 (a) IOHC/ICFF (arrowed) is occasionally visible on a craniocaudal radiograph if the X-ray beam is within 5 degrees of the orientation of the fissure. Lack of evidence of a fissure on plain radiographs does not rule out the possibility of IOHC/ICFF. (b–d) Variable appearance of IOHC/ICFF on CT; partial fissuring, cavitation and complete fissures may be present each with varying degrees of sclerotic change. (e–f) Incongruency may be present which can comprise either a shortened ulna or shortened radius (double-headed arrows), but some dogs do not demonstrate any evidence of incongruency. H = humerus; R = radius; U = ulna.

Surgical management

Currently the most common transcondylar implant employed is a screw (Figure 19.24). The surgeon has several options to consider regarding implant selection and method of application when placing a screw. The screw may be used as a lag or positional implant and inserted from either the medial or lateral aspect. It is likely that fusion of the fissure occurs infrequently following placement of the screw, thus as large a screw as possible should be used to maximize the area moment of inertia (AMI) – a measure of the implant's resistance to bending – which is proportional to the fourth power of the core radius. Cortical screws have a larger core diameter than cancellous screws and are therefore preferred. Assuming an implant is chosen of a size approximately 50% of the diameter of the condyle, then a 4.5 mm cortical screw is appropriate for most spaniels and Labrador Retrievers, this screw having a significantly greater AMI than either a 3.5 mm cortical or a 4.5 mm cancellous screw. The 4.5 mm shaft screw (Veterinary Instrumentation, UK) is a partially threaded screw that has a smooth shaft as wide as the thread over more than half its length, offering five times the bending strength of a 4.5 mm cortical screw. In a reported case series (Moores *et al.*, 2014), shaft screw breakage did not occur in any case with a mean follow-up of approximately 2 years. Elsewhere, the incidence of 3.5 mm or 4.5 mm screw failure in a recent publication was 2.5% (Hattersley *et al.*, 2011). A potential disadvantage of the shaft screw is that it has always to be placed in lag fashion with the glide hole crossing the IOHC area to penetrate into the far condyle. Lag screw placement allows compression of the fissure, which is speculated to reduce the risk of implant failure, with reduced infection rates reported with lag *versus* position screw placement (Hattersley *et al.*, 2011). The compression induced by a lag

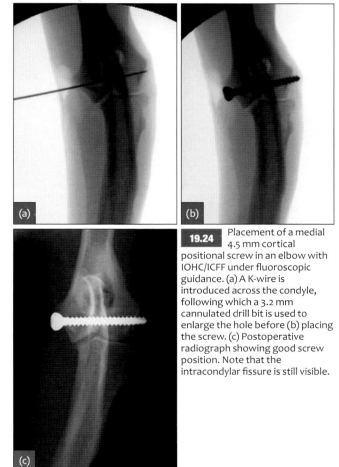

19.24 Placement of a medial 4.5 mm cortical positional screw in an elbow with IOHC/ICFF under fluoroscopic guidance. (a) A K-wire is introduced across the condyle, following which a 3.2 mm cannulated drill bit is used to enlarge the hole before (b) placing the screw. (c) Postoperative radiograph showing good screw position. Note that the intracondylar fissure is still visible.

screw may, however, induce joint incongruence (Charles *et al.*, 2009) and anecdotally there are reports of worsening lameness following lag screw placement in a proportion of cases. A complication rate of approximately 60% has been reported with screw placement, the most common being seroma formation (43%) and sepsis (42%) (Hattersley *et al.*, 2011). Both of these complications appear reduced when the screw was inserted from medial to lateral across the condyle (Clarke *et al.*, 2012). However, placement of a screw from medially may carry an increased risk of inadvertent joint penetration (Barnes *et al.*, 2014).

Placement of a self-compressing (Acutrak®, Acumed) screw in parallel with an autogenous dowel of bone has been described as an alternative to screw placement alone (Fitzpatrick *et al.*, 2009c). However, it is unclear histologically if the graft can vascularize and confer any meaningful strength across the fissure, avoiding fatigue fracture. Forage of the condyle in an attempt to facilitate healing across the fissure is not effective and cannot be recommended (Butterworth and Innes, 2001).

Placement of a transcondylar implant does nothing to address medial compartment disease (26–44% of cases), joint incongruity (0–75% of cases) or osteoarthritis (60–79% of cases) that may be concurrently present in these joints. The presence of incongruity may be significantly correlated with lameness (Moores *et al.*, 2012) as well as theoretically increasing the risk of implant failure via persistent shear force across the condylar implant. Thus if incongruence due to an axial mismatch in radioulnar length is present, the author would advocate concomitant proximal ulnar osteotomy/ostectomy in an effort to reduce shear force on the condylar screw.

Management of condylar fracture secondary to IOHC/ICFF

As these fractures are articular, prompt rigid internal fixation with accurate anatomical reconstruction is mandatory to minimize residual joint incongruity and promote primary bone healing. The reader is referred to the *BSAVA Manual of Canine and Feline Fracture Repair and Management*, for further details on the management of humeral condylar fracture subsequent to IOHC/ICFF.

Flexor enthesiopathy

Aetiology and pathogenesis

Mineralization in the region of the medial epicondyle of the humerus was originally described in 1966 (Ljunggren *et al.*) and has since been described under numerous pseudonyms including ununited medial epicondyle, traumatic avulsion of the humeral medial epicondyle, osseous metaplasia/dystrophic calcification of the flexor tendons, medial humeral condylar OCD and medial epicondylar spur. The precise cause of these mineralizations is currently unclear but possibilities include primary formation following a local increase in stress and microtrauma and secondary to incongruity, elbow dysplasia and osteoarthritis. It is unclear to what extent mineralizations in this region contribute to lameness, as they often coexist with other joint pathology and can be incidental findings (Figure 19.25).

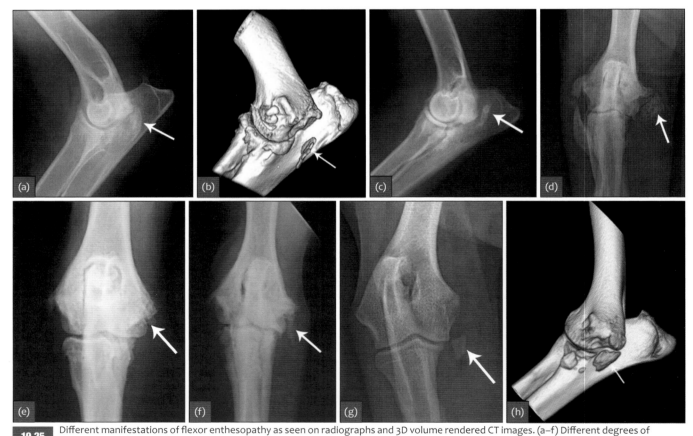

19.25 Different manifestations of flexor enthesiopathy as seen on radiographs and 3D volume rendered CT images. (a–f) Different degrees of mineralization (arrowed) are evident in the vicinity of the medial epicondyle and origin of the flexor tendons. Changes tend to be more advanced when concomitant elbow joint disease is present, most commonly elbow dysplasia with secondary osteoarthritis. (g–h) Region of mineralization distal to the medial epicondyle (arrowed); this was previously termed 'ununited medial epicondyle' but histological studies do not support a failure of fusion of the epicondyle.

Medial epicondylar mineralization is present in 40% of dogs with elbow lameness (de Bakker *et al.*, 2012). Mineralizations can be subdivided into those with a 'primary flexor enthesopathy' (15%), i.e. medial epicondylar changes with no other identifiable elbow disease and those with 'concomitant flexor enthesopathy' (85%), i.e. primary joint pathology is identified which in the majority of cases is MCPD. Generally, concomitant flexor enthesopathy lesions often appear more extensive on diagnostic imaging, which suggests their propensity to develop is accelerated by pre-existing joint disease. Specific breed predilections do not appear to exist but reported breeds (which may in part reflect the geographic area of study) include the Great Swiss Mountain Dog, Rottweiler, Labrador Retriever and Newfoundland, with an increased propensity in males (65%).

Diagnosis

Plain radiographs are advocated as a primary screening method for detection of enthesopathy but cannot distinguish between primary and concomitant forms (de Bakker *et al.*, 2013). A mediolateral and a 15-degree oblique craniolateral–caudomedial view are both necessary to adequately assess for mineralization. CT and MRI detect flexor pathology with high sensitivity, and either of these combined with arthroscopy are effective in screening for concomitant disease. A recent study categorized four distinct lesions comprising epicondylar spurring with or without a calcified body, a calcified body in isolation or an irregular outline of the epicondyle (de Bakker *et al.*, 2012) (see Figure 19.25).

Treatment

If mineralization is an incidental finding, lameness is not identified and elbow pain is not present, then no treatment is required. If lameness and elbow pain, or pain on palpation of the origin of the flexor tendons in the area of mineralization is identified, advanced imaging is required to differentiate between primary or concomitant flexor enthesopathy. It has been suggested that for dogs with primary flexor enthesopathy, joints are injected with 0.5–2 mg/kg of methylprednisolone acetate or that the origins of the flexor muscles are surgically transected (Van Ryssen *et al.*, 2012). However, case numbers are limited and long-term efficacy of such therapies is currently unknown. Concomitant flexor enthesopathy has been treated by both surgical resection of calcified tissue and treatment of concomitant intra-articular lesions (Meyer-Lindenberg *et al.*, 2004).

Salvage procedures for the elbow joint

Elbow replacement

Canine elbow replacement has evolved over the last 25 years in an attempt to provide a functional salvage procedure in dogs with intractable lameness due to primary articular disease or end-stage osteoarthritis. Arthroplasty systems may be stemmed or stemless, cemented or cementless, partial (replacing part of the joint, e.g. medial compartment) or complete, the latter being subdivided into constrained, semi-constrained or non-constrained depending on the degree of linkage between components.

The first system, developed in 1996 by Lewis, was a constrained system implanted into research dogs and was associated with a high complication rate; the project was subsequently abandoned. Conzemius *et al.* (2001) described a semi-constrained cemented system implanted in normal research dogs and subsequently in 20 dogs with severe elbow osteoarthritis (2003). Force plate analysis in this latter study revealed 'satisfactory' outcomes in 80% of dogs; however, up to 20% of patients were reported to experience serious complications including infection, luxation and humeral or ulnar fracture (Conzemius *et al.*, 2003; Innes, 2011). Discontent with the clinical reliability of this system prompted development of several new systems, including the TATE Elbow® (BioMedtrix) 1st and 2nd generation (Acker *et al.*, 2008) (Figure 19.26) and Sirius (Osteogen) (Lorenz *et al.*, 2015), as well as hemi-arthroplasty systems from Kyon (Wendelburg and Tepic, 2011) and the CUE (Arthrex) (Schulz *et al.*, 2011). The long-term clinical efficacy of all of these new systems remains to be reported.

Ex vivo validation of the TATE system's ability to conserve elbow range of motion (Burton *et al.*, 2013) has been reported but no extensive clinical results have yet been published. A case series of 39 dogs receiving first and second generation components has, however, recently been presented (Dejardin and Guillou, 2012). Force plate

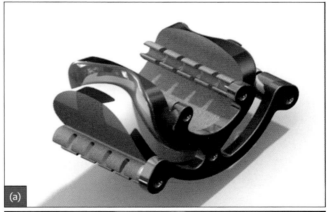

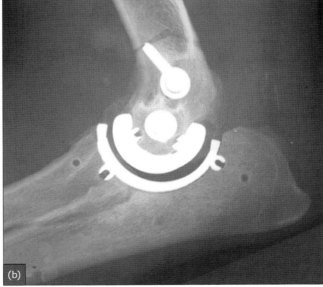

19.26 (a) The BioMedtrix TATE Elbow® 2nd generation prosthesis. The arthroplasty system is an unlinked, semi-constrained, cementless, stemless implant. (b) Postoperative mediolateral radiograph showing the implant in place.
(a, Reproduced with permission of BioMedtrix)

data are limited, but in six cases with 3-year follow-up, peak vertical force was greater than in the contralateral limb and continued to improve up to 2 years postoperatively. Reported complications include infection, ulnar nerve damage, ulnar fracture, humeral fracture and implant instability.

Suitability of a patient for elbow arthroplasty should comprise a careful clinical evaluation coupled with comprehensive owner counselling regarding the surgical procedure, potential for complications, perceived outcome, postoperative management and rehabilitation. There should also be a discussion on the mechanical limitations of alternative salvage via arthrodesis, along with discussion on the feasibility of amputation as both an alternative to and as a salvage for total joint replacement should catastrophic complication occur. This ensures a thorough and fair disclosure of management options to the client prior to embarking on this surgery.

Elbow arthrodesis

Arthrodesis can be considered if elbow replacement is simply not possible, following failed replacement, or in the cases of severe non-reconstructable articular fracture. Following elbow arthrodesis, a significant gait anomaly is induced, with patients tending to circumduct the limb when walking. Acceptable function has been reported but some dogs may only use the limb intermittently or not at all (de Haan *et al.*, 1996). Surgical technique is critical to optimizing outcome, with internal fixation using a plate and screws applied to the caudal aspect of the humerus and ulna at an angle of 130–140 degrees being advocated (de Haan *et al.*, 1996).

Arthrodesis of the elbow has also been described in three cats, two with a caudal bone plate and one with a transarticular external fixator (Moak *et al.*, 2000). However, this surgery was poorly tolerated and arguably better mobility may be achieved with amputation.

Amputation

In cases of failure of elbow replacement, arthrodesis or as a primary treatment modality for financial reasons, forequarter amputation can be considered as a means of palliation of intractable pain due to elbow osteoarthritis. Subjectively the results of forequarter amputation are good in the majority of cases (Carberry and Harvey, 1986). A key consideration as to the suitability of this surgery is concurrent disease in other limbs, particularly the contralateral thoracic limb, given that elbow osteoarthritis is frequently present bilaterally.

References and further reading

Acker R, Van Der Meulen G and Sidebotham CA (2008) Preliminary evaluation of the TATE Elbow total arthroplasty system in client owned dogs. *Proceedings of the 14th ESVOT Congress, 10–14th September*, Munich, p. 13

Barnes DM, Morris AP and Anderson AA (2014) Defining a safe corridor for transcondylar screw insertion across the canine humeral condyle: a comparison of medial and lateral surgical approaches. *Veterinary Surgery* **43**, 1020–1031

Barr ARS and Denny HR (1985) The management of elbow instability caused by premature closure of the distal radial growth plate in dogs. *Journal of Small Animal Practice* **26**, 427–435

Billings LA, Vasseur PB, Todoroff RJ et al. (1992) Clinical results after reduction of traumatic elbow luxations in nine dogs and one cat. *Journal of the American Animal Hospital Association* **28**, 137–142

Bingel SA and Riser WH (1977) Congenital elbow dislocations in the dog. *Journal of Small Animal Practice* **18**, 445–456

Blond L, Dupuis J, Beauregard G et al. (2005) Sensitivity and specificity of radiographic detection of canine elbow incongruence in an *in vitro* model. *Veterinary Radiology and Ultrasound* **46**, 210–216

Böhmer E, Matis U and Waibl H (1987) Zur Operativen Darstellung der Processus anconaeus ulnae beim Hund (Modifikation des Zunganges von Chalman und Slocum) *Tierärztliche Praxis* **15(4)**, 425–429

Bongartz A, Carofiglio F, Piaia T et al. (2008) Traumatic partial elbow luxation in a dog. *Journal of Small Animal Practice* **49**, 359–362

Böttcher P, Bräuer S and Werner H (2013) Estimation of joint incongruence in dysplastic canine elbows before and after dynamic proximal ulnar osteotomy. *Veterinary Surgery* **42**, 371–376

Bouck GR, Miller CW and Taves CL (1995) A comparison of surgical and medical treatment of fragmented coronoid process and osteochondritis dissecans of the canine elbow (1995). *Veterinary and Comparative Orthopaedics and Traumatology* **8**, 177–183

Bräuer S and Böttcher P (2015) Focal humero-ulnar impingement following subtotal coronoid ostectomy in six dogs with fragmented medial coronoid process. *Tierärztliche Praxis Kleintiere* **43**, 156–160

Burton NJ, Ellis JR, Burton KJ et al. (2013) An *ex vivo* investigation of the effect of the TATE canine elbow arthroplasty system on kinematics of the elbow. *Journal of Small Animal Practice* **54**, 240–247

Burton NJ, Owen MR, Colborne GR et al. (2009) Can owners and clinicians assess outcome in dogs with fragmented medial coronoid process? *Veterinary and Comparative Orthopaedics and Traumatology* **22**, 183–189

Burton NJ, Owen MR, Kirk LS et al. (2011) Conservative *versus* arthroscopic management for medial coronoid process disease in dogs: a prospective gait evaluation. *Veterinary Surgery* **40**, 972–980

Burton NJ, Warren-Smith CMR, Roper DP et al. (2013) CT assessment of the influence of dynamic loading on physiological incongruency of the canine elbow. *Journal of Small Animal Practice* **54**, 291–298

Butterworth SJ and Innes JF (2001) Incomplete humeral condylar fractures in the dog. *Journal of Small Animal Practice* **42**, 394–398

Campbell JR (1969) Non-fracture injuries to the canine elbow. *Journal of the American Veterinary Medical Association* **155**, 735–744

Campbell JR (1971) Luxation and ligamentous injuries of the elbow in the dog. *Veterinary Clinics of North America: Small Animal Practice* **1**, 429–440

Campbell JR (1979) Congenital luxation of the elbow of the dog. *Veterinary Annual* **19**, 229–236

Carberry CA and Harvey HJ (1986) Owner satisfaction with limb amputation in dogs and cats. *Journal of the American Animal Hospital Association* **23**, 227–232

Carrera I, Hammond GJC and Sullivan M (2008) Computed tomographic features of incomplete ossification of the canine humeral condyle. *Veterinary Surgery* **37**, 226–231

Charles EA, Ness MG and Yeadon R (2009). Failure mode of transcondylar screws used for treatment of incomplete ossification of the humeral condyle in 5 dogs. *Veterinary Surgery* **38**, 185–191

Clarke SP, Levy J and Ferguson J (2012) Peri-operative morbidity associated with medio-lateral positional screw placement for humeral intra-condylar fissure. *BVOA proceedings, Birmingham Hilton Metropole NEC, 12th April*, pp. 31–32

Collins KE, Cross AR, Lewis DD et al. (2001) Comparison of the radius of curvature of the ulnar trochlear notch of Rottweilers and Greyhounds. *American Journal of Veterinary Research* **62**, 968–973

Conzemius MG, Aper, RL and Corti LB (2003) Short-term outcome after total elbow arthroplasty in dogs with severe, naturally occurring osteoarthritis. *Veterinary Surgery* **32**, 545–552

Conzemius MG, Aper RL and Hill CM (2001) Evaluation of a canine total-elbow arthroplasty system: A preliminary study in normal dogs. *Veterinary Surgery* **30**, 11–20

Cuddy LC, Lewis DD, Kim SE et al. (2012) Contact mechanics and three-dimensional alignment of normal dog elbows. *Veterinary Surgery* **7**, 818–828

Danielson KC, Fitzpatrick N, Muir P and Manley PA (2006) Histomorphometry of fragmented medial coronoid process in dogs: a comparison of affected and normal coronoid processes. *Veterinary Surgery* **35**, 501–509

Dassler CL and Vasseur PB (2003) Elbow luxation. In: *Textbook of Small Animal Surgery, 3rd edn, Vol 2*, ed. DH Slatter, pp. 1919–1927. WB Saunders, Philadelphia

de Bakker E, Saunders J, Gielen I et al. (2012) Radiographic findings of the medial humeral epicondyle in 200 canine elbow joints. *Veterinary and Comparative Orthopaedics and Traumatology* **25**, 359–365

de Bakker E, Saunders JH, van Bree H, Gielen I and Van Ryssen B (2013) Radiographic features of primary and concomitant flexor enthesopathy in the canine elbow. *Veterinary Radiology and Ultrasound* **54**, 107–113

DeCamp C E, Hauptman J, Knowlen G et al. (1986) Periosteum and the healing of partial ulnar osteotomy in radius curvus of dogs. *Veterinary Surgery* **15**, 185–190

de Haan JJ, Roe SC and Lewis DD (1996) Elbow arthrodesis in twelve dogs. *Veterinary and Comparative Orthopaedics and Traumatology* **3**, 25–28

Dejardin LM and Guillou RP (2012) Total elbow replacement in dogs. *Proceedings from the 16th ESVOT Congress 2012*, Bologna (Italy), pp. 147–149

Denny HR (1995) Elbow dysplasia – conservative and surgical treatment. *Proceedings of VI Nordic Symposium on Small Animal Disease together with the 30th Annual Meeting of the Finnish Association of Veterinary Practitioners Naabtali Finland. Section 1*, pp. 17–19

Farrell M, Draffan D, Gemmill T et al. (2007) In vitro validation of a technique for assessment of canine and feline elbow joint collateral ligament integrity and description of a new method for collateral ligament prosthetic replacement. Veterinary Surgery 36, 548–556

Farrell M, Thomson DG and Carmichael S (2009) Surgical management of traumatic elbow luxation in two cats using circumferential suture prosthesis. Veterinary and Comparative Orthopaedics and Traumatology 22, 66–69

Farrell M, Trevail T, Marshall W, Teadon R and Carmichael S (2011) Computed tomographic documentation of the natural progression of humeral intracondylar fissure in a Cocker Spaniel. Veterinary Surgery 40, 966–971

Fitzpatrick N, Bertran and Solano MA (2015) Sliding humeral osteotomy: medium-term objective outcome measures and reduction of complications with a modified technique. Veterinary Surgery 44, 137–149

Fitzpatrick N, Caron A and Solano MA (2013a) Bi-oblique dynamic proximal ulnar osteotomy in dogs: reconstructed computer tomographic assessment of radioulnar congruence over 12 weeks. Veterinary Surgery 42, 727–738

Fitzpatrick N, Garcia-Nolan T and Daryani A (2011) Structural analysis of canine medial coronoid disease by micro CT: Radial incisure verses tip fragmentation. Veterinary Surgery 40, E26

Fitzpatrick N, Smith TJ, Evans RB, O'Riordan J and Yeadon R (2009a) Subtotal coronoid ostectomy for treatment of medial coronoid disease in 263 dogs. Veterinary Surgery 38, 233–245

Fitzpatrick N, Smith TJ, Evans RB and Yeadon R (2009b) Radiographic and arthroscopic findings in the elbow joints of 263 dogs with medial coronoid disease. Veterinary Surgery 38, 213–223

Fitzpatrick N, Smith TJ, O'Riordan J and Yeadon R (2009c) Treatment of incomplete ossification of the humeral condyle with autogenous bone grafting techniques. Veterinary Surgery 38, 173–184

Fitzpatrick N, Yeadon R and Farrell M (2013b) Surgical management of radial head luxation in a dog using an external skeletal traction device. Veterinary and Comparative Orthopaedics and Traumatology 26, 140–146

Fitzpatrick N, Yeadon R and Smith TJ (2009d) Early clinical experience with osteochondral autograft transfer for treatment of osteochondritis dissecans of the medial humeral condyle in dogs. Veterinary Surgery 38, 246–260

Fitzpatrick N, Yeadon R, Smith TJ and Shulz K (2009e) Techniques of application and initial clinical experience with sliding humeral osteotomy for treatment of medial compartment disease of the canine elbow. Veterinary Surgery 38, 261–278

Fitzpatrick N and Yeadon R (2009) Working algorithm for treatment decision making for developmental disease of the medial compartment of the elbow in dogs. Veterinary Surgery 38, 285–300

Fox SM, Burbridge HM, Bray JC et al. (1996) Ununited anconeal process: lag screw fixation. Journal of the American Animal Hospital Association 32, 52–56

Gasch EG, Labruyere JJ and Bardet JF (2012) Computed tomography of ununited anconeal process in the dog. Veterinary and Comparative Orthopaedics and Traumatology 25(6), 498–505

Gemmill T and Clements D (2016) BSAVA Manual of Canine and Feline Fracture Repair and Management, 2nd edn. BSAVA Publications, Gloucester

Gemmill TJ, Mellor DJ, Clements DN et al. (2005) Evaluation of elbow incongruency using reconstructed CT in dogs suffering fragmented coronoid process. Journal of Small Animal Practice 46, 327–333

Gilson SD, Piermattei DL and Schwarz PD (1989) Treatment of humeroulnar subluxation with a dynamic proximal ulnar osteotomy: A review of 13 cases. Veterinary Surgery 18, 114–122

Groth AM, Benigni L, Moores AP et al. (2009) Spectrum of computed tomographic findings in 58 canine elbows with fragmentation of the medial coronoid process. Journal of Small Animal Practice 50(1), 15–22

Guillou RP, Dejargin LM, Bey MJ et al. (2011) Three dimensional kinematics of the normal elbow at the walk and trot. Veterinary Surgery 40, E30

Guthrie S (1989) Some radiographic and clinical aspects of ununited anconeal process. Veterinary Record 124, 661–662

Hare WCD (1961) The age at which the centres of ossification appear roentgenographically in the limb bones of the dog. American Journal of Veterinary Research 22, 825–835

Hattersley R, McKee M, O'Neill T et al. (2011) Postoperative complications after surgical management of incomplete ossification of the humeral condyle in dogs. Veterinary Surgery 40, 728–733

Haudiquet PR, Marcellin-Little DJ and Stebbins ME (2002) Use of the distomedial-proximolateral oblique radiograph view of the elbow joint for examination of the medial coronoid process in dogs. American Journal of Veterinary Research 63, 1000–1005

Hayes HM Jr, Selby LA, Wilson GP et al. (1979) Epidemiologic observations of canine elbow disease (emphasis on dysplasia). Journal of the Small Animal Hospital Association 15, 449–453

Huibregtse BA, Johnson AL, Muhlbauer MC et al. (1994) The effect of treatment of fragmented coronoid process on the development of osteoarthritis of the elbow. Journal of the American Animal Hospital Association 30, 190–195

Hulse D, Young B, Beale B et al. (2010) Relationship of the biceps-brachialis complex to the medial coronoid process of the canine ulna. Veterinary and Comparative Orthopaedics and Traumatology 23, 173–176

Innes JF (2011) Complications with Iowa State TER and how this has informed development of the Sirius TER. Complications in Orthopaedic Surgery. British Veterinary Orthopaedic Association November 2011, Bristol, UK. pp 18–20

Jaeger GH, Marcellin-Little DJ, DePuy V et al. (2007) Validity of goniometric joint measurement in cats. American Journal of Veterinary Research 68, 822–826

Jaeger GH, Marcellin-Little DL and Levine D (2002) Reliability of goniometry in Labrador Retrievers. American Journal of Veterinary Research 63, 979–986

Jungius K-P, Schmid MR, Zanetti M et al. (2006) Cartilaginous defects of the femorotibial joint: accuracy of coronal short inversion time inversion-recovery MR sequence 1. Radiology 240, 482–488

Kene ROC, Lee R and Bennett D (1982) The radiological features of congenital elbow luxation/subluxation in the dog. Journal of Small Animal Practice 23, 621–630

Klumpp S, Ondreka N, Amort K et al. (2010) Diagnostic value of CT and MRI for the diagnosis of coronoid pathology in the dog. Tieraerztliche Praxis Ausgabe Kleintiere Heimtiere 38(1), 7–14

Kramer A, Holsworth IG, Wisner ER et al. (2006) Computed tomographic evaluation of canine radioulnar incongruence in vivo. Veterinary Surgery 35, 24–29

Langley-Hobbs SJ and Carmichael S (1996) Management of a caudolateral radial head luxation in a five-month-old Shih Tzu. Veterinary and Comparative Orthopaedics and Traumatology 9, 186–189

Larsen LJ, Roush JK and McLaughlin RM (1999) Microangiography of the humeral condyle in Cocker Spaniel and non-Cocker Spaniel dogs. Veterinary and Comparative Orthopaedics and Traumatology 12, 134–137

Lau SF, Wolschrijn CF, Siebelt M et al. (2013) Assessment of articular cartilage and subchondral bone using EPID-MicroCT in Labrador retrievers with incipient medial coronoid disease. The Veterinary Journal 198, 116–121

Lavrijsen ICM, Heuven HCM, Voorhout G et al. (2012) Phenotypic and genetic evaluation of elbow dysplasia in Dutch Labrador Retrievers, Golden Retrievers and Bernese Mountain dogs. The Veterinary Journal 193, 486–492

Lewis RH (1996) Development of an elbow arthroplasty (canine) clinical trials. Proceedings from the 6th Annual ACVS Symposium, October 1996, San Francisco, CA, USA, p. 110

Lhermette P and Sobel D (2008) BSAVA Manual of Canine and Feline Endoscopy and Endosurgery. BSAVA Publications, Gloucester

Ljurggren G, Cawley AJ and Archibald J (1966) The elbow dysplasias in the dog. Journal of the American Veterinary Medical Association 148, 887–891

Lorenz ND, Channon S, Pettitt R, Smirthwaite P and Innes JF (2015) Ex vivo kinematic studies of a canine unlinked semi-constrained hybrid total elbow arthroplasty system. Veterinary and Comparative Orthopaedics and Traumatology 28, 39–47

Lowry JE, Carpenter LG, Park RD et al. (1993) Radiographic anatomy and technique for arthrography of the cubital joint in clinically normal dogs. Journal of the American Veterinary Medical Association 203(1), 72–77

Macpherson GC, Lewis DD, Johnson KA et al. (1992) Fragmented coronoid process associated with premature distal radial physeal closure in four dogs. Veterinary and Comparative Orthopaedics and Traumatology 5, 93–99

Marcellin-Little DJ, DeYoung DJ and Ferris KK (1994) Incomplete ossification of the humeral condyle in spaniels. Veterinary Surgery 23, 475–487

Marti JM, Miller A (1994) Delimitation of safe corridors for the insertion of external fixator pins in the dog 2: Forelimb. Journal of Small Animal Practice 35, 78–85

Mason DR, Schulz KS, Fujita Y, Kass PH and Stover SM (2005) In vitro force mapping of normal canine humeroradial and humeroulnar joints. American Journal of Veterinary Research 66, 132–135

Mason DR, Schulz, KS, Samii VF et al. (2002) Sensitivity of radiographic evaluation of radio-ulnar incongruence in the dog in vitro. Veterinary Surgery 31, 125–132

Mason TA and Baker MJ (1978) The surgical management of elbow joint deformity with premature growth plate closure in dogs. Journal of Small Animal Practice 19, 639–645

Matis U (1992) Treatment of ununited anconeal process. Proceedings of the 6th Congress of the European Society of Veterinary Orthopaedics and Traumatology, p. 16

Meyer-Lindenberg A, Fehr M and Nolte I (1991) Zur Luxation antebrachii traumatica des Hundes – Häufigkeit, Symptome, Therapie und Ergebnisse. (In German) Kleintierpraxis 36, 607–616

Meyer-Lindenberg A, Fehr M and Nolte I (2001) Short and long term results after surgical treatment of an ununited anconeal process in the dog. Veterinary and Comparative Orthopaedics and Traumatology 14, 101–110

Meyer-Lindenberg A, Fehr M and Nolte I (2006) Co-existence of ununited anconeal process and fragmented medial coronoid process of the ulna in the dog. Journal of Small Animal Practice 47, 61–65

Meyer-Lindenberg A, Heinen V, Hewicker-Trautwein M (2004) Occurrence and treatment of bone metaplasia arising from the medial epicondyle of the humerus flexor tendons in the dog (In German). Tierärztliche Praxis 32, 276–85

Meyer-Lindenberg A, Langhann A, Fehr M et al. (2003) Arthrotomy versus arthroscopy in the treatment of the fragmented medial coronoid process of the ulna (FCP) in 421 dogs. Veterinary and Comparative Orthopaedics and Traumatology 16, 204–210

Milton JL, Horne RD, Bartels JE et al. (1979) Congenital elbow luxation in the dog. Journal of the American Veterinary Medical Association 175, 572–582

Milton JL and Montgomery RD (1987) Congenital elbow dislocations. Veterinary Clinics of North America: Small Animal Practice 17, 873–888

Mitchell KE (2011) Traumatic elbow luxation in 14 dogs and 11 cats. Australian Veterinary Journal 89, 213–216

Moak, PC, Lewis DD, Roe SC et al. (2000) Arthrodesis of the elbow in three cats. Veterinary and Comparative Orthopaedics and Traumatology 13, 149–153

Montgomery M and Tomlinson J (1985) Two cases of ectrodactyly and congenital elbow luxation in the dog. *Journal of the American Animal Hospital Association* **21**, 781–785

Moores AP, Agthe P and Schaafsma IA (2012) Prevalence of incomplete ossification of the humeral condyle and other abnormalities of the elbow in English Springer Spaniels. *Veterinary and Comparative Orthopaedics and Traumatology* **25(3)**, 211–216

Moores AP, Benigni L and Lamb CR (2008) Computed tomography *versus* arthroscopy for detection of canine elbow dysplasia lesions. *Veterinary Surgery* **37**, 390–398

Moores AP, Tivers MS and Grierson J (2014) Clinical assessment of a shaft screw for stabilisation of the humeral condyle in dogs. *Veterinary and Comparative Orthopaedics and Traumatology* **27**, 179–185

Ness MG (1998) Treatment of fragmented coronoid process in young dogs by proximal ulnar osteotomy. *Journal of Small Animal Practice* **39**, 15–18

O'Brien MG, Boudrieau RJ and Clark GN (1992) Traumatic luxation of the cubital joint (elbow) in dogs: 44 cases (1978–1988) *Journal of the American Veterinary Medical Association* **201**, 1760–1765

Olsson SE (1977) Osteochondrosis in the dog. In: *Current Veterinary Therapy VI*, ed. RW Kirk, pp. 880–886. Saunders, Philadelphia

Pettitt RA, Tattersall J, Gemmill T *et al.* (2009) Effect of surgical technique on radiographic fusion of the anconeus in the treatment of ununited anconeal process. *Journal of Small Animal Practice* **50**, 545–548

Pfeil I, Böttcher P and Starke A (2012) Proximal abduction ulnar osteotomy (PAUL) for medial compartment disease in dogs with elbow dysplasia. *16th ESVOT Congress Bologna (Italy) 12–15th September*, pp. 314–318

Phillips A, Burton NJ, Warren Smith CMR *et al.* (2015) Topographic bone density of the radius and ulna in Greyhounds and Labrador Retrievers with and without medial coronoid process disease. *Veterinary Surgery* **44**, 180–190

Piola V, Posch B, Radke H *et al.* (2012) Magnetic resonance imaging features of canine incomplete humeral condyle ossification *Veterinary Radiology and Ultrasound* **53(5)**, 560–565

Presnell K (1990) Ununited anconeal process of the elbow. In: *Current Techniques in Small Animal Surgery*, ed. MJ Bojrab, pp. 778–782. Lea and Febiger, Philadelphia

Preston CA, Schulz KS and Kass PH (2000) *In vitro* determination of contact areas in the normal elbow joint of dogs. *American Journal of Veterinary Research* **61**, 1315–1321

Rahal SC, De Biasi F, Vulcano *et al.* (2000) Reduction of humeroulnar congenital elbow luxation in 8 dogs by using a transarticular pin. *The Veterinary Journal* **41**, 849–853

Ramadan RO and Vaughan LC (1978) Premature closure of the distal ulnar growth plate – a review of 58 cases. *Journal of Small Animal Practice* **19**, 647–667

Read RA, Armstrong SJ, O'Keefe JD *et al.* (1990) Fragmentation of the medial coronoid process of the ulna in dogs: a study of 109 cases. *Journal of Small Animal Practice* **31**, 330–334

Robins GM (1987) The management of distal radial growth plate closure. *Australian Veterinary Practitioner* **17**, 143–144

Samoy Y, Van Vynckt D, Gielen I *et al.* (2012) Arthroscopic findings in 32 joints affected by severe elbow incongruity with concomitant fragmented medial coronoid process. *Veterinary Surgery* **41(3)**, 355–361

Schmidt TH, Fisher M and Bottcher P (2012) Fluoroscopic kinematography of the sound and dysplastic canine elbow. *Proceedings of the 16th ESVOT Congress, Bologna, Italy 12–15th September*, p. 91

Schulz KS, Cook JL and Karnes J (2011) Canine unicompartmental elbow arthroplasty system. *Proceedings of the 21st Annual American College Veterinary Surgeons Symposium, November 3–5th Chicago, Illinois*, pp. 123–125

Skinner O, Burton NJ, Warren-Smith C *et al.* (2015) Computed tomographic evaluation of elbow congruity during arthroscopy in a canine cadaveric model. *Veterinary and Comparative Orthopaedics and Traumatology* **28**, 19–24

Sinibaldi KR and Arnoczky SP (1975) Surgical removal of the ununited anconeal process in the dog. *Journal of the American Animal Hospital Association* **11**, 192–198

Sjostrum L, Kasstrom H and Kallberg M (1995) Ununited anconeal process in the dog: Pathogenesis and treatment by osteotomy of the ulna. *Veterinary and Comparative Orthopaedics and Traumatology* **8**, 10–16

Staiger BA and Beale BS (2005) Use of arthroscopy for debridement of the elbow joint in cats. *Journal of the American Veterinary Medical Association* **226**, 401–403

Strickland AL and Sprinz H (1973) Studies of the influence of oestradiol and growth hormone on the hypophysectomised, immature rat epiphyseal cartilage growth plate. *American Journal of Obstetrics and Gynaecology* **115**, 471–477

Temwichitr J, Leegwater PA and Hazewinkel HA (2010) Fragmented coronoid process in the dog: A heritable disease. *The Veterinary Journal* **185**, 123–129

Tirgari M (1980) Clinical, radiological and pathological aspects of ununited medial coronoid process of the elbow joint in dogs. *Journal of Small Animal Practice* **21**, 595–608

Trostel CT, McLaughlin RM and Pool RR (2003) Canine elbow dysplasia: Anatomy and Pathogenesis. *The Compendium on Continuing Education for the Practicing Veterinarian* **25**, 754–762

Turner BM, Abercromby RH, Innes J *et al.* (1998) Dynamic proximal ulnar osteotomy for the treatment of ununited anconeal process in 17 dogs. *Veterinary and Comparative Orthopaedics and Traumatology* **22**, 76–79

Vandewater A and Olmstead ML (1983) Premature closure of the distal radial physis in the dog. *Veterinary Surgery* **12**, 7–12

Van Ryssen B, de Bakker E, Beaumlin Y *et al.* (2012) Primary flexor enthesiopathy of the canine elbow: imaging and arthroscopic findings in eight dogs with discrete radiographic changes. *Veterinary and Comparative Orthopaedics and Traumatology* **25(3)**, 239–245

Van Ryssen B, van Bree H and Simonens P (1993) Elbow arthroscopy in clinically normal dogs. *American Journal of Veterinary Research* **54**, 191–198

Vermote KA, Bergenhuyzen AL, Gielen I *et al.* (2010) Elbow lameness in dogs of six years and older: arthroscopic and imaging findings of medial coronoid disease in 51 dogs. *Veterinary and Comparative Orthopaedics and Traumatology* **23**, 43–50

Viehmann B, Waibl H and Brunnberg L (1999) Computer assisted interpretation of radiographs for elbow dysplasia in dogs (I). Trochlear incisures of the ulna. *Kleintierpraxis* **44**, 595–606

Wagner K, Griffon DJ, Thomas MW *et al.* (2007) Radiographic, computed tomographic, and arthroscopic evaluation of experimental radio-ulnar incongruence in the dog. *Veterinary Surgery* **36**, 691–698

Walker RG and Hickman J (1958) Injury to the elbow joint in the dog. *Veterinary Record* **70**, 1191–1194

Wendelburg K and Tepic S (2011) Kyon Elbow prosthesis project. *Kyon Symposium, 15–17th April*, Boston, Massachusetts, USA

Wind AP (1986) Elbow Incongruity and Developmental Elbow Diseases in the dog: Part 1. *Journal of the American Animal Hospital Association* **22**, 711–724

Wind AP and Packard ME (1986) Elbow Incongruity and Developmental Elbow Diseases in the dog: Part 2. *Journal of the American Animal Hospital Association* **22**, 725–730

Witte PG, Bush MA and Scott HW (2010) Propagation of a partial incomplete ossification of the humeral condyle in an American Cocker Spaniel. *Journal of Small Animal Practice* **51**, 591–593

Wucherer KL, Ober CP and Conzemius MG (2012) The use of delayed gadolinium enhanced magnetic resonance imaging of cartilage and t2 mapping to evaluate articular cartilage in the normal canine elbow. *Veterinary Radiology and Ultrasound* **53(1)**, 57–63

IMAGING TECHNIQUES

Thomas W. Maddox

Much of the pathology affecting the elbow joint is osseous in nature and so, in principle, radiography should be well suited to imaging elbow disease. This is true to an extent, but many of the lesions concerned can be located in regions that are difficult to clearly visualize on conventional radiographs. Consequently, coupled with its wider availability, computed tomography (CT) is being increasingly used for examination of the elbow.

RADIOGRAPHY

Standard views

The standard orthogonal views are the mediolateral extended and craniocaudal views. The use of a radiographic grid is not required.

Mediolateral view

This view allows assessment of major elbow incongruity and osteophyte formation on the cranial aspect of the joint. The subchondral bone of the trochlear notch of the elbow can be evaluated for evidence of sclerosis. The medial coronoid process can be seen, but superimposition of the radial head can hinder examination.

* The animal is placed in lateral recumbency with the target limb dependent against the cassette/plate and the contralateral limb retracted caudally; slight extension of the head and neck is beneficial (Figure 19.27).
* For a neutral view, the joint angle should be approximately 90–120 degrees.
* The primary beam is centred on the medial humeral epicondyle.
* Collimate to include approximately one-third of the length of the humerus and radius/ulna.

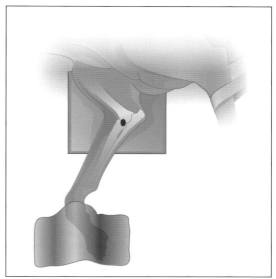

19.27 Patient positioning for a mediolateral view of the elbow.

Craniocaudal view

This view allows outline assessment of the articular surface of the humeral condyle and osteophyte formation on the medial and lateral humeral epicondyles. It is essential for evaluation of the minority of humeral condylar fissures/IOHC which are detectable radiographically and for fractures involving the humeral condyle. It should be noted that although part of the medial coronoid can be seen, this is only the most abaxial part and not the axial apical region where fragmentation typically occurs. However, osteophyte formation on the margin of the coronoid can be assessed.

* The animal is placed in sternal recumbency with the target limb extended, ensuring the humerus and radius/ulna are aligned in a straight line (Figure 19.28).
* Foam wedges/sandbags can be placed under the axilla of the contralateral limb to slightly rotate the animal to the side of interest.
* The head and neck are slightly elevated and flexed away from the side of interest.
* The primary beam is centred on the medial and lateral humeral epicondyles.
* Collimate to just beyond the medial and lateral skin margins and approximately one-third of the length of the humerus and radius/ulna.

Special views

The main additional views required of the elbow are the flexed mediolateral and craniocaudal oblique views. Contrast arthrography of the elbow is technically possible (Lowry et al.,

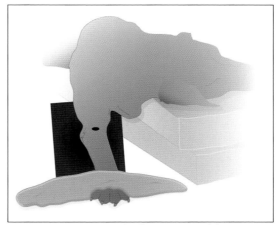

19.28 Patient positioning for a craniocaudal view of the elbow.

→ **IMAGING TECHNIQUES CONTINUED**

1993), but can be difficult and unrewarding, and is infrequently performed as it offers no benefit over advanced imaging techniques such as CT or magnetic resonance imaging (MRI).

Flexed mediolateral view

This view is useful as it allows evaluation of the anconeal process without superimposition from the medial humeral epicondyle, permitting assessment for an ununited anconeal process, early osteophyte formation and flexor enthesopathy.

- The leg of the animal is placed in maximal flexion (joint angle <60 degrees) and held in place with sandbags or ties (Figure 19.29).
- Positioning, primary beam centring and collimation are otherwise as for the standard mediolateral view; however, placing a foam wedge under the carpus can help to minimize the rotation that this view is prone to.

Craniolateral–caudomedial oblique view

This view allows clearer visualization of the medial coronoid process and the medial part of the humeral condyle, although the wider availability of advanced imaging techniques means that this view is now infrequently required.

- The animal is positioned as for the standard craniocaudal view and the limb is pronated approximately 15–45 degrees (Figure 19.30).
- Positioning, primary beam centring and collimation are otherwise as for the standard craniocaudal view.

Craniomedial–caudolateral oblique view

This view is useful as it more often aligns the primary X-ray beam with the orientation of an intracondylar fissure in cases of incomplete ossification (the optimal angle to achieve this is approximately 15 degrees). As with the other oblique view, the wider availability of advanced imaging techniques means that this view is now infrequently required.

- The animal is positioned as for the standing craniocaudal view and the limb is supinated approximately 15–45 degrees (Figure 19.31).
- Positioning, primary beam centring and collimation are otherwise as for the standard craniocaudal view.

COMPUTED TOMOGRAPHY

CT is a very useful imaging modality for the elbow joint. The main advantage is the acquisition of images in a transverse plane (and reconstruction in sagittal and dorsal/frontal planes), which eliminates the superimposition of structures that limit radiological interpretation. In addition, the increased contrast resolution compared with radiography (primarily relating to soft tissues) is also beneficial.

Most of the significant musculoskeletal conditions that affect the elbow can be imaged well using CT (Groth *et al.*, 2009; Gasch *et al.*, 2012; Moores *et al.*, 2012; Samoy *et al.*, 2012). The exceptions to this are lesions wholly restricted to cartilage; as with radiography, cartilage cannot be confidently identified without the use of intra-articular contrast media. However, under normal circumstances, cartilage lesions such as osteochondrosis invariably lead to some changes in the subchondral bone and, even if these are subtle, they can usually be detected on CT.

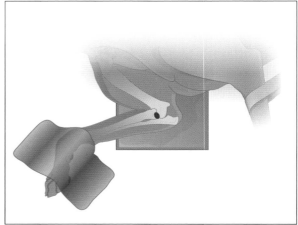

19.29 Patient positioning for a flexed mediolateral view of the elbow.

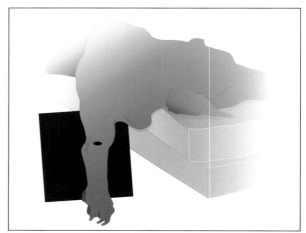

19.30 Patient positioning for a craniolateral–caudomedial oblique (Cr15°L-CdMO) view of the elbow.

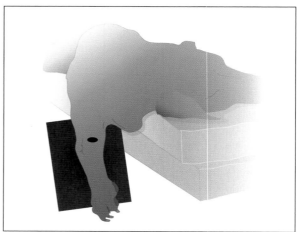

19.31 Patient positioning for a craniomedial–caudolateral oblique (Cr15M°-CdLO) view of the elbow.

→ **IMAGING TECHNIQUES CONTINUED**

Standard technique

The rapid acquisition times of multidetector CT means that examination can normally be carried out under sedation.

- The animal is placed in sternal recumbency with the thoracic limbs fully extended (Figure 19.32).
- In order to obviate the effects of beam hardening and streak artefacts, it is advisable to flex the head and neck laterally so they are outside the scan field.
- Both elbows can be scanned concurrently.
- The scan margins should extend from slightly proximal to the olecranon to include the proximal one-quarter of the radius/ulna.
- Once acquired the separate images of both elbows should be reconstructed with as small a field of view as feasible.

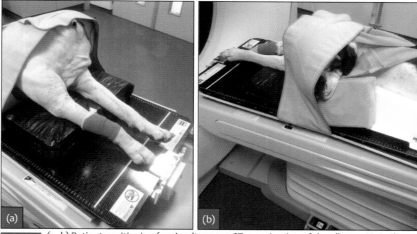

19.32 (a–b) Patient positioning for simultaneous CT examination of the elbows. Note the head and neck are flexed out of the primary area of interest.

- Alternatively, the animal can be placed in lateral recumbency with one limb retracted and both elbows scanned separately.
- Reconstruction of images using bone and soft tissue algorithms is advisable.

The use of multiplanar reformatting into sagittal and frontal/dorsal planes is recommended, particularly for identification of an osteochondrosis lesion, which can be hard to evaluate on transverse images (Figure 19.33). Similarly, evaluation of elbow congruency is almost impossible without reformatting (Figure 19.34). The use of 3D volume or surface rendering is rarely of diagnostic value, except in cases of elbow fractures. Intravenous (system) contrast media is rarely required unless neoplastic or inflammatory soft tissue lesions are suspected. As with radiography, positive-contrast arthrography is possible but rarely deemed necessary.

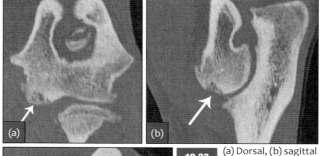

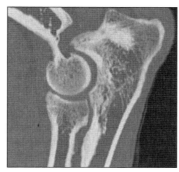

19.33 (a) Dorsal, (b) sagittal and (c) transverse multiplanar reconstructed CT images of the elbow of a dog. The reformatting allows easier observation of the osteochondrosis lesion (arrowed) of the medial part of the humeral condyle and the surrounding sclerosis.

MAGNETIC RESONANCE IMAGING

MRI offers similar advantages to CT in that its cross-sectional nature eliminates superimposition and images can be acquired in multiple planes. In addition, it offers far higher soft tissue contrast, and whilst the resolution of bone is lower than CT, it is still adequate for the detection of the bony lesions likely to be encountered (Klumpp et al., 2010), including IOHC (Piola et al., 2012). Furthermore, there is the potential for direct detection of cartilage lesions (Wucherer et al., 2012). However, the higher cost and longer acquisition times (requiring the use of general anaesthesia) are amongst the reasons why MRI is currently less commonly used for evaluation of the elbow.

As a consequence of its less frequent use, a standardized protocol for MRI studies has yet to be developed and a variety of approaches have been used. Dogs are generally scanned in lateral recumbency with the target limb dependent and extended cranially, and the contralateral limb retracted caudally. The use of a small flexible coil is advised and T1- and T2-weighted images should be acquired in a minimum of three standard orthogonal planes.

19.34 Sagittal reconstructed CT image of the elbow of a dog. Moderately severe elbow incongruence can be easily appreciated affecting the radioulnar (step) and humeroulnar (uneven joint width) articulations.

→ **IMAGING TECHNIQUES CONTINUED**

ULTRASONOGRAPHY

Although ultrasonography is rarely used in evaluation of the elbow joint, it is a useful technique for assessment of soft tissue lesions. Soft tissue lesions are relatively uncommon, but ultrasonography can allow evaluation of mineralization of the flexor muscles adjacent to the medial epicondyle (Van Ryssen *et al.*, 2012). The medial and lateral collateral ligaments can also be seen ultrasonographically.

Osseous lesions, such as UAP and fragmented medial coronoid process, can also be observed, but no further information is provided over radiographs, particularly for UAP. Fissures of the medial coronoid process cannot be detected reliably and osteophyte formation on the margins of the coronoid can be confused for fragmentation.

OPERATIVE TECHNIQUE 19.1

Arthroscopy of the elbow

There are many variations in all aspects of arthroscopic technique for the elbow. These include the use of fixed limb positioning aids *versus* a freely held limb, motorized fluid pumps *versus* a pressure cuff bag, variation in the access used for insufflation and in techniques for examination and instrument use. The relative advantages and disadvantages of these variables are outwith the scope of this guide and discussed elsewhere – see Chapter 15 and the *BSAVA Manual of Canine and Feline Endoscopy and Endosurgery*. The author's preferred technique is presented simply as a guide; however, arthroscopy is a specialized practical skill with a steep learning curve that is best learnt through attendance at a technique-specific course.

INDICATIONS

Diagnosis of elbow lameness, quantification of severity of medial/lateral compartment cartilage damage, removal of cartilage flaps or medial coronoid fragments, lavage for infective arthritis and synovial biopsy.

POSITIONING AND PREPARATION

Dorsal recumbency to prepare and drape, moving into lateral recumbency for each elbow. Hair is clipped across the chest, joining medially in bilateral cases. Clipping should extend distally to the level of the carpus. A sandbag placed under the drape under the lateral aspect of the elbow is useful to act as a fulcrum to open the medial joint compartment. In unilateral cases, lateral recumbency with affected limb lowermost and the upper limb tied away.

ASSISTANT

Essential. Alternatively, use of a limb positioning guide, if available, can hold the elbow suitably abducted for single surgeon arthroscopy.

EQUIPMENT EXTRAS

1.9 mm or 2.4 mm 30-degree fore-oblique arthroscope with appropriate cannula and blunt obturator; 5 litres of Hartmann's fluid in positive pressure infuser system and sterile giving set; light source; video camera and control box; monitor; image archiving system; arthroscopic instrumentation; switching stick; cannulae of varying diameters for use as instrument portals; hooked probe; hand burr; fragment graspers; (motorized shaver system); 5 ml and 10 ml syringes (see Chapter 14).

SURGICAL APPROACH

Medial portal sites for egress needle, arthroscope and instruments (Figure 19.35).

SURGICAL TECHNIQUE

The limb is held at a mid-stance angle of approximately 135 degrees by the assistant, using the sandbag as a fulcrum to open the medial joint compartment. A 50 mm (2 inch) 19 G needle is placed into the caudomedial joint pouch. This is oriented craniodistally, entering through the skin at a point equidistant between the corner of the medial epicondylar ridge and the olecranon. A 5 ml syringe is attached to the needle and aspirated to confirm the

→

→ **OPERATIVE TECHNIQUE 19.1 CONTINUED**

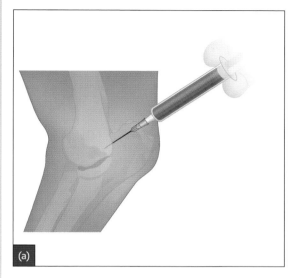
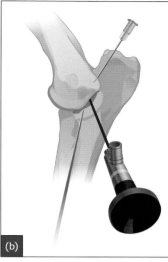

19.35 Portal positions for medial elbow arthroscopy. (a) An egress needle is placed first to insufflate the joint with Hartmann's solution; this needle is oriented in a craniodistal orientation and enters the caudomedial joint pouch at a point equidistant between the medial epicondyle and the olecranon. (b) The arthroscope portal is established at the level of the mid-trochlear notch of the ulna and the instrument portal is placed cranial to the arthroscope at the level of the apex of the medial coronoid process.

needle is in the joint. This syringe is removed and a new syringe containing 10 ml Hartmann's solution is connected and 5–10 ml of fluid is injected to distend the joint (which should be both visible medially and palpable). A 50 mm (2 inch) 19 G needle is then placed into the joint at a point distal and slightly caudal to the medial epicondyle. Egress of Hartmann's solution through the needle confirms articular placement. A No. 11 scalpel blade is oriented proximodistally relative to the limb and used to incise immediately caudal to the needle, along its path into the joint. The arthroscopic sleeve with blunt obturator is passed into the joint, this is normally associated with a defined 'clunk' as the cannula engages between the humeral trochlea and and trochlear notch of the ulna. The obturator is removed and the arthroscope inserted. The joint is inspected in a systematic fashion with a combination of movement of the arthroscope and rotation of the light post as follows:

1 Anconeal process (light post (LP) at 3 o'clock (L) or 9 o'clock (R)).

2 Ulnar trochlear notch.

3 Lateral coronoid process and radial head (LP at 12 o'clock position).

4 Lateral portion of the humeral condyle.

5 Medial portion of the humeral condyle (LP at 9 o'clock (L) or 3 o'clock (R)).

6 Medial coronoid process (LP at 9 o'clock (L) or 3 o'clock (R)).

7 Medial collateral ligament.

Should an instrument portal need to be established, triangulation is achieved by use of a hypodermic needle placed approximately 1 cm cranial to the arthroscope portal. Entry of the needle into the joint is observed through the arthroscope and the optimal angle of needle entry assessed such as to permit an instrument to reach the desired region of the joint without undue stress. A No. 11 scalpel blade is used to establish a portal along the line of this needle, following which a switching stick is introduced. An appropriately sized cannula is placed over the stick and the stick withdrawn, or alternatively instrumentation can be placed via an open portal with no cannula. Instrumentation is placed through the cannula as appropriate. Removal of osteochondral fragments affecting either the medial portion of the humeral condyle or medial coronoid process is achieved with fragment graspers.

Closure

Single skin sutures are placed in each portal site.

POSTOPERATIVE CARE

A protective adhesive dressing is placed over the portal sites.

OPERATIVE TECHNIQUE 19.2

Caudolateral approach to the elbow

Geoff Robins and John Innes

POSITIONING

Lateral recumbency with the affected limb uppermost.

ASSISTANT

Optional, depending on the procedure.

EQUIPMENT EXTRAS

Gelpi-style self-retaining retractors or small stifle distractor; two pairs of Senn hand-held retractors, if working with an assistant.

SURGICAL TECHNIQUE

A curved skin incision is made behind the caudal edge of the lateral condyle of the humerus centred on the easily palpable lateral epicondylar process (Figure 19.36a). The fascia is divided along the cranial edge of the lateral head of the triceps muscle. Retraction of the fascia will reveal the anconeus muscle, which is then divided across its fibres in its mid-section (Figure 19.36b). Alternatively, the anconeus muscle can be sharply incised and elevated from its attachment to the lateral epicondylar ridge (Figure 19.36c). Retraction of the muscle with the underlying joint capsule exposes the caudal joint compartment, the lateral condyle of the humerus and the anconeal process. This approach can be extended caudodistally if a proximal ulnar osteotomy is to be undertaken in combination with a procedure necessitating caudolateral approach.

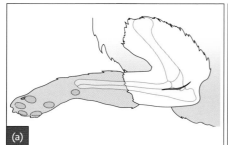

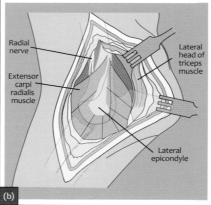

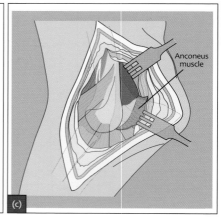

19.36 (a) The curvilinear skin incision is made just caudal to the lateral epicondylar ridge. (b) The anconeus muscle can be incised along its fibres or (c) elevated from its origin on the lateral epicondylar ridge.

PRACTICAL TIP

Full flexion of the elbow is necessary to explore the anconeal process thoroughly. However, with the joint in this position, the surrounding muscles can make visibility difficult. Enough exposure is gained by this approach to remove the anconeal process easily, but if internal fixation is to be conducted, then the modified approach (see below) is preferred

Modified approach

If internal fixation of the separated anconeal process is anticipated, a modification of the caudolateral approach is recommended to provide better access to the anconeal process in the flexed position (Böhmer *et al.*, 1987). The area is exposed by separating between the lateral and long heads of the triceps muscle along a line which is caudal to, but parallel with the humerus. Distally the attachment of the lateral head of the triceps is separated from the olecranon, leaving some of the tendon behind to facilitate closure later (Figure 19.37). The anconeus muscle

→ **OPERATIVE TECHNIQUE 19.2 CONTINUED**

is then bluntly dissected from the long head of the triceps muscle. The periosteal insertion of the anconeus muscle is incised on the ulna, the olecranon and the lateral epicondylar crest of the humerus. Retraction of the anconeus muscle cranially and the long head of the triceps caudally achieves superior exposure of the caudal compartment of the elbow joint.

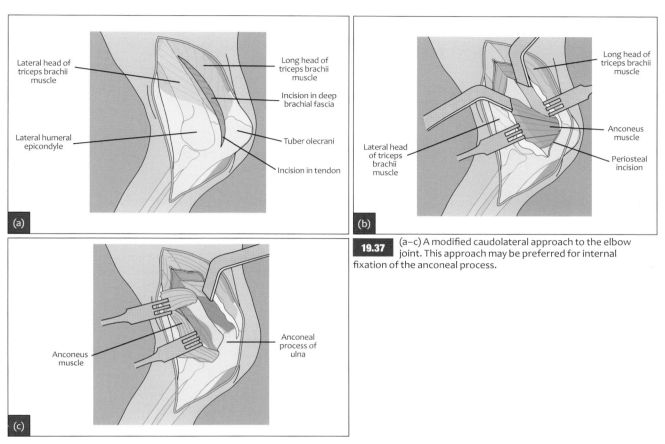

19.37 (a–c) A modified caudolateral approach to the elbow joint. This approach may be preferred for internal fixation of the anconeal process.

Closure

The joint capsule and the divided anconeus muscle are closed with a simple continuous pattern using absorbable monofilament sutures, followed by the fascia, subcutaneous tissue and skin.

POSTOPERATIVE CARE

The joint is protected with a light dressing for 5–7 days. If internal fixation has been performed then more support is provided with a Robert Jones bandage for 2 weeks.

OPERATIVE TECHNIQUE 19.3

Medial approach to the elbow

Geoff Robins and John Innes

POSITIONING

Lateral recumbency with the affected limb lowermost. The upper leg is pulled caudally. A small sandbag or folded towel is positioned under the affected elbow to act as a fulcrum, which will help with exposure.

ASSISTANT

Essential to help with manipulation of the joint to gain adequate exposure of the interior of the joint through this limited approach.

EQUIPMENT EXTRAS

Gelpi self-retaining retractors or small stifle distractors; Senn hand-held retractors.

SURGICAL TECHNIQUE

A curved 3–4 cm skin incision is centred over the medial epicondyle (Figure 19.38a). Numerous layers of subcutaneous fascia are divided to expose the medial epicondyle and the flexor muscles of the antebrachium (Figure 19.38b).

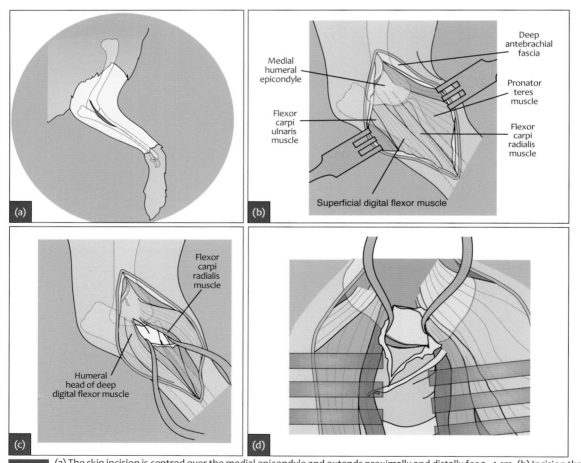

19.38 (a) The skin incision is centred over the medial epicondyle and extends proximally and distally for 3–4 cm. (b) Incision through the underlying fascia and subsequent retraction exposes the origin of the flexor tendons. (c) Blunt dissection between the deep digital flexor tendon and the flexor carpi radialis tendon exposes the joint capsule. (An alternative approach is to separate between the flexor carpi radialis and pronator teres tendons.) (d) The joint capsule is incised. Internal rotation of the elbow joint can aid inspection of the medial coronoid process. If necessary, the caudal aspect of the medial collateral ligament can be incised to increase exposure.

→ **OPERATIVE TECHNIQUE 19.3 CONTINUED**

> **WARNING**
>
> The ulnar nerve is located at the proximal end of the incision and care should be taken when the fat in this area is divided. The proximity of the brachial artery and vein and the median nerve to the underside of the pronator teres muscle should be recognized

Exposure of the joint is achieved by muscle separation, either between the pronator teres and the flexor carpi radialis or between the flexor carpi radialis and the deep digital flexor that lies caudal to it (Figure 19.38c). If more exposure is required the insertions of the relevant muscles can be partially transected.

The joint capsule and, if necessary, the medial collateral ligament are divided parallel with the joint surface (Figure 19.38d). Retraction of the joint capsule will reveal the medial part of the humeral condyle and the outer aspect of the medial coronoid process. Better exposure of the deeper aspects of the joint can be achieved by abduction and pronation of the radius and ulna or alternatively by flexing the carpus and using the sandbag as a fulcrum to lever the joint open. The elbow joint is a close-fitting joint and this approach provides limited but adequate exposure.

Closure

The joint capsule, collateral ligament and muscles are repaired with absorbable sutures. Slight elevation of the limb may facilitate tying the sutures. The fascial layers and skin are closed in separate layers with continuous absorbable sutures.

POSTOPERATIVE CARE

The joint is supported in a padded bandage for 5–7 days. Exercise is restricted for 2–3 weeks.

OPERATIVE TECHNIQUE 19.4

Subtotal coronoidectomy

POSITIONING

Lateral recumbency with the affected limb lowermost. The upper limb is pulled caudally and affixed to the operating table with a tie. A small sandbag can be positioned under the elbow to act as a fulcrum if additional exposure is required.

ASSISTANT

Essential to fulcrum open the medial aspect of the joint.

EQUIPMENT EXTRAS

Small sagittal saw (e.g. 3M microdriver) with small blade or small osteotome and mallet; small Gelpi retractors x 2; Hohmann retractors; saline for lavage; small fragment forceps; suction unit.

SURGICAL TECHNIQUE

If arthroscopic evaluation of the medial compartment has been performed then a 2 cm curvilinear incision is made to enlarge the arthroscope portal over the craniomedial aspect of the condyle. Subcutaneous tissues are bluntly dissected with care to avoid damage to the ulnar nerve caudally and median nerve cranially. Take care when placing Gelpi retractors that these nerves are not inadvertently stretched.

The flexor carpi radialis (FCR) and superficial and deep digital flexor muscles are identified and blunt dissection between these bellies or between the FCR and pronator teres muscles exposes the medial joint capsule caudal to the medial collateral ligament (MCL) and proximal to the insertion of the biceps brachii muscle. The MCL is not transected. The joint capsule is incised parallel to the MCL with a No. 11 scalpel blade. The Gelpi retractors are carefully repositioned inside the joint caudal to the MCL. It is necessary for the assistant to hold the flexed carpus and distal limb fully pronated to improve visualization of the medial elbow joint space.

→

→ **OPERATIVE TECHNIQUE 19.4 CONTINUED**

A small sagittal saw is used to osteotomize the medial coronoid process from its medial border to the caudal extent of the radial incisures cranial to the sagittal ridge of the ulnar trochlear notch, as shown by the green line in Figure 19.39. A small sharp osteotome can also be used but care must be taken to avoid inadvertent fracture. The fragment is removed *en bloc* together with any loose coronoid fragments (Figure 19.40). The joint is lavaged to remove any osteochondral debris.

> **WARNING**
>
> The ulnar nerve is located at the proximal end of the incision and the brachial artery, vein and medial nerve on the underside of the pronator teres

> **WARNING**
>
> Care should be exercised when performing the osteotomy that the radial head is not inadvertently damaged by an overzealous cut. When the osteotomy is nearly complete a small osteotome can be substituted for the saw blade. Gentle advancement and twisting of the osteotome will encourage the coronoid fragment to separate

Closure

The joint capsule, intramuscular and subcutaneous tissues are closed in separate layers with a continuous pattern using absorbable sutures.

POSTOPERATIVE CARE

Perioperative opioid and non-steroidal anti-inflammatory medication should be administered based on individual postoperative assessment. A 2–6 week course of postoperative non-steroidal anti-inflammatory medication, followed by reassessment, is appropriate.

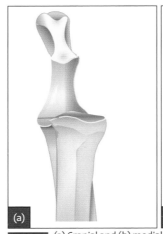
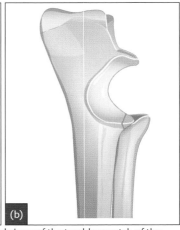

19.39 (a) Cranial and (b) medial views of the trochlear notch of the ulna. The green line shows the recommended orientation of the osteotomy.

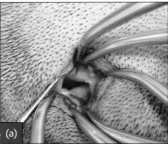
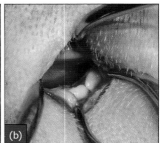
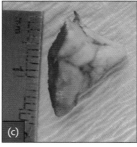

19.40 (a) A limited arthrotomy is made to the medial joint compartment. (b) The medial coronoid process is ostectomized and removed. (c) The ostectomized fragment.
(Courtesy of Noel Fitzpatrick)

OPERATIVE TECHNIQUE 19.5

OCD flap removal by medial arthrotomy

POSITIONING

Lateral recumbency with the affected limb lowermost. The unaffected limb is pulled caudally and secured with a tie. A small sandbag can be positioned under the affected elbow to act as a fulcrum.

ASSISTANT

Essential to help with manipulation of the joint.

→ **OPERATIVE TECHNIQUE 19.5 CONTINUED**

EQUIPMENT EXTRAS

Suction; small Gelpi retractors x 2.

SURGICAL APPROACH

A curved 3–4 cm incision is centred over the medial epicondyle (Figure 19.41a). Numerous layers of subcutaneous fascia are divided to expose the medial epicondyle and the flexor muscles of the antebrachium (Figure 19.41b).

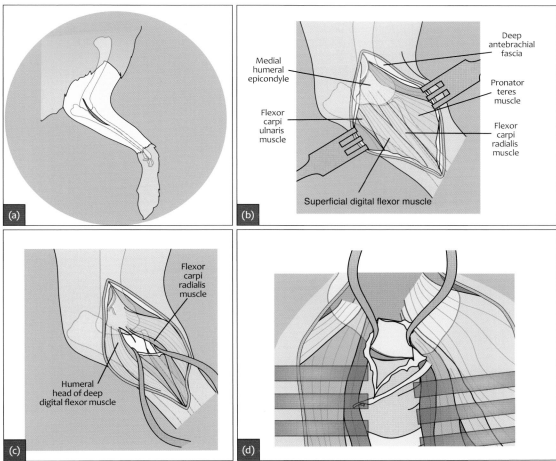

19.41 (a) The skin incision is centred over the medial epicondyle and extends proximally and distally for 3–4 cm. (b) Incision through the underlying fascia and subsequent retraction exposes the origin of the flexor tendons. (c) Blunt dissection between the deep digital flexor tendon and the flexor carpi radialis tendon exposes the joint capsule. (An alternative approach is to separate between the flexor carpi radialis and pronator teres tendons.) (d) The joint capsule is incised. Internal rotation of the elbow joint can aid inspection of the medial coronoid process. If necessary, the caudal aspect of the medial collateral ligament can be incised to increase exposure.

WARNING

The ulnar nerve is located at the proximal end of the incision and care should be taken when the fat in this area is divided. The proximity of the brachial artery and vein and the median nerve to the underside of the pronator teres muscle should be recognized

Exposure of the joint is achieved by muscle separation, either between the pronator teres and the flexor carpi radialis muscles or between the flexor carpi radialis and the deep digital flexor muscles that lie caudal to it (Figure 19.41c). If more exposure is required, the insertions of the relevant muscles can be transected.

The joint capsule and, if necessary, the medial collateral ligament are divided parallel with the joint surface (Figure 19.41d). Retraction of the joint capsule will reveal the medial part of the humeral condyle and the outer aspect of the medial coronoid process. Better exposure of the deeper aspects of the joint can be achieved by abduction and pronation of the radius and ulna or, alternatively, by flexing the carpus and using a sandbag as a fulcrum to lever the joint open. The elbow joint is a close-fitting joint and this approach provides limited but adequate exposure. →

→ **OPERATIVE TECHNIQUE 19.5 CONTINUED**

SURGICAL TECHNIQUE

Following exposure of the medial joint compartment, the OCD flap is identified on the trochlea of the humerus; systematic flexion and extension of the joint in combination with the assistant applying valgus pressure to the antebrachium will allow optimum observation of the flap. The flap is grasped with a fine pair of haemostats and a No. 11 blade is used to release the flap for removal.

PRACTICAL TIP

There is currently insufficient evidence to substantiate that debridement of the flap bed results in any tangible difference in clinical outcome; thus surgery should be undertaken with appropriate informed owner consent and only in dogs that have failed to respond to conservative management. Curettage, forage (drilling) and microfracture techniques for the underlying subchondral bone have been described in an effort to promote fibrocartilage formation, but it is unclear how effective these techniques are clinically, or how this influences postoperative lameness and function

The medial coronoid process is inspected concurrently. The joint is flushed to remove osteochondral debris and then closed.

Closure

The joint capsule, collateral ligament and muscles are repaired with absorbable sutures. Slight elevation of the limb may facilitate tying the sutures. The fascial layers and skin are closed in separate layers with continuous absorbable sutures.

POSTOPERATIVE CARE

The joint is supported in a padded bandage for 5–7 days. Exercise is restricted for 2–3 weeks.

OPERATIVE TECHNIQUE 19.6
Closed reduction of traumatic lateral luxation

POSITIONING

Lateral recumbency with the affected limb uppermost.

ASSISTANT

Useful for medium to large-breed dogs.

TECHNIQUE

Palpation prior to manipulation allows delineation of the radial head, trochlear notch of the ulna and humeral condyle, and orthogonal radiographs/CT of the joint allow assessment of whether complete or partial luxation is present.

Significant pressure may need to be applied to reduce the elbow and as such, manipulations should be performed with care to minimize the risk of iatrogenic fracture

Where luxation is partial, the anconeal process remains on the axial surface of the lateral epicondylar ridge and only steps 5 and 6 are required. The following sequence of manoeuvres is performed for complete lateral luxation (Figure 19.42):

→ **OPERATIVE TECHNIQUE 19.6 CONTINUED**

1 The elbow is fully flexed and held for a period to fatigue the periarticular musculature.

2 The joint is then extended to an angle of just less than 90 degrees.

3 With the carpus flexed to 90 degrees, the antebrachium is rotated inwardly (pronation) using the metacarpus as a handle, pushed away from the body (i.e the carpus is rotated externally), while the thumb of the other hand is used to manipulate the anconeal process towards the lateral epicondyle.

4 Medial pressure is then applied to the lateral aspect of the olecranon to force the anconeal process into the axial recess of the lateral epicondylar ridge, engaging the tip of the anconeal process in the direction of the olecranon fossa of the humerus.

5 Maintaining medial pressure on the olecranon, the elbow is then extended to lock the anconeal process in this position.

6 Thumb pressure is then changed to the radial head and internal rotation of the antebrachium further increased to reduce the radial head.

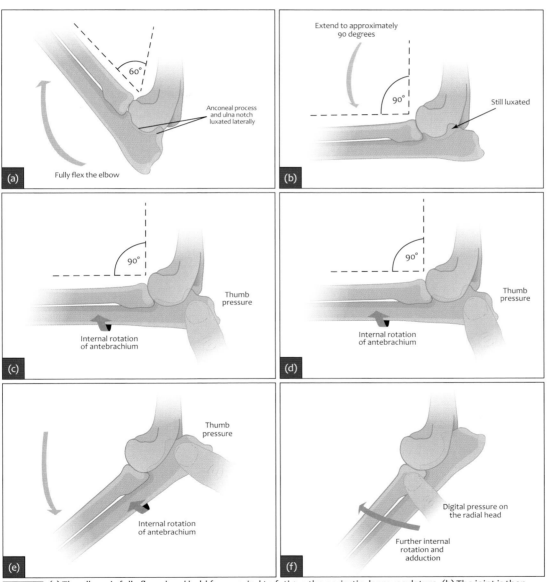

19.42 (a) The elbow is fully flexed and held for a period to fatigue the periarticular musculature. (b) The joint is then extended to an angle of just less than 90 degrees. (c) The antebrachium is rotated inwardly while the thumb of the other hand is used to manipulate the anconeal process towards the lateral epicondyle. (d) Medial pressure is applied to the lateral aspect of the olecranon to force the anconeal process into the axial recess of the lateral epicondylar ridge. (e) Medial pressure is maintained on the olecranon and the elbow is extended to lock the anconeal process in this position. (f) Thumb pressure on the radial head and internal rotation of the antebrachium are applied to reduce the radial head.

→ **OPERATIVE TECHNIQUE 19.6 CONTINUED**

Successful reduction is usually accompanied by an instant return to normal range of motion and restoration of normal topographical anatomy. Orthogonal radiographs are obtained to assess reduction and the collateral ligament integrity is then assessed (see text for details).

POSTREDUCTION CARE

The joint is supported in extension with a Spica splinted dressing for 10–14 days.

OPERATIVE TECHNIQUE 19.7
Collateral ligament repair

POSITIONING

Lateral recumbency with the affected limb positioned so that the affected collateral ligament is uppermost. If both collateral ligaments are ruptured then the patient should be placed in dorsal recumbency with a hanging limb preparation.

ASSISTANT

Not essential.

EQUIPMENT EXTRAS

Self-retaining retractors; drill with appropriate drill bits; screws or bone anchors; washers; depth gauge; screwdriver and orthopaedic wire; nylon leader line or alternative suture material (e.g. FiberWire®, Arthrex).

SURGICAL APPROACH

This depends on whether the lateral, medial or both collateral ligaments require repair/replacement. A lateral approach should extend between the lateral epicondyle of the humerus and neck of the radius; a medial approach should extend between the medial epicondyle of the humerus and the ulna immediately caudodistal to the ulnar trochlear notch. The reader is referred to the text on traumatic elbow luxation for a detailed description of the origin and insertion of the collateral ligaments.

SURGICAL TECHNIQUE

This depends on the surgical stabilization technique being employed:

1   Primary repair: the ends of the ligament are identified and if sufficient ligament is present, a locking loop/three loop pulley suture with appropriate suture material is placed (Figure 19.43). Augmentation of this repair as described in Step 2 should then be considered.

2   The origin/insertion of the collateral ligament(s) are identified and bone anchors or self-tapping screws with washers inserted at these points. Non-absorbable suture material is then placed between the anchors in a figure-of-eight pattern (Figure 19.44). On rare occasions where an origin or insertion avulsion fracture of the ligament has occurred, it may be possible to reattach the bone with a spiked washer and bone screw.

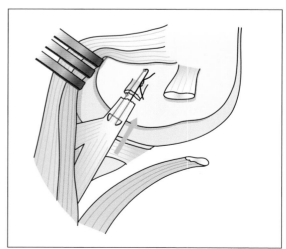

19.43   Repair of a torn lateral collateral ligament with a locking loop suture pattern.

→ OPERATIVE TECHNIQUE 19.7 CONTINUED

3 If both collateral ligaments are ruptured, the author would advocate placement of a Farrell suture (Farrell *et al.*, 2007) (see Figure 19.9); this is where a bilateral approach is made to the collateral ligaments, transverse bone tunnels are drilled in the humeral condyle, proximal radius and ulna, and then non-absorbable suture material (e.g. FiberWire®) or leader line and crimps are placed. Polydioxanone has also been used successfully in cats.

Closure

The joint capsule, intermuscular and subcutaneous tissues are closed in separate layers with a continuous pattern, using absorbable sutures.

POSTOPERATIVE CARE

Regardless of the stabilization technique employed, the elbow should be supported in extension with a Spica splint dressing for 10–14 days. Passive range of motion exercise is important after splint removal. Implants are usually left *in situ*.

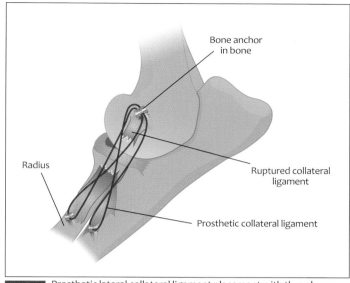

19.44 Prosthetic lateral collateral ligament placement with three bone anchors and figure-of-eight FiberWire®.

OPERATIVE TECHNIQUE 19.8

Dynamic proximal ulnar osteotomy/ostectomy

PREOPERATIVE CONSIDERATIONS

Owners should be counselled preoperatively that exuberant callus formation is a common sequela in young dogs and may result in a palpably/visibly thickened proximal ulna; this usually remodels and regresses with time. Non-union with persistent instability at the osteotomy site may also occur in a proportion of cases, as may debilitating radiohumeral instability in a minority of cases. A distal ulnar ostectomy/osteotomy may be considered as an alternative to avoid such serious complications.

PLANNING

The position of the osteotomy/ostectomy can be planned from a mediolateral radiograph. The osteotomy/ostectomy runs from caudoproximal to craniodistal on the ulna. The cut should begin on the caudal aspect of the ulna, 1–3 cm (depending on the size of the dog) distal to the level of the radial head. This point can be measured on the radiograph relative to the olecranon.

POSITIONING

Dorsal recumbency with the affected limb cranially or lateral recumbency with the affected limb uppermost.

ASSISTANT

Ideally needed to assist with retraction and lavage during osteotomy.

EQUIPMENT EXTRAS

Two Hohmann retractors or self-retaining retractors (if no assistant); periosteal elevator; sagittal saw; osteotome.

→ **OPERATIVE TECHNIQUE 19.8 CONTINUED**

SURGICAL APPROACH

The lateral epicondyle and radial head are palpated. A caudolateral skin incision is made over the point on the caudal ulna determined by measurements made on the preoperative radiograph. Dissection is performed through the caudal subcutaneous tissues and the periosteum on the caudal ulna is incised using a scalpel blade. The flexor carpi ulnaris and extensor carpi ulnaris muscles are elevated from medially and laterally, respectively. Two Hohmann retractors are placed laterally and medially to retract the musculature.

SURGICAL TECHNIQUE

The osteotomy is commenced on the caudal aspect of the ulna with the sagittal saw which is then advanced craniodistally at an angle of 45 degrees. In addition, the osteotomy can be orientated bi-obliquely proximocaudolateral to distocraniomedial in an attempt to further minimize potential for malalignment associated with soft tissue traction. Copious lavage should be used to minimize thermal damage to the bone. Care should be taken not to make the osteotomy too proximal or too short oblique as this may increase the risk of delayed or non-union as well as elbow subluxation. The oblique orientation of the osteotomy coupled with the direction of the pull of the muscles results in lengthening of the ulna and self-stabilization of the fragments, but its effect on ultimate elbow joint congruity is somewhat unpredictable (Figures 19.45, 19.46 and 19.47).

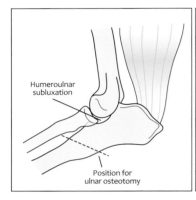
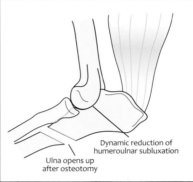

19.45 To lengthen the ulna, a cut is made in a distocranial to proximocaudal direction. The triceps muscle should pull the bone proximally.

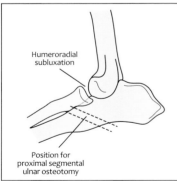
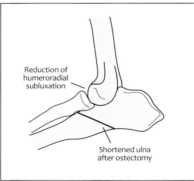

19.46 To shorten the ulna, a segmental ulnar ostectomy is performed equivalent to or slightly greater in size than the humeroradial gap.

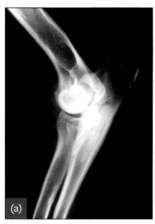
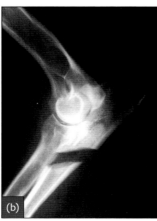

19.47 (a) Preoperative mediolateral radiograph of the elbow of a German Shepherd Dog with a humeroradial subluxation (and panosteitis). (b) Postoperative mediolateral radiograph showing reduction of the joint subluxation after a proximal segmental ulnar ostectomy.

→ **OPERATIVE TECHNIQUE 19.8 CONTINUED**

In skeletally immature dogs with significant physeal growth potential, a distal ulnar ostectomy may be performed instead (Figure 19.48). This may be associated with reduced patient morbidity, and a relatively elastic interosseous ligament may permit a degree of axial proximal shift of the ulna relative to the radius. During surgery, the second transverse osteotomy cut can be started prior to completing the first cut while the ulna is still palpably stable.

PRACTICAL TIP
Care should be taken as the cut is completed to avoid damage to the radius. Radial damage can be avoided by advancing the osteotomy to near completion and then substituting the saw for an osteotome. Careful tapping and twisting of the osteotome will then complete the cut without any risk of radial damage. Iatrogenic damage of the radius predisposes to synostosis formation at this site

Closure

The fascia is apposed with a simple continuous suture of polydioxanone. Routine closure of the subcutaneous tissue and skin is performed.

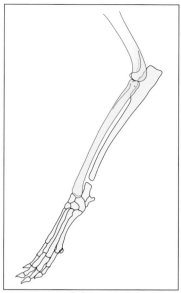

19.48 Distal ulnar osteotomy is an alternative in young dogs and causes less postoperative morbidity.

POSTOPERATIVE CARE

A firm padded bandage is applied for 3–5 days postoperatively. Room rest is indicated until follow-up radiographs are performed. Radiographs are performed after 8 weeks to assess osteotomy healing. Dogs will often remain lame until the osteotomy/ostectomy site is stable, which may take 8–16 weeks depending on the position of the osteotomy and the age and size of the patient.

OPERATIVE TECHNIQUE 19.9

Ununited anconeal process internal fixation or removal

PLANNING

If proximal ulnar osteotomy (PUO) and internal fixation are to be performed then preoperative scaled radiographs are useful for planning the surgery. The craniocaudal cross-sectional diameter of the ulna at the level of the anconeal process is measured to assess likely screw length. The craniocaudal width of the UAP is similarly measured. The caudal length of the ulna from the olecranon to the intended start position of the PUO is measured.

POSITIONING

Lateral recumbency with the affected limb uppermost.

ASSISTANT

Unnecessary if the process is being removed and self-retaining retractors are available. Essential if internal fixation or concurrent proximal ulnar osteotomy is to be performed.

EQUIPMENT EXTRAS

Small Gelpi retractors x 2; Senn retractor; small pair of pointed reduction forceps; oscillating saw; appropriate sized cortical screws; drill bits; K-wires; drill insert sleeve; tap; screwdriver; a pair of small Hohmann retractors; air/electric drill or K-wire driver; cannulated drill bits of appropriate diameter are desirable and an adjustable drill 'C-guide'.

→ **OPERATIVE TECHNIQUE 19.9 CONTINUED**

PRACTICAL TIP

It may be advantageous to use conventional cortical screws as opposed to self-tapping screws. Self-tapping screws have a fluted tip that will be less secure in the UAP than a conventional screw

SURGICAL APPROACH

Caudolateral approach (see Operative Technique 19.2) for UAP removal or internal fixation. Full flexion of the joint improves visualization of the UAP. PUO requires extension of the caudolateral approach or a separate caudal approach to the ulnar shaft at the level of proposed osteotomy with medial elevation of the flexor carpi ulnaris muscle and lateral elevation of the extensor carpi radialis muscle.

SURGICAL TECHNIQUE

Internal fixation and PUO

Should be performed concurrently as fusion rates are higher, implant failure is reduced and progression of osteoarthritis is minimized. Osteotomy of the ulna is performed prior to internal fixation of the UAP to eliminate any influence of shear force on reduction and compression of the process. A caudal approach to the ulna is performed at the level of proposed osteotomy (the osteotomy should be level with the radial head caudally on the ulna and cranially will finish above the interosseus ligament). Following the skin incision, medial elevation and retraction of the flexor carpi ulnaris muscle and lateral elevation and retraction of the extensor carpi ulnaris muscle are performed. Hohmann retractors are slid down the lateral and medial aspects of the ulna and the tips engaged with each other on the cranial aspect of the ulna. The musculature is then retracted with the Hohmann retractors and a sagittal saw used to osteotomize the ulna at a 45- degree angle from proximocaudal to distocranial. The direction of the osteotomy and direction of pull of the triceps muscle results in dynamic lengthening of the ulna. Stabilization of the ulna with an intramedullary pin is not necessary.

PRACTICAL TIP

Take care when completing the osteotomy not to damage the radius as this may predispose to synostosis formation or fracture

Internal fixation of the UAP can be performed in one of two ways:

- The C-guide device is placed with its tip on the anconeal process. An anti-rotational K-wire is then placed from the caudal aspect of the ulna, through the C-guide towards its tip, engaging the anconeal process. The K-wire is placed either slightly cranial or caudal to the tip of the UAP so as not to interfere with the position of the screw. The C-guide is then repositioned over the apex of the UAP and a glide hole, pre-measured from the radiograph, is drilled from the caudal aspect of the ulna towards the UAP, parallel with the K-wire. The hole should stop at the base of the UAP fragment, as pre-measured from the radiograph. The drill is then removed and a drill sleeve placed in the hole. The lag part of the hole is drilled into the ulna from caudally, again a pre-measured distance as assessed on the radiograph. The depth of the hole is measured and the hole is tapped. A non-self-tapping screw is then placed (Figure 19.49)

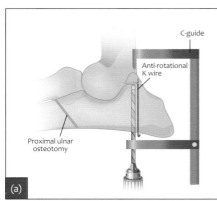 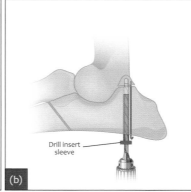 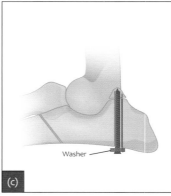

19.49 (a) Following proximal ulnar osteotomy, the C-guide is used to place an anti-rotational K-wire into the UAP. The C-guide is then positioned over the apex of the UAP and the glide hole for the lag screw drilled into the ulna. The depth of this hole is pre-measured from preoperative radiographs. (b) A drill insert sleeve is placed into the glide hole and the drill bit for the lag part of the hole advanced into the UAP. The depth of this hole is again measured from preoperative radiographs. (c) The depth of the hole is measured and the hole is tapped a pre-measured distance (1–2 mm less than the depth). The screw is then placed and carefully tightened, taking care not to strip the threads; 1–2 washers can be placed if the depth of the hole is between screw sizes.

→ **OPERATIVE TECHNIQUE 19.9 CONTINUED**

PRACTICAL TIP

The pilot hole in the tip of the anconeus may be carefully drilled to only just exit cranially (within the joint). This allows accurate screw length measurement using a standard depth gauge. Should the depth fall between screw sizes, the longer length screw can be placed with one or two washers placed at the insertion site, against the caudal ulnar cortex. These have the effect of offsetting the length of the screw on the caudal aspect of the ulna, functionally shortening the length within the UAP

- Should an appropriate sized cannulated drill bit be available, then a K-wire can be introduced in the joint, into the tip of the anconeal processed and directed caudally to exit the caudal aspect of the bone. An anti-rotational K-wire is introduced from the caudal aspect of the ulna parallel to the first K-wire as described above. A cannulated drill bit is then introduced from caudally over the first K-wire and the glide part of the hole drilled to the base of the UAP fragment, as measured from the radiographs. The drill and first K-wire are then removed, a drill sleeve placed in the hole from caudally and the lag part of the hole drilled into the anconeal process a distance pre-measured from the radiograph. The depth of the hole is measured and the hole is tapped. A non-self-tapping screw is then placed. This technique ensures that the lag screw is perfectly centred in the UAP (Figure 19.50).

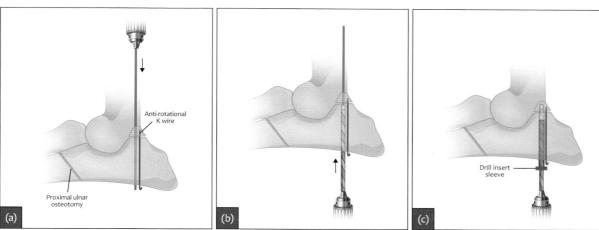

19.50 (a) Following placement of the anti-rotational K-wire, a second K-wire is advanced from the apex of the anconeal process to exit the ulna gradually. (b) A cannulated drill bit of appropriate size is then advanced over the K-wire to form the glide hole for the lag screw. The depth of the hole is pre-measured from preoperative radiographs. (c) The second K-wire is then removed, a drill insert sleeve placed into the glide hole and the drill bit for the lag part of the hole advanced into the UAP. The depth of this hole is again measured from preoperative radiographs. Fixation is then completed as per Figure 19.49.

Process removal

The anconeus muscle and joint capsule are sharply incised with a curvilinear incision following the contour of the humeral condyle. Gelpi and Senn retractors are used to retract the muscle to expose the process. Fragment forceps can be used to grab the process. Fibrous attachments of the process to the ulna can be released with a scalpel blade or osteotome (Figure 19.51).

Closure

The anconeus muscle is reattached with a continuous absorbable suture. Skin is closed routinely.

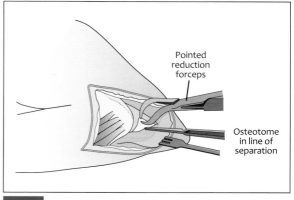

19.51 Removal of an ununited anconeal process.

POSTOPERATIVE CARE

- The joint should be immobilized in a padded bandage for 4–7 days to reduce postoperative swelling.
- Room rest for 6 weeks.
- Analgesia should be provided as required. Non-steroidal anti-inflammatories are often required for several weeks.
- Radiographs should be performed 6 weeks postoperatively to assess healing and implants.

OPERATIVE TECHNIQUE 19.10

Lengthening of the radius

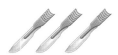

PREOPERATIVE CONSIDERATIONS

It is very challenging to achieve restoration of acceptable elbow joint congruity. Joint tolerances are small and significant lameness may be induced if lengthening is imprecise or the final 'resting' position of the radial head is axially/abaxially malaligned relative to the humerus and ulna. Particularly in more mature patients, radial head shape will be abnormal due to a lack of prior loading and contact with the humeral condyle. The medial joint compartment should be evaluated concurrently in all cases since there is a significant risk of concomitant medial coronoid process disease.

Lengthening can either be 'static', by the application of a plate to the dorsal radius, or 'dynamic', by the application of linear, hybrid or circular external skeletal fixation incorporating linear distraction. Plating has the advantage of being a single procedure; however, postoperative adjustment in length is not possible and thus this surgery should be performed only once the patient is nearing/at skeletal maturity.

Dynamic lengthening has the advantage of allowing fine postoperative adjustment but the disadvantage of morbidity associated with the use of the frame. This surgery (using a linear external skeletal fixator (ESF)) is described below, but should be undertaken only by experienced surgeons with a solid understanding of the techniques and following appropriate training.

PLANNING

Orthogonal radiographs of both antebrachii and additional radiographs/CT centred on the elbow are performed. The size of the humeroradial gap is calculated. The need for adjunctive angular or rotational correction is assessed by clinical examination of the dog and from CT images or radiographs.

STATIC LENGTHENING

Positioning

Dorsal recumbency with the affected limb pulled caudally. As with all lengthening or angular correction surgery, the entire limb including the shoulder joint should be visible within the sterile field.

Assistant

Essential.

Equipment extras

Sagittal saw; appropriate plate and screws; bending irons; curettes for harvesting autogenous bone graft; Gelpi retractors or two Hohmann retractors; suction; equipment for temporary ESF placement if desired.

Surgical approach

Autogenous bone graft is harvested from the ipsilateral proximal humerus. A craniomedial skin incision is then performed over the mid-diaphysis of the radius (protecting the cephalic vein) and dissection performed down to the radius.

Surgical technique

Two Hohmann retractors or Gelpi retractors are placed cranially and caudally to reflect and protect the antebrachial flexor and extensor muscles. A line is then scored transversely across the dorsal radius as a reference point for measuring the degree of lengthening required following osteotomy. An osteotomy of the radius is performed, either transversely or in a 'Z' configuration to help maintain some bone to bone contact. Copious lavage is used during bone cutting to minimize thermal necrosis. The proximal radius is then advanced proximally by an amount that is predetermined by preoperative imaging, and the osteotomy is temporarily stabilized with K-wires or through placement of a temporary two-pin, type II ESF. Intraoperative radiographs or fluoroscopy are useful to assess whether the radial lengthening is sufficient. The gaps between the osteotomized bone ends are packed with bone graft and a plate is then contoured and applied to the dorsal radius using standard AO/ASIF techniques. A locking plate is advantageous, both because juvenile bone is soft, and because less precise contouring of the plate to the bone is needed. Bone graft is packed at the osteotomy site. A minimum of three screws proximal and distal to the radial osteotomy are recommended as this is a bridging fixation.

→ **OPERATIVE TECHNIQUE 19.10 CONTINUED**

Closure

Subcutaneous tissues and skin are closed in a routine fashion.

Postoperative care

A compression dressing is applied to the limb for 5–10 days. Strict room rest is required for 6 weeks, followed by repeat radiographs to assess bone healing.

DYNAMIC LENGTHENING (USING A LINEAR ESF)

Positioning

Dorsal recumbency with leg pulled caudally.

Assistant

Very useful.

Equipment extras

Oscillating saw; Gelpi retractors or two Hohmann retractors; periosteal elevator; battery drill and drill bits; linear distractor; ESF pins and sliding clamps.

Surgical approach and technique

A centrally threaded ESF pin is placed in the proximal radius. A second pin is placed in the distal radius. A small skin incision is made centred on the mid-diaphysis of the radius, and Gelpi retractors or two Hohmann retractors are placed cranially and caudally to reflect and protect the antebrachial flexor and extensor muscles. The radius is osteotomized using a sagittal saw with copious saline lavage. Sliding clamps are placed on threaded bars. Additional half pins are added through the spare clamps and sliding clamps (Figure 19.52). All pins on clamps are tightened.

> **PRACTICAL TIP**
>
> Pins should be placed in safe corridors wherever possible (Marti and Miller, 1994)

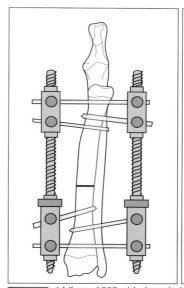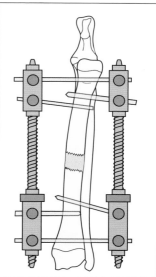

19.52 A bilateral ESF with threaded bars, knurled nuts and sliding clamps is applied in order to distract the bones and increase radial length.

Closure

The periosteum and fascia are closed over the osteotomy site with an absorbable suture material. Subcutaneous tissue and skin are closed in a routine fashion.

Postoperative care

In the skeletally immature animal, the frame is left for a 24–48 hour consolidation period (consider longer, up to 4 or 5 days in mature dogs) before distraction is commenced. Distraction of 0.5 mm twice a day is normally appropriate; however, this can be increased should premature consolidation of callus occur, or reduced if lack of regenerative bone is observed on sequential radiographs. The limb is radiographed regularly (initially weekly) to assess humeroradial congruity and regenerative bone. Once elbow subluxation is reduced and confirmed on radiographs, the ESF can be left *in situ* with the clamps tightened until sufficient consolidation of bone has occurred to permit removal.

Chapter 20

The carpus

Stephen Clarke and Jonathan Pink

Conditions affecting the structure and function of the carpus are not uncommon in small animal practice and can have debilitating consequences for thoracic limb function. Trauma can result in fractures or damage to the supporting soft tissues of the carpus leading to instability and lameness, while the carpus can also be a site for degenerative or inflammatory arthropathies. Localization of lameness to the carpus can be straightforward if gross instability or pain are present. However, selection of an appropriate management plan can be challenging and the surgical options available can be unforgiving if technical errors are not avoided.

Anatomy

The carpus is a complex joint and a sound understanding of functional anatomy is imperative for accurate interpretation of both the clinical and diagnostic imaging findings. The seven carpal bones in cats and dogs are arranged into proximal and distal rows (Figure 20.1). The carpus is a composite ginglymus or hinge joint made up of antebrachiocarpal, middle carpal, and carpometacarpal joints that permit flexion (100 degrees) and extension (10 degrees) together with limited medial and lateral movement (15 degrees valgus and 5 degrees varus). Of the three joints, the antebrachiocarpal and middle carpal joints provide the greatest range of motion (70% and 25%, respectively) with the carpometacarpal joint contributing minimally to carpal

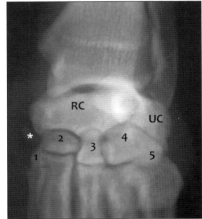

20.1 Radiograph of the canine carpus showing the position of the radial (RC), ulnar (UC) and small numbered carpal bones (1–5). There is a sesamoid bone (∗) medial to the middle carpal joint within the tendon of insertion of the abductor pollicis longus muscle.

motion (5%). The anatomical arrangement of carpal bones and carpal stability is maintained by a complex array of dorsal, palmar and collateral ligamentous structures (Figure 20.2) of which the collateral ligaments, palmar fibrocartilage, palmar radiocarpal ligament, palmar ulnocarpal ligament and the flexor mechanism are the main supporting structures. The palmar fibrocartilage is a development of the fibrous component of the palmar joint capsule and incorporates the palmar intercarpal ligaments. It has attachments to all the carpal bones and attaches distally to the bases of metacarpals 3–5. The flexor mechanism of the carpus is provided by the flexor carpi ulnaris

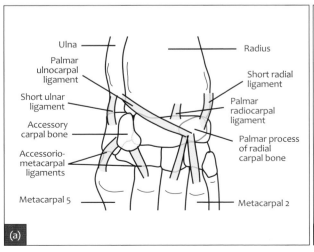

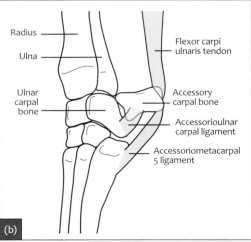

20.2 (a) Ligaments of the palmar aspect of the carpus. The palmar fibrocartilage is not shown. (b) Lateral aspect of the carpus showing the main soft tissue attachments of the accessory carpal bone.

muscle which inserts on to the proximopalmar aspect of the accessory carpal bone. Distally, the accessory carpal bone provides a point of attachment for the accessoriometacarpal ligaments (inserting on the base of metacarpals 4 and 5). These proximal and distal soft tissue structures form a natural tension band that helps to limit carpal hyperextension. Despite anatomical differences in individual carpal bones, there has been little direct anatomical comparison between the feline and canine carpus. One known disparity between the species is that the canine carpal radial collateral ligament has both deep oblique and straight superficial portions, while only a single broad oblique component is present in the cat.

Investigations

Examination

As well as gait assessment (see Chapters 1 and 2), it is important to visually assess the patient's forelimb conformation for carpal deformity such as hyperextension, valgus or varus. The absence of substantial soft tissue coverage around the carpus facilitates palpation of some underlying ligaments, tendons and bony structures. Focal or generalized soft tissue thickening and swelling may be readily detected and pain may be elicited on point palpation over specific structures. Manipulation of the carpus allows for assessment of both pain and range of motion. Irrespective of the underlying cause, as carpal pathology becomes chronic, reduction in range of flexion is a common finding. Instability of the carpus may or may not be readily apparent on conscious examination and thorough assessment with the patient sedated or anaesthetized may be required to appreciate subtle loss of normal carpal stability.

Diagnostic imaging

Radiography is the predominant imaging technique, although computed tomography (CT) examination allows for more detailed and superimposition-free cross-sectional imaging and is increasingly available. Magnetic resonance imaging (MRI) and ultrasonography have only limited and specific indications.

Specific details on appropriate imaging techniques for the carpus are provided in the imaging section at the end of this chapter. For more general information on imaging techniques and their application, see Chapter 3.

Arthrocentesis

Arthrocentesis, if indicated, is performed at the level of the antebrachiocarpal joint (see Chapter 4) primarily to differentiate between inflammatory and non-inflammatory arthropathies.

Congenital abnormalities

Congenital abnormalities of the carpus are extremely rare in both the dog and cat. When present they may be the result of a primary carpal abnormality such as agenesis or malformation of the carpal bones, or secondary to a more complex abnormality such as radial agenesis or ectrodactyly. In most situations, obvious limb deformity and poor or absent limb function will be readily evident on examination. Radiographic or CT evaluation is required to fully define the underlying condition. Most of these conditions require either amputation or salvage surgery, such as partial or pancarpal arthrodesis with or without concomitant limb lengthening.

Developmental abnormalities

Flexural deformity and hyperextension – carpal laxity syndrome

Carpal flexural deformity can develop between 6 and 12 weeks of age in puppies of any breed. Affected puppies can be of either sex and are otherwise generally active, healthy and usually growing well on a suitable plane of nutrition. Malnutrition may be a feature in some affected puppies but trauma is not. Flexural deformity is a physiological rather than a pathological phenomenon which has been proposed to result from a transient disparity in the rate of growth between the skeletal and soft tissues leading to relative shortening of muscles and tendons (Vaughan, 1992). Puppies can be affected either unilaterally or bilaterally with the deformity generally developing suddenly, resulting in a typical posture demonstrating a variable degree of carpal hypoextension. Digit posture can also be affected and the paw can appear to deviate into varus (Figure 20.3). Pain is not a feature on orthopaedic examination and in most cases the carpus can be manipulated into a normal position although tautness of the flexor carpi ulnaris tendon is apparent. Radiographs show no obvious skeletal abnormality. Conservative management is successful in almost all cases with the signs generally resolving within 2 to 4 weeks. Ensuring appropriate nutrition and providing moderated activity on a surface which facilitates traction is advised; slippery surfaces should be avoided. If the deformity does not resolve within 4 weeks, surgical intervention should be considered as persistence of the deformity could lead to secondary skeletal malformation. Transection of the tendons of both the humeral and ulnar heads of the flexor carpi ulnaris proximal to their insertion on the accessory carpal bone is effective in resolving the deformity.

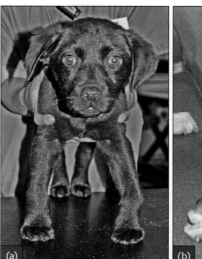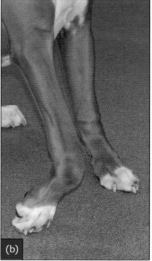

20.3 (a) A 12-week-old Labrador Retriever with carpal flexural deformity. Note the altered digit posture.
(b) Carpal flexural deformity in a 17-week-old Boxer.

Carpal hyperextension can develop in puppies from 1 to 6 months of age (Cetinkaya *et al.*, 2007) and has been suggested to be due to reduced flexor muscle tone resulting in a palmigrade posture. This condition shares many similarities with carpal flexural deformity in terms of predisposing factors, sudden onset of signs and either uni- or bilateral involvement, and should similarly be seen as a temporary physiological abnormality. Pain is absent on examination and resolution of clinical signs is expected within 2 to 4 weeks with conservative management. Regular controlled exercise to facilitate normal muscle tone is appropriate and splinted or support dressings are counterproductive as they protect the soft tissues from the normal loading required for proper development. Indeed, carpal hyperextension may be seen in puppies as a consequence of prolonged bandage or splint support of the carpus.

Antebrachial growth deformity

Disruption of growth of the distal ulnar and/or radial physes can result in abnormal carpal joint development and dysfunction as part of a more complex antebrachial abnormality. The reader is referred to Chapter 8 for more detailed information of such abnormalities.

Traumatic carpal injuries

Traumatic injuries of the carpus are common and can result in fracture, luxation or subluxation of individual carpal bones and carpal joints. More than one joint level may be affected and careful examination in the conscious and sedated or anaesthetized animal in conjunction with diagnostic imaging (often utilizing stress radiography) can be necessary to determine the position or positions and nature of the injuries present. Only some fractures of the carpus are briefly mentioned within this chapter; the reader is referred to the *BSAVA Manual of Canine and Feline Fracture Repair and Management* for further information on these injuries.

Antebrachiocarpal joint luxation

Luxation of the antebrachiocarpal joint (Figure 20.4) in dogs involves complete disruption of the supporting structures, potentially on all aspects of the joint. This is a devastating injury for joint function and management necessitates pancarpal arthrodesis.

In common with the majority of traumatic feline carpal injuries, antebrachiocarpal joint luxation is usually seen following a fall from a height (Nakladal *et al.*, 2013). The presence of only a single broad oblique medial collateral ligament in the cat can permit antebrachiocarpal joint luxation without multiple ligamentous involvement (Voss *et al.*, 2003). Consequently, this can be a less devastating injury than in the dog and it may be possible to manage antebrachiocarpal luxation in cats by ligament repair or placement of a prosthetic ligament.

Antebrachiocarpal joint subluxation

Antebrachiocarpal joint subluxation can occur in dogs following rupture of the short (oblique) and long (straight) components of the radial collateral ligament without multiligamentous involvement. This results in medial instability and valgus deviation of the paw (Figure 20.5). Ligament repair and prosthetic support using either synthetic or

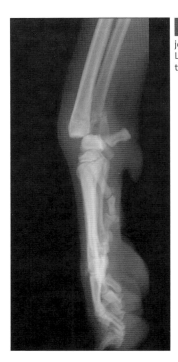

20.4 Traumatic luxation of the antebrachiocarpal joint in a 2-year-old working Labrador Retriever. A fracture of the distal ulna is also present.

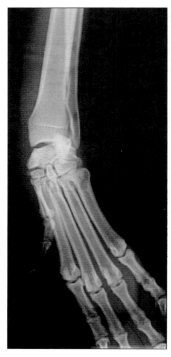

20.5 Antebrachiocarpal joint subluxation associated with a traumatic grade III sprain of the radial collateral ligaments in a 4-year-old German Shepherd Dog, sustained in a road traffic accident.

autogenous tissues have been reported. However, in the authors' experience, medium to long-term outcomes can be variable and more predictable function can be achieved with pancarpal arthrodesis.

Radial carpal bone luxation

Disruption of radial collateral, dorsal and intercarpal ligaments allows rotation of the radial carpal bone through a combination of hyperextension and pronation followed by supination (Miller *et al.*, 1990). The luxated radial carpal bone lies caudal or caudomedial to the distal radius with its proximal surface oriented palmaromedially (Figure 20.6).

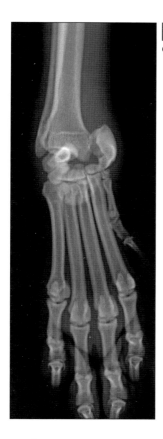

20.6 Luxation of the radial carpal bone in a 3-year-old Border Collie.

Open reduction through a medial or dorsal midline approach with repair or reconstruction of the medial collateral ligament has been reported. Additional stabilization with an arthrodesis wire placed mediolaterally through the radial carpal bone and into the ulnar carpal bone has been described (Miller *et al.*, 1990; Pitcher, 1996); postoperative adjunctive support is recommended. Although only a limited number of cases have been described in the literature, it would seem that a favourable outcome can be achieved with surgical reduction and stabilization of the radial carpal bone. However, pancarpal arthrodesis could be considered as an alternative management option at the outset.

Luxation of the second carpal bone

Luxation of the second carpal bone has been reported in a Staffordshire Bull Terrier. This injury was seen in conjunction with wider carpal trauma following a road traffic accident and was managed by pancarpal arthrodesis. Subluxation of the second carpal bone has been described in two racing Greyhounds. These dogs showed mild to moderate lameness, and differing degrees of focal discomfort, swelling and carpal bone displacement were reported. Both were managed by internal fixation, and, although implant removal was subsequently felt to be necessary, both dogs returned to racing (Guilliard and Mayo, 2001).

Shearing injuries

Shearing injuries typically occur when the limb is caught between a vehicle's moving wheel and the road, resulting in a heavily contaminated abrasion injury with loss and devitalization of variable amounts of soft tissue and bone. The medial (tension) aspect of joint as opposed to limb is generally affected and the radial styloid process, radial collateral ligament and abaxial aspect of the base of metacarpal 2 can be lost, resulting in gross instability and exposure of

the medial joint spaces. Considerable amounts of debris may be embedded into the exposed tissues and degloving can result in the skin defect initially appearing substantially larger than is truly the case.

Shearing injuries present two main challenges: wound management and joint instability. The wound should be lavaged and debrided to remove necrotic and foreign material. The extent of non-viable soft tissues is often not immediately apparent and sequential debridement may be required over several days. If possible, the skin margins at the limits of the wound may then be approximated without tension to reduce the area of exposed tissue. It is important to allow for continued drainage of exudate from the wound, rather than being tempted to fully appose skin margins. Most wounds will heal by second intention though occasionally skin grafting may be required to reduce healing time and create a more durable, functional and cosmetic result.

Transarticular external skeletal fixation (TESF) has greatly simplified the management of these cases and is used in preference to external coaptation where significant instability is present (Figure 20.7). TESF is applied as soon as the patient's condition is stable enough for anaesthesia. This technique immobilizes the joint in a weight-bearing position and facilitates revascularization of traumatized soft tissues while allowing appropriate wound management. Once a healthy granulation bed is present, a decision can be made as to whether prosthetic ligaments should be placed in order to optimize stability of the joint; in most cases the development of periarticular fibrosis results in satisfactory joint stability over a 6 to 8 week period. Arthrodesis can subsequently be considered for those individuals with a suboptimal outcome. In dogs with marked instability, immediate arthrodesis with external fixator stabilization can offer good outcomes, although this would not generally be the authors' preferred option.

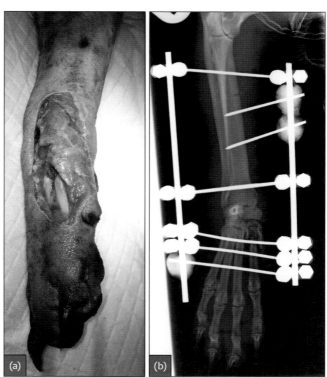

20.7 (a) Shearing injury affecting the medial aspect of the distal antebrachium, carpus and metacarpus. (b) The carpus has been stabilized using a transarticular external skeletal fixator. (Courtesy of Simon Gilbert)

Carpal sprain/strain injuries

Non-specific carpal sprains and strains are not uncommon injuries in working and athletic dogs but specific soft tissue injuries are also seen, with a number being identified predominantly in performance or athletic animals (Figure 20.8). Acute injuries tend to be associated with soft tissue swelling, variable lameness and, in some cases, joint instability.

Radial carpal bone fracture

Acute traumatic fractures of the radial carpal bone occur uncommonly. Fracture types include dorsal chip or slab fractures, palmar process fractures and parasagittal fractures; management of these fractures is discussed in the *BSAVA Manual of Canine and Feline Fracture Repair and Management*. More commonly, radial carpal bone fractures present as insidious chronic and progressive lameness cases in the skeletally mature dog without a history of associated trauma. A variety of breeds can be affected and in the UK, Boxers appear over-represented. A parasagittal fracture configuration is most common (Figure 20.9a) although in some cases a concomitant dorsal slab fracture is present, creating a T- or Y-shaped comminuted configuration. Although the aetiopathogenesis of these fractures remains uncertain, an underlying failure of normal ossification within the radial carpal bone has been proposed. The fracture configurations closely approximate to the planes of fusion of the three centres of ossification of the radial carpal bone and histopathology from affected cases has been supportive of incomplete ossification

(Gnudi *et al.*, 2003). This may result in zones of natural weakness within the radial carpal bone that predispose it to fracture. There may be breed differences in patterns of ossification within the radial carpal bone, which could explain why particular breeds are disproportionately affected. An alternative, though less likely, possibility is that the pathology represents a stress fracture.

Lameness, reduced range of motion, firm soft tissue swelling and carpal pain are common examination findings (Tomlin *et al.*, 2001); some patients may have bilateral pathology. Diagnosis can be confirmed in most cases with radiography. Concomitant osteoarthritis is a common feature. In some cases, CT may be beneficial to better define the abnormalities present (Figure 20.9b). Conservative management can be considered but in clinically affected dogs, lameness of variable severity persists and osteoarthritis progresses. External coaptation and dorsal fragment excision appear to provide similar outcomes to conservative management (Li *et al.*, 2000). Internal fixation in patients with only parasagittal radial carpal bone fractures can result in resolution of lameness (Perry *et al.*, 2010), although such an outcome is not consistently reported between studies and some patients have required subsequent pancarpal arthrodesis (Li *et al.*, 2000; Tomlin *et al.*, 2001). Where T-shaped comminuted fractures are present, primary repair is not recommended. From the available evidence it would appear that pancarpal arthrodesis (Figure 20.9c) is an effective and predictable way to manage chronic radial carpal bone fracture (Li *et al.*, 2000; Tomlin *et al.*, 2001) and is the authors' treatment of choice.

Injury	Clinical signs	Management and prognosis	Reference
Carpal sprain injury	Mild to moderate lameness after racing. Range of flexion may be reduced and pain is present on joint manipulation. No gross instability is present. A grade I or II sprain injury is suspected, but no specific diagnosis is made	Rest and appropriate support dressing if indicated. Prognosis for return to the previous racing form is guarded as recurrence is common	Guilliard, 2006
Dorsal radiocarpal ligament sprain	Chronic low-grade lameness of variable severity. A characteristic soft tissue swelling is visible and palpable from the dorsal radial rim of the antebrachiocarpal joint to a point 1–2 cm distally, and pain is elicited on carpal flexion. Radiography should be performed as an associated small avulsion fracture of the origin of the ligament may be present	Surgical excision of small avulsion fracture fragments if present and external coaptation of the limb in a weight-bearing position for 3 weeks using a splinted bandage. The prognosis is considered to be good	Guilliard, 1997
Short radial collateral ligament sprain	Acute onset lameness and associated soft tissue swelling on the dorsomedial aspect of the carpus; pain can be elicited on point palpation of the ligament	Kennel rest and/or carpal support bandaging for 6 weeks. With an appropriate rehabilitation programme, the prognosis for return to racing has been reported to be good	Guilliard and Mayo, 2000; Guilliard, 2006
Flexor carpi ulnaris strain	Variable lameness. Not exclusive to the racing Greyhound. Obvious tendon thickening is present. In some patients the tendon is avulsed completely from its insertion and in some cases an associated type IV accessory carpal bone fracture can be present; as such, radiography should be performed	Surgical management of bone or tendon avulsions is indicated. Bone fragments are small and are rarely amenable to internal fixation; therefore, the avulsed tendon is reattached to the accessory carpal bone and adjacent soft tissues. Postoperatively, the repair is protected by use of a carpal flexion splint, with gradual extension of the carpus over a 6-week period. The prognosis for pet dogs is excellent but is more guarded for performance animals	Guilliard, 2006

20.8 Summary of specific carpal soft tissue injuries in the racing Greyhound.

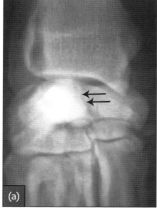

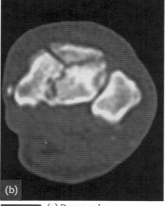

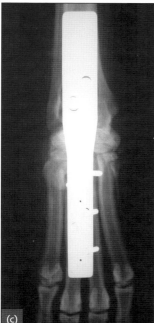

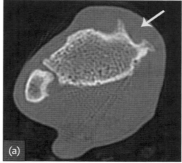

20.9 (a) Dorsopalmar radiograph of the carpus in a 4-year-old Boxer. A parasagittal radial carpal bone fracture (arrowed) is present. (b) Transverse CT image of a Y-shaped fracture in the radial carpal bone of a 6-year-old Brittany Spaniel, subsequently managed by pancarpal arthrodesis. (c) The Boxer in (a) was also managed with pancarpal arthrodesis using a CastLess pancarpal arthrodesis plate.

(b, Courtesy of Gordon Brown)

shows bony remodelling of the distomedial radius (Figure 20.10cd). Medical management involves injection of a long-acting preparation of methylprednisolone (acetate) around the tendon. Surgical resection of proliferative soft tissue and bone to free the tendon and tenotomy have been described for cases that fail to respond to medical management (Grundmann and Montavon, 2001).

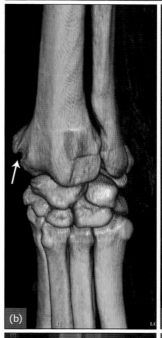

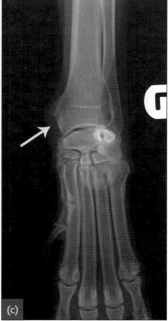

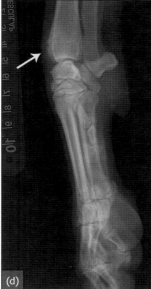

20.10 (a) Computed tomographic cross-sectional image of the distal antebrachium of a 6-year-old Irish Setter with stenosing tenosynovitis of the abductor pollicis longus tendon. There is bony remodelling (arrowed) of the margins of the medial sulcus of the radius through which the tendon passes. (b) CT 3D volume rendered reconstruction showing the remodelled and protruding groove (arrowed) on the craniomedial aspect of the same radius. The bone remodelling is much easier to appreciate on the CT images. (c–d) Dorsopalmar and mediolateral radiographs of the carpus of a dog with the same condition showing bone remodelling of the cranial and medial aspects of the distal radius (arrowed).

(c, d, Courtesy of Gareth Arthurs)

Tenosynovitis of the abductor pollicis longus tendon

The abductor pollicis longus muscle originates on the lateral aspect of the distal ulna and radius and passes obliquely across the cranial aspect of the radius such that its tendon of insertion runs along the medial sulcus of the cranial radius to insert on the base of the first metacarpal. The muscle serves to abduct and extend the first digit, but given that this digit is vestigial in dogs, it is reasonable to consider its primary role (and hence its relatively substantial size) to be adduction of the paw.

Stenosing tenosynovitis describes the proliferation of soft tissue and bone resulting in impingement of the abductor pollicis longus tendon at the level of the medial sulcus and can be a cause of chronic lameness in affected dogs. A firm swelling is present on the medial aspect of the antebrachiocarpal joint and discomfort can be elicited on carpal flexion. Advanced imaging provides detailed information, in particular relating to bony changes (Figure 20.10ab), while ultrasound examination by an experienced operator can demonstrate the soft tissue changes. In more advanced cases, radiography

Chronic sprain of the lateral collateral ligament complex

This uncommon condition reported by Langley-Hobbs *et al.* (2007) is thought to involve a chronic grade I or II sprain injury and is manifested by abnormal forelimb conformation. Dobermanns appear to be over-represented and affected dogs present with carpal varus, often with concomitant carpal hypoextension, pronation, limb abduction and elbow varus. Paw posture is also affected with more weight borne on the lateral aspect of digits 3, 4 and 5. Despite the abnormal conformation, lameness and functional impairment may not be present; when they are, lameness is insidious in onset but progressive in nature, being associated with chronic progressive joint instability and the development of associated degenerative joint disease. Affected carpi are thickened, may have a reduced range of motion in flexion, and are variably painful. Radiography typically shows periarticular soft tissue swelling and periarticular osteophyte and enthesophyte formation on the base of metacarpal 5 and the fifth metacarpophalangeal joint. Bone formation and soft tissue mineralization are often present in the region of the first carpometacarpal joint, potentially associated with concurrent abductor pollicis longus tendon pathology. Stressed radiographs highlight the varus deformity. Treatment is dependent on the degree of limb dysfunction; appropriate medical management should be considered initially in clinically affected patients, with pancarpal arthrodesis indicated for those that fail to respond.

Carpal hyperextension

With the exception of carpal laxity syndrome in pups, carpal hyperextension develops as a consequence of inflammatory arthritis, degenerative joint disease or, most commonly, trauma. Carpal hyperextension has been defined as extension exceeding 190 degrees, although there can be significant variation between individuals and between breeds. Management decisions are clinically driven and determined by the degree of lameness, dysfunction or exercise intolerance that is present and not solely on the load-bearing angle of the carpus.

Traumatic hyperextension injuries involve disruption of the palmar supporting structures (palmar ligaments, palmar fibrocartilage and to a lesser extent the short collateral ligaments) typically following a fall or jump from a height. Their disruption can result in hyperextension (Figure 20.11) at the level of the antebrachiocarpal, middle carpal or carpometacarpal joints, or a combination of these. The distribution of joint involvement in the dog varies considerably in the literature, though it would seem that the antebrachiocarpal joint is unaffected in over 50% of cases (Piermattei *et al.*, 2006), while in the cat the antebrachiocarpal joint is most commonly affected (Nakladal *et al.*, 2013). In some cases it may be possible to determine which joint is involved based on stressed mediolateral radiographs; proximal displacement of the ulnar carpal bone suggests middle carpal joint disruption, while proximal tilting of the accessory carpal bone indicates rupture of its distal ligamentous attachments, and loss of the normal appearance of the dorsal aspect of the distal row of carpal bones suggests carpometacarpal disruption.

Conservative management of traumatic hyperextension injuries involving ligamentous damage is highly unlikely to be effective and progressive instability, degenerative joint disease and lameness are to be expected. Surgical techniques to restore normal anatomy and function have been

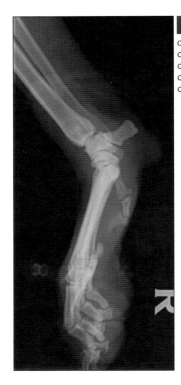

20.11 Stressed mediolateral radiograph of the carpus of a 3-year-old Dalmatian showing carpal hyperextension as a result of carpometacarpal instability, in this case resulting from a fall from a cliff.

described though have largely fallen from favour due to their unpredictable results and the problematic surgical approach to the palmar aspect of the carpus. Consequently carpal arthrodesis, either partial or pancarpal, is generally recommended for management of hyperextension injuries.

In addition to the soft tissue injuries described above, fractures of the accessory carpal bone or the base of the fifth metacarpal can also lead to carpal hyperextension (Figure 20.12). The ulnaris lateralis muscle and accessoriometacarpal ligaments attach to the base of the fifth

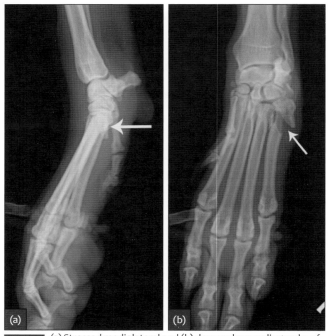

20.12 (a) Stressed mediolateral and (b) dorsopalmar radiographs of the carpus of a 2-year-old Border Collie. The hyperextension in this case is associated with a fracture of the base of the fifth metacarpal (arrowed).

metacarpal and fractures can therefore result in both hyperextension and varus instability. Type III accessory carpal bone fracture disrupts the attachment of the accessoriometacarpal ligaments resulting in hyperextension, but this injury is less common in pet dogs than fifth metacarpal fractures. Provided injuries to other supporting structures are not present, rigid internal stabilization of the fracture has the potential to result in good function. However, it is hard to rule out concurrent injury to the palmar fibrocartilage and other palmar ligaments and pancarpal arthrodesis provides a more predictable outcome in these cases.

Arthrodesis

Pancarpal arthrodesis or occasionally partial carpal arthrodesis is undertaken to salvage a pain-free, functional outcome where previous medical or surgical management has failed, or is likely to fail. Irrespective of the fixation system used the principles of arthrodesis should be adhered to, in particular meticulous articular cartilage debridement, use of bone grafts and rigid stabilization at a functional arthrodesis angle.

Pancarpal arthrodesis

Pancarpal arthrodesis (PCA) can be considered for pathology affecting any of the carpal joints (see Operative Technique 20.1). Stabilization for PCA is most commonly achieved using internal fixation with a bone plate and screws applied to the dorsal aspect of the carpus (Figure 20.13). In theory, palmar plating (on the tension side of the joint) is biomechanically superior but is rarely performed due to the challenges of the surgical approach. Medial or orthogonal bone plating (Figure 20.14) or use of cross pins with a dorsal bone plate can be considered as alternative

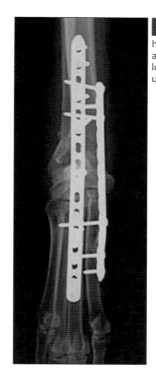

20.14 A 6-year-old Greyhound with a distal radial articular fracture has been managed with pancarpal arthrodesis; orthogonally placed 2.7 mm locking compression plates have been used.

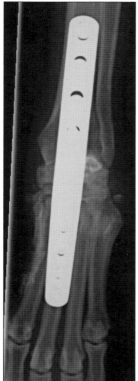

20.13 Dorsal placement of a hybrid dynamic compression (3.5/2.7 mm) plate for pancarpal arthrodesis.

techniques offering a biomechanical advantage. The dorsal approach allows best access for articular cartilage debridement and provides the most straightforward location for bone plate placement. This has led to the development of a large selection of PCA-specific plates with the two most commonly used implants being the hybrid dynamic compression plate (HDCP) and the CastLess plate (CLP) (Bristow et al., 2015).

External support involving a period of bandaging in the immediate postoperative period followed by cast or splint application for approximately 6 weeks is commonplace following PCA, having been considered a necessity for many years. Recently, the use of cast application in particular has become an area of increasing debate. Although a mechanical study to assess the effect of cast application on HDCP strain did show a protective effect, the difference was considered unlikely to be of clinical significance (Woods et al., 2012). Bristow et al. (2015) reported that following a period of initial bandaging, casting was used in 56% (HDCP) and 11.4% (CLP) of cases, with cast-associated complications occurring in 43% and 17%, respectively. When both bandaging and casting were considered together, the associated complication rates were 32% (HDCP) and 18% (CLP). The study also concluded that external coaptation had no measurable clinical benefit. In the authors' opinion a soft support bandage, maintained for 3–7 days after surgery without further external coaptation is appropriate for the vast majority of PCA procedures.

In addition to morbidity from bandages or casts, postoperative complications are common following PCA surgery. Infection is the most commonly documented complication with others including screw loosening, metacarpal fracture and failure to achieve arthrodesis; plate failure rarely occurs. Multiple complications can occur concurrently. At present there does not appear to be a significant difference in intra- or postoperative complication rates or in outcome between the HDCP or CLP (Bristow et al., 2015). Appropriate preoperative planning, strict asepsis and good surgical technique are all paramount in attempting to minimize the postoperative complication rate.

Despite being a major intervention, the outcome following PCA is good in most patients; no or mild lameness was reported in 73% and 83% of dogs using a HDCP or CLP respectively (Bristow *et al.*, 2015). PCA can be considered in active working dogs; Jerram *et al.* (2009) reported 83% of such dogs to resume most or all of their working duties normally. Calvo *et al.* (2009) described PCA in 18 cats. A dorsally placed HDCP, dynamic compression plate or veterinary cuttable plate was used, with some cases having supplementary cross pin fixation; external coaptation was used in eight cases. A satisfactory or excellent outcome was reported in those cats that had long-term follow-up.

Partial carpal arthrodesis

Partial carpal arthrodesis (PaCA) is less commonly performed but can be considered when the antebrachiocarpal joint is spared from the pathological process affecting the carpus. Determining that this is the case can be challenging as antebrachiocarpal joint pathology may not be readily apparent at the outset. Preservation of the joint which provides the majority of mobility is an attractive idea and has been proposed to facilitate limb function particularly on rough/uneven terrain. Andreoni *et al.* (2010) found that following partial carpal arthrodesis, carpal extension angles were maintained during weight-bearing although the range of motion in flexion was reduced to approximately half of normal values. The same study reported largely comparable objective outcome measures of limb function between patients who had either partial or pancarpal arthrodesis.

Various fixation systems for PaCA have been described. Multiple intramedullary K-wires can be placed from the distal aspect of multiple metacarpal bones and driven across the carpometacarpal and middle carpal joints to be seated in the radial carpal bone, or cross K-wires can be used. Alternatively plate fixation using either a dynamic compression plate (DCP) or T-plate can be used. A novel canine CastLess partial carpal arthrodesis plate (Figure 20.15) has recently been developed; an *ex vivo* biomechanical study showed that both this novel partial arthrodesis plate and T-plate fared similarly, being superior to cross pinning in some but not all respects (Burton *et al.*, 2013). To date there have been no clinical studies describing the use of the CastLess partial arthrodesis plate but it is hoped that its design features will help

overcome the challenges that have been associated with straight or T-plate application (see Operative Technique 20.2) and reduce the postoperative morbidity that can be seen with other fixation systems. Unlike PCA, there is currently no evidence to indicate whether adjunctive external coaptation is required in the early postoperative period. However, this may be dependent on the fixation system used. PaCA complications can include infection, implant problems, morbidity associated with external coaptation and development of antebrachiocarpal pathology.

From the small number of PaCA case series that have been published, a substantial variation in outcome has been reported. Despite a high postoperative complication rate, Haburjak *et al.* (2003) reported good to excellent outcome with cross pin fixation. Willer *et al.* (1990) reported resolution of lameness in 70% of patients who had predominately transarticular, intramedullary K-wire and, less commonly, T-plate fixation, while Denny and Barr (1991) reported a satisfactory outcome in only 50% of patients when a DCP was used. A suboptimal outcome may in part be due to the development of degenerative pathology in the antebrachiocarpal joint. This may be secondary to residual or developing antebrachiocarpal hyperextension, an undetected concurrent low-grade soft tissue injury (Willer *et al.*, 1990; Denny and Barr, 1991; Haburjack *et al.*, 2003), subsequent overloading of the antebrachiocarpal joint, or impingement of the dorsal aspect of the antebrachiocarpal joint by the proximal edge of a bone plate.

Given the challenges that PaCA presents and given the difficulty in excluding possible concomitant antebrachial carpal joint pathology, many surgeons prefer to perform a PCA at the outset.

References and further reading

Andreoni AA, Rytz U, Vannini R and Voss K (2010) Ground reaction force profiles after partial and pancarpal arthrodesis in dogs. *Veterinary and Comparative Orthopaedics and Traumatology* **23**, 1–6

Benson JA and Boudreau RJ (2002) Severe carpal and tarsal shearing injuries treated with an immediate arthrodesis in seven dogs. *Journal of the American Animal Hospital Association* **38**, 370–380

Bristow PR, Meeson RL, Thorne RM *et al.* (2015) Clinical comparison of the hybrid dynamic compression plate and the CastLess Plate for pancarpal arthrodesis in 219 dogs. *Veterinary Surgery* **44**, 70–77

Burton NJ, Miles AW and Pollintine P (2013) Biomechanical comparison of a novel CastLess arthrodesis plate with T-plate and cross pin techniques for canine partial carpal arthrodesis. *Veterinary and Comparative Orthopaedics and Traumatology* **26**, 165–171

Calvo I, Farrell M, Chase D *et al.* (2009) Carpal arthrodesis in cats. Long-term functional outcome. *Veterinary and Comparative Orthopaedics and Traumatology* **22**, 498–504

Cetinkaya MA, Yardimci C and Sağlam M (2007) Carpal laxity syndrome in forty-three puppies. *Veterinary and Comparative Orthopaedics and Traumatology* **20**, 126–130

Clarke SP, Ferguson JF and Miller A (2009) Clinical evaluation of pancarpal arthrodesis using a CastLess plate in 11 dogs. *Veterinary Surgery* **38**, 852–860

Comerford EJ, Doran IC and Owen MR (2006) Carpal derangement and associated carpal valgus in a dog. *Veterinary and Comparative Orthopaedics and Traumatology* **19**, 113–116

Denny HR and Barr ARS (1991) Partial and pancarpal arthrodesis in the dog: a review of 50 cases. *Journal of Small Animal Practice* **32**, 329–334

Earley TD and Dee JF (1980) Trauma to the carpus, tarsus and phalanges of dogs and cats. *Veterinary Clinics of North America: Small Animal Practice* **10**, 717–747

Gemmill TJ, Clarke SP and Carmichael S (2004) Carpal agenesis in a domestic short haired cat. *Veterinary and Comparative Orthopaedics and Traumatology* **17**, 163–166

Gemmill T and Clements D (2016) *BSAVA Manual of Canine and Feline Fracture Repair and Management, 2nd edn.* BSAVA Publications, Gloucester

Gnudi G, Mortellaro CM, Bertoni G *et al.* (2003) Radial carpal bone fracture in 13 dogs. *Veterinary and Comparative Orthopaedics and Traumatology* **16**, 178–183

Grundmann S and Montavon PM (2001) Stenosing tenosynovitis of the abductor pollicis longus muscle in dogs. *Veterinary and Comparative Orthopaedics and Traumatology* **14**, 95–100

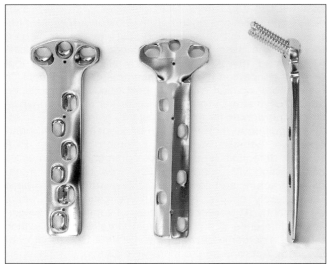

20.15 The CastLess partial carpal arthrodesis plate.
(Courtesy of Neil Burton)

Guilliard MJ (1997) Dorsal radiocarpal ligament sprain causing intermittent lameness in high activity dogs. *Journal of Small Animal Practice* **38**, 463–466

Guilliard MJ (1998) Enthesiopathy of the short radial collateral ligaments in racing greyhounds. *Journal of Small Animal Practice* **39**, 227–230

Guilliard MJ (2006) The carpus. In: *BSAVA Manual of Canine and Feline Musculoskeletal Disorders*, ed. J Houlton, J Cook, J Innes and S Langley-Hobbs, pp. 281–288. BSAVA Publications, Gloucester

Guilliard MJ and Mayo AK (2000) Sprain of the short radial collateral ligament in a racing greyhound. *Journal of Small Animal Practice* **41**, 1169–1171

Guilliard MJ and Mayo AK (2001) Subluxation/luxation of the second carpal bone in two racing greyhounds and a Staffordshire bull terrier. *Journal of Small Animal Practice* **42**, 356–359

Haburjak JJ, Leneham TM, Davidson CD *et al.* (2003) Treatment of carpometacarpal and middle carpal joint hyperextension injuries with partial carpal arthrodesis using a cross pin technique: 21 cases. *Veterinary and Comparative Orthopaedics and Traumatology* **16**, 105–111

Hittmair KM, Groessl V and Mayrhofer E (2012) Radiographic and ultrasonographic diagnosis of stenosing tenosynovitis of the abductor pollicis longus muscle in dogs. *Veterinary Radiology and Ultrasound* **53**, 135–141

Innes JF, McKee WM, Mitchell RAS, Lascelles BDX and Johnson KA (2001) Surgical reconstruction of ectrodactyly deformity in four dogs. *Veterinary and Comparative Orthopaedics and Traumatology* **14**, 201–209

Jerram RM, Walker AM, Worth AJ and Kuipers Von Lande RG (2009) Prospective evaluation of pancarpal arthrodesis for carpal injuries in working dogs in New Zealand, using dorsal hybrid plating. *New Zealand Veterinary Journal* **57**, 331–337

Langley-Hobbs SJ, Hamilton MH and Pratt JNJ (2007) Radiographic and clinical features of carpal varus associated with chronic sprain of the lateral collateral ligament complex in 10 dogs. *Veterinary and Comparative Orthopaedics and Traumatology* **20**, 324–330

Li A, Bennett D, Gibbs G *et al.* (2000) Radial carpal bone fractures in 15 dogs. *Journal of Small Animal Practice* **41**, 74–79

McKee WM and Reynolds J (2007) Ulnocarpal arthrodesis and limb lengthening for the management of radial agenesis in a dog. *Journal of Small Animal Practice* **48**, 591–595

Miller A, Carmichael S, Anderson TJ and Brown I (1990) Luxation of the radial carpal bone in four dogs. *Journal of Small Animal Practice* **31**, 148–154

Nakladal B, vom Hagen F, Brunnberg M *et al.* (2013) Carpal joint injuries in cats – an epidemiological study. *Veterinary and Comparative Orthopaedics and Traumatology* **26**, 333–339

Nordberg CC and Johnson KA (1999) Magnetic resonance imaging of normal canine carpal ligaments. *Veterinary Radiology and Ultrasound* **40**, 128–136

Perry K, Fitzpatrick N, Johnson J and Yeadon R (2010) Headless self-compressing cannulated screw fixation for treatment of radial carpal bone fracture or fissure in dogs. *Veterinary and Comparative Orthopaedics and Traumatology* **23**, 84–101

Piermattei DL, Flo, GL and DeCamp CE (2006) Fractures and other orthopaedic conditions of the carpus, metacarpus, and phalanges. In: *Brinker, Piermattei and Flo's Handbook of Small Animal Orthopedics and Fracture Repair*, pp. 382–428. Saunders, Philadelphia

Pitcher GD (1996) Luxation of the radial carpal bone in a cat. *Journal of Small Animal Practice* **37**, 292–295

Shires PK, Hulse DA and Kearney MT (1985) Carpal hyperextension in two-month-old pups. *Journal of the American Veterinary Medical Association* **186**, 49–52

Slocum D and Devine T (1982) Partial carpal fusion in the dog. *Journal of the American Veterinary Medical Association* **180**, 1204–1208

Tomlin JL, Pead MJ, Langley Hobbs SJ and Muir P (2001) Radial carpal bone fracture in dogs. *Journal of the American Animal Hospital Association* **37**, 173–180

Vaughan LC (1992) Flexural deformity of the carpus in puppies. *Journal of Small Animal Practice* **33**, 381–384

Voss K, Geyer H and Montavon PM (2003) Antebrachiocarpal luxation in a cat. A case report and anatomical study of the medial collateral ligament. *Veterinary and Comparative Orthopaedics and Traumatology* **16**, 266–270

Whitelock R (2001) Conditions of the carpus in the dog. *In Practice* **23**, 2–13

Willer RL, Johnson KA, Turner TM and Piermattei DL (1990) Partial carpal arthrodesis for third degree carpal sprains. A review of 45 carpi. *Veterinary Surgery* **19**, 334–340

Woods S, Wallace RJ and Mosley JR (2012) The effect of external coaptation on plate deformation in an *ex vivo* model of canine pancarpal arthrodesis. *Veterinary and Comparative Orthopaedics and Traumatology* **25**, 439–444

IMAGING TECHNIQUES

Thomas W. Maddox

The complex anatomy of the carpus makes imaging a challenge; even purely osseous disease can be difficult to evaluate fully on radiographs and special views are frequently required. There is a large number of supporting ligamentous structures and no currently available imaging modality is able to depict all of these with a high degree of clarity.

RADIOGRAPHY

Standard views

Standard views of the carpus are the mediolateral and dorsopalmar views. Radiographic grids are not required and a high detail system should be used if available. The cassette or image detector should be placed on the table immediately under the carpus.

Mediolateral view

There is much superimposition of the carpal bones and joints on this view, but some of the antebrachiocarpal joint can be assessed, along with the dorsal surfaces of the carpal bones. Dorsal and palmar soft tissue swelling is also well assessed on this view.

* The animal is placed in lateral recumbency with the target limb protracted cranially and dependent against the cassette/plate and the contralateral limb retracted caudally (Figure 20.16).
* The carpus should be in a neutral to mildly extended position.
* The primary beam is centred on the carpal joint.
* Collimate to include one-third of the distal antebrachium and most of the metacarpals.

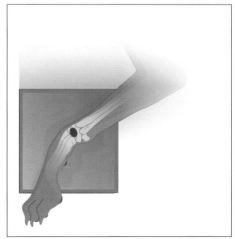

20.16 Patient positioning for a mediolateral view of the carpus.

➡

→ **IMAGING TECHNIQUES CONTINUED**

Dorsopalmar view

This view is useful for assessment of the carpal joints and the carpal bones are relatively well separated; medial and lateral soft tissue swelling is also well appreciated.

- The animal is placed in sternal recumbency with the target limb extended; radiographic positioning aids can be placed under the contralateral axilla to rotate the animal slightly to the side of interest (Figure 20.17).
- Foam pads or sandbags can be used to stabilize the elbow and ensure a straight position.
- The primary beam is centred on the carpal joint.
- Collimate to include one-third of the distal antebrachium and most of the metacarpals.

Special views

The complex anatomy means that oblique views are sometimes necessary to develop a three-dimensional appreciation of any changes seen (although where available, the use of CT has largely supplanted this). Stressed views of the carpus can be obtained in both orthogonal planes. As is always the case for stressed views, radiographs of the contralateral limb should be obtained for comparison.

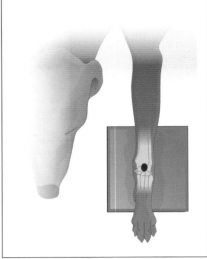

20.17 Patient positioning for a dorsopalmar view of the carpus.

PRACTICAL TIP

For stressed views, the limb proximal to the joint being stressed needs to be held firmly with respect to the distal limb where 'stress' is being applied. Two ties or tapes applied parallel to each other a short distance apart in the proximal segment and one distally (below the level of interest) pulling in the opposite direction are recommended

Dorsolateral–palmaromedial oblique view

- The animal is positioned as for the dorsopalmar view and the distal limb pronated to rotate the dorsal surface of the carpus medially by approximately 45 degrees.
- Positioning, centring and collimation are otherwise as for the standard dorsopalmar view.

Dorsomedial–palmarolateral oblique view

- The animal is positioned as for the dorsopalmar view and the distal limb supinated to rotate the dorsal surface of the carpus laterally by approximately 45 degrees.
- Positioning, centring and collimation are otherwise as for the standard dorsopalmar view.

Stressed extended view

While this view is useful for radiographic confirmation of clinically evident carpal hyperextension, it can be difficult to achieve.

- The animal is positioned as for the mediolateral view.
- Dorsally secured (distally) and caudally secured (proximally) tapes or ties are used to maintain the carpus in maximal extension (Figure 20.18).
- Positioning, centring and collimation are otherwise as for the standard mediolateral view.

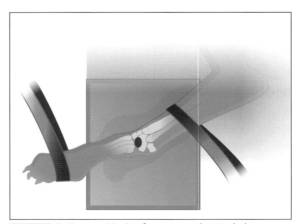

20.18 Patient positioning for a stressed extended mediolateral view of the carpus.

→ **IMAGING TECHNIQUES CONTINUED**

Flexed mediolateral view

This view allows evaluation of the dorsal surface of the carpal bones and can help identify small fractures involving their margins.

- The animal is positioned as for the mediolateral view.
- Tapes or ties across the angle of the joint are used to maintain the carpus in maximal flexion (Figure 20.19).
- Positioning, centring and collimation are otherwise as for the standard mediolateral view.

Medially and laterally stressed dorsopalmar views

These views are useful to demonstrate insufficiency of the collateral ligaments. The antebrachium is stabilized with ties and an opposing shearing force is applied distal to the carpus. Standard dorsopalmar radiographs are obtained (Figure 20.20).

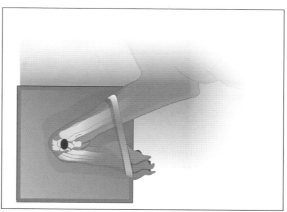

20.19 Patient positioning for a flexed mediolateral view of the carpus.

COMPUTED TOMOGRAPHY

While few new lesions not apparent on high quality radiographs will be seen, the tomographic (slice-based) nature of CT removes superimposition. Lesions will often be better characterized and the extent of changes more fully appreciated. Occasionally, subtle minimally displaced fractures or small avulsion fractures of the articular margins will be identified. Chronic, minimally or non-displaced radial carpal bone fractures are readily evaluated by CT.

Standard technique

- The animal should be placed in sternal recumbency with the thoracic limbs fully extended.
- The scan margins should extend from the distal quarter of the radius/ulna to include the metacarpals.
- Once acquired it is imperative that separate images of both carpi are reconstructed with as small a field of view as feasible.
- Reconstruction using bone and soft tissue algorithms is advisable.

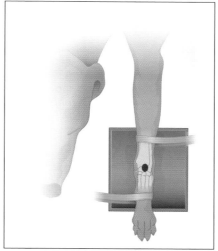

20.20 Patient positioning for stressed dorsopalmar views of the carpus; placing the ties as shown will stress the lateral aspect of the joint.

MAGNETIC RESONANCE IMAGING

In theory, MRI should be well placed to evaluate the soft tissue structures of the carpus, but the small size of this region in most cases can mean that imaging of the carpus is less rewarding than might be expected. However, images of acceptable quality can be acquired with the use of small flexible coils (Nordberg and Johnson, 1999).

ULTRASONOGRAPHY

Ultrasonography is relatively infrequently used in imaging of the carpus, but is useful in evaluating tenosynovitis of the abductor pollicis longus muscle (Hittmair *et al.*, 2012).

OPERATIVE TECHNIQUE 20.1

Pancarpal arthrodesis

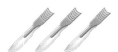

PREOPERATIVE CONSIDERATIONS

Attention should be given to appropriate plate selection as dictated by patient size. Particular attention should be given to selecting a plate of suitable length to span at least 50% of the metacarpus; this is recommended to reduce the risk of postoperative metacarpal fracture. The hybrid dynamic compression plate (HDCP) and the CastLess plate (CLP) are most commonly used; most HDCPs and all CLPs share the advantage of allowing placement of smaller diameter screws in the radial carpal bone and metacarpus than those used in the radius. Strict asepsis is paramount; the authors recommend clipping and aseptic preparation of the entire limb down to the paw for inclusion within the surgical field. The limb can be suspended using a sterile towel clamp placed into either a digit pad or nail. Drapes are placed to isolate the limb, including the proximal humerus if an autogenous cancellous bone graft is to be harvested. Either an adhesive drape or, alternatively, a sterile cohesive bandage can be used to cover the foot, carpus and antebrachium and can be sutured to the edges of the surgical wound. The cohesive bandage has the advantage of assisting in retraction of the wound edges once sutured to them.

If autogenous cancellous bone graft is to be used, it is usually harvested from the ipsilateral proximal humerus. Alternatively, allograft, e.g. demineralized bone matrix, can be used (see the *BSAVA Manual of Canine and Feline Fracture Repair and Management*).

POSITIONING

The patient can be positioned in lateral recumbency with the affected limb uppermost, sternal recumbency with the limb drawn cranially, or dorsal recumbency with the limb drawn caudally. Draping of the limb can be more challenging with the patient in sternal recumbency, and additional care is required to maintain rotational alignment of the limb if the patient is positioned in lateral recumbency.

ASSISTANT

Not essential if the surgeon is experienced and familiar with the technique but very helpful, especially with the patient in dorsal rather than lateral recumbency.

EQUIPMENT EXTRAS

Appropriately sized bone plate and screw kits; bone burr; Gelpi self-retaining retractors; drill; Volkmann curette(s) for bone graft collection.

SURGICAL TECHNIQUE

A dorsal midline skin incision is made (Figure 20.21a) starting proximally over the distal third of the radius, extending distally over the carpus and ending in the distal metacarpal region; the incision is curved towards the medial aspect of the metacarpus so that it does not lie directly over the plate. The extensor carpi radialis tendon is transected at its insertion on to metacarpals 2 and 3, and the common digital extensor tendons are protected and retracted laterally (Figure 20.21b). Transection of the abductor pollicis longus muscle is generally required to facilitate exposure of the distal radius. Following exposure of the dorsal aspect of the carpus, the dorsal joint capsule is excised to expose the antebrachiocarpal, middle carpal and carpometacarpal joints. Articular cartilage can now be debrided from all three joints using a high-speed bone burr (Figure 20.22).

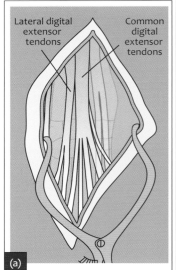
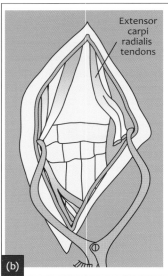

20.21 (a) Mid-dorsal skin incision over the carpus parallel to the cephalic vein. (b) The extensor carpi radialis tendons are sectioned and the common digital extensor tendon is retracted.

→

→ **OPERATIVE TECHNIQUE 20.1 CONTINUED**

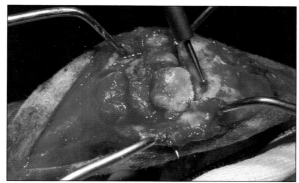

20.22 Removal of the articular cartilage from the radial carpal bone using a high-speed bone burr.

HDCP application

There will undoubtedly be differences in screw insertion sequence and execution of plate and bone graft application between surgeons; the following represents the authors' preferred technique. The HDCP is centred over metacarpal 3 so that the central round hole is positioned over the radial carpal bone; an appropriate pilot hole is drilled through the radial carpal bone and the screw is inserted. This is followed by the most distal metacarpal screw, proximal metacarpal screw, distal radial screw and proximal radial screw. The proximal metacarpal and distal radial screws are placed as compression screws. The bone plate is removed and bone graft placed into the joint spaces. The HDCP is replaced and reinsertion of the previously placed screws is followed by placement of the remaining radial and metacarpal screws (Figure 20.23).

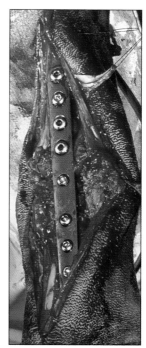

20.23 Placement of a 3.5/2.7 mm hybrid dynamic compression plate.

CastLess plate application

The distal component of the plate is centred over metacarpals 3 and 4; this is facilitated by placing a 0.9 mm K-wire or small hypodermic needle through each alignment hole and between metacarpals 3 and 4; screw hole 5 is centred over the radial carpal bone. The radial carpal screw is placed first. Subsequently screws 8 and 9 are placed as compression screws, followed by screws 3 and 4, again as compression screws. The authors' order of placement for the remaining screws is 6, 7, 10, 11, 1 then 2 (Figure 20.24). Readers are directed to the paper by Clarke *et al.* (2009) for more information about CLP application.

Closure

The tendons of the extensor carpi radialis are sutured to the remnant of the joint capsule; the subcutaneous tissues and the skin are closed routinely.

POSTOPERATIVE CARE

Following postoperative radiography, a soft dressing is applied for 48 hours before being changed; the duration of bandaging is generally in the region of 2–7 days. The authors do not routinely place a dressing, splinted or otherwise, after this time. However, if a palmar splint or a bi-valve cast is used, it should be placed once the soft tissue swelling has resolved. Meticulous splint/cast management is required in an attempt to avoid complications; the frequency of changes should be at least weekly, although ultimately the frequency will be dictated by individual patient requirement. When used, the cast or splinted dressing usually remains in place for about 6 weeks. The patient should be strictly rested until follow-up at 6 weeks after surgery. Radiography should be performed at that time; assuming arthrodesis is progressing satisfactorily, limited controlled lead activity should be allowed for a further 6 weeks, followed by a gradual return to normal activity.

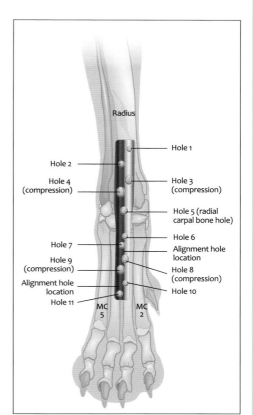

20.24 Positioning and screw hole numbering for CastLess pancarpal arthrodesis (PCA) plate application. MC = metacarpal.

→ **OPERATIVE TECHNIQUE 20.1 CONTINUED**

PRACTICAL TIPS

- Meticulous debridement of all the articular cartilage is required; the most common reason for failure of arthrodesis is inadequate cartilage removal. Use of a small bone burr and fully flexing the carpal joints facilitates removal of the articular cartilage; a small Freer periosteal or Hohmann retractor inserted into the joint spaces also facilitates access.
- Drill holes into the distal radius and the proximal metacarpal bones from their respective articular surfaces to create channels for neovascularization.
- Achieving an appropriate arthrodesis angle is important; an excessively straight distal forelimb conformation will result in increased wear of the nails of digits 3 and 4 during protraction of the limb. An HDCP provides an inherent 5 degrees of carpal hyperextension; a CastLess plate will provide 8 degrees, without plate contouring. Based on the carpal conformation of the contralateral forelimb the surgeon may occasionally elect to contour the plate to increase the arthrodesis angle obtained, but this is usually unnecessary.
- Burring bone from the dorsal aspect of the base of metacarpal 3 (and 4 if using the CLP) and the dorsal aspect of the distal radius facilitates seating of the bone plate.
- A hypodermic needle can be placed into the space between metacarpals 2 and 3, and 3 and 4; this helps centralize the distal component of the HDCP on metacarpal 3. Accurate placement of metacarpal screws is very important. In most patients, the screw used in the metacarpal will be relatively oversized and eccentric placement can predispose to metacarpal fracture. Particular attention should be paid to the angle of screw insertion in the distal portion of the CLP.
- Once the start point for the radial carpal bone pilot hole is marked, removal of the bone plate allows for more accurate pilot hole drilling. The radial carpal bone is concave on its distal aspect so the hole should be oriented in a distodorsal–proximopalmar direction to optimize the bone/screw interface.
- The radial carpal bone screw should be the last one to be fully tightened. This should help preserve the normal anatomical relationship between the radial carpal bone and the distal radius.
- If a splint or cast is used, ensure appropriate client education regarding its management.

OPERATIVE TECHNIQUE 20.2

Partial carpal arthrodesis

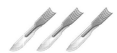

PREOPERATIVE CONSIDERATIONS

Attention must be given to ensuring appropriate case selection; thorough clinical and radiographic assessment is essential. If there is any doubt that the antebrachiocarpal joint may be involved then pancarpal arthrodesis should be performed. Application of a standard T-plate is described in this text; readers are directed to the appropriate literature regarding alternative fixation techniques.

Aseptic preparation of the surgical field and the use of autogenous or allogenic bone graft/substitutes are as described in Operative Technique 20.1

POSITIONING

See Operative Technique 20.1.

ASSISTANT

See Operative Technique 20.1.

EQUIPMENT EXTRAS

Appropriately sized bone plate and screw kits; bone burr; Gelpi self-retaining retractors; drill; Volkmann curette(s) for bone graft collection.

➜ **OPERATIVE TECHNIQUE 20.2 CONTINUED**

SURGICAL TECHNIQUE

A dorsal midline skin incision is made starting proximally over the distal radial metaphysis and extending distally over the carpus to end at the distal metacarpal region; the incision is curved towards the medial aspect of the metacarpal region so that it does not lie directly over the plate. Following exposure of the dorsal aspect of the carpus, the dorsal joint capsule is excised to expose the middle carpal and carpometacarpal joints, which are meticulously debrided of articular cartilage using a high-speed bone burr. Following placement of autogenous or allogenic bone graft, an appropriately sized T-plate is then secured to the dorsal aspect of the carpus, i.e. the radial carpal bone, and the third metacarpal bone. As with pancarpal arthrodesis, accurate centring of the plate on metacarpal 3 is important. One radial carpal bone screw is placed first followed by the most distal screw in metacarpal 3. The second radial carpal bone screw is then placed followed by the remainder of the screws in metacarpal 3. If possible, a screw should be placed in the third carpal bone (Figure 20.25).

Closure

See Operative Technique 20.1.

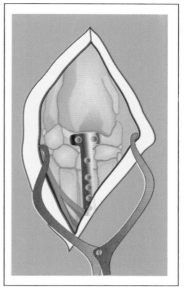

20.25 A T-plate has been placed on the dorsal aspect of the carpus, centred on metacarpal 3.

POSTOPERATIVE CARE

Following postoperative radiography, a soft dressing is applied for 48 hours before being changed; the duration of bandaging is likely to be in the region of 2–7 days. The use of external coaptation is at the surgeon's discretion with the considerations similar to those for PCA. The patient should be strictly rested until follow-up at 6 weeks postoperatively. Radiography should be performed at that time; assuming arthrodesis is progressing satisfactorily, limited controlled lead activity should be allowed for a further 6 weeks followed by a gradual return to normal activity.

PRACTICAL TIPS

- Accurate plate position with respect to screw position and placement relative to the radial carpal bone are challenging but imperative for success. The plate should be attached distally on the dorsal aspect of the radial carpal bone; too proximal and it will impinge on the distal radius when the antebrachiocarpal joint is extended during weight-bearing; too distal and the proximal two screws may not engage the radial carpal bone adequately. Given the position of the plate, the screws must be oriented in a distopalmar– proximodorsal direction within the radial carpal bone to ensure maximal bone purchase.
- The novel design of the CastLess partial arthrodesis plate is such that it may help ameliorate some of the challenges associated with plate application on the radial carpal bone; it also allows for screw placement in both the radial and ulnar carpal bones as well as in metacarpals 3 and 4.
- Opening of the antebrachiocarpal joint capsule allows for visual assessment of the dorsal aspect of the radial carpal bone; this can facilitate accurate radial carpal bone screw placement.
- As well as orthogonal postoperative radiographs, a stressed radiograph of the carpus to mimic weight-bearing is useful as it may highlight plate impingement.
- Ensure appropriate client education regarding splint/cast management if appropriate.

Chapter 21

The distal limb

Mike Guilliard

Lameness associated with conditions found in the distal limbs is common in first opinion practice. During an examination for lameness, it is important that a thorough clinical assessment is made of the metacarpus/metatarsus and paw including the pads, nails and skin.

A number of conditions of traumatic, infectious, multifactorial or unknown aetiology may specifically affect the pads and skin of the distal limb and cause lameness. Some of these conditions are dermatological in nature but are included here as the main presenting sign may be lameness.

Animals with distal limb lameness often hold the affected foot off the ground with the limb in partial flexion. Walking and trotting on hard or irregular surfaces may exacerbate the degree of lameness. Sight hounds are prone to corns and in these breeds, a thorough examination of the digital paw pads should be made before making further investigations.

Anatomy

The distal limb comprises the metacarpus/metatarsus and the foot and includes the metacarpal/metatarsal and phalangeal bones, the metacarpophalangeal (MCP) or metatarsophalangeal (MTP) and interphalangeal joints, together with the articular ligaments and flexor and extensor tendons (Figure 21.1). The integument of the foot comprises the skin, paw pads and nails. There are four weight-bearing digits on each foot numbered medially to laterally from 2 to 5. Digit 1 is the dewclaw and in the pelvic limbs is usually vestigial.

The metacarpal and metatarsal bones, numbered 2 to 5, lie between the carpometacarpal and tarsometatarsal joints and the MCP/MTP joints. Each digit consists of three bones: the first, second and third phalanges. The nail grows around the ungual process which is an extension of the third phalanx. The main function of the nail is to grip the ground during acceleration, deceleration and turning.

Between the phalangeal bones are the proximal and distal interphalangeal joints. The MCP/MTP joints each have large paired sesamoid bones attached to the palmar/plantar aspect of the joints by a complex arrangement of ligaments. The sesamoid bones are numbered medially to laterally from 1 to 8, and are within the tendons of insertion of the interosseous muscles. There are also small sesamoid bones within the extensor tendons on the dorsal aspect of both the MCP/MTP joints and the proximal interphalangeal (PIP) joints.

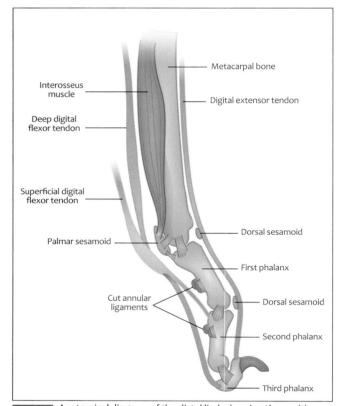

21.1 Anatomical diagram of the distal limb showing the positions of the bones, main ligaments and tendons. The annular ligaments are shown cut in the illustration, so that the superficial and deep superficial digital flexor tendons can be better seen.

The weight-bearing paw pads comprise a large metacarpal/metatarsal pad and smaller digital pads. The epidermis has a rough surface to increase grip and the base consists largely of fibro-adipose tissue that acts as cushioning during load bearing. The interdigital skin is referred to as the webbing.

On the palmar/plantar aspect of the distal limb run the deep digital flexor tendon, which inserts on the flexor process of the third phalanx, and the superficial digital flexor tendon, which inserts on the proximal part of the second phalanx. At the MCP/MTP joint, the deep digital flexor tendons pass through the tubular sheath formed by the branches of the superficial digital flexor tendon. The digital flexor tendons are held in close proximity to the digits by annular ligaments. The weaker lateral and common digital extensor tendons combine to run down the dorsal aspect of the digits and insert on the third phalanx. The interdigital joints are maintained in flexion by the flexor tendons and the interosseous muscles. More detailed surgical anatomy is given with the description of each specific injury.

Clinical examination and diagnostics

A thorough examination of the entire distal limb should be made as part of a wider orthopaedic examination. The dog should be observed in its normal stance and then during walking and trotting. The physical examination is then made in a thorough, specific and repeatable order so that any potential abnormalities are detected and nothing is missed. This could begin with the nails followed by the pads, interdigital skin, phalangeal joints, etc. The examination should include the dewclaw.

Visual examination, which may require clipping of the coat in long-haired breeds, can detect:

- Swelling, either local or more general
- Abnormal posture, such as a raised nail or abnormal weight-bearing
- Wounds
- Dermatitis, particularly interdigital, on the palmar or plantar aspect of the foot
- Fractured nails.

Manual examination can detect:

- Focal pain, by the application of digital pressure
- Joint instability, checked in the mediolateral plane with the joint in both flexion and extension; dorsopalmar/dorsoplantar instability is uncommon
- Decreased range of motion of the joints
- Crepitus
- Swelling
- Loose nail.

> It is important to compare clinical findings with other digits on both the same and the contralateral foot, as changes can be subtle

Further tests:

- Synoviocentesis, cytology, and culture and sensitivity testing
- Radiography: orthogonal and stressed views
- Computed tomography (CT) including contrast studies
- Fine-needle aspiration and biopsy.

> It is important to realize that lameness may originate from an associated primary injury elsewhere in the paw and not necessarily directly from the pathology that is visible. For example, chronic subluxation of the PIP joint causing a rotational deformity of the distal digit can result in painful dermatological changes to the pad and interdigital skin

Synoviocentesis

It is possible to aspirate synovial fluid from the MCP/MTP joints and the proximal and distal interphalangeal joints using a 23 G hypodermic needle and 2 ml syringe. The approach to the MCP/MTP joints is dorsolateral with the joint in 45 degrees of flexion, and in the proximal and distal interphalangeal joints, the approach is lateral with the joint in a neutral position and the distal end of the digit distracted away from the operator to open the joint (see Chapter 4).

An effusion in one of the joints of the digit will have a small volume and may only fill the needle's hub. This is sufficient to make a smear for cytological staining, but insufficient for bacterial culture. In contrast, any useful volume of synovial fluid can rarely be withdrawn from a normal digital joint.

The presence of effusion confirms joint pathology. A raised white cell count that is predominantly neutrophilic is indicative of a joint infection or immune-mediated polyarthritis (see Chapter 6).

Surgical preparation

Adequate aseptic preparation of the pads and nails is challenging. Isolation of these areas from the surgical site can be achieved by the application of a sterile cohesive bandage to cover the entire foot that can also be extended to use as a tourniquet around the distal antebrachium/tibia. An incision can then be made through the dressing directly over the surgical site. However, an autoclaved cohesive bandage is not necessarily sterile (see Chapter 13). A bloodless site is useful for most surgical procedures of the distal limbs. Haemostasis of the distal phalanx can also be achieved by an assistant applying mediolateral digital pressure behind the digital pad, thus occluding the artery.

Cohesive bandages, such as Vetrap, are not waterproof; therefore, an additional sterile glove or impermeable paper drape can be used over the foot and under a sterile cohesive dressing to prevent strike-through.

External coaptation and wound dressings

Some form of support or postoperative protective dressing is recommended for a number of conditions. It is advisable to apply orthopaedic padding between the digits to prevent nail-induced ischaemic wounds from impinging on adjacent digits, and to adequately cover pressure points such as the point of the calcaneus and the abaxial aspects of the base of metacarpal/metatarsal bones 2 and 5.

To minimize the potential for dressing induced injuries, the author advises the following measures:

- Apply adequate orthopaedic padding with a conforming bandage under an elastic bandage
- Apply padding between the toes
- Change the dressing regularly, at least every 7 days
- Keep the dressing dry using a protective covering when outdoors. Remember that male dogs can urinate on thoracic limb foot dressings.

> **WARNING**
>
> Foot or distal limb casts can cause ischaemic injury and should be used with care. They require frequent monitoring. Adequate support can be obtained with a gutter spoon splint, thus allowing simple dressing changes

Metacarpophalangeal and metatarsophalangeal joint injury

This can result from trauma, osteoarthritis, immune-mediated disease and bacterial infective arthritis.

Anatomy

The MCP/MTP joints lie between the metacarpal/metatarsal bones and the first phalanx. On the palmar/plantar aspect of each joint is a pair of sesamoid bones that are separated from each other by a prominent sagittal ridge of bone. Each pair is embedded in the tendon of insertion of its respective interosseous muscle and articulates primarily with the distal metacarpal/metatarsal bone, with a small secondary articulation to the first phalanx. There is a thick fibrous band connecting each pair, the intersesamoidean ligament, forming a groove in which the superficial and deep digital flexor tendons run. Further ligaments attach the sesamoids to the metacarpal/metatarsal bones and the first phalanx (Figures 21.2 and 21.3).

The joint is also supported by collateral ligaments and the joint capsule. A small, palpable sesamoid is present in the common digital extensor tendon dorsal to the joint.

Subluxation and luxation

The majority of instabilities occur in abaxial digits 2 or 5, and are most commonly rotational subluxations classified as axial rotational instability (AxRI) where the digital pad is rotated axially (Figure 21.4), or abaxial rotational instability (AbRI) where the digital pad is rotated abaxially (Figure 21.5) (Guilliard, 2012). The joint can also subluxate laterally with rupture of the medial ligaments. Avulsion of a small bone fragment attached to a collateral ligament occurs occasionally.

Abaxial luxation of the first phalanx can occur with a concomitant luxation of one or both sesamoid bones (Figure 21.6). These injuries are common in the racing Greyhound. Subluxation of more than one joint is uncommon but can be a debilitating injury (Figures 21.7 and 21.8).

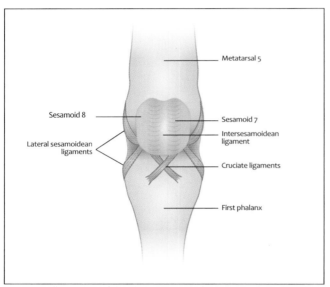

21.2 Illustration of the plantar aspect of metatarsophalangeal joint 5 showing the relationship of the sesamoidean ligaments to the joint. The large intersesamoidean sagittal ridge lies under the intersesamoidean ligament.

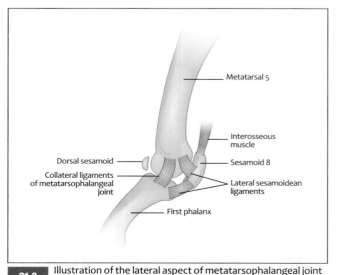

21.3 Illustration of the lateral aspect of metatarsophalangeal joint 5 showing the relationship of the ligaments to the bones.

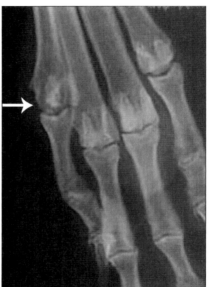

21.4 A dorsoplantar radiograph of the pelvic limb paw of a Greyhound showing axial rotational deformity of digit 5. Torsion of the metatarsophalangeal joint is evident from the axial rotation of the sesamoids (arrowed). Diagnosis of concomitant instability is made by palpation, but cannot be made from this radiograph. Abaxial soft tissue swelling is apparent.

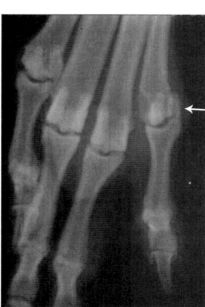

21.5 A stressed dorsoplantar radiograph of the pelvic limb paw of a Greyhound showing abaxial rotational instability of digit 2 causing abaxial displacement of the digit. Note the abaxial subluxation of both sesamoid bones (arrowed).

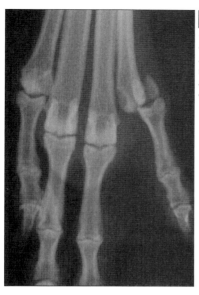

21.6 A dorsoplantar radiograph of a pelvic limb paw of a Greyhound showing abaxial luxation of the metatarsophalangeal joint and sesamoid bones of digit 5.

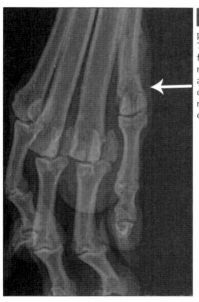

21.7 A dorsoplantar radiograph of the pelvic foot of a Greyhound. There is an old healing fracture of the distal second metatarsal bone (arrowed) and rotational subluxations of MTP joints 3, 4 and 5 resulting from a subsequent dog fight.

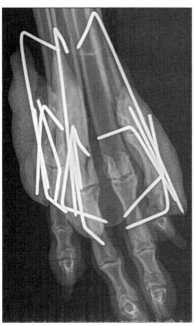

21.8 A dorsoplantar radiograph of the dog in Figure 21.7 following the application of transarticular external skeletal fixators across the reduced joints. 1.4 mm pins in a 2:2 configuration were applied to the metatarsal and first phalangeal joints.

Axial rotational instability

This is commonly seen in the MTP joint of the fifth digit of the racing Greyhound and is not limb specific. A common predisposing factor for subluxation is torsion of the fifth metatarsal bone; this is detected from a dorsoplantar radiographic view giving the erroneous appearance of the sesamoid bones being displaced axially. The large sagittal ridge prevents true displacement.

External rotation of the digit will reduce the subluxation but it will re-subluxate on weight-bearing. It is difficult to appreciate this instability on stressed radiographs. Diagnosis is by observation of the subluxation, the presence of periarticular soft tissue swelling, and inducement of the instability and its reduction by manipulation.

The lameness resolves rapidly with conservative management but the joint remains permanently subluxated with a reduced range of movement. Many Greyhounds will return to successful racing, but for some lameness will persist. The author recommends that acute injuries are treated with the application of a transarticular external skeletal fixator (see Operative Technique 21.1).

An uncommon sequel in the chronic case is impingement of the nail of the fifth digit on to the fourth digit. Permanent nail removal (ungual crest ostectomy) is then necessary (see Operative Technique 21.3)

Abaxial rotational instability and lateral subluxation/luxation

In the racing Greyhound, AbRI and lateral instability occur mainly in the fifth MTP joint; this is over-represented in the left pelvic limb. As the dog leans into the bend to counteract the centrifugal forces, the lateral aspects of the left paws of both the thoracic and pelvic limbs, i.e. the fifth digits, are subjected to the greatest loads.

AbRI and lateral subluxation result in a more profound lameness than AxRI. Diagnosis is by observation of periarticular swelling with or without abnormal positioning of the digit. Palpation will detect instability that may be rotational or lateral. Radiography may detect avulsion fractures of the collateral ligament, sesamoid displacement and luxation. Stressed radiographs show joint incongruity.

Treatment involves maintaining the joint in normal congruity for several weeks and allowing the development of periarticular fibrosis to stabilize the joint. Inherently stable joints can be treated with external coaptation for 3 weeks, but more unstable joints require surgical intervention. Techniques involving ligament reconstruction and the use of prosthetic ligaments have been described but are difficult to perform well. The application of a transarticular external skeletal fixator gives excellent results (Guilliard, 2012). Small periarticular avulsion fractures can be left to form a fibrous union with no adverse result (see Operative Technique 21.1).

Sprain of metacarpophalangeal/ metatarsophalangeal joints 3 and 4

Acute injury to these joints is uncommon as there is support from the adjacent digits. Palmar/plantar luxation of the first phalanx in these joints is rare and can be difficult to reduce. Conservative management of joint sprain usually results in lameness resolution but if lameness persists, application of a transarticular external skeletal fixator should be considered to achieve joint immobilization.

Osteoarthritis of the metacarpophalangeal/metatarsophalangeal joints

This is a common finding in older dogs and can affect multiple joints. It is significantly more common in the MCP as opposed to the MTP joints. It may be seen as an incidental finding or as a cause of lameness. In one study (Franklin *et al.*, 2009) it was the primary cause of lameness in only 14/49 affected dogs. It is seen in many working dogs and in non-working dogs that have been active ball or stick chasers. When clinically significant, it presents with an exercise-induced lameness that often resolves with rest. Typically there is a reduced range of motion and an observable thickening of the joint(s) with pain (a key sign in clinically relevant cases) on firm flexion. Radiography shows periarticular osteophyte deposition and spur (enthesophyte) formation (Figure 21.9).

If multiple joints are involved, synoviocentesis and cytology should be undertaken to eliminate immune-mediated polyarthritis as a differential diagnosis.

The majority of cases can be managed conservatively with weight loss, reduced exercise and the use of non-steroidal anti-inflammatory drugs (NSAIDs) as necessary, depending on the severity of clinical signs. Severe vigorous forms of exercise such as ball chasing may need to be discouraged. If there is persistent lameness originating from one joint, a surgical salvage procedure may be considered. Examples of salvage techniques include arthrodesis, excision arthroplasty and digital amputation (see Operative Technique 21.2).

Arthrodesis of the metacarpophalangeal/metatarsophalangeal joint

Arthrodesis of single or multiple joints can be an effective salvage procedure for chronic debilitating osteoarthritis or joint subluxation when other treatment measures have been unsuccessful. Some degree of gait abnormality may result. If a single digit is involved, digit amputation should be considered as an alternative (see Operative Technique 21.2).

Excision arthroplasty of the metacarpophalangeal/metatarsophalangeal joint

There is little published literature regarding this procedure but it should be considered as an alternative to arthrodesis or digit amputation, the latter being retained as a future salvage option. In the author's limited experience, excision arthroplasty is straightforward and well tolerated. A dorsal approach allows the removal of the articular surface of the first phalangeal bone with bone cutters and the removal of metacarpal/metatarsal bone articular cartilage with a curette.

Conditions of the palmar and volar sesamoid bones

Acute fractures

Fracture of a sesamoid bone is occasionally found in the racing Greyhound and other high activity breeds. It can affect any of the sesamoids although sesamoids 2 and 7 are over-represented. There is acute onset lameness with pain on joint manipulation, especially with dorsopalmar/dorsoplantar digital pressure. Sharp demarcation of the fracture margins is apparent on radiography (Figure 21.10).

It is important not to confuse fracture with bi- or multipartite sesamoids that can be an incidental finding identified during the work-up of joint sprain. With the latter there is little response to digital pressure and the lameness will resolve rapidly over 2 weeks, compared to the fracture case that will remain lame for several weeks.

Treatment of sesamoid fracture can be conservative or surgical (see the *BSAVA Manual of Canine and Feline Fracture Repair and Management*).

Bipartite or multipartite sesamoids

These are a common finding in certain breeds, such as the Rottweiler (Figure 21.11) and the Greyhound (Figure 21.12), usually affecting sesamoids 2 or 7. It has been suggested that the cause is a result of excess pressure from the flexor tendons that lie eccentrically over these sesamoids because of the distal divergence of metacarpal bones 2 and 5.

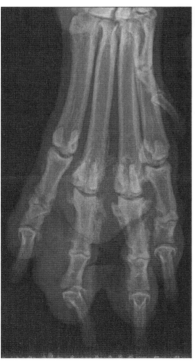

21.9 A dorsopalmar radiograph of the foot of a Labrador Retriever showing osteoarthritis of the MCP joints 3 and 4. There is also marked irregular periosteal new bone on the distal metacarpal and proximal first phalangeal bones.

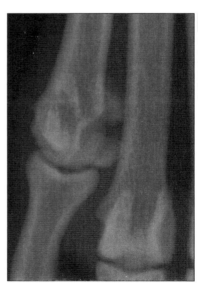

21.10 A dorsopalmar radiograph of the metacarpophalangeal joint of a Greyhound showing a fracture of the sesamoid bone. Note the distraction of the proximal fragment and the sharp fracture margins.

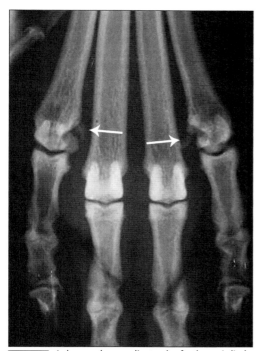

21.11 A dorsopalmar radiograph of a thoracic limb paw of a Rottweiler. Sesamoid bones 2 and 7 are fragmented (arrowed). This was a coincidental finding and not the cause of lameness.

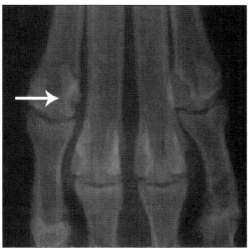

21.12 A dorsopalmar radiograph of the thoracic limb paw of a Greyhound. Sesamoid bone 2 is bipartite (arrowed).

These changes are not associated with lameness and are coincidental radiographic findings. In dogs with extensive changes, there may be some periarticular thickening and reduced flexion.

Sesamoid disease of young dogs

In Australia, there is a recognized syndrome of chronic pain in the MCP joints of adolescent dogs, particularly the Rottweiler and Australian Cattle Dog. The dog is presented with an acute or chronic lameness with a synovial effusion and radiographic changes to the sesamoids that include enlargement, lytic changes and multiple fragments within the sesamoid. The cause has not been determined but vascular compromise has been suggested because, histologically, the affected bones show varying stages of fracture repair with extensive areas of bone necrosis (Robins and Read, 1998).

Treatment is conservative management with NSAIDs or, in refractory cases, steroids can be used.

> Note: radiographic signs of sesamoid disease should always be treated with caution when investigating thoracic limb lameness. Other causes of lameness such as elbow dysplasia are common especially in the Rottweiler

> Note: sesamoidectomy has been suggested as treatment for conditions of the MCP/MTP joints where there is evidence of sesamoid disease. The author recommends this procedure only for cases of sesamoid fracture that do not resolve with rest, or for those seen in the racing Greyhound (see Operative Technique 21.7)

The proximal interphalangeal joint

Anatomy

The PIP joint is the articulation between the first and second phalanges. It is supported abaxially by broad collateral ligaments and the joint capsule. On the dorsal aspect, the joint capsule is thickened by a small cartilaginous sesamoid that lies within the digital extensor tendon. On the palmar/plantar aspects, the superficial and deep digital flexor tendons are held in close proximity to the joint by a strong annular ligament distal to the joint (see Figure 21.1).

Instability

Instability of the joint can be classified as 'stable on reduction' where the joint can be manually subluxated but reverts back to normal congruity, or 'unstable' where the joint subluxates during weight-bearing. The degree of instability is dependent on the degree of damage to the collateral ligament and joint capsule. If there is an avulsion fracture associated with the collateral ligament, the joint will be unstable. Complete luxation is rare and is associated with global soft tissue damage.

Damage to the joint is associated with varying degrees of lameness and possible rotational deformity of the distal digit. There is periarticular soft tissue swelling. Diagnosis is made by manually examining the joint for instability in the mediolateral plane, usually under general anaesthesia; note that in the normal joint, a small degree of mediolateral instability is present when the joint is in 45 degrees of flexion.

Avulsion fractures are diagnosed by radiography; similarly, subluxation is confirmed by stress radiography.

The stable joint can be treated by external coaptation for 3 weeks, together with shortening of the nail to reduce the lever arm on the joint. The nail can safely be cut back to the corium causing some haemorrhage, but excision at the skin interface risks the development of osteomyelitis in the third phalanx. This is followed by restricted exercise for 4 weeks.

Historically, the treatment of the unstable PIP joint has followed this chronology:

- Pin firing
- Blistering
- Periarticular injection of sclerosing agents
- Prosthetic ligament replacement using wire or nylon suture materials
- Ligament reconstruction
- Placement of a transarticular external skeletal fixator.

The first three techniques have welfare implications and should not be used. Prosthetic ligament replacement has lost favour and most surgeons now reconstruct the ligament or apply an external fixator.

In the author's experience, all the techniques give inconsistent results except for external skeletal fixation. The collateral ligaments are broad and the isometric points vary with joint flexion and extension, making it impossible to replicate with a linear prosthesis. Ligament reconstruction with synthetic suture material (polydioxanone) is difficult to achieve accurately as the ruptured ligament is invariably frayed and often avulsed from the bone. Note that all of these techniques rely on periarticular fibrosis to stabilize the joint; this is only achievable if the joint is held in normal congruency during the convalescent period.

The application of a transarticular external skeletal fixator holds the joint in normal congruency allowing stabilizing fibrosis to develop (see Operative Technique 21.1). In the racing Greyhound this technique has given excellent results, even where there is avulsion fracture or complete luxation (Guilliard, 2003; Guilliard, 2012). The application of an external fixator may result in an enlarged joint with reduced range of motion. If articular damage is severe, including from an avulsion fracture, then ankylosis may develop but this has no detrimental effect on outcome.

Permanent nail removal (ungual crest ostectomy) (see Operative Technique 21.3) is essential to reduce the lever arm in many cases. The criteria for ungual crest ostectomy are:

- An unstable joint
- A 'stable on reduction' joint of digits 3 and 4
- Multiple digit involvement. Occasionally the PIP joints of digits 3 and 4 are affected resulting in a severe rotational deformity.

Salvage surgery of the proximal interphalangeal joint

Ankylosis

The application of a transarticular external skeletal fixator is the procedure of choice as it is a simple technique that creates no residual damage to the digit (see Operative Technique 21.1). It can be successfully used in the management of articular fractures (see the BSAVA Manual of Canine and Feline Fracture Repair and Management) and in cases of chronic instability with joint infection. Treatment of these more severe cases will result in a reduced range of joint motion or often ankylosis but this is unlikely to have any clinical implication.

Arthrodesis

Two techniques are described in the literature and are outlined below. The PIP joint should be arthrodesed in a semi-extended position to allow for extension of the digit when galloping.

Dorsal bone plate: After joint preparation and reflection of the extensor tendon, a small plate is applied to the dorsal aspect of the digit. The foot is supported in a spoon splint for several weeks postoperatively.

Pin and tension-band wire: After removal of all the articular cartilage and application of a bone graft, a fine arthrodesis wire is driven from the dorsal aspect of the condyles of the first phalanx, through the joint and into the medullary cavity of the second phalanx. A tension-band wire is placed across the joint around the pin and through the second phalanx. With this technique, rotational instability can occur. In addition, the cut ends of the pin and the wires can easily erode the overlying skin leading to infection and failure of the arthrodesis. The author does not recommend this procedure.

Excision arthroplasty

Excision arthroplasty has been described for the treatment of fractures of digits 3 and 4 as an alternative to amputation, with a successful outcome (de Rooster *et al.*, 2007).

Amputation

Severe or chronic injury to the joint occurring in only one digit can be successfully managed by amputation of the digit at the level of the MCP/MTP joint. Alternatively, a salvage procedure (as above) may be used with the option of amputation in the future if it is unsuccessful. If the joints of more than one digit are affected then digit-sparing salvage surgery should be performed, as amputation of two or more digits will most likely cause a residual lameness.

> **WARNING**
>
> Digit amputation through the diaphysis of the first phalanx is likely to lead to a chronic lameness from concussive injury over the bone stump. A sliding graft using the digital pad is unlikely to prevent this happening

The distal interphalangeal joint

Anatomy

The distal interphalangeal (DIP) joint lies between the second and third phalanges. It is supported by strong, broad collateral ligaments and the joint capsule. On the dorsal aspect is the extensor tendon and the dorsal elastic ligament, both inserting on the third phalanx in close proximity to the joint. On the palmar/plantar aspect runs the deep digital flexor tendon, which inserts on the flexor process of the third phalanx.

Instability

Instability can be classified as 'stable' where the joint can be manually subluxated but reverts back to normal congruity, and 'unstable' where the joint subluxates during weight-bearing (Figure 21.13); this depends on the degree of damage to the collateral ligament and joint capsule.

Mild joint sprain presents as a swollen joint with little palpable instability and 4 weeks of restricted exercise is usually curative.

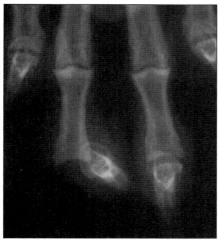

21.13

A stressed dorsopalmar radiograph of the thoracic limb paw of a Greyhound. The distal interphalangeal joint is luxated and unstable.

A stable joint injury requires removal of the nail lever arm, either by cutting short the nail or by permanent nail removal (see Operative Technique 21.3).

An unstable joint requires ungual crest ostectomy and a tacking suture of polydioxanone across the collateral ligament to hold the joint in normal congruency. No attempt is made to repair the damaged ligament; the suture is attached to periarticular fibrous tissue and ligament remnants. External support dressings are unnecessary. The prognosis is excellent.

Open subluxation of the distal interphalangeal joint

This is a condition seen primarily in the thoracic limb of the racing and pet Greyhound. There is a small dorsopalmar cut in the skin on the lateral aspect of the joint in the second digit associated with mild lameness (Figure 21.14); the wound heals rapidly with routine wound management, but on exercise it always recurs. Under general anaesthesia, subluxation of the joint can be induced with the lateral condyle of the second phalanx tearing open the fibrous tissue over the joint.

Treatment by removing the lever arm of the nail with an ungual crest ostectomy is generally very successful (see Operative Technique 21.3). Rarely, this condition affects the PIP joint or the dewclaw.

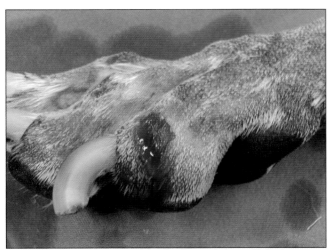

21.14 Open subluxation of the distal interphalangeal joint in a pet Greyhound.

Chronic degenerative changes in the distal interphalangeal joint

Distal digital ostectomy is the preferred treatment for chronic degenerative changes as it preserves the digit (see Operative Technique 21.4). Otherwise some form of digital amputation is necessary.

Tendon injuries

On the dorsal aspect of the metacarpus/metatarsus and foot are the weak digital extensor tendons, which insert on the dorsal aspect of the third phalanx. On the palmar/plantar aspect run the superficial and deep digital flexor tendons. Injury to these structures can be either extrinsic from bites, traffic accidents and cuts or intrinsic as a result of mechanical overload.

Severance of the digital tendons

Severance of the extensor tendons is generally well tolerated, causing few clinical problems. Damage to the flexor tendons causes a postural deformity of the digits that can result in lameness from abnormal weight-bearing on the digital pads.

Where a flexor tendon has been severed, surgical repair may be possible using horizontal mattress or baseball (continuous cruciate) suture patterns, but protection of the repair is necessary and challenging as the tensile strength of the healing tendon is only 50% after 6 weeks (Woo *et al.*, 1994). Casting the foot risks ischaemic necrosis and infection as common complications. It is possible to construct a walking frame with circular fixators applied to the carpus/tarsus and a final distal ring forming a shoe that prevents any weight-bearing on the digits.

Rupture of the superficial digital flexor tendon

The tendon inserts on the proximal end of the palmar/plantar aspect of the second phalanx. Rupture of the tendon results in a flattened toe known as a 'dropped toe' but with the nail still in contact with the ground as the deep digital flexor tendon is still intact. This rarely causes a clinical problem and no treatment is necessary.

Rupture of the deep digital flexor tendon

The tendon inserts on the flexor process of the third phalanx. Rupture of the tendon causes the nail to be elevated with weight-bearing on the caudal aspect of the digital pad; this is known as a 'knocked-up toe' (Figure 21.15)

Some dogs tolerate this injury with no lameness while others develop a concussive lameness on the caudal pad and adjacent skin. It usually results from tendon overload with no external trauma; surgical repair is generally not indicated. If lameness persists then a distal digital ostectomy is necessary (see Operative Technique 21.4).

Contracture of the digits

Rupture of the common calcaneal tendon causes hock hyperflexion and an increase in the distance the flexor tendons have to span. This, and possibly an adaptive contracture of the digital flexor tendons as the dog strives to maintain posture, causes hyperflexion of the interphalangeal joints.

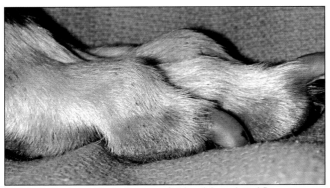

21.15 Rupture of both the superficial and deep digital flexor tendons in a central digit. Note the extended 'dropped' PIP joint resulting from rupture of the superficial tendon, as well as the cranial positioning of the nail compared with digit 4, and the 'knocked-up' DIP joint with elevated nail resulting from rupture of the deep tendon rupture.

Permanent contracture of the superficial digital flexor tendon can be a sequel to dressing injuries over the point of the calcaneus, or from repair of calcaneal fractures or proximal intertarsal subluxation especially where a tension-band wire technique has been used, resulting in adhesions to the tendon.

This results in a debilitating deformity (Figure 21.16). Treatment involves severing the affected tendons distal to the adhesions. The prognosis is good and surprisingly does not result in hyperextended digits.

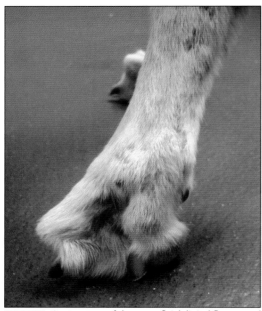

21.16 Contracture of the superficial digital flexor tendons as a sequel to failed tarsal fracture surgery and ischaemia from an overtight dressing over the attachment of the common calcaneal tendon to the calcaneus.

Rupture of the metacarpal superficial digital flexor tendon in the racing Greyhound

This is an injury to the tendon of either digit 5 of the left thoracic limb or digit 2 of the right thoracic limb as a result of increased load as the dog leans into the bends running in an anticlockwise direction. The dog presents with a mild forelimb lameness and a marked linear swelling over the palmar aspect of the metacarpus extending to the sesamoids of the MCP joint.

Conservative management rapidly resolves the lameness but leaves a palpable fibrous band. Some dogs continue to feel discomfort when racing and surgical removal of the fibrous mass is indicated. This procedure is often done at initial presentation and results in a successful return to racing (Prole, 1971).

A linear incision is made over the enlarged tendon and careful dissection frees it from the surrounding tissues allowing excision. A tourniquet around the distal antebrachium is useful. A postoperative dressing is applied for 5 days with the dog returning to work after 3 weeks. Removal of this tendon does not affect the posture of the digit as this is maintained by the interosseous muscles through the two sesamoid bones that have ligamentous insertions on the proximal palmar aspect of the first phalanx.

Conditions of the digital pads and integument of the paw

A number of conditions of traumatic, infectious, multifactorial or unknown aetiology may specifically affect the pads and skin of the distal limb and cause lameness (Figure 21.17). Some of these conditions are dermatological in nature but are included here as the main presenting sign may be lameness.

• Fracture of the second or third phalanges
• Fracture of the ungual process
• Nail bed injuries
• Symmetrical lupoid onychodystrophy
• Bacterial infective arthritis
• Osteomyelitis of the third phalanx
• Joint sprain with or without subluxation
• Neoplasia
• Osteoarthritis
• Dermatological conditions

21.17 Differential diagnosis of a swollen distal digit.

Hyperplastic pads

Abnormal weight-bearing on digital pads can result in hyperkeratosis or hyperplasia. Hyperkeratosis also arises when the pad is not subjected to wear, but this in itself is unlikely to cause lameness. However, excessive wear may occur on the opposite margin of the pad, and if weight-bearing occurs on the adjacent skin, this may become hyperplastic and appear as an extension of the normal pad tissue (Figure 21.18). This can result in pedal dermatitis (Figure 21.19) or a concussive lameness with digital pressure across this tissue resented. Hyperplasia is over-represented in the fifth digital pad.

Hyperkeratosis and hyperplasia can cause a secondary bacterial or yeast dermatitis that results from the creation of excessive skin folds; careful examination of the foot will show these abnormalities. Medical treatment is often prolonged and unrewarding, with common recurrence. The aim of surgical treatments is to eliminate any skin folds together with the hyperplastic skin or pad. Surgical excision of diseased tissue can be combined with a separation podoplasty procedure that permanently splits the interdigital skin (webbing) allowing the digits to spread, thus preventing the formation of skin pockets (see Operative Technique 21.5).

Hyperplastic areas of the pad can be treated by excisional separation podoplasty to remove the excess pad

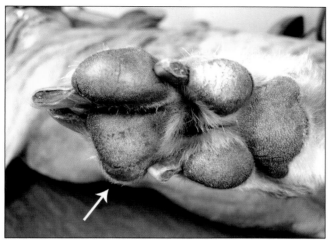

21.18 A hyperplastic digital pad (arrowed) that has developed from abnormal weight-bearing on the distal digit.

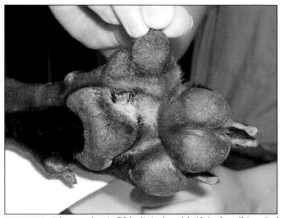

21.19 A hyperplastic fifth digital pad (a 'false' pad) in a Dobermann with skin fold pedal dermatitis. Resection of the hyperplastic pad combined with incisional separation podoplasty of the adjacent interdigital webbing resolved the lameness.

tissue, leaving a normal-sized digital pad. This should alter the weight-bearing area of the pad and prevent recurrence. Suturing the palmar/plantar skin to the pad will result in healing by secondary intention which can take up to 6 weeks. The dog will be lame until healing is complete.

Conjoined pads

This is a congenital condition in which two or more digital pads are joined together with no interposing interdigital skin. It can result in hyperplasia of the pad/skin margins and can be treated by separation of the pads by an incisional separation podoplasty; this also removes secondary skin folds.

Corns

A corn is a circumscribed area of hyperkeratitis on the digital pad (Figure 21.20). It is found almost exclusively in sight hounds and can cause a profound lameness that is worse on hard ground.

Diagnosis is by visual examination of the pad, dorsopalmar/plantar digital pressure producing a pain response and mediolateral digital palpation detecting a thickening of

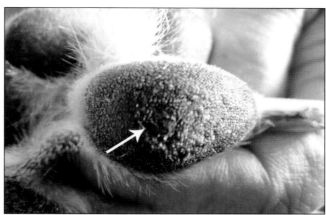

21.20 A corn (arrowed) on the digital pad of a Greyhound. This is a circumscribed area of hyperkeratosis that protrudes above the surface of the pad.

the pad. Some corns have an exuberance of hard cornified tissue while others are confluent with the pad. There can be a central dark area from bruising, giving the appearance of a foreign body puncture wound. The majority of corns occur in the pads of digits 3 and 4 in the thoracic limbs. A mediolateral radiographic view of the pad will eliminate radiopaque foreign bodies.

There is much speculation as to the cause, but evidence suggests a mechanical cause as seen in humans with tight-fitting shoes or hammer toes. In one survey 40% of cases had concomitant anatomical deformity, the most common being an elongation of the deep digital flexor tendon causing elevation of the nail during full limb extension (Guilliard et al., 2010). A penetrating wound of the pad has been suggested as a contributing cause but the author has never found a foreign body or observed corn formation as a sequel to pad penetration. However, the histological appearance of the 'root' lined with epithelial cells is suggestive of a penetration (Figure 21.21). Several studies have discounted a viral aetiology (Balara et al., 2009).

Treatment can be conservative management with regular paring and the application of softening agents, or surgical. There are a number of techniques but the author prefers surgical excision (see Operative Technique 21.6). Whatever procedure is used, the chance of recurrence is high unless the underlying mechanical cause is addressed. In one survey, 75% of dogs were free of lameness after 1 year but by 5 years the recurrence rate was over 50% (Guilliard et al., 2010); surgical excision can be repeated.

Management of the persistently recurrent corn can be conservative using specialized boots, or by digital amputation usually at the MCP/MTP joint. Occasionally, distal digital ostectomy can be successful in preserving the pad by altering the weight-bearing area.

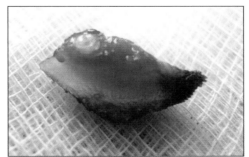

21.21 An excised corn showing thickened pad tissue and a cylindrical 'root' extending into the subdermis.

> When investigating lameness in sight hounds, always examine the feet before undertaking extensive radiographic studies of the entire limb

> Corns can be very painful and become a welfare issue. Consider digit amputation if other treatments fail

Foreign body in the paw pad

This is a common injury seen in first opinion practice. Digital pressure will isolate the affected pad and careful examination of the pad will show either an entry wound that usually exudes serum, or the blunt end of a thorn. Careful shaving of the superficial dermis with a scalpel blade detects thorns and superficial foreign bodies. Wound margins can be prised apart but indiscriminate digging into the wound should be avoided.

A mediolateral radiographic view taken with the affected pad isolated by adhesive tape detects radiopaque foreign bodies such as grit and glass (Figure 21.22)

If no foreign body is detected then the assumption is that a penetrating wound has occured and a protective dressing is applied for 7 days to stop further foreign body penetration. Other imaging techniques, such as contrast fistulogram, or advanced imaging, such as CT or contrast CT, can also be very helpful to investigate pad foreign bodies. If lameness persists, the tract can also be surgically excised or explored and while this may detect a foreign body, it can also be unrewarding. If a foreign body is present then a linear proximodistal full thickness incision is made through the pad, the foreign body is removed and the pad sutured. If the foreign body cannot be found then thoroughly flushing with saline may dislodge and reveal it.

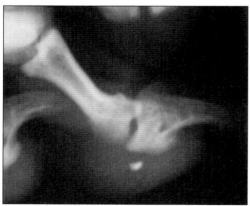

21.22 A mediolateral radiograph of a digital pad containing a glass foreign body.

> Some corns have soft centres that hold superficial grit particles (secondary penetration) as well as bruise marks

Nail conditions

Nails can crack, splinter, fracture or shell, exposing the corium. Loose fragments of nail are painful and require removal, usually under anaesthesia. The exposed corium rapidly granulates allowing nail regrowth. If the ungual process is fractured, then the distal fragment with the overlying nail should be removed. Nail clippers or bone cutters are suitable for this procedure. Haemorrhage can be controlled with a caustic pencil or potassium permanganate.

If the ungual process is fractured within the overlying skin, then ungual crest ostectomy should be considered.

Symmetrical lupoid onychodystrophy

This condition is characterized by some or all of the following nail disorders which usually affect most of the nails, although initially it may occur in a single nail (Auxilia *et al.*, 2001):

* Malformation of the nail
* Pain in a nail
* Separation of the nail from the underlying corium
* Sloughing of nails
* Spontaneous breaking or splitting of a nail
* Inflammation of the nail fold
* Pus in the nail fold.

Most dogs can be managed by the removal of loose nail fragments and appropriate antibiosis if pus is present. If this fails, more aggressive long-term medical therapy may be necessary (see the *BSAVA Manual of Canine and Feline Dermatology*). Ungual crest ostectomy can be performed on nails that are unresponsive to therapy.

Interdigital skin lesions

Lameness from interdigital dermatitis (pododermatitis, furunculosis, chronic fibrosing interdigital pyoderma and pedal folliculitis) in dogs is a multifaceted disease that is often recurrent and difficult to diagnose and treat (Duclos, 2013). Pockets of bacteria become entrapped in fibrous tissue that can be impenetrable to antibiotics. Medical management can be prolonged, expensive and often only palliative. Surgical excision in some cases can be curative (Figure 21.23).

A simple surgical excision technique may be adequate for small lesions, but where there is likely to be extensive skin loss, either a fusion or a separation podoplasty procedure can be used.

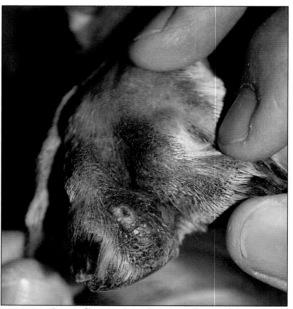

21.23 Chronic fibrosing interdigital pyoderma after antibiotic treatment but prior to excisional separation podoplasty.

Interdigital foreign bodies

Foreign bodies in the interdigital skin, such as grass awns and thorns, can be surgically removed by an incision through the dorsal skin over the suspected area. Advanced imaging such as CT can be very helpful in identifying and precisely localizing the foreign body, facilitating accurate removal. The presenting signs can mimic other conditions such as chronic fibrosing interdigital pyoderma; for these, excisional separation podoplasty should be considered.

Webbing injuries

The interdigital webbing is the skin separating and in between the digits. In the racing Greyhound two conditions are seen:

Split web

This is a split in the cranial edge of the web that can extend to the metacarpal/metatarsal pad. The split will rapidly heal by secondary intention but will almost invariably open again on exercise. Careful reconstruction can be successful but the author's preference is incisional separation podoplasty (see Operative Technique 21.5).

Split foot

A split foot occurs exclusively in the pelvic limbs and is a full thickness split of the plantar skin overlying the digital flexor tendons (Figure 21.24). A precursor is a sand burn where there is a partial abrasion of the dermis. The webbing over the third digit of the right pelvic limb is over-represented. The aetiology is thought to be sand abrasion of the taut skin over the flexor tendons.

Suturing or healing by secondary intention results in rapid healing, however, the split will recur every time the dog races on sand. Treatment is by incisional separation podoplasty of the abaxial webbing; this decreases the tautness of the skin over the tendons. It is important to extend the incision to the metatarsal pad. The incisional margins and the original split are sutured. This is successful in the majority of cases. If the split recurs, the webbing between digits 3 and 4 should be excised; this is usually successful.

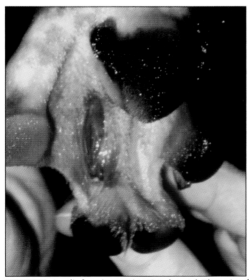

21.24 A split foot in a racing Greyhound. There is a full thickness split of the dermis overlying the flexor tendons to digit 3 or digit 4 in the pelvic limb paw.

Fusion podoplasty

This procedure is described for the treatment of chronic fibrosing interdigital pyoderma and other pedal conditions in the dog and cat (Swaim *et al.*, 1991; Papazoglou *et al.*, 2011). It involves removal of affected tissues of the paw and fusing together one or more digits by suturing together the dorsal and palmar/plantar skin incision. This in effect unites the digital paw pads. If not correctly performed, complications include abnormal pad wear and dermal clefts with persistent ongoing dermatitis.

> The author does not recommend this procedure as separation podoplasty is simpler and has far fewer complications

Separation podoplasty

Separation podoplasty can be incisional or excisional (see Operative Technique 21.5). It involves cutting back the interdigital skin (webbing) from its cranial border to the metacarpal or metatarsal pad. The dorsal skin is then sutured to the palmar/plantar skin to form a permanent 'V' (Figure 21.25).

This is a common procedure in the racing Greyhound and does not increase the incidence of fractures or subluxations in the adjacent digits (Guilliard, 2012). If necessary more than one interdigital web can be incised.

Using this technique it is possible to create a sliding skin graft to cover a dorsal digital skin deficit. Interdigital lesions can be excised leaving sufficient peripheral skin for closure over adjacent digits.

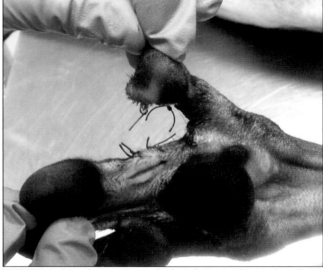

21.25 Incisional separation podoplasty being used to treat a split foot in a racing Greyhound.

Infection of the paw

Infections involving the soft tissues of the paw are common as a result of penetrating wounds, foreign bodies, dermatological disease and as a complication of surgical intervention. In addition, dogs may present lame as a result of bacterial infections deep within the bone or joints of the paw.

Bacterial (septic) arthritis

Bacterial joint infection can occur in any of the joints of the digits; usually this originates from haematogenous bacteraemia. It is most commonly found in the distal interphalangeal joint; the patient presents with lameness and joint swelling/effusion. Usually there are no signs of external penetration. A tentative diagnosis is made from the finding of high numbers of polymorphonuclear leucocytes in aspirated joint fluid. Due to the low volume of joint fluid aspirated, there is rarely sufficient quantity to attempt culture.

A 4-week course of an appropriate antibiotic usually results in a rapid reduction of clinical signs and carries a good long-term prognosis.

Osteomyelitis of the third phalanx

This presents as a very swollen, painful distal digit, often with an exudate from the nail bed, and can be a sequel to nail bed trauma such as fracture of the ungual process. Radiography is generally unhelpful in the diagnosis.

Treatment can be by distal digital ostectomy, or preferably by ungual crest ostectomy removing all the soft necrotic bone. A 3-week course of the appropriate antibiotic is prescribed which usually equates to continuation for 2 weeks after the clinical signs have abated. Note that antibiotic therapy alone is not curative.

Other conditions of the distal limb

Neoplasia

Squamous cell carcinoma and malignant melanoma are the most common tumours affecting the distal digits in the dog. Diagnosis is by biopsy; palliative or curative treatment is by amputation of the digit but initially the tumour needs to be staged (for further details, see the *BSAVA Manual of Canine and Feline Oncology*).

In the cat, metastasis from a primary pulmonary carcinoma is the most common tumour found in the digits; cases present with lameness and not pulmonary signs. The prognosis is very guarded; this emphasizes the importance of thoracic radiography in such cases. Squamous cell carcinoma is the second most common digital tumour in cats (Gottfried *et al.*, 2000).

Papilloma virus (warts)

These can be found on the palmar/plantar skin. They appear as cauliflower-like growths of keratin and, if the cause of lameness, are surrounded by oedematous skin; surgical excision is curative. Very rarely are they found on the pads.

Histiocytoma

Occasionally, this benign self-limiting tumour is found on the foot, resulting in lameness. Surgical excision can be undertaken but natural regression occurs in about 2 months. It is common in the Greyhound.

Musladin–Leuke syndrome (Chinese Beagle syndrome)

Musladin–Leuke syndrome is a genetic disease in Beagles that affects the development and structure of connective tissue and is found in multiple body systems. Typically, puppies have slant narrowed eyes and very tight skin with little scruff. They tend to be small in stature and have a stiff ballerina-type gait (Figure 21.26).

On examination, it is not possible to extend the MCP/MTP joints. The gait deformity stabilizes at maturity and some dogs cope well. A genetic test is available. Note that flexor tendinotomy does not improve the stature.

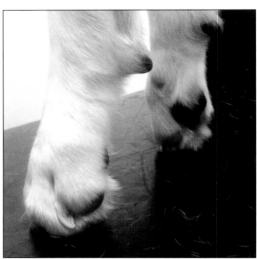

21.26 Musladin–Leuke syndrome in a Beagle. Note the ballerina-type stance.

Hypertrophic osteopathy (Marie's Disease)

Pallisading periosteal new bone develops on the bones of the distal limb and can result in lameness and swollen metacarpal/metatarsal bones and digits. The cause is related to a space-occupying lesion in the thorax or, occasionally, the abdomen (see Chapter 7).

References and further reading

Auxilia ST, Hill PB and Thoday KL (2001) Canine symmetrical lupoid onchodystrophy: a retrospective study with particular reference to management. *Journal of Small Animal Practice* **42**, 82–87

Balara JM, McArthy RJ, Kiupel M *et al.* (2009) Clinical, histologic, and immunohistochemical characterization of wart-like lesions on the paw pads of dogs: 24 cases (2000–2007). *Journal of Animal Veterinary Medicine* **274**, 1555–1558

de Rooster H, Risselada M and van Bree H (2007) Excision arthroplasty of the interphalangeal joint as an alternative to digit amputation in two dogs. *Journal of Small Animal Practice* **48**, 169–173

Dobson J and Lascelles D (2011) *BSAVA Manual of Canine and Feline Oncology, 3rd edn.* BSAVA Publications, Gloucester

Duclos D (2013) Canine pododermatitis. *Veterinary Clinics of North America: Small Animal Practice* **43**, 57–87

Franklin SP, Park RD and Egger EL (2009) Metacarpophalangeal and metatarsophalangeal Osteoarthritis in 49 dogs. *Journal of the American Animal Hospital Association* **45**, 112–117

Gemmill T and Clements D (2016) *BSAVA Manual of Canine and Feline Fracture Repair and Management, 2nd edn.* BSAVA Publications, Gloucester

Gottfried SD, Popovitch CA, Goldschmidt MH and Schelling C (2000) Metastatic digital carcinoma in the cat: a retrospective study of 36 cats (1992–1998). *Journal of the American Animal Hospital Association* **36**, 501–509

Guilliard MJ (2003) Proximal interphalangeal joint instability in the dog. *Journal of Small Animal Practice* **44**, 399–403

Guilliard MJ (2012) *The nature, incidence and response to treatment of injuries to the distal limbs in the racing greyhound.* Royal College of Veterinary Surgeons Diploma of Fellowship by Thesis, London

Guilliard MJ, Sedboerg I and Shearer DH (2010) Corns in dogs; signalment, possible aetiology and response to treatment. *Journal of Small Animal Practice* **51**, 162–168

Jackson H and Marsella R (2012) *BSAVA Manual of Canine and Feline Dermatology, 3rd edn.* BSAVA Publications, Gloucester

Kaufman KL and Mann FA (2013) Short- and long-term outcomes after digit amputation in dogs: 33 cases (1999–2011). *Journal of the American Veterinary Medical Association* **242**, 1249–1254

Ober CP and Freeman LE (2009) Computed tomographic, magnetic resonance imaging, and cross-sectional anatomic features of the manus in cadavers of dogs without forelimb disease. *American Journal of Veterinary Research* **70**, 1450–1458

Ober CP, Jones JC, Larson MM *et al.* (2008) Comparison of ultrasound, computed tomography, and magnetic resonance imaging in detection of acute wooden foreign bodies in the canine manus. *Veterinary Radiology and Ultrasound* **49**, 411–418

Papazoglou LG, Ellison GW, Farese JP *et al.* (2011) Fusion podoplasty for the management of chronic pedal conditions in seven dogs and one cat. *Journal of the American Animal Hospital Association* **47**, 199–205

Prole JHB (1971) Superficial flexor tendon injuries in the greyhound. *Veterinary Record* **89**, 437–438

Robins GM and Read RA (1998) Diseases of the sesamoid bones. In: *Canine Sports Medicine and Surgery*, ed. MS Bloomberg, JF Dee and RA Taylor, pp. 255–264. WB Saunders Company, Philadelphia

Rochat MC and Mann FA (1998) Metatarsophalangeal arthodesis in three dogs. *Journal of the American Veterinary Medical Association* **34**, 158–163

Swaim SF, Lee AH, MacDonald JM *et al.* (1991) Fusion podoplasty for the treatment of chronic fibrosing interdigital pyoderma in the dog. *Journal of the American Hospital Association* **27**, 264–274

Woo SL-Y, An K-N, Arnoczky SP *et al.* (1994) Anatomy, biology and biomechanics of tendon, ligament and meniscus. In: *Orthopaedics Basic Science*, ed. SS Simon, pp. 45–88. American Academy of Orthopaedic Surgeons, Philadelphia

IMAGING TECHNIQUES

Thomas W. Maddox

The distal limb can be difficult to image satisfactorily, as the structures involved are small and the changes seen may be subtle. Bony lesions are well characterized on radiographs, particularly if high detail systems are used. Similarly, CT is also useful. Although the spatial resolution is lower than radiography, its cross-sectional nature is advantageous and the use of contrast media can provide increased soft tissue contrast.

RADIOGRAPHY

Standard views

The standard views of the manus and pes are the mediolateral and dorsopalmar/plantarodorsal views.

Mediolateral view

The digits and metacarpals/metatarsals are largely superimposed on this view.

- The patient is placed in lateral recumbency with the target limb dependent against the cassette/plate and the contralateral limb retracted (Figure 21.27).
- The carpus/tarsus should be in a neutral to mildly extended position.
- The primary beam is centred on the distal metacarpals/metatarsals.
- Collimate to include the digits and carpus/tarsus.

21.27 Patient positioning for a mediolateral view of the manus.

Dorsopalmar/plantarodorsal views

These views afford the best images of the digits and there is no bony super-imposition (except for the sesamoids).

- The patient is placed in sternal recumbency with the target limb extended. Radiographic positioning aids can be placed under the contralateral limb to rotate the body slightly to the side of interest (Figures 21.28 and 21.29). The primary beam is centred on the distal metacarpals/metatarsals.
- Collimate to include the digits and carpus/tarsus.

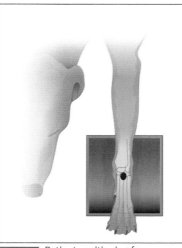

21.28 Patient positioning for a dorsopalmar view of the manus.

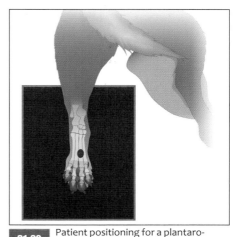

21.29 Patient positioning for a plantaro-dorsal view of the pes. Note the use of wedges or sandbags to elevate the contralateral limb to facilitate positioning.

→ **IMAGING TECHNIQUES CONTINUED**

Special views

Splayed toe mediolateral view

The splayed digit view is the only special view routinely acquired. This view separates out the digits well if performed correctly, but the metacarpals/metatarsals are still largely superimposed (except distally).

- The patient is positioned as for the mediolateral view.
- Tape is applied to at least the most medial and most lateral digits, which are then pulled in a dorsal and palmar/plantar direction (Figure 21.30).
- Collimation and centring is as for the standard mediolateral view.

COMPUTED TOMOGRAPHY

CT can be useful to characterize subtle changes not readily apparent on radiographs (such as mild periosteal reaction associated with a foreign body, fragmentation of the palmar metatarsophalangeal (MTP) sesamoids or osteophyte/ethesophyte formation of the MTP joints), or to better define previously identified pathology (Figure 21.31). Some soft tissue structures can be seen, but the small amount of fat present in the distal limb means that there is little natural contrast. The use of systemic or intravenous contrast medium will increase the visible soft tissue contrast.

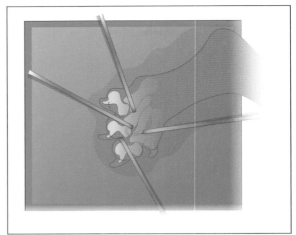

21.30 Patient positioning for a splayed toe mediolateral view of the digits; note the use of tape to separate the toes.

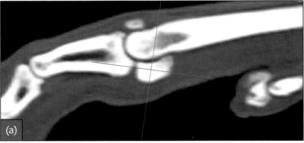
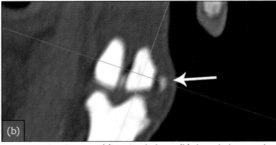
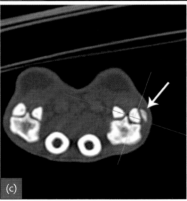

21.31 Multiplanar CT reconstruction images: (a) sagittal plane, (b) dorsal plane and (c) transverse plane. These reconstructions show a medial sagittal fracture of (medial) palmar sesamoid 1 of the MCP/MTP joint of digit 2 (arrowed). This 5-year-old Labrador Retriever had exercise-induced acute onset thoracic limb lameness clinically localized to this joint, but radiographs were inconclusive.
(Courtesy of Gordon Brown)

Standard technique

- The patient is positioned as for views of the carpus (manus) or tarsus (pes).
- The scan margins should extend from the carpus/tarsus to the distal extent of the digits.
- The small size of the regions of interest means that separate images of both distal limbs are reconstructed with as small a field of view as feasible.
- Reconstruction using bone and soft tissue algorithms is advisable (particularly the latter if contrast medium is administered).

→ **IMAGING TECHNIQUES CONTINUED**

Systemic contrast studies

The use of intravenous contrast agents can allow identification of regions of soft tissue inflammation and increase the conspicuity of changes associated with foreign bodies.

* A plain study of the region is acquired first.
* Approximately 600 mg/kg iodine of a non-ionic, lower osmolar contrast agent is rapidly administered (via the saphenous vein if the manus is being imaged, and via the cephalic vein for the pes).
* Images of the region are acquired after a short delay (typically 20–40 seconds).

MAGNETIC RESONANCE

MRI imaging offers some of the advantages of CT in imaging the distal limb, although the low contrast between tendon and cortical bone can cause problems, and sesamoid bones may not be distinguishable from the tendons that contain them (Ober and Freeman, 2009). Additionally, the small size of the distal limb can result in images of relatively low signal or require a compensatory decrease in spatial resolution or increase in scan acquisition times.

ULTRASONOGRAPHY

Ultrasonography is infrequently used for imaging of the distal limb, but can be useful in the identification of foreign material (Ober *et al.*, 2008).

OPERATIVE TECHNIQUE 21.1

The application of a digital external skeletal fixator

POSITIONING

* Thoracic limb digits: sternal recumbency with the limb extended cranially.
* Pelvic limb digits: dorsal recumbency with the limb extended caudally.

ASSISTANT

Not necessary.

EQUIPMENT EXTRAS

Orthopaedic drill; 1.4 mm and 1.6 mm arthrodesis wire; parallel action pliers; pin cutters; acrylic putty.

SURGICAL TECHNIQUE

Proximal interphalangeal joint instability

Two pins are inserted into the first phalanx, ideally at the proximal and distal ends of the diaphysis, and two pins are similarly placed into the second phalanx (Figure 21.32). For medium to large-breed dogs, 1.4 mm is an appropriate pin size.

The skin is tensioned and the pin inserted with a low speed, high torque drill. Pre-drilling is not necessary. The operator should feel the penetration of the medullary cavity and the exit from the far cortex. The point of the exited pin should just be palpable. The angle of insertion is 10 to 20 degrees from the sagittal plane to avoid the digital tendons and the pins are placed on the abaxial aspect of the digit. Using pliers, the pins are bent at right-angles about 1 cm from the skin to overlie each other. The putty is applied and moulded around the pins (Figure 21.33).

> Ensure normal joint congruity as the putty hardens

→ **OPERATIVE TECHNIQUE 21.1 CONTINUED**

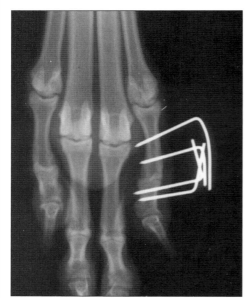

21.32 A dorsoplantar radiograph of a pelvic limb paw of a Greyhound with a transarticular external skeletal fixator placed for treatment of PIP joint instability. The acrylic putty was applied after the joint was aligned.

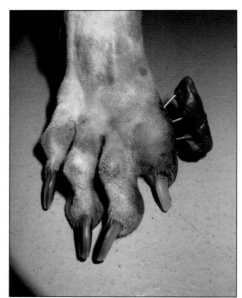

21.33 A transarticular external skeletal fixator *in situ*. It is important that the acrylic putty is not too close to the skin.

MCP/MTP joint instability

Two pins are inserted in the first phalanx and two or three pins in the metacarpal/metatarsal bone; 1.6 mm is an appropriate pin size for the latter.

> **WARNING**
>
> The proximal metacarpal/metatarsal pin should be inserted at the proximal end of the diaphysis, otherwise it can produce a stress riser leading to fracture

POSTOPERATIVE CARE

Postoperative dressings are not necessary even when a concomitant ungual crest ostectomy is performed. An Elizabethan collar or muzzle should be considered. The dog should be exercised on the lead and not taken over ground that might snag the fixator.

The frame is usually removed 3 weeks after application, with exercise restricted for a further 4 weeks. Premature frame removal due to complications can still result in a successful outcome.

COMPLICATIONS

These are very common; the frequency increases with time elapsed postoperatively and include:

- Pin tract exudation and infection
- Pin loosening
- Osteomyelitis
- Pin impingement from over insertion
- Acrylic impingement on adjacent tissues
- Dog biting and removing the frame.

When necessary, antibiotics may be used to control complications related to pin tract infection, although most of these are relatively minor and quickly resolve following frame removal.

OPERATIVE TECHNIQUE 21.2

Amputation of the digit

POSITIONING

- Thoracic limb digit: sternal recumbency with the limb extended cranially.
- Pelvic limb digit: dorsal recumbency with the limb extended caudally.

ASSISTANT

Useful.

EQUIPMENT EXTRAS

Bone cutters or small oscillating saw.

SURGICAL TECHNIQUE

Amputation through the distal metacarpal/metatarsal bone of digits 2 or 5

A sterile elastic dressing is applied from the paw to either the distal antebrachium or distal tibia to act as a tourniquet (see Chapter 13). The skin incision is made from the distal metacarpal/metatarsal bone to run dorso-abaxially over the joint. One incision runs over the first phalanx through the dorsal skin of the webbing up to its cranial margin. A second incision is made from the bifurcation at the joint to run over the palmar/plantar skin over the first phalanx and through the skin of the webbing to join the first incision (Figure 21.34).

The dorsal aspect of the MCP/MTP joint is exposed and incised allowing the joint to be disarticulated and the entire digit to be excised. The distal end of the metacarpal/metatarsal bone is dissected free of soft tissue and the condyles removed with an oblique cut using bone cutters or a small oscillating saw (Figure 21.35). The sesamoid bones and exposed flexor tendons are then excised.

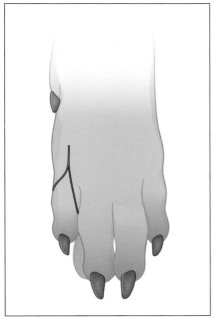

21.34 Illustration showing the dorsal skin incisions for amputation of an abaxial digit 2 or 5.

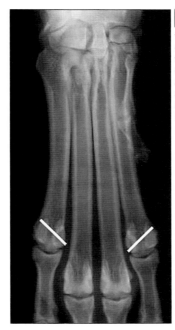

21.35 A dorsopalmar radiograph of the metacarpus. The diagonal white lines show the positions of the osteotomies for amputation of digits 2 and 5. Digits 3 and 4 are amputated through the MCP/MTP joints.

Closure

The tourniquet is released, bleeding vessels tied off and the soft tissues are closed over the excision site with a continuous suture of polyglycolic acid followed by intradermal sutures.

→ **OPERATIVE TECHNIQUE 21.2 CONTINUED**

Amputation through the MCP/MTP joint of digits 3 or 4

After the application of the tourniquet, a skin incision is made over the dorsal aspect of the distal metacarpal/metatarsal bone, continuing over the joint and then bifurcating to incise both the dorsal and palmar/plantar skin of the webbing on either side of the digit. The joint is incised on its dorsal aspect and disarticulated allowing the digit to be excised. The sesamoids are left *in situ* and the articular cartilage is not removed.

Closure

After the release of the tourniquet, the bleeding vessels are tied off. The dorsal incision is sutured and the soft tissues are sutured and apposed over the excision site.

POSTOPERATIVE CARE

A light dressing is applied for 5 days. Exercise is restricted until healing is complete. Postoperative morbidity is mild for amputation involving digits 2 and 5, but for amputation through the joint of digits 3 and 4, lameness can be expected for several weeks; therefore, care and caution should be taken in making the decision to amputate as these central two digits are the main weight-bearing digits of the pes (Kaufman and Mann, 2013).

OPERATIVE TECHNIQUE 21.3

Ungual crest ostectomy (permanent nail removal)

POSITIONING

Lateral recumbency.

ASSISTANT

Useful for positioning and haemostasis.

EQUIPMENT EXTRAS

Bone cutters and rongeurs.

SURGICAL TECHNIQUE

The assistant holds the distal digit firmly between forefinger and thumb just proximal to the digital pad. The skin and digital pad are incised about 3 mm proximal to the nail (Figure 21.36). Careful dissection of the subcutaneous tissues will reveal the dorsal joint capsule of the distal interphalangeal joint and the nail bed. Bone cutters are used to remove the nail and ungual process (Figure 21.37). The excision should be made approximately 2 mm distal to the distal interphalangeal joint.

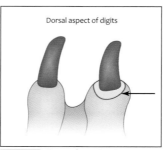

Dorsal aspect of digits

21.36 Ungual crest ostectomy showing the skin incision circumscribing the nail (arrowed).

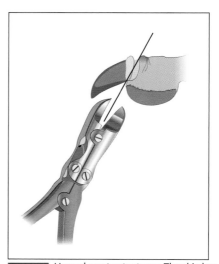

21.37 Ungual crest ostectomy. The skin has been retracted from the ungual process allowing its removal with bone cutters.

→ **OPERATIVE TECHNIQUE 21.3 CONTINUED**

Using rongeurs, all of the nail bed and remaining ungual process and crest have to be removed (Figure 21.38). This will destroy the attachments of the digital extensor tendon and the dorsal elastic ligament. Entering the joint should be avoided but removal of a small amount of the dorsal articular bone usually has no clinical consequence. At this point the skin margins should easily cover the exposed bone. Skin tension implies insufficient bone removal. Bleeding is usually minimal.

Closure

Only the skin requires suturing with three or four simple sutures of monofilament nylon.

POSTOPERATIVE CARE

A light protective dressing for 3 days.

> If remnants of the germinal layer of the nail remain then regrowth recurs and can lead to osteomyelitis of the third phalanx. Aggressive removal is necessary

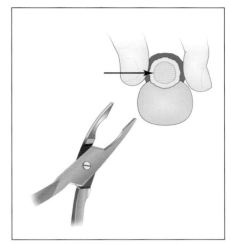

21.38 Ungual crest ostectomy. The remnants of the nail and ungual crest are removed with rongeurs.

OPERATIVE TECHNIQUE 21.4

Distal digit (phalanx 3) ostectomy

POSITIONING

Lateral recumbency.

ASSISTANT

Necessary for positioning and haemostasis.

EQUIPMENT EXTRAS

Bone cutters and rongeurs.

SURGICAL TECHNIQUE

The assistant holds the distal digit firmly between forefinger and thumb just proximal to the digital pad. The skin and digital pad are incised about 3 mm proximal to the nail (see Figure 21.36). Careful dissection of the subcutaneous tissues will reveal the dorsal joint capsule of the distal interphalangeal joint. Sharp dissection of the joint capsule will enable the joint to be entered and opened by nail flexion. From within the joint, the lateral collateral ligaments and joint capsule are severed revealing the deep digital flexor tendon attached to the flexor process of the third phalanx (P3). The tendon is cut and P3, together with the nail, is dissected free of any attachments and discarded. The deep digital flexor tendon is trimmed. The digital pad must be preserved.

The distal condyles of the second phalanx (P2) are exposed and removed with bone cutters to allow better pad positioning. Rongeurs are used to remove any sharp bone fragments. The incision is closed with simple non-absorbable sutures placed through the pad and skin.

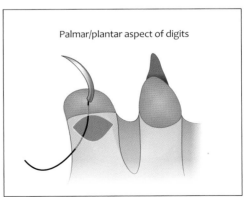

Palmar/plantar aspect of digits

21.39 Distal digital ostectomy. An eliptical area of skin is excised proximal/dorsal to the digital pad. The defect is closed using simple interrupted sutures so that the pad is pulled over the bone stump. →

→ **OPERATIVE TECHNIQUE 21.4 CONTINUED**

This rotates the pad dorsally.

An elliptical area of palmar/plantar skin is excised just proximal/dorsal to the digital pad. Suturing the pad to the skin margin 'walks' the pad over the bone stump of P2 (Figure 21.39). The pad should now have little mobility over the stump. If there is excessive mobility, then further skin excision may be necessary. It is important that the bone stump is completely covered by the pad to prevent future concussive injuries.

POSTOPERATIVE CARE

A light protective dressing for 7 days. Restricted exercise for 4 weeks.

> In sight hounds a corn can develop in the pad if it is not correctly positioned

---

OPERATIVE TECHNIQUE 21.5

Incisional and excisional separation podoplasty

POSITIONING

The dog is positioned in lateral, ventral or dorsal recumbency dependent on the perceived access to the webbing and lesion.

ASSISTANT

Very useful.

EQUIPMENT EXTRAS

None.

SURGICAL TECHNIQUE

The assistant holds apart the nails of the digits either side of the affected web. If the lesion requires excision this is performed by careful dissection, preserving as much adjacent skin as possible. The interdigital webbing is incised through both the dorsal and palmar/plantar skin from the cranial border to the metacarpal/metatarsal pad (Figure 21.40). The positioning of the incision can be crafted to create addition skin to cover a defect as a sliding graft or as a means of relieving tension.

Closure

Closure is by suturing the dorsal skin to the palmar/plantar skin to form a permanent 'V'. Simple sutures are used with the first placed at the caudal extremity of the incision by the pad. The author's preferred suture material is polyglactin 910 (see Figure 21.25).

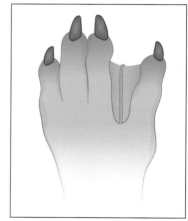

21.40 Incisional separation podoplasty. Illustration showing the position of the incision.

POSTERATIVE CARE

For simple incisional podoplasty, a light dressing is applied for 5 days. Excisional podoplasty where partial pad removal has also been carried out may need dressing for longer periods, with frequent changes. Sutures can be removed from 10 days onwards or may be left to be absorbed.

> As it is not possible to suture skin to pad without leaving some exposed pad tissue, healing of this exposed pad tissue is by second intention and areas of granulation tissue are common. This can be painful until epithelialization is complete. Suture removal may require sedation

OPERATIVE TECHNIQUE 21.6

Corn excision

POSITIONING

Lateral recumbency with the affected pad uppermost.

ASSISTANT

Essential.

EQUIPMENT EXTRAS

None.

SURGICAL TECHNIQUE

Haemostasis is achieved by the assistant holding the digit between thumb and forefinger on the caudal margins of the pad. A full thickness, proximal to distal incision of the pad is made around the axial and abaxial aspects of the corn. This allows the 'root' of the corn to be gently freed from the subcutaneous fibro-adipose tissues.

Closure

The wound is closed with several sutures of 2.0 metric (3/0 USP) polyglactin 910 with the sutures placed well away from the margins of the wound (Figure 21.41).

POSTOPERATIVE CARE

A protective dressing is applied to the foot and changed at weekly intervals for a total of 3 weeks.

> It is very important that the dressing is kept dry

   The sutures wear through once the dressing has been removed. Lameness should resolve in about 6 weeks when the scar tissue has grown out.

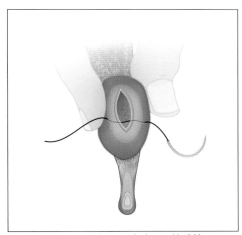

21.41 Corn excision. With the pad held between the thumb and forefinger by an assistant, the corn is excised and the wound closed with simple interrupted sutures.

OPERATIVE TECHNIQUE 21.7

Sesamoidectomy

POSITIONING

- Thoracic limb – the dog is positioned in dorsal recumbency.
- Pelvic limb – the dog is positioned in dorsal or sternal recumbency depending on surgeon preference.

ASSISTANT

Useful.

EQUIPMENT EXTRAS

None.

SURGICAL TECHNIQUE

A surgical approach is made over the affected sesamoid bone with a longitudinal skin incision running abaxially to the metacarpal/metatarsal pad. The annular ligament is transected and the underlying digital flexor tendons are displaced to expose the palmar/plantar aspect of the sesamoid (Figure 21.42). The fragment or the entire bone can then be dissected from the interosseous tendon proximally and the sesamoidean ligaments.

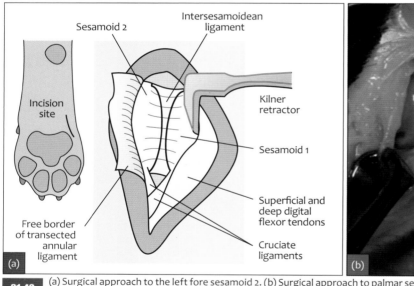
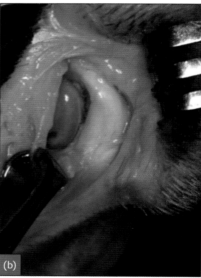

21.42 (a) Surgical approach to the left fore sesamoid 2. (b) Surgical approach to palmar sesamoid 7.
(b, Courtesy of JEF Houlton)

Closure

Closure of the subcutaneous tissues is with a synthetic suture material. Skin closure is routine.

POSTOPERATIVE CARE

The foot should be bandaged for 10 days to protect the wound.

Chapter 22

The hip

Toby J. Gemmill and Bill Oxley

Conditions affecting the hip, or coxofemoral joint, are common in small animal practice, especially in younger animals where a variety of developmental conditions can be encountered. In older patients, degenerative osteoarthritis of the hip is also common; other conditions such as neoplasia affecting the hip are seen less frequently. Many diseases affecting the hip joints are extremely debilitating, and successful treatment can be very rewarding for the veterinary surgeon, owner and the patient.

Clinical anatomy

The hip is a diarthrodial ball and socket joint, the spherical head of the femur being accommodated by the concave acetabulum. Although the contours of the articular surfaces of the acetabulum and the femoral head are closely matched, subtle physiological incongruence has been identified, the radius of curvature of the acetabulum being slightly smaller than that of the femoral head. During loading of the hip, the bone and cartilage of the acetabulum deform slightly, making the articular surfaces more congruent; this mechanism optimizes cartilage loading during weight-bearing (Greenwald and Connor, 1971).

The acetabulum is covered by articular hyaline cartilage on its cranial, dorsal and caudal surfaces; collectively these load-bearing regions are known as the lunate surface (Figure 22.1). The non-load-bearing acetabular fossa, situated ventromedially, is the origin of the ligament of the femoral head, also known as the round or teres ligament.

Ventrally, the acetabular fossa is bordered by the transverse acetabular ligament, which extends between the cranioventral and caudoventral poles of the acetabulum. The acetabulum does not face perfectly laterally, but instead is angled slightly caudally, or retroverted; this corresponds to the orientation of the femoral neck, which is anteverted by around 20 degrees in the normal dog (Figure 22.2). The neck of the femur is inclined with respect to the femoral diaphysis by about 140 degrees.

The hip is a highly constrained and inherently stable joint. Primary stabilizers of the hip include the ligament of the femoral head and the sock-like joint capsule; secondary stabilizers include the fibrocartilagenous dorsal extension of the acetabular margin known as the acetabular labrum, and the regional muscles inserting around the hip including the gluteals, iliopsoas, gemelli, internal and external obturators, and the rectus femoris.

The main blood supply to the femoral head and neck is derived from the proximal femoral circumflex vessels. These enter the femur via the metaphysis, and course proximally through the femoral neck. In mature animals, these vessels contribute to the vascularity of the femoral head. However, in immature animals these vessels do not

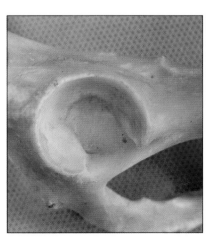

22.1 Cadaveric image of the acetabulum of a dog, showing the weight-bearing lunate surface and the ventromedially located acetabular fossa. The fossa is the origin of the ligament of the femoral head.

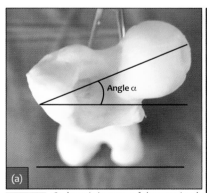
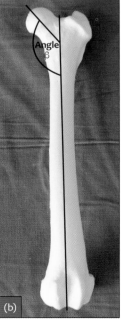

22.2 Cadaveric images of the proximal femur of a dog. (a) The neck is anteverted by around 15–20 degrees (angle α), which corresponds to the retroversion of the acetabulum. (b) The femoral neck is inclined with respect to the femoral diaphysis by about 140 degrees (angle β).

cross the proximal femoral physis; instead the femoral head is supplied entirely by capsular vessels inserting around the periphery of the epiphysis (Figure 22.3). Any vessels within the ligament of the femoral head do not provide a meaningful contribution in the dog, although may do so in the cat. The peripheral capsular vessels can be damaged during trauma or iatrogenically during surgery; in juvenile animals this can lead to avascular necrosis of the femoral head.

The sciatic nerve courses dorsal and caudal to the hip (Figure 22.4) and can be damaged during surgery; adequate precautions must be taken to identify and protect this nerve to avoid iatrogenic neural injury, especially when making an extensive dorsal approach to the hip.

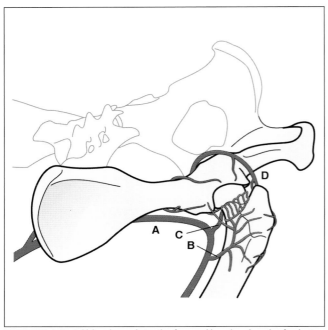

22.3 Arterial blood supply to the femoral head and neck of a dog, showing the femoral artery (A), lateral circumflex femoral artery (B), medial circumflex femoral artery (C), and caudal gluteal artery (D). Note the capsular vessels inserting around the periphery of the epiphysis which supply the femoral head in the juvenile animal.
(Reproduced from the *BSAVA Manual of Small Animal Fracture Repair and Management*)

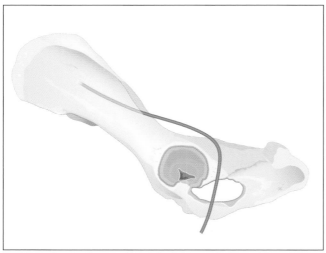

22.4 The sciatic nerve (green line) crosses the ilium at the sciatic notch and runs caudodorsal to the hip.

Clinical examination of the hip

The majority of clinically significant conditions affecting the hip will lead to discomfort and lameness. A loss of range of motion is also commonly encountered, especially with chronic conditions, and secondary muscle atrophy affecting the entire limb can develop. However lameness may not be obvious in all cases, especially when patients are affected bilaterally by conditions such as hip dysplasia. In such cases owners may complain that their pets have difficulty rising from rest, pelvic limb stiffness and exercise intolerance rather than overt lameness.

Initially, a careful assessment of the animal's gait should be performed by observing ambulation at different speeds from either side, from the front and from behind the patient. Unilateral lameness can often be confirmed; bilaterally affected animals may exhibit swaying of the hips or bunny-hopping when trotting. Pelvic limb muscle atrophy can be appreciated by careful palpation and comparison of left and right. In bilaterally affected cases, thoracic limb musculature may appear overdeveloped in comparison with relatively poorly muscled pelvic limbs.

If a condition affecting the hip is suspected, a thorough examination of all other joints should first be performed to exclude other conditions. The hips can then be examined in more detail. With the patient either standing or in lateral recumbency, each hip in turn can be manipulated through flexion, extension and abduction to assess range of motion, pain, and the presence of crepitus. The normal range of motion of the hip joint is approximately 160 degrees in flexion and extension, 90 degrees in abduction and adduction, and 90 degrees in internal and external rotation. Many animals with hip pathology exhibit pain on firm extension of the joint. However caution is required as hip extension can exacerbate caudal lumbar pain or discomfort associated with regional soft tissues such as the hip flexor muscles. Animals with genuine hip pain will usually exhibit pain on both extension and abduction of the hip; pain associated with the hip flexor muscles is usually apparent on hip extension but not abduction; animals with caudal lumbar pain will often tolerate abduction of the hip but exhibit discomfort on palpation of the affected region of the spine. A brief neurological examination should always be performed to exclude any neurological deficits, which would be more suggestive of a spinal condition or a peripheral nerve lesion.

The relative location of different bony landmarks should be assessed. Animals with severe hip dysplasia or dorsal luxation of the hip often have particularly prominent greater trochanters, which may be displaced dorsally (Figure 22.5). If only one hip is affected, dorsal displacement of the femur can also be appreciated by assessing the relative heights of the stifles during stance. If an animal has a ventral luxation of the hip it often possible to appreciate distal and medial translation of the greater trochanter, and distal displacement of the stifle.

The 'thumb displacement test' is a useful manoeuvre to detect dorsal luxation of the hip. In a normal hip, if the femur is internally and externally rotated the bone pivots around the femoral head, and the greater trochanter will move cranially and caudally. Therefore if the examiner's thumb is placed between the trochanter and the tuber ischium and the limb externally rotated, the thumb should be forced laterally as the space between the trochanter and the tuber ischium narrows. If the hip is dorsally luxated, external rotation of the femur leads to movement of the femoral head rather than the trochanter; a thumb placed between the trochanter and the tuber ischium is not displaced (Figure 22.6).

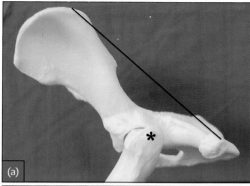

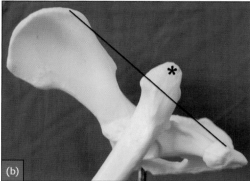

22.5 (a) The palpable greater trochanter (∗) in a normal dog is located ventral to an imaginary line between the wing of the ilium and the tuber ischium (black line). (b) If a dorsal luxation of the hip has occurred, the greater trochanter is located further dorsally.

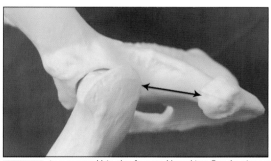

22.6 In a normal hip the femoral head is a fixed point; caudal rotation of the femur leads to narrowing of the gap between the greater trochanter and the tuber ischium (black arrow), which causes displacement of the examiner's thumb from the sciatic notch. If a dorsal luxation of the hip has occurred, caudal rotation of the femur leads to cranial movement of the unrestrained femoral head; the greater trochanter does not move caudally, and the examiner's thumb is not displaced.

Differential diagnoses for apparent pain affecting the hip joint

- Hip dysplasia
- Hip luxation (dorsal or ventral)
- Fractures of the femoral head, neck or acetabulum
- Avascular necrosis of the femoral head (ANFH, or Legg–Calvé–Perthes disease)
- Atraumatic slipped femoral capital epiphysis (SFCE)
- Neoplasia (bone or soft tissue)
- Osteoarthritis
- Inflammatory arthritis (infection or immune-mediated disease)
- Heterotopic osteochondrofibrosis
- Iliopsoas myopathy
- Caudal lumbar spinal conditions

Diagnostic investigations

Having localized a condition to the hip, further investigations should be performed. These may include:

- Examination under sedation or anaesthesia
- Radiography
- Advanced imaging using computed tomography (CT) or magnetic resonance imaging (MRI)
- Arthrocentesis
- Arthroscopy
- Biopsy by blind needle aspiration, ultrasound- or CT-guided, or open surgical approach.

Examination under sedation or anaesthesia

Having localized a problem to the hip joint based on examination of the conscious patient, further manipulations performed with the animal deeply sedated or under anaesthesia can be useful. The Ortolani manoeuvre (Figure 22.7) is used to assess hip laxity and can be performed with the patient in either lateral or dorsal recumbency. With the hip held at a standing angle, the stifle is grasped and an axial force applied along the length of the femur in a distal to proximal direction. If the hip is lax, this causes the femoral head to subluxate from the acetabulum. The axial force is then maintained as the limb is slowly abducted. At a critical point the femoral head will reduce back into the acetabulum, usually with a perceptible 'clunk'. A 'good quality' Ortolani sign, akin to the sensation of shutting a car door, indicates a lax hip with relatively normal bony anatomy. A 'poor quality' sign with a poorly defined 'clunk' indicates more advanced degeneration, often associated with flattening of the dorsal acetabular rim, bony remodelling of the joint and infilling of the acetabulum with soft tissue or bone. In very chronic cases the Ortolani sign may be lost as the acetabulum fills in completely; this should not be confused with a normal hip.

Other manoeuvres have also been described to assess hip laxity. Barlow's test is performed in conjunction with the Ortolani test, and refers to detection of subluxation of the femoral head as an axial force is applied to the femur with the limb held in a weight-bearing position. Barden's test is performed less commonly. The thigh is grasped and lifted laterally with a hand placed over the greater trochanter to detect any lateral hip movement. Lateral displacement of greater than 0.5 cm is considered positive for hip laxity.

Radiography

After clinical examination, radiography is the 'first line' diagnostic procedure for most cases. Useful views include the lateral, hip-extended ventrodorsal, and hip-flexed or 'frog-legged' ventrodorsal views (see Imaging Techniques section and the *BSAVA Manuals of Canine and Feline Radiography and Radiology* and *Canine and Feline Musculoskeletal Imaging*). A comparison of hip-extended and hip-flexed ventrodorsal views is useful for detection of conditions such as SFCE and early ANFN.

Radiographs should be perfectly positioned to avoid artefact and allow complete assessment, especially for the ventrodorsal views. Prior to interpretation, the radiographs should be scrutinized for malpositioning; the wings of the ilia and the obturator foramina should be perfectly symmetrical (Figure 22.8). If there is any evidence of rotation, it is best to repeat the radiographs.

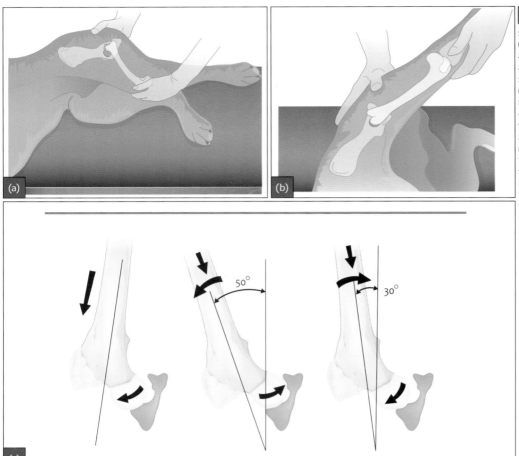

22.7 The Ortolani manoeuvre performed under heavy sedation or general anaesthesia. (a) With the hip held at a standing angle, an axial force is applied along the femur which causes subluxation of the dysplastic hip. (b) While the axial force is maintained the limb is abducted, eventually causing reduction of the femoral head; this is the reduction angle (with respect to the vertical). (c) The axial force is maintained and the limb is adducted, and the femoral head subluxates; this is the luxation angle (with respect to the vertical). Note that in (a) and (b) the dog is shown in lateral recumbency and in (c) the dog is shown in dorsal recumbency.

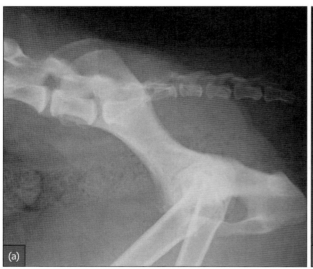
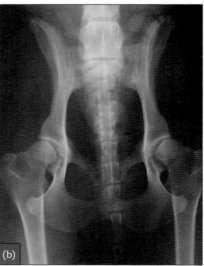

22.8 (a) Lateral and (b) ventrodorsal hip-extended radiographs of the pelvis of a Labrador Retriever. Note that the wings of the ilia and the obturator foramina are symmetrical on the ventrodorsal view, indicating perfect positioning. Mild degenerative changes can be appreciated affecting the hips.

Assessment of the proximal femora can be challenging in chronic cases where full extension of the hips is not possible. To evaluate this region in detail, a caudocranial view can be obtained which allows the femur to be positioned parallel to the radiographic cassette (Figure 22.9). It is important with this view that the crus is drawn cranially to avoid superimposition of the lower limb over the distal femur.

It has been shown that in some cases hip laxity may not be apparent on a standard hip-extended view due to torsional tightening of the joint capsule. Various special views have been described to circumvent this problem. The PennHIP (Pennsylvania hip improvement program) view uses a distraction device to force the femoral heads laterally, inducing subluxation. With the patient in dorsal recumbency, a radiolucent device is placed between the thighs. An operator then grasps the stifles and forces them together, subluxating the hips. The resultant image (Figure 22.10) allows hip laxity to be quantified using a 'distraction index' (DI).

An alternative to PennHIP radiography is the use of dorsolateral subluxation radiography to obtain a dorsolateral subluxation score (DLSS). For this procedure, the patient is positioned in sternal recumbency in a custom-made trough, with the femurs in a weight-bearing position (Farese *et al.*, 1998). Because weight is borne by the stifles, subluxation of the hips is induced. A dorsoventral radiograph can then be obtained. The degree of subluxation of the hips can then be assessed from the radiograph, and a 'subluxation index' calculated, in a similar fashion to the DI.

Computed tomography

CT images can be rapidly acquired and give excellent cross-sectional imaging of the hip joints (Figure 22.11). Use of different 'window levels' can allow assessment of bone and, to a lesser extent, soft tissues; soft tissue assessment can be improved by the use of intravenous contrast enhancement. Post-acquisition data manipulation can allow production of images in different planes, as well as three-dimensional images. Although CT is useful for assessment of neoplastic processes and planning surgery for complex fractures, it is unnecessary for the majority of routine cases.

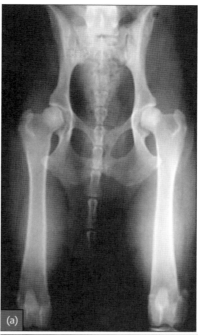
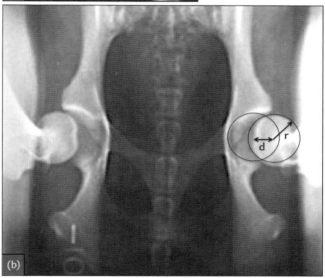

22.10 (a) Ventrodorsal hip-extended radiograph and (b) PennHIP view of the same dog. Hip laxity is more easily appreciated on the PennHIP view. The distraction index (DI) is calculated after drawing circles around the femoral head and over the acetabulum. The distance between the centres of the two circles 'd' is then measured and compared with the radius of the femoral head; DI = d/r.
(Courtesy of Professor Gail Smith)

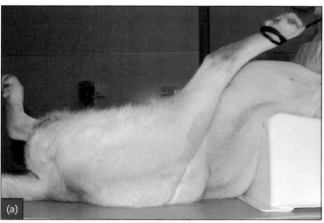
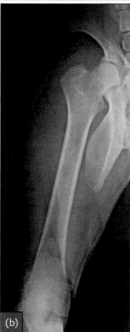

22.9 (a) Labrador Retriever positioned for a caudocranial radiograph of the femur. This view allows the femur to be positioned parallel to the radiographic cassette, avoiding foreshortening of the bone on (b) the radiograph.

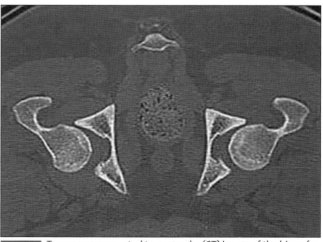

22.11 Transverse computed tomography (CT) image of the hips of a dog. The morphology of the joints can be evaluated in detail.

Magnetic resonance imaging

MRI is slower and more expensive to acquire than CT and in most instances is inferior for assessment of bone. However, it allows excellent soft tissue assessment. Its main indication is the detailed assessment of neoplastic processes, especially smaller lesions such as peripheral nerve tumours that cannot be imaged using other modalities. It is also the modality of choice for assessment of the lumbar spinal cord, and is useful in cases where iliopsoas myopathy is suspected.

Arthrocentesis

Synovial fluid analysis is useful for investigation of any arthropathy, and is essential for diagnosis of inflammatory arthritis such as infection or immune-mediated disease. The main anatomical landmark for arthrocentesis of the hip is the greater trochanter. Following aseptic preparation of the skin, a hypodermic needle can be introduced immediately craniodorsal to the proximal aspect of the trochanter and aimed towards the joint (Figure 22.12). A 25–75 mm (1–3 inch) needle is used, depending on the size of the patient. Synovial fluid is aspirated, and following gross assessment can be submitted for cytology and bacteriology (see Chapter 4).

Arthroscopy

Arthroscopy of the hip joint can provide diagnostic information including assessment of articular cartilage and the integrity of the acetabular labrum, and facilitates biopsy of intra-articular lesions. Treatment of certain lesions can be undertaken, such as removal of small chip fractures of the femoral head. Hip arthroscopy is technically challenging and is performed uncommonly.

Biopsy

Biopsy can be useful for investigation of suspected neoplastic lesions as well as obtaining tissue for bacteriology if an infectious process is suspected. Biopsy of tumours should be planned carefully based on imaging; CT and MRI are especially useful in this respect as they allow improved spatial assessment of lesions compared with radiography.

For further information on sampling techniques, see Chapter 4.

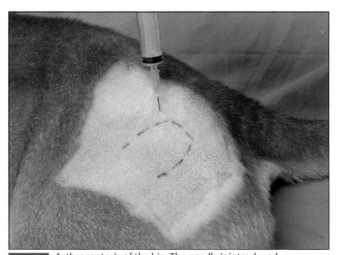

22.12 Arthrocentesis of the hip. The needle is introduced craniodorsal to the greater trochanter (indicated by the dotted line on the cadaver) and directed towards the joint.

Conditions affecting the hip

Hip dysplasia

Hip dysplasia is one of the most frequently diagnosed orthopaedic developmental conditions in the dog, and also occurs in the cat. There is considerable variation in both the prevalence of the condition between breeds, and the severity of clinical signs in affected individuals, which range from completely absent to severe dysfunction. Clinical efforts have focused firstly on screening programmes which aim to reduce the prevalence of the condition via elimination of affected dogs from the breeding population, and secondly on the treatment of affected individuals. Hip dysplasia has a genetic basis, with a complex polygenetic mode of inheritance; the phenotype of any individual is the result of the interaction between several genes and the environment. Unfortunately, despite the implementation of screening and breeding programmes in many countries, the rate of reduction in the prevalence of hip dysplasia has been slow. The development of management strategies for affected individuals has been more successful, with the prognosis generally considered good following implementation of appropriate treatment.

Aetiology

Genetically predisposed puppies are born with normal hips; however, early in life they develop joint laxity, synovitis and effusion. These changes permit lateral subluxation of the femoral head, which manifests as clinically detectable passive joint laxity as early as 8 weeks of age. The underlying cause of joint laxity remains unknown, although numerous theories have been proposed including relatively poor pelvic muscle mass, hormonal influences, and primarily increased joint fluid volume. Regardless of the initial cause, the development of joint laxity results in abnormal loading of the coxofemoral joint. Joint reaction forces are concentrated within reduced areas of contact at the dorsomedial femoral head and adjacent dorsal acetabular rim, leading to microfracture of subchondral bone and articular cartilage overloading. Altered joint loading also modifies epiphyseal development leading to flattening of the femoral head, relative underdevelopment of the dorsal acetabular rim, and acetabular infilling (Figure 22.13). Chronic, progressive cartilage overloading overwhelms the early anabolic chondrocytic response to extracellular matrix injury, initiating a self-perpetuating cycle of matrix degeneration, inflammation and cartilage loss that is characteristic of osteoarthritis. This phase is characterized by osteophyte formation, thickening of the joint capsule and remodelling of the acetabulum and femoral head. These features progressively reduce joint instability, which is typically clinically unapparent by 12–18 months of age; often there is a concurrent reduction in joint pain as capsular stretching, microfracturing, and gross instability resolve. Clinical function may therefore improve, although a variable degree of discomfort associated with osteoarthritis can develop. This sequence of events explains the typical bimodal age distribution of dogs presented with hip dysplasia.

Clinical signs

Young dogs are usually presented between 5 months and 1 year of age. A variable degree of pelvic limb lameness is frequently reported; however, since bilateral lameness may be less obvious to owners, presenting complaints may include unwillingness to exercise, frequent sitting during

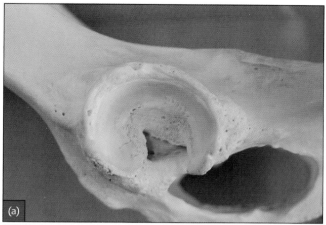

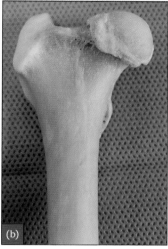

22.13 Cadaveric images of a crossbreed dog with hip dysplasia. New bone has formed (a) within the acetabular fossa and on the dorsal acetabular rim, and (b) around the margin of the femoral head.

Given the potential for hip dysplasia to be present but associated with minimal or no functional impairment in patients of any age, clinical assessment of the hips should always be performed as part of a comprehensive ortho-paedic examination to exclude concurrent clinically signifi-cant pathology elsewhere. In one study, the cause of lameness in almost one-third of dogs referred for manage-ment of hip dysplasia was actually cranial cruciate ligament disease, despite 94% of these cases having radiographic evidence of hip dysplasia (Powers et al., 2005).

Diagnostic investigations

A potentially bewildering range of investigations has been described for the diagnosis of hip dysplasia including con-ventional radiographic views, stress radiographic tech-niques, measurements derived from CT and MRI studies, ultrasonography, and clinical assessments of joint laxity. However, orthogonal radiographic views of the pelvis are adequate for diagnosis in most patients; more complex techniques are usually reserved for early diagnosis in young asymptomatic dogs for screening programmes, or early preventative surgery.

Diagnostic approach in the symptomatic patient: Lateral and hip-extended ventrodorsal radiographs of the pelvis are obtained as previously described with careful attention to good positioning to maximize diagnostic value. Radiographs should be assessed for evidence of joint lax-ity, remodelling and osteophyte formation.

* Joint laxity may be assessed subjectively by how well the femoral heads sit within the acetabulum, or by measurement of the Norberg angle (NA) and quantification of the percentage femoral head coverage (%FHC). The NA is the angle between a line connecting the centre of the femoral head and the cranial effective acetabular rim, and a line between the centres of the femoral heads (Figure 22.14). The NA decreases with

walks, reluctance to jump or run, and gait abnormalities such as a hip sway and a shortened, stiff or bunny-hopping gait. Problems are usually insidious in onset, with stiffness after rest often reported as an early feature; sudden onset lameness occurs less frequently, most likely following microfracturing of subchondral bone or acute tearing of the joint capsule or the ligament of the femoral head.

A variable degree of gluteal muscle atrophy is a com-mon feature, and a prominent greater trochanter may be apparent due to dorsolateral subluxation and loss of surrounding muscle mass. These features are easier to appreciate when asymmetry exists but bilateral pathology often results in approximately symmetrical changes. Manipulation of the hip is typically resented, especially during extension. Instability may be apparent if a hand is placed over the greater trochanter as the animal walks. In young dogs, the Ortolani test is specific but insensitive, thus the absence of gross coxofemoral instability does not preclude a diagnosis of hip dysplasia.

In the older dog, clinical signs are typically associated with osteoarthritis. Pelvic limb lameness may be a feature; however, in many cases owners report less specific prob-lems such as reduced exercise tolerance, reluctance to run or jump, and stiffness after rest (especially following extended exercise). These signs are typically insidious in onset; acute onset lameness should prompt consideration of alternative differential diagnoses. Palpation frequently reveals gluteal muscle atrophy although this is often quite mild. Manipulation is usually resented, especially in exten-sion, and there may be a reduced range of motion and crepitus. Gross coxofemoral instability is rarely present.

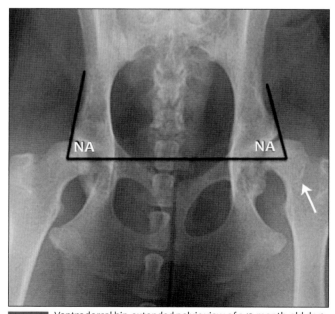

22.14 Ventrodorsal hip-extended pelvic view of a 12-month-old dog with hip dysplasia. The Norberg angle (NA) for each hip is the angle between a line connecting the centres of the femoral heads, and lines drawn from the centre of each femoral head to the ipsilateral cranial effective acetabular rim. A 'Morgan's line' can also be appreciated (arrowed); this is caused by early osteophyte formation at the insertion of the joint capsule.

greater subluxation; values greater than 105 degrees are considered normal. The %FHC (Figure 22.15) represents the proportion of the femoral head medial to the dorsal acetabular edge; values above 50% are considered normal.

- Remodelling may include blunting of the cranial effective acetabular rim, loss of the dorsal acetabular edge, flattening of the femoral head, and thickening of the femoral neck.
- Osteophyte formation may be noted at the cranial, dorsal and caudal acetabular edges, within the acetabular fossa, and affecting the femoral neck. The earliest changes are often noted at the attachment of the joint capsule on the femoral neck causing a fine, radiopaque line termed the caudal curvilinear osteophyte or Morgan's line (see Figure 22.14).

In the young symptomatic dog with hip dysplasia, evidence of joint laxity and osteophyte formation are typically apparent by the time radiography is performed. However, since osteoarthritis occurs secondary to laxity, osteophytes may be absent or subtle. In such cases, radiographic diagnosis may be dependent on demonstration of joint laxity, which can itself appear subtle due to tightening of the joint during limb extension for radiographic positioning.

In the older dog, subluxation, osteophytosis and remodelling are usually obvious (Figure 22.16) but the extent of radiographic evidence of osteoarthritis correlates poorly with the severity of joint pain or functional impairment. As such, and regardless of radiographic appearance, the hip joint must always be confirmed as the source of pain and lameness, especially if the presenting history is inconsistent with hip dysplasia (for example acute, severe lameness).

Diagnostic approach in the asymptomatic patient: A hip-extended ventrodorsal (VD) radiograph of the pelvis is used in the UK for the British Veterinary Association/Kennel Club (BVA/KC) hip dysplasia scoring scheme. Dogs over 12 months of age are eligible. Joint laxity is scored objectively according to the NA, with eight further subjective scores attributed according to the degree of subluxation, remodelling and osteophytosis at specific locations. Scores for

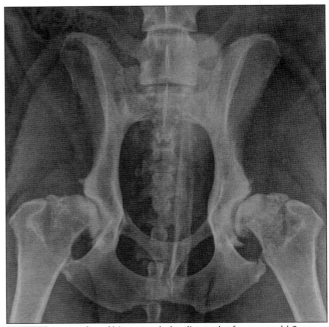

22.16 Ventrodorsal hip-extended radiograph of a 4-year-old German Shepherd Dog with severe hip dysplasia. Note the marked subluxation, remodelling of the acetabulum and femoral head, and extensive osteophyte formation.

each hip range from zero (normal) to 53; the score for each hip is added to give the overall score. Current recommendations are that only dogs with a total score lower than the breed median score, and without radiographic evidence of osteophyte formation, should be used for breeding. Two other major scoring schemes are administered by Orthopaedic Foundation for Animals (OFA) in the USA, and the Fédération Cynologique Internationale (FCI) in Belgium. Similar to the BVA/KC scheme, scoring is predominantly subjective; the OFA scheme has seven grades (1 to 7; excellent, good, fair, borderline, and mild, moderate and severe dysplasia), and the FCI five grades (A to E; normal, near normal, and mild, moderate and severe dysplasia). In both schemes breeding is not recommended from dogs with any of the dysplastic grades.

Although these subjective scoring systems have been in existence for several decades (the BVA/KC scheme was introduced for all breeds in 1983), the resultant rate of improvement in hip scores has been slow, albeit measurable. In one study, the mean OFA hip score reduced from 2.00 in the period 1970–1984, to 1.92 in the period 2001–2007 (Hou *et al.*, 2010). An important factor is the relatively low heritability of the hip dysplasia phenotype as measured by the VD hip-extended radiograph. Heritability is an estimate of the extent to which environmental factors determine the phenotype in dogs genetically predisposed to a condition. The higher the heritability index (minimum 0, maximum 1), the more accurately the phenotype reflects the genotype, and the more effective a breeding programme based on phenotypic measurement can be in reducing the prevalence of the unwanted genotype. Two recent analyses of large data sets from the OFA and BVA/KC schemes have estimated heritability of hip dysplasia, as quantified using a hip-extended VD radiograph, at 0.21 and 0.35 respectively (Hou *et al.*, 2010; Lewis *et al.*, 2010). Such low values reflect the environmental influences, and the diagnostic inaccuracy of the hip-extended VD radiograph. In a recent study, 55% of dogs graded suitable for breeding

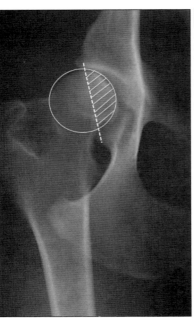

22.15 The percentage femoral head coverage (%FHC) (shaded area) is the proportion of the femoral head medial to the dorsal acetabular rim (dotted line). Values less than 50% are considered abnormal.

using the OFA scheme at 2 years of age were later graded as dysplastic using the same criteria (Smith *et al.*, 2012); this high false-negative rate was attributed to the late development of osteophytes (especially when lean bodyweight, a key environmental factor, was maintained), and tightening of the joint during limb extension for radiographic positioning. The precision of subjective scoring systems has also been questioned.

These factors prompted development of more objective phenotypic measurements based on the quantification of passive hip laxity; examples include the DI (the PennHIP method) and the dorsolateral subluxation score (DLSS). A number of potential advantages over traditional ventrodorsal hip-extended radiographs have been proposed, both for breeding schemes and for early diagnosis in individual dogs. Firstly, the degree of passive laxity is directly quantified; this has been shown to be proportional to the risk of development of osteoarthritis (Smith *et al.*, 2001). Secondly, the assessment of osteophyte formation is not key; this may be minimal in affected dogs when young, or where environmental features are favourable. Thirdly, the objectivity of these measurements is associated with high precision. These features contribute to the much higher estimated heritability of hip dysplasia as measured by the DI of between 0.56 and 0.83 (Smith *et al.*, 2012). A hands-free PennHIP technique has recently been validated for use in the UK, although there is currently no official UK breeding programme incorporating DI values (Guilliard, 2014).

Treatment

Treatment options for the symptomatic animal include conservative treatment, preventative surgical techniques such as juvenile pelvic symphysiodesis (JPS) or triple pelvic osteotomy (TPO), palliative surgical techniques where the joint is preserved, such as denervation, and salvage surgical techniques such as femoral head and neck excision (FHNE) and total hip replacement (THR). Selection of the most appropriate treatment in any individual depends on numerous factors including age, severity of presenting signs, financial constraints, and in most cases the response to initial non-invasive treatment.

Conservative treatment: An initial conservative approach should be considered for most patients. Frequently conservative treatment is successful in alleviating presenting signs to a level where good clinical function can be achieved and maintained in the long term. In other cases, attention to key features such as appropriate bodyweight will minimize the risk of complications following palliative or salvage surgery. In the young dog, hip pain is associated with instability and many individuals will show significant clinical improvement if comfort and function can be maintained until 12–15 months of age as joint stability improves. Studies have shown that approximately 50–75% of young dogs achieve satisfactory long-term function with this approach (Barr *et al.*, 1987; Farrell *et al.*, 2007). However, early surgical intervention is considered for young dogs with very painful hips because pain, muscle atrophy and instability may progress in these cases. In the older dog, hip pain is typically due to osteoarthritis, and with very few exceptions non-surgical treatment should be attempted initially, even where advanced radiographic changes are present.

A comprehensive non-surgical treatment strategy should include maintenance of lean bodyweight, exercise management and analgesic treatment.

Lean bodyweight: Achieving and maintaining lean bodyweight is a key element of non-surgical management of hip dysplasia in dogs of all ages. As a complex trait, the phenotype of a genetically predisposed individual is modified by environmental factors, of which bodyweight is a particularly important example. In a long-term study of paired Labrador Retriever littermates, ad-lib fed puppies developed osteoarthritis at a younger age, of greater severity and higher overall prevalence than puppies fed a restricted ration (Smith *et al.*, 2006). In older dogs where hip pain is primarily associated with osteoarthritis, excessive bodyweight may adversely affect the function of a joint via altered biomechanics (increased loading) and systemic pro-inflammatory effects. In one study of overweight dogs with hip dysplasia, lameness scores improved significantly when bodyweight reduced by 11–18% following calorie restriction (Impellizeri *et al.*, 2000).

Exercise management: Dogs of any age with hip dysplasia will benefit from an appropriate amount of exercise. Many dogs are presented having been rested by their owners for variable periods, an approach which may establish a cycle of weight gain, muscle atrophy, and reduced range of joint motion, all leading to increased lameness. In the young dog, muscle mass and function are important to maximize joint stability, while in dogs of any age, lean bodyweight is important to limit forces exerted on the compromised joint. The benefits of exercise must, however, be balanced against the obvious potential adverse effect of overuse of a joint compromised by laxity or osteoarthritis. In general, low-impact activity such as lead walks should be recommended; frequent short walks are usually better tolerated, with the duration gradually increased over a period of several weeks. Precise recommendations will depend on the individual patient's exercise tolerance at presentation and response to early treatment. High impact activities such as running and jumping should be prevented until the clinical situation has improved. Additional strategies such as underwater treadmill exercise and a structured physiotherapy programme are often useful. A recent study found longer daily exercise duration to be associated with reduced lameness in dogs with hip dysplasia and osteoarthritis (Greene *et al.*, 2013). In cases where even moderate low-impact exercise is poorly tolerated (usually young dogs with painful subluxation), early surgical intervention should be considered.

Analgesia: The use of non-steroidal anti-inflammatory drugs (NSAIDs) is indicated, both in young dogs for the control of pain associated with hip joint laxity, and in the older dog where they can be effective for the reduction of clinical signs of osteoarthritis. If well tolerated by the patient, treatment should be continued for a sufficient period for the more slowly achieved benefits of weight loss and exercise increase to become apparent. Ability to exercise will be promoted by reduced joint pain, and NSAID treatment should be continued if doubt exists; this may be several weeks or months. If progress is good, the response to a reduced dose and then withdrawal of treatment can be tested. However, some dogs require continuous treatment or tactical dosing (for example following a longer walk, or in the colder months).

Dietary omega-3 fatty acid supplementation can improve lameness scores and reduce the NSAID requirement of dogs with osteoarthritis, probably as a result of decreased pro-inflammatory eicosanoid synthesis, and should be considered in the management of dogs with hip dysplasia. The use of other nutraceuticals such as glucosamine and chondroitin can also be considered although the evidence surrounding their efficacy is limited.

Surgical treatment: Surgical intervention is most frequently indicated when conservative management has been unsuccessful, regardless of age. No single definition of success exists but key criteria include significant mitigation of pain and restoration of acceptable function; this is itself highly variable between patients based on lifestyle and owner expectations. To complicate decision-making further, the relative advantages and risks of different interventions must be weighed against the severity and nature of presenting signs to allow selection of the most appropriate approach in each individual case.

Surgery may also be indicated when a conservative approach is felt unlikely to be effective from the outset, most frequently in young dogs presenting with marked hip pain and instability.

Less frequently, preventative surgery may be considered in both asymptomatic and mildly symptomatic dogs. JPS and TPO aim to increase dorsal acetabular coverage of the femoral head, improving loading and reducing the progression of osteoarthritis. Since candidate dogs could potentially be managed successfully with non-surgical treatment, or alternative surgery with a good prognosis (such as THR), these approaches require careful preoperative assessment and fully informed discussion with owners.

Preventative surgery:

- **Triple pelvic osteotomy** improves acetabular coverage of the femoral head via rotation of the acetabulum following osteotomies of the pubis, ischium and ilium (Figure 22.17). Although passive joint laxity is unaltered, capture of the femoral head is improved and subluxation mitigated. TPO is usually considered only in young, symptomatic dogs with mild to moderate hip joint laxity, but without radiographic evidence of osteoarthritis. This is because TPO is less effective when significant pre-existing degenerative joint disease is present (usually by 9–10 months of age) or, similarly to JPS, if severe laxity is present. This is typically assessed by measurement of the Ortolani angle of reduction, which should be less than 30 degrees, and 10 degrees more than the angle of subluxation (Vezzoni *et al.*, 2005).

- The TPO procedure has evolved considerably since its original description by Hohn and Janes (1969). Key changes have included the use of TPO-specific plates, limitation of the acetabular rotation angle to 20 degrees, and strategies to reduce the incidence of cranial screw loosening, a common complication when three cortical screws were used. These include application of a second ventral plate, increased sacral screw purchase, the use of locking screws, placement of four cranial screws, and preservation of the ischium (double pelvic osteotomy (DPO)). The DPO relies on bending of the ischium and pelvic symphysis to allow acetabular rotation, a process facilitated by an osteotomy of the dorsal ischial cortex (the 2.5 PO; Petazzoni *et al.*, 2012).Good or excellent clinical outcomes following TPO are reported in between 76% and 92% of cases (McLaughlin *et al.*, 1991; Rasmussen *et al.*, 1998). Despite this, TPO remains a relatively infrequently performed procedure as a result of the narrow criteria for candidacy, the potential for progressive osteoarthritis due to persistent joint laxity and altered loading, the risk of complications, the potential for successful conservative management in many candidate dogs, and the very good outcomes associated with similarly invasive interventions such as THR.

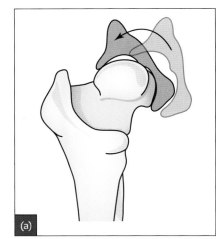
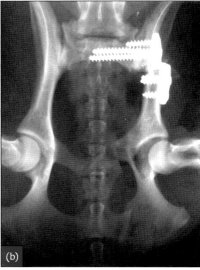

22.17 Triple pelvic osteotomy. (a) The acetabular fragment is acutely rotated along its long axis (arrowed) thus improving dorsal coverage of the femoral head. (b) The ilial osteotomy is stabilized using a plate and bone screws.

- **Juvenile pubic symphysiodesis** takes advantage of the normal growth potential of the pelvis to improve acetabular coverage of the femoral head. Thermal injury to the pubic symphysis (using electrocautery) results in premature closure, effectively tethering the ventral aspect of the acetabulum. Continued growth of the remainder of the pelvis causes the acetabula to rotate ventrally (Figure 22.18), in the same way as is achieved acutely during TPO. It follows that JPS will only be effective where sufficient growth potential exists; 16 weeks of age (18 weeks in giant breeds) is considered the **maximum age**. In practice most symptomatic dogs present later than this, thus JPS is typically performed in asymptomatic dogs following screening for passive hip joint laxity. This should include measurement of the DI, firstly due to the moderate false-negative rate associated with the Ortolani sign at this age, and secondly since very lax hips do not benefit sufficiently to warrant the procedure. An optimal DI range for JPS of 0.3–0.5 has been recommended, although significant reduction in the progression of hip osteoarthritis has been demonstrated in dogs with a DI between 0.3 and 0.7 (Dueland *et al.*, 2010). Dogs undergoing JPS and TPO should be neutered, since despite an improved phenotype they otherwise retain the ability to perpetuate a dysplastic genotype. Although long-term functional outcomes are unknown, JPS appears likely to prove a beneficial intervention in young dogs with mild to moderate hip laxity.

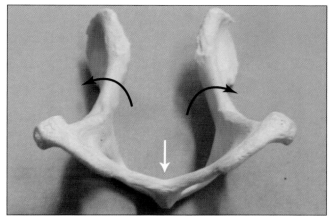

22.18 Juvenile pubic symphysiodesis. Thermal injury to the pubic symphysis (straight arrow) prevents further widening of the ventral aspect of the pelvis. As the dorsal aspect continues to grow, the acetabulae rotate ventrally (curved arrows), improving dorsal femoral head coverage.

Palliative and salvage surgery: Outcomes following palliative surgery such as hip denervation are somewhat variable, and these procedures are rarely performed. Salvage surgery, such as FHNE and THR, can be considered in dogs that have failed to respond to conservative management or where preventative procedures such as TPO or JPS are inappropriate. Further details of these procedures are given at the end of this chapter (see Salvage surgery).

Avascular necrosis of the femoral head

ANFH is a relatively common condition in small-breed dogs, especially terriers and Miniature Poodles. An equivalent condition was described in humans in 1910 by three authors simultaneously, Legg, Calvé and Perthes, so ANFH is also commonly known as Legg–Calvé–Perthes disease. An autosomal recessive mechanism of inheritance with a high heritability has been demonstrated in Manchester Terriers (Vasseur *et al.*, 1989) and West Highland White Terriers (Robinson, 1992), and is suspected in other breeds; therefore, affected animals should not be used for breeding. The condition is unilateral in around 85% of cases and there is no obvious sex predisposition.

The precise aetiopathogenesis is poorly understood. The epiphysis in growing dogs receives its blood supply from circumferential vessels that enter the bone at the attachment of the joint capsule close to the capital physis. It is thought that a temporary vascular compromise occurs rather than permanent destruction of vessels; this may be secondary to other factors such a temporary elevation in intra-articular pressure. The initial necrotic phase is followed by attempts to repair the bone by a process of remodelling, known as creeping substitution. Excessive resorption of bone leads to a loss of support for subchondral bone and subsequent collapse of the overlying articular cartilage. The resultant loss of articular congruence leads to the rapid development of osteoarthritis.

Clinical examination

Dogs are usually first affected at 4–11 months of age. An insidious, progressive lameness is typical, although more acute onset can occur in some cases. On presentation, most dogs are severely lame and often exhibit periods of non-weight-bearing. Gluteal and pelvic limb muscle atrophy is usually marked. Obvious discomfort is apparent on manipulation of the affected hip, and crepitus may be appreciated in chronic cases.

Diagnosis

Diagnosis is usually straightforward based on plain radiographs. Ventrodorsal hip-extended and frog-legged views are most useful. In the early stages irregular areas of radiolucency affecting the femoral head can be appreciated (Figure 22.19). These changes can be subtle; advanced imaging such as CT and MRI can be helpful although these are rarely required. The joint space is often widened, giving an appearance of coxofemoral subluxation. In later stages, the femoral head is remodelled and adopts an irregular shape characterized by flattening of the femoral head, lucency of the femoral neck and often sclerosis of the proximal femoral metaphysis (Figure 22.20). Osteoarthritis leads to the development of osteophytes in more chronic cases.

Treatment

Rarely, dogs can be presented with a mild lameness and minimal radiographic changes. These patients can be managed conservatively with a fair prognosis; however, owners should be warned that many animals will develop significant osteoarthritis in the long term. Dogs that are more severely lame, or where conservative treatment has been ineffective, are candidates for salvage surgery. Surgical options include FHNE and THR (see below and Operative Technique 22.8).

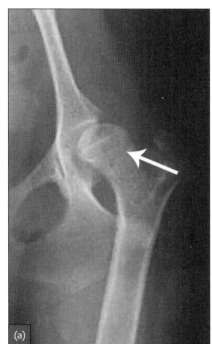

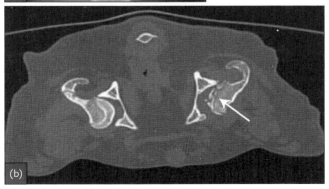

22.19
(a) Ventrodorsal view of the left hip of an 8-month-old West Highland White Terrier. Subtle radiolucency of the femoral head can be appreciated, indicative of early avascular necrosis of the femoral head (ANFH); in addition, the joint space appears slightly widened (arrowed).
(b) Subchondral bone loss (arrowed) is much more obvious on a CT scan.

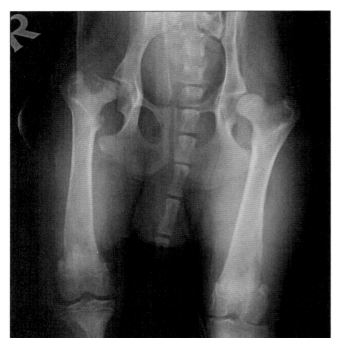

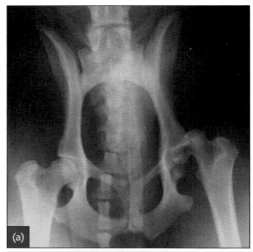

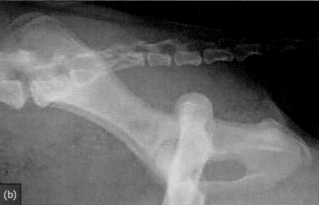

22.20 Ventrodorsal pelvic radiograph of an 11-month-old Yorkshire Terrier with advanced ANFH showing marked remodelling of the right femoral head and neck.

Coxofemoral luxation

Dislocation of the hip is the most commonly encountered luxation in dogs and cats. In the majority of cases there will be a history of significant trauma such as a road accident, a fall, or a fight with another dog. Spontaneous hip luxation can occur, secondary to either underlying hip dysplasia or presumed connective tissue disorders. Affected animals are usually skeletally mature; in juvenile animals the forces required to cause a hip luxation more commonly result in fracture of the relatively weak proximal femoral physis. In adult animals, hip luxation can often occur in conjunction with small avulsion fractures of the femoral head, associated with the attachment of the ligament of the femoral head (Figure 22.21).

Most commonly the femoral head luxates in a dorsal direction, usually craniodorsally. Ventral luxation is less common; in these patients initial discomfort can be severe due to impingement of the obturator nerve, but the discomfort often resolves rapidly. Affected animals can sometimes ambulate surprisingly well as the femoral head impacts into the obturator foramen giving some degree of mechanical support to the limb.

Clinical examination

Patients are usually presented with pelvic limb lameness of variable severity, ranging from moderate to non-weight-bearing.

Animals with a craniodorsal luxation usually hold the limb externally rotated and slightly adducted. The femur is displaced proximally, resulting in prominence of the greater trochanter. The stifle will be located slightly proximally compared to the normal contralateral limb and apparent limb length is relatively short; this can usually be appreciated when the animal is standing. Manipulation of the hip is painful, and crepitus is often present. The thumb displacement test can be performed; if the hip is dorsally luxated the examiner's thumb is not forced out of the depression caudal to the hip when the femur is externally rotated.

22.21 (a) Ventrodorsal pelvic radiograph of a 3-year-old Staffordshire Bull Terrier. The left hip is luxated and an avulsion fracture of the femoral head is present. (b) The lateral view shows the luxation is in a dorsal direction.

Caudodorsal luxation often results in slight internal rotation of the limb. Ventral luxation results in a distally displaced femur and a stifle that is located distally compared to the normal contralateral limb. The trochanter may be difficult to appreciate as it is displaced ventrally and medially. For ventral luxations the thumb displacement test is unreliable.

Radiography

Diagnosis of hip luxation is straightforward using plain radiographs (see Figure 22.21). Mediolateral and ventrodorsal views should be obtained to allow confirmation of the direction of luxation and the presence of complicating factors such as avulsion fractures of the femoral head or underlying hip dysplasia.

Treatment

A variety of factors can influence the choice of treatment. In most cases closed reduction is attempted in the first instance. This is more likely to be successful if performed promptly, as soon as the patient can be safely anaesthetized, and if there is no pre-existing hip dysplasia or osteoarthritis. In more chronic cases, hypertrophy of the torn ligament of the femoral head will often preclude stable reduction, necessitating surgery. The presence of fractures of the femoral head will also necessitate surgery, since these must be either removed (if small) or stabilized. Animals with underlying hip dysplasia have a significantly increased risk of re-luxation of the hip following both closed and open reduction, and consideration should be given to immediate salvage surgery in these cases (FHNE or THR, see later).

Closed reduction: To achieve closed reduction, the animal is anaesthetized and placed in lateral recumbency with the affected limb uppermost. A sling is placed around the dependent limb and anchored dorsally to provide countertraction.

- For a craniodorsal luxation, the affected limb is externally rotated to lift the femoral head clear of the dorsal acetabular rim, and then pulled distally. The limb is then internally rotated to engage the femoral head in the acetabulum (Figure 22.22). Vigorous manipulation and firm medial pressure have been advocated to expel any residual haematoma from the joint.
- Closed reduction of ventral luxations is more challenging as the femoral head is frequently impacted into the obturator foramen. The femur is pulled distally and laterally; it can be helpful to place pointed forceps on the greater trochanter to aid traction in certain

cases. The femur is then externally rotated and pulled proximally, before being internally rotated to reduce the femoral head into the acetabulum.

- Following closed reduction, it is obligatory to obtain post-manipulation orthogonal radiographs of the pelvis to confirm and document reduction of the hip. For a dorsal luxation, a frog-legged ventrodorsal view (rather than a hip-extended view) is less likely to cause re-luxation of the hip. For a ventral luxation a hip-extended view should be obtained.

Various procedures have been described to maintain the hip in reduction while capsular healing occurs. These include application of an Ehmer sling (Figure 22.23), use of an 'off-weight-bearing' sling where the hock is bandaged in a flexed position to prevent the paw contacting the ground, and surgical techniques such as closed application of a transarticular pin or a hinged external skeletal fixator (ESF) applied from the pelvis to the proximal femur. The Ehmer sling can be successful for dorsal luxations but great care is needed to avoid the development of dressing sores on the cranial aspect of the thigh, and the dressing is prone to slippage. The off-weight-bearing sling is safer but may not force the femoral head into the acetabulum as effectively; this sling can also be used for ventral luxations, as can simple hobbles placed between the pelvic limbs. Closed application of a transarticular pin or use of an ESF are used uncommonly since if a surgical procedure is to be employed, most surgeons opt for open reduction and internal stabilization. Use of an ischio-ilial (DeVita) pin driven from caudally to cranially dorsal to the femoral head has also been described; however, this technique has been associated with a high rate of complications including sciatic nerve damage.

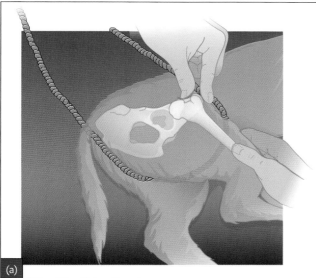

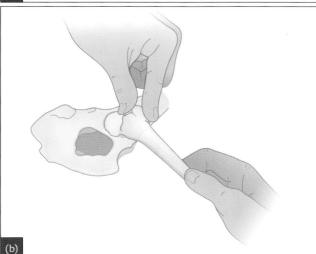

22.22 (a–b) Closed reduction of a dorsal hip luxation. The patient is secured on the table using a sling placed around the pelvis and dependent limb. The affected limb is externally rotated and pulled distally and then internally rotated to reduce the hip.

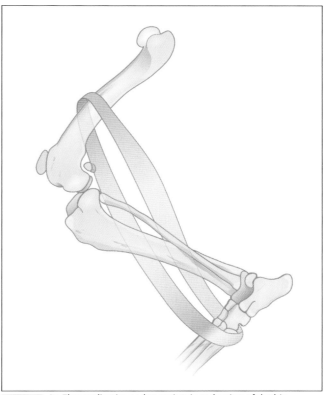

22.23 An Ehmer sling is used to maintain reduction of the hip. Adhesive dressing material is placed between the distal thigh and metatarsus, passing medially to the crus in both directions.

Open reduction: Indications for surgical (open) intervention include:

- Failure to achieve closed reduction, or re-luxation of the hip
- Fractures of the femoral head
- Pre-existing hip dysplasia or osteoarthritis
- Injuries to other limbs that preclude the use of a sling or that would lead to excessive early weight-bearing on the hip.

A plethora of surgical techniques have been described to achieve stabilization of the joint, reflecting the fact that perfect results have not been reported for any single technique. Common to all techniques, the acetabulum and femoral head are exposed and any remnants of the ligament of the femoral head excised to allow complete reduction. If the capsule is folded into the acetabulum, this is carefully reflected but preserved to allow suturing following reduction; this can add significantly to the stability of the joint.

Techniques that have been described to maintain hip stability following reduction include:

- Hip toggle
- Iliofemoral suture
- Transarticular pin
- Dorsal capsular sling
- TPO.

Hip toggle: The toggle technique (see Operative Technique 22.4) is used to create a prosthetic ligament of the femoral head (McLaughlin, 1995). Following a craniolateral approach, a tunnel is drilled through the acetabular fossa and the femoral head and neck. The toggle is placed into the pelvic canal to anchor the prosthetic ligament to the pelvis. Heavy gauge suture material is passed from the toggle, across the joint, and through the femoral bone tunnel, and is anchored on the lateral aspect of the femur by tying to another toggle pin, a screw or a plastic button. Closed fluoroscopically guided toggle pin placement has also been described (Serdy *et al.*, 1999).

In most cases, non-absorbable suture material is used. Monofilament nylon is popular but can break at the point it passes through the toggle; in addition this material can lead to osteolysis of the femoral neck. Braided materials such as polyester or polyethylene are strong and are resistant to abrasion; however, these materials can be associated with an increased risk of postoperative infection.

The toggle technique is relatively robust, can be used in all sizes of patient and can be used to treat dorsal and ventral luxations. The surgical technique can be challenging, but is made much easier by careful planning and appropriate surgical assistance.

Iliofemoral suture: The iliofemoral suture (IFS) technique causes internal rotation of the femur and prevents lateral translation of the femoral head (Martini *et al.*, 2001) (see Operative Technique 22.5). The suture is placed between the greater trochanter and the pelvis in the vicinity of the origin of the rectus femoris muscle, immediately cranioventral to the hip (see Operative Technique 22.4). Numerous variations on the technique have been described; most commonly bone tunnels are drilled through the greater trochanter and through the ventral aspect of the ilium, and sutures looped through these tunnels. It can be difficult to pass the suture through the tunnel in the ilium in some cases; alternative techniques include use of a toggle rod or suture anchor, or placement of the suture through the tendon of origin of the rectus femoris muscle.

Either absorbable or non-absorbable heavy gauge suture material can be used; use of multiple strands may be superior to use of a single strand. In most cases, the patient walks with the limb slightly internally rotated for 1–2 weeks, but then a more normal posture is regained. It is probable that the suture either stretches or snaps at this point, and is unlikely to provide long-term stability; therefore, absorbable sutures such as polydioxanone may be the most appropriate material to use.

The IFS technique is relatively simple to perform but may be less robust than other techniques, especially in larger patients.

Deep gluteal tenodesis: Tenodesis of the deep gluteal tendon using a screw and spiked washer with the reduced hip slightly internally rotated has a similar stabilizing effect. Good outcomes have been reported in cats and dogs up to 50 kg (Rochereau and Bernarde, 2012).

Transarticular pin: A stainless steel pin can be temporarily placed across the joint to maintain reduction while capsular healing occurs (Hunt and Henry, 1985; Sissener *et al.*, 2009). The size of the pin may range from 1.6–2.0 mm in a cat, up to 3.8 mm in a large dog. A pilot hole is drilled through the femoral head and neck, and a pin then placed from the lateral aspect of the femur to exit the bone at the fovea capitis on the femoral head. The hip is then reduced and held slightly internally rotated and abducted before the pin is driven across the joint, through the acetabular fossa and into the pelvic canal (Figure 22.24). The pin is left in place for around 3 weeks, and then removed (see Operative Technique 22.6).

The transarticular pin technique is relatively simple and can be used for dorsal and ventral luxations. However, complications can occur including pin breakage, migration and femoral neck fracture. In addition, a second surgical procedure is obligatory to remove the pin.

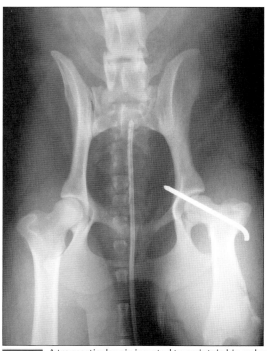

22.24 A transarticular pin inserted to maintain hip reduction in a dog.

Dorsal capsular sling: Following suturing of any remaining joint capsule, a prosthetic dorsal capsule can be created to prevent lateral translation of the femoral head (Braden and Johnson, 1988) (see Operative Technique 22.7). Screws or suture anchors are placed in the dorsal acetabular rim and sutures passed between these and bone tunnels drilled in the femoral neck (Figure 22.25). It is unlikely the sutures provide long-term support, and hence multiple strands of heavy gauge absorbable material such as polydioxanone should be used. Suture anchors have a lower profile than screws and washers but often have relatively sharp edges; partially threaded cancellous screws and smooth washers may cause less abrasion to the sutures.

The implants can be placed via a craniolateral or, more commonly, a dorsal approach. If a dorsal approach is made incorporating a trochanteric osteotomy, the greater trochanter can be transposed distally and caudally during closure; this increases tension in the gluteal muscles and may improve hip stability.

The dorsal sling technique can provide secure reduction of the hip, and is most applicable to dorsal luxations. The technique is relatively technically demanding and, should re-luxation of the hip occur, any protruding screw heads can cause significant damage to the femoral head.

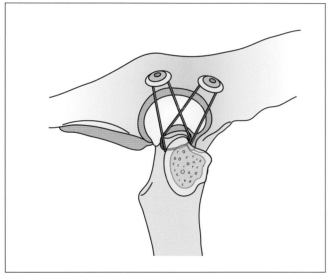

22.25 Dorsal capsular sling. Screws are placed in the dorsal acetabular rim, and sutures passed from these screws to bone tunnels drilled in the femoral neck. The joint is usually approached via a trochanteric osteotomy.

Triple pelvic osteotomy: For dorsal luxations, TPO causes ventroversion of the acetabulum, which improves 'capture' of the femoral head and hip stability (Haburjak *et al.*, 2001). This technique has been described for anatomically normal or slightly dysplastic hips. It can be combined with other techniques such as an iliofemoral suture, or can be used as a sole procedure. Although not specifically described for management of hip luxations, variations on the technique such as double pelvic osteotomy could also be used.

Although good results have been reported for management of hip luxations including those with mild underlying osteoarthritis, TPO is a technically demanding procedure that should only be undertaken by experienced surgeons. Complications are common; these can include implant failure, sciatic nerve damage and incisional problems.

Ventral plate stabilization for ventral luxations: Following a ventral approach and reduction of the luxation, a plate can be applied across the ventral aspect of the acetabulum between the ilium and the ischium, effectively augmenting the ventral acetabular ligament (Venzin and Montavon, 2007). Alternatively a prosthetic sling can be used to achieve the same effect, placed through bone tunnels or attached by screws. The procedure is technically demanding but can be very effective. It is used most commonly to manage recurrent ventral luxation following THR (Figure 22.26).

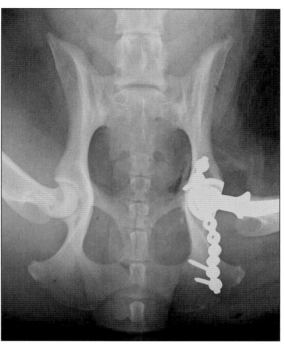

22.26 Postoperative radiograph showing placement of a ventral acetabular plate to maintain reduction following ventral luxation as a complication of total hip replacement.

Prognosis

Following closed reduction, re-luxation of the hip occurs in around 40% of cases; the prognosis may be slightly better in cats. Following surgery, re-luxation occurs in around 10–20% cases irrespective of which technique has been used to maintain stability. Re-luxation following surgical treatment is usually an indication for salvage surgery.

Detailed comparison of different techniques is challenging due to small case numbers and a lack of suitable controls in different studies. The authors' preferred technique in most cases is the hip toggle; iliofemoral sutures can be useful for small patients where limited bone stock can make drilling tunnels through the femoral neck challenging. In the long term, owners should be warned that some degree of osteoarthritis is common and will require ongoing management.

Management of hip luxation with pre-existing hip dysplasia

The presence of pre-existing hip disease such as hip dysplasia will dramatically increase the risk of re-luxation of the hip following either closed or surgical reduction; this is because of pre-existing poor dorsal acetabular coverage. In addition, joint function and comfort may already be suboptimal due the to the pre-existing dysplasia. In these cases salvage procedures should be considered from the outset. FHNE is simple to perform but recovery periods can be prolonged and long-term lameness is common, especially in larger patients. THR is an effective technique for management of hip luxation in animals of all sizes with pre-existing osteoarthritis or concurrent hip fractures; in one small case series, 100% of dogs had no observable lameness at long-term follow-up (Pozzi et al., 2004). THR can be performed following failure of other surgical techniques, but the risk of complications including infection may be increased.

Fractures affecting the hip

Fractures affecting the acetabulum and proximal femur are relatively common. Most animals have a history of significant trauma, but on occasions fractures can occur in the absence of trauma, for example acetabular stress fractures in racing greyhounds. Surgery to stabilize the fractures or perform a salvage procedure is indicated in almost all cases. Further information regarding fracture repair can be found in the *BSAVA Manual of Canine and Feline Fracture Repair and Management*; information on salvage surgery for the hip is given below.

Slipped femoral capital epiphysis

Traumatic femoral capital physeal fractures are encountered occasionally in dogs and cats, and are generally treated by open reduction and internal fixation using small pins (see the *BSAVA Manual of Canine and Feline Fracture Repair and Management*). A subgroup of patients has been reported in which separation of the capital epiphysis appears to occur in the absence of any significant trauma (McNicholas et al., 2002; Moores et al., 2004). This condition has been described as epiphysiolysis or SFCE. Analogous conditions have been reported in pigs and humans.

The aetiology of SFCE is not fully understood. The condition in cats is more common in overweight adolescent males and has been associated with early neutering which can delay physeal closure. It has been suggested that affected animals have of a form of physeal dysplasia causing an inherent weakness in the physis (Craig, 2001), leading to progressive structural failure under normal weight-bearing loads. The condition is often bilateral, although this is not always the case.

Diagnosis

Affected animals are usually presented with a chronic, insidious onset of lameness that can become severe. Marked muscle atrophy is often present, and affected animals exhibit significant discomfort on manipulation of the hip. In the early stages radiographic abnormalities affecting the proximal femur can be very subtle; careful comparison of hip-extended and 'frog-legged' ventrodorsal radiographs can allow identification of physeal instability (Figure 22.27). Advanced imaging such as CT can be helpful, although this is rarely required. In the later stages, marked remodelling of the femoral neck occurs leading to more obvious radiographic changes (Figure 22.28).

Treatment

In the majority of patients, marked remodelling of the femoral neck at the time of presentation precludes open reduction and internal fixation, and salvage procedures are

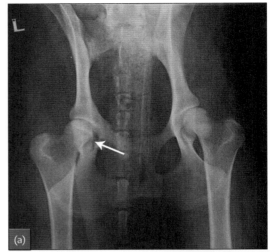
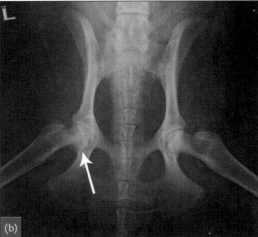

22.27 (a) Ventrodorsal hip-extended and (b) 'frog-legged' pelvic radiographs showing a slipped femoral capital epiphysis on the left. Subtle widening of the left capital physis is evident on the hip-extended view (arrowed); the lesion is more obvious on the flexed view (arrowed). The lesions are subtle but comparison of the affected left to the normal right hip shows that the appearance of the anatomical relationship between the femoral head and neck is different.

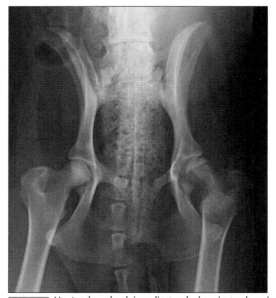

22.28 Ventrodorsal pelvic radiograph showing a chronic slipped femoral capital epiphysis. Marked lytic remodelling of the femoral neck on the right can be appreciated.

indicated. FHNE can give acceptable outcomes but THR is preferred if available (Gemmill *et al.*, 2012), since functional outcomes after joint replacement are superior; this applies to all sizes of dogs and cats, not only larger patients.

Heterotopic osteochondrofibrosis

This is an uncommon cause of lameness seen predominantly in the Dobermann. The condition is characterized by the development of a soft tissue mass, which later becomes mineralized, in the muscles caudal to the hip such as the external hip rotator muscles and the origin of the hamstrings.

The aetiology is unclear. It has been proposed that the mineralization occurs following spontaneous intramuscular haemorrhage secondary to haemostatic disorders; indeed, the condition has been described as von Willebrand's associated heterotopic osteochondrofibrosis. However, the condition has also been identified in animals that are negative for von Willebrand's disease. Another possibility is that the condition occurs secondary to minor repetitive trauma. Affected animals, especially Dobermanns, are also predisposed to other degenerative conditions, such as Achilles tendinopathy, and it is possible that these patients could have a more generalized disease affecting connective tissues. Chondroid and osseous metaplasia appear to occur following initial fibrosis.

Clinical examination

Affected animals are presented with chronic progressive pelvic limb lameness. Discomfort is apparent on extension of the hip and the range of motion is often decreased. Abduction is generally well tolerated. In some cases, a mass can be palpated caudal to the greater trochanter.

Radiography

In later stages, the mineralized mass can be identified radiographically (Figure 22.29). In earlier cases this can be more challenging and advanced imaging, such as CT or MRI, may be helpful.

Treatment

Many cases can be managed conservatively, but if the lameness persists, surgical resection of the mass should be considered. This usually results in an immediate improvement in the range of motion of the hip. The use of corticosteroids following surgery has been suggested to limit subsequent fibrosis, but there is no published evidence regarding efficacy. Owners should be made aware of the possibility of recurrence.

Iliopsoas myopathy

The psoas muscle groups arise from the ventral surfaces of the caudal thoracic and lumbar vertebrae and run caudally. The psoas minor muscle inserts on the cranioventral aspect of the ilium; the psoas major courses caudally and forms a common tendon with the iliacus muscle, which arises from the ventral aspect of the ilium. The common iliopsoas tendon inserts on the lesser trochanter and acts to flex the hip. Various conditions have been reported affecting the iliopsoas muscle group including traumatic strains, inflammatory conditions such as myositis, chronic conditions such as fibrotic myopathy, and neoplasia. These conditions are relatively uncommon; in the authors' experience, the most frequently encountered is myositis secondary to migrating foreign bodies such as grass awns.

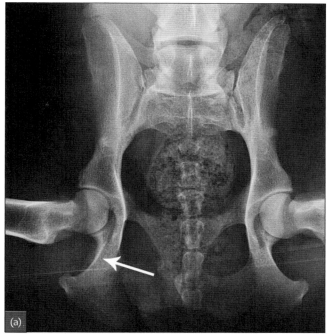

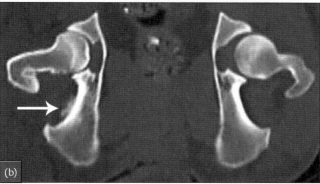

22.29 (a) Ventrodorsal pelvic radiograph of a 5-year-old Dobermann with heterotopic osteochondrofibrosis, showing irregular mineralization of the ischium (arrowed). (b) The changes are more obvious on a CT scan (arrowed).

Affected animals are usually presented with pelvic limb lameness of variable severity. Patients can be affected bilaterally, which can result in a stiff, stilted gait but with less obvious lameness. On clinical examination, discomfort is usually apparent on extension of the hip with concurrent internal rotation of the pelvic limb; abduction of the hip is generally well tolerated. The range of motion of the hip may be decreased in extension. Neurological examination may reveal a diminished or absent patellar reflex; this is because the femoral nerve runs through the psoas muscles and secondary neuritis can be encountered. Important differential diagnoses for diminished patellar reflexes include myelopathies affecting the L4–L6 spinal cord segments, and primary peripheral femoral nerve conditions such as neoplasia.

Diagnosis of conditions affecting the iliopsoas muscle can be challenging. Ultrasonography can reveal pockets of fluid and an abnormal appearance to muscle bellies, but the modality is highly operator dependent. More reliable imaging can be achieved using contrast-enhanced CT or MRI. Fine-needle aspirates of regional tissues can be obtained under ultrasound guidance, but they are often non-diagnostic. Larger samples can be obtained by open surgical biopsy; a lateral trans-ilial approach can be performed.

Treatment depends on the underlying primary cause, but is often medical in the first instance. If medical treatment is unsuccessful or if irreversible fibrosis is present, a ventromedial approach can be made to the lesser trochanter and iliopsoas tenotomy performed. Based on small case numbers, the prognosis for management of iliopsoas fibrotic myopathy by tenotomy appears to be associated with a favourable prognosis (Ragetly et al., 2009).

Neoplasia

Neoplastic conditions affecting the hip are uncommon. Tumours can arise from various tissues including bone, the joint itself and regional soft tissues. Osteosarcoma affecting the pelvis or the proximal femur and soft tissue sarcomas are encountered most frequently. Round cell tumours such as lymphoma or myeloma can also affect tissues adjacent to the hip. Metastatic disease, especially from carcinomas, is rare.

Animals are presented with pelvic limb lameness of variable severity. Discomfort is often elicited on hip manipulation or palpation of regional tissues. Bony lesions can usually be identified using radiography; soft tissue lesions may require the use of advanced imaging, such as contrast-enhanced CT or MRI.

Patients should be thoroughly staged for metastatic disease, and biopsy of the tumour considered; this can be done under ultrasound guidance using Trucut needles, or via an open surgical approach. Cytology following fine-needle aspiration can be helpful in some cases. Lesions affecting bone can be biopsied using Jamshidi™ needles; these can be passed into the femoral head and neck from laterally if necessary, entering the femur immediately distal to the greater trochanter.

Treatment of neoplasia depends on the histological diagnosis and tumour staging; further information can be found in the *BSAVA Manual of Canine and Feline Oncology*. Surgical procedures that may be considered include limb amputation by hip disarticulation, and hemipelvectomy. THR was successfully performed to treat a dog with a fibrosarcoma affecting the femoral head (Scherrer et al., 2005).

Inflammatory conditions of the hip

Although uncommon, inflammatory arthritis, such as infection or immune-mediated disease can occasionally be encountered affecting the hip. The typical clinical picture is an animal with a persistently painful hip joint but with normal radiographic findings, although osteoarthritic joints are predisposed to haematogenous infection and sudden, marked lameness in such cases should prompt consideration of this problem. In chronic cases erosive changes may be seen. Advanced imaging such as MRI can allow identification of a joint effusion and synovial thickening, and can help to exclude other conditions such as neoplasia. Arthrocentesis and synovial fluid analysis allows confirmation of inflammatory arthritis. If infection is present, bacteriology may reveal an underlying aetiological agent. Septic arthritis can usually be treated medically although surgical debridement and placement of topical antibiotics may be indicated in some cases. Most cases of immune-mediated arthritis are treated using immunosuppressive drugs; in rare cases salvage procedures, such as FHNE, or preferably THR, can be considered if cartilage destruction results in an intractably painful joint. Further information can be found in Chapter 6.

Salvage procedures for the hip

Irrespective of the primary cause, chronic hip osteoarthritis is relatively common. In some cases this can be successfully managed with multimodal conservative treatment. If conservative treatment is ineffective, then salvage or palliative surgical procedures should be considered. Salvage surgery includes FHNE and THR; palliative surgery includes acetabular denervation.

Salvage surgery

FHNE (see Operative Technique 22.8) and THR are the most frequently performed surgical interventions for hip dysplasia. Both techniques aim to alleviate joint pain by elimination of bone-on-bone contact between the abnormal femoral head and acetabulum, and can therefore be employed in young dogs with marked hip pain and older dogs with osteoarthritis. The mechanical stability afforded by THR is superior to that following FHNE, a difference that contributes significantly to the overall factor in outcomes between the procedures. Functional outcome following THR is usually excellent, with a return to normal limb loading and gait anticipated (Budsberg et al., 1996). Outcomes following FHNE are less predictable. Although traditionally considered successful in cats and dogs less than 15 kg, a recent study found over 66% of such dogs exhibited long-term lameness, and that 25–33% of these dogs and cats had pain on hip manipulation (Off and Matis, 2010). Outcomes in heavier dogs are perceived to be less favourable, although the procedure can still be successful and should be considered if THR is not possible due to financial constraints or clinical reasons. Indeed, a high rate of owner satisfaction has been reported despite the less than optimal functional outcome following FHNE (Off and Matis, 2010).

Femoral head and neck excision: FHNE was adapted for use in small animals from the original Girdlestone procedure in humans. The femoral head and neck are resected (Figure 22.30), leaving the femur connected to the pelvis by only capsular and muscular attachments. Healing occurs by fibrosis and a pseudarthrosis forms. The process of fibrosis can take several months. Ultimately animals often regain acceptable limb function and owner satisfaction is high, although limb function is unlikely to be normal; most animals will have a decreased range of hip motion, effective limb shortening, muscle atrophy, and a variable level of lameness associated with residual hip instability and/or pain (Off and Matis, 2010). Most patients also exhibit pain on manipulation of the hip in the long term. However, the procedure is relatively straightforward, complications other than imperfect outcome are rare, the procedure can give acceptable results especially if intensive postoperative physiotherapy and aggressive analgesia are provided, and the procedure is much less costly than alternatives such as THR.

A range of factors can influence outcome following FHNE including bodyweight, duration of disease prior to surgery, postoperative care and surgical technique. Patient bodyweight appears to be especially important; animals less than 15 kg often have an acceptable though rarely perfect outcome, whereas in heavier patients the recovery is less predictable. Postoperative care also appears to be important; aggressive analgesia, physiotherapy and hydrotherapy can all lead to improved functional results in the long term. Good surgical technique will improve outcomes, specifically a well oriented osteotomy to minimize the risk

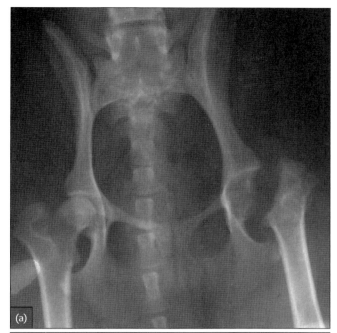

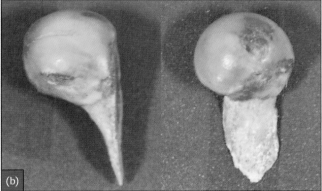

22.30 (a) Postoperative ventrodorsal pelvic radiograph following femoral head and neck excision. (b) The excised portion of bone viewed from a caudal direction (left) and a medial direction (right). Note the obliquity of the osteotomy at the femoral neck.

of postoperative bone-on-bone contact, and a well executed, minimally traumatic surgical approach. Modifications to the surgical technique such as biceps muscle flap interposition between the femur and the pelvis do not appear to improve outcomes and can be associated with an increased risk of complications; therefore such modifications are not currently recommended.

Total hip replacement: As in humans, total joint replacement is considered the gold standard for surgical salvage of the hip in cats and dogs. The procedure involves replacement of both the acetabulum and the femoral head and neck with prosthetic components. The components can be attached to the bone using polymethylmethacrylate (PMMA, or bone cement) or can be implanted in a cementless fashion. For cemented fixation, irregular cavities are created in the pelvis and the femur. PMMA is injected into these cavities, pressurized, and the implant is then placed into the cement. The PMMA hardens and creates a grout that locks the implant to the bone. For cementless fixation precise cavities are created and the implants impacted into these recipient beds. Initial stability is provided by friction or screw fixation; in the long term stability is provided by bone ingrowth into the implants.

Considerable controversy exists regarding cemented and cementless fixation systems. Although cementless systems were first developed in humans to reduce long-term complications such as aseptic loosening of the implants, modern cemented systems often have equivalent or improved results compared with cementless systems. For medium-sized and larger dogs, cemented and cementless systems are available. Comparison of different systems is hampered by weak study design, but in general the outcomes using different systems appear to be largely similar. Hybrid fixation, using a cementless acetabular cup with a cemented femoral stem, is also possible (Figure 22.31); this approach avoids the complications associated with cemented acetabular and cementless femoral components (Gemmill *et al.*, 2011). In veterinary practice at the time of writing, cementless systems are not available for smaller patients such as cats or small dogs although cemented micro and nano systems can be used in these patients. Outcomes using these systems are very good in the hands of experienced surgeons; recovery rates are very rapid and the requirement for postoperative physiotherapy compared with FHNE is decreased. Long-term function is generally excellent (Jankovits *et al.*, 2012).

Complications of THR can include luxation, infection, aseptic loosening, femoral fracture and sciatic neuropraxia. These complications can usually be successfully managed although further surgery may be necessary. Complication rates are somewhat variable but can be as low as 5% in the hands of experienced surgeons.

In contrast to FHNE, THR is more predictable in all sizes of patients and can restore normal kinetic function of the hip and limb. The major determinant of success appears to be the avoidance of complications; this is strongly associated with increased surgeon experience.

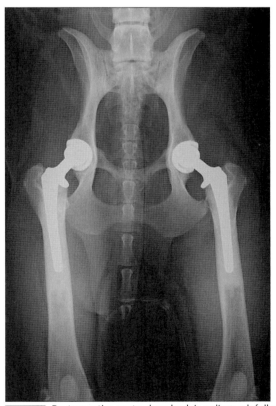

22.31 Postoperative ventrodorsal pelvic radiograph following bilateral hybrid total hip replacement in a Springer Spaniel. The acetabular components are cementless, the femoral components are cemented.

Palliative hip surgery

Hip denervation: Joint denervation has been used successfully for many years to treat articular diseases of the hands and feet in humans and the distal limb in horses. Innervation of the hip joint is by periosteal branches of the cranial gluteal and sciatic nerves craniolaterally, the obturator nerve caudolaterally, the femoral nerve ventrally, and branches from periarticular muscles. It has been proposed in dogs that hip denervation can be achieved by elevation of the periosteum on the craniolateral aspect of the hip via a craniolateral approach. The procedure is relatively simple, has a low risk of complications, and can be performed bilaterally on a single occasion. Although favourable outcomes have been reported for the management of osteoarthritis of the canine hip (Kinzel et al., 2002), a more recent study was less encouraging and demonstrated no improvement in limb function as assessed by force plate (Lister et al., 2009). There are also concerns that denervation may accelerate the progression of osteoarthritis, and that re-innervation of the joint may occur in the long term.

Other palliative techniques: A number of additional techniques have been described including augmentation of the dorsal acetabular rim (e.g. the biocompatible osteoconductive polymer shelf arthroplasty and the dorsal acetabular rim arthroplasty), pectineal my otomy, and intertrochanteric osteotomy. There is currently insufficient evidence to support the use of these techniques and they are not recommended.

References and further reading

Barr ARS, Denny HR and Gibbs C (1987) Clinical hip dysplasia in growing dogs: the long-term results of conservative management. *Journal of Small Animal Practice* **28**, 243–252

Braden TD and Johnson ME (1988) Technique and indications of a prosthetic capsule for repair of recurrent and chronic coxofemoral luxations. *Veterinary and Comparative Orthopaedics and Traumatology* **1**, 26–29

Breur GJ and Blevins WE (1997) Traumatic injury of the iliopsoas muscle in three dogs. *Journal of the American Veterinary Medical Association* **210**, 1631–1634

Budsberg SC, Chambers JN, Lue SL, Foutz TK and Reece L (1996) Prospective evaluation of ground reaction forces in dogs undergoing unilateral total hip replacement. *American Journal of Veterinary Research* **57**, 1781–1785

Caughlan A and Miller A (1998) *BSAVA Manual of Small Animal Fracture Repair and Management*. BSAVA Publications, Gloucester

Craig LE (2001) Physeal dysplasia with slipped capital femoral epiphysis in 13 cats. *Veterinary Pathology* **38**, 92–97

Dobson J and Lascelles D (2011) *BSAVA Manual of Canine and Feline Oncology, 3rd edn*. BSAVA Publications, Gloucester

Dueland RT, Patricelli AJ, Adams WM, Linn KA and Crump PM (2010) Canine hip dysplasia treated by juvenile pubic symphysiodesis. Part II: two year clinical results. *Veterinary and Comparative Orthopaedics and Traumatology* **23**, 318–325

Farese JP, Todhunter RJ, Lust G, Williams AJ and Dykes NL (1998) Dorsolateral subluxation of hip joints in dogs measured in a weight-bearing position with radiography and computed tomography. *Veterinary Surgery* **27**, 393–405

Farrell M, Clements DN, Mellor D et al. (2007) Retrospective evaluation of the long-term outcome of non-surgical management of 74 dogs with clinical hip dysplasia. *Veterinary Record* **160**, 506–511

Gemmill T and Clements D (2016) *BSAVA Manual of Canine and Feline Fracture Repair and Management, 2nd edn*. BSAVA Publications, Gloucester

Gemmill TJ, Pink J, Clarke SP and McKee WM (2012) Total hip replacement for the treatment of atraumatic slipped femoral capital epiphysis in dogs. *Journal of Small Animal Practice* **53**, 453–458

Gemmill TJ, Pink J, Renwick A et al. (2011) Hybrid cemented/cementless total hip replacement in dogs: seventy-eight consecutive joint replacements. *Veterinary Surgery* **40**, 621–630

Greene LM, Marcellin-Little DJ and Lascelles BDX (2013) Associations among exercise duration, lameness severity, and hip joint range of motion in Labrador Retrievers with hip dysplasia. *Journal of the American Veterinary Medical Association* **242**, 1528–1533

Greenwald AS and O'Connor JJ (1971) The transmission of load through the human hip joint. *Journal of Biomechanics* **4(6)**, 507–512

Guilliard M (2014) The Penn Hip method of predicting canine hip dysplasia. *In Practice* **36**, 66–74

Haburjak JJ, Lenehan TN, Harari J et al. (2001) Treatment of traumatic coxofemoral luxation with triple pelvic osteotomy in 19 dogs (1987–1999). *Veterinary and Comparative Orthopaedics and Traumatology* **14**, 69–77

Hohn RB and Janes JM (1969) Pelvic osteotomy in the treatment of canine hip dysplasia. *Clinical Orthopaedics and Related Research* **62**, 70–78

Hoolaway A and McConnell F (2013) *BSAVA Manual of Canine and Feline Radiography and Radiology: A Foundation Manual*. BSAVA Publications, Gloucester

Hou Y, Wang Y, Lust G et al. (2010) Retrospective analysis for genetic improvement of hip joints of cohort Labrador Retrievers in the United States: 1970–2007. *PLoS One* **5**, e9410

Hunt CA and Henry WB Jr. (1985) Transarticular pinning for repair of hip dislocation in the dog: a retrospective study of 40 cases. *Journal of the American Veterinary Medical Association* **187**, 828–833

Impellizeri JA, Tetrick MA and Muir P (2000) Effect of weight reduction on clinical signs of lameness in dogs with hip osteoarthritis. *Journal of the American Veterinary Medical Association* **216**, 1089–1091

Jankovits DA, Liska WD and Kalis RH (2012) Treatment of avascular necrosis of the femoral head in small dogs with micro total hip replacement. *Veterinary Surgery* **41**, 143–147

Kinzel S, Von Scheven C, Buecker A, Stopinski T and Kupper W (2002) Clinical evaluation of denervation of the canine hip joint capsule: a retrospective study of 117 dogs. *Veterinary and Comparative Orthopaedics and Traumatology* **15**, 51–56

Kirberger RM and McEvoy FJ (2016) *BSAVA Manual of Canine and Feline Musculoskeletal Imaging, 2nd edn*. BSAVA Publications, Gloucester

Lewis TW, Blott SC and Woolliams JA (2010) Genetic evaluation of hip score in UK Labrador Retrievers. *PLoS One* **5**, e12797

Lister SA, Roush JK, Renberg WC and Stephens CL (2009) Ground reaction force analysis of unilateral coxofemoral denervation for the treatment of canine hip dysplasia. *Veterinary and Comparative Orthopaedics and Traumatology* **22**, 137–141

Martini FM, Simonazzi B and Del Bue M (2001) Extra-articular absorbable suture stabilization of coxofemoral luxation in dogs. *Veterinary Surgery* **30**, 468–475

McLaughlin RN (1995) Traumatic joint luxations in small animals. *Veterinary Clinics of North America: Small Animal Practice* **25**, 1175–1196

McLaughlin RN, Miller CW, Taves CL et al. (1991) Force plate analysis of triple pelvic osteotomy for the treatment of canine hip dysplasia. *Veterinary Surgery* **20**, 291–297

McNicholas Jr WT, Wilkens BE, Blevins WE et al. (2002) Spontaneous femoral capital physeal fractures in adult cats: 26 cases (1996–2001). *Journal of the American Veterinary Medical Association* **221**, 1731–1736

Moores AL, Moores AP, Brodbelt DC, Owen MR and Draper ERC (2007). Regional load bearing of the canine acetabulum. *Journal of Biomechanics* **16**, 3732–3737

Moores AP, Owen MR, Fews D et al. (2004) Slipped capital femoral epiphysis in dogs. *Journal of Small Animal Practice* **45**, 602–608

Off W and Matis U (2010) Excision arthroplasty of the hip joint in dogs and cats. *Veterinary and Comparative Orthopaedics and Traumatology* **23**, 297–305

Petazzoni M, Tamburro R, Nicetto T and Kowaleski MP (2012) Evaluation of the dorsal acetabular coverage obtained by a modified triple pelvic osteotomy (2.5 pelvic osteotomy): an ex vivo study on a cadaveric canine codel. *Veterinary and Comparative Orthopaedics and Traumatology* **25**, 385–389

Powers MY, Martinez SA, Lincoln JD, Temple CJ and Arnaiz A (2005) Prevalence of cranial cruciate ligament rupture in a population of dogs with lameness previously attributed to hip dysplasia: 369 cases (1994–2003). *Journal of the American Veterinary Medical Association* **227**, 1109–1111

Pozzi A, Kowaleski MP, Dyce J and Johnson KA (2004) Treatment of traumatic coxofemoral luxation by cemented total hip arthroplasty. *Veterinary and Comparative Orthopaedics and Traumatology* **17**, 198–203

Ragetly GR, Griffon DJ, Johnson AL, Blevins WE and Valli VE (2009) Bilateral iliopsoas muscle contracture and spinous process impingement in a German shepherd dog. *Veterinary Surgery* **38**, 946–953

Rasmussen LM, Kramek BA and Lipowitz AJ (1998) Preoperative variables affecting long-term outcome of triple pelvic osteotomy for treatment of naturally developing hip dysplasia in dogs. *Journal of the American Veterinary Medical Association* **213**, 80–85

Robinson R (1992) Legg-Calve-Perthes disease in dogs: genetic aetiology. *Journal of Small Animal Practice* **33**, 275–276

Rochereau P and Bernarde A (2012) Stabilization of coxo-femoral luxation using tenodesis of the deep gluteal muscle. Technique description and reluxation rate in 65 dogs and cats (1995–2008). *Veterinary and Comparative Orthopaedics and Traumatology* **25**, 49–53

Scherrer W, Holsworth I, Goossens M and Schulz K (2005) Coxofemoral arthroscopy and total hip arthroplasty for management of intermediate grade fibrosarcoma in a dog. *Veterinary Surgery* **34**, 43–46

Serdy MB, Schulz KS, Hornof W et al. (1999) Closed toggle pinning for canine traumatic coxofemoral luxation. *Veterinary and Comparative Orthopaedics and Traumatology* **12**, 6–14

Sissener TR, Whitelock RG and Langley-Hobbs SJ (2009) Long-term results of transarticular pinning for surgical stabilisation of coxofemoral luxation in 20 cats. *Journal of Small Animal Practice* **50**, 112–117

Smith GK, Karbe GT, Agnello KA and McDonald-Lynch MB (2012) Pathogenesis, Diagnosis and Control of Canine Hip Dysplasia. In: *Veterinary Surgery Small Animal, Volume 1*, ed. KM Tobias and SA Johnston, pp. 824–848. Elsevier, St Louis, Missouri

Smith GK, Lawler DF, Biery DN *et al.* (2012) Chronology of hip dysplasia development in a cohort of 48 Labrador Retrievers followed for life. *Veterinary Surgery* **41**, 20–33

Smith GK, Mayhew PD, Kapatkin AS *et al.* (2001) Evaluation of risk factors for degenerative joint disease associated with hip dysplasia in German Shepherd Dogs, Golden Retrievers, Labrador Retrievers, and Rottweilers. *Journal of the American Veterinary Medical Association* **219**, 1719–1724

Smith GK, Paster ER, Powers MY *et al.* (2006) Lifelong diet restriction and radiographic evidence of osteoarthritis of the hip joint in dogs. *Journal of the American Veterinary Medical Association* **229**, 690–693

Vasseur PB, Foley P, Stevenson S and Heitter D (1989) Mode of inheritance of Perthes' disease in Manchester Terriers. *Clinical Orthopaedics* **244**, 281–292

Venzin C and Montavon PM (2007) Augmentation of the transverse acetabular ligament in canine caudoventral hip luxation. *Veterinary and Comparative Orthopedics and Traumatology* **20**, 320–323

Vezzoni A, Dravelli G, Corbari A *et al.* (2005) Early diagnosis of canine hip dysplasia. *The European Journal of Companion Animal Practice* **15**, 173–184

IMAGING TECHNIQUES

Thomas W. Maddox

Much of the musculoskeletal pathology affecting the hip is related to the osseous components and so radiography is the main modality employed for imaging, although CT is equally valuable and offers some advantages. Most of the significant conditions will be adequately observed on MRI, but this is not often used specifically for imaging of the hip.

RADIOGRAPHY

Standard views

The standard radiographic views obtained of the hips/pelvis are the extended ventrodorsal and lateral views.

Ventrodorsal view (extended)

This view is the standard for assessment of the coxofemoral joints, especially with regard to subluxation.

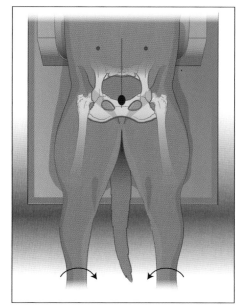

* The animal is placed in dorsal recumbency and stabilized with a trough, sandbags or wedges; care should be taken to ensure the animal is as straight as possible (Figure 22.32).
* A grid should be used for any animal larger than a cat or small dog.
* Both pelvic limbs are fully and symmetrically extended with the femora parallel.
* The stifles should be internally rotated so the patellae are positioned centrally over the distal femora and then secured with tape or ties.
* The primary beam is centred on the midline at the level of the greater trochanters.
* Collimate to include the iliac crests cranially, caudally to the mid-femur or stifles and laterally to the skin margins.

The resultant radiograph should be carefully scrutinized for evidence of axial rotation as malpositioning is common and can exaggerate or minimize the appearance of disease. The shape and size of the obturator foramina and iliac wings can be compared for symmetry. Axial rotation can be corrected by raising the side of the pelvis with the smaller obturator foramen and wider iliac wing. Palpation of the greater trochanters to assess height from the table top during radiography is useful to assess for symmetrical positioning.

22.32 Patient positioning for a ventrodorsal view of the hip and pelvis; the black dot indicates the centring point.

Lateral view

This view results in superimposition of the coxofemoral joints but is the orthogonal projection for the ventrodorsal view. If one side is affected, then this side is placed against the cassette/plate in order to minimize magnification and maximize sharpness.

* The patient is placed in lateral recumbency with the pelvic limbs in a neutral position and foam padding between the stifles (Figure 22.33).
* A wedge can be placed underneath the sternum to minimize rotation of the body.

→ IMAGING TECHNIQUES CONTINUED

- The primary beam is centred on the greater trochanter.
- Collimate to include the iliac crest cranially and dorsally, the ischiatic tuberosity caudally and the proximal third of the femur ventrally/distally.

Special views

Flexed ventrodorsal view

Also known as the 'frog-legged' view, this is useful if the animal is in too much pain to allow full extension or if the hip joints only have a limited range of motion. Assessment of coxofemoral subluxation is less reliable, but it provides good visualization of the femoral head and neck and is valuable for the detection of fractures of these structures and other articular fractures.

- The animal is positioned as for an extended ventrodorsal view but the pelvic limbs are allowed to relax into a neutral position (limbs should still be symmetrically positioned) (Figure 22.34).
- Centre and collimate as for the extended ventrodorsal view.

If there is clinical evidence of significant hip pain and no abnormalities are detected on the extended ventrodorsal view, then it is recommended to obtain the flexed view.

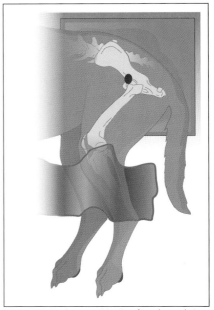

22.33 Patient positioning for a lateral view of the hip and pelvis.

Lateral view of index hip

This overcomes the problem of superimposition of the coxofemoral joints.

- The animal is positioned as for the lateral view, with the target limb against the cassette/plate.
- The unaffected limb is abducted out of the primary beam (Figure 22.35).
- Centre and collimate approximately as for the lateral view; it is normally possible to palpate the hip joint and centre directly on it.

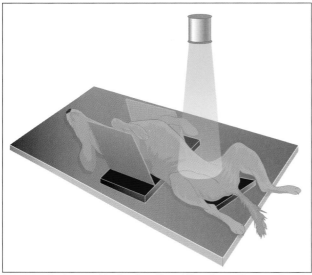

22.34 Patient positioning for a flexed (frog-legged) ventrodorsal view of the hip and pelvis.

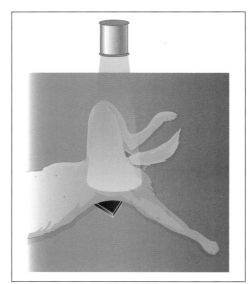

22.35 Patient positioning for a lateral view of one hip joint.

COMPUTED TOMOGRAPHY

CT will allow excellent assessment of bony lesions, although unfamiliarity can initially make assessment of conditions such as hip dysplasia more difficult. The ability to reformat images means that positioning is less critical than for radiography, although gross malpositioning will still compromise assessment. The availability of multiplanar and three-dimensional reconstructions can significantly enhance the understanding of the morphology of pelvic fractures.

→ **IMAGING TECHNIQUES CONTINUED**

Standard technique

Acquisition times are sufficiently short that examination may normally be carried out under sedation, but animals with very painful hips may require the use of general anaesthesia.

- The animal can be placed in ventral or dorsal recumbency and the hip joint flexed or mildly extended (orientation of the entirety of the femora in the same plane as the coxofemoral joints should be avoided as it can result in significant photon starvation artefact).
- The scan margins should extend from the iliac crest to the caudal perineum.
- Reconstruction using a bone (and usually soft tissue) algorithm is recommended.

  Transverse planes images are usually the most useful, but multiplanar reconstructions may also be beneficial.

Magnetic resonance imaging and ultrasonography

The hips can be adequately evaluated with MRI, but the modality is rarely used solely for this purpose. Both MRI and ultrasonography have more value in assessing the surrounding muscles and soft tissues, such as the iliopsoas muscle (Breur and Blevins, 1997; Ragetly *et al.*, 2009).

OPERATIVE TECHNIQUE 22.1

Craniolateral approach to the hip

INDICATIONS

Fractures of the femoral head and neck, and the cranial aspect of the acetabulum; open reduction of dorsal or ventral hip luxation; femoral head and neck excision; total hip replacement.

POSITIONING

Lateral recumbency with the affected limb uppermost. It can be useful to secure the patient to the surgical table using tape and a sling passed around the dependent limb and pelvis; this allows traction to be placed on the affected limb during surgery. The hair should be clipped dorsally beyond the midline and distally to at least the level of the tarsus. The limb is draped in a four-quarter fashion and the paw wrapped in a sterile shroud.

ASSISTANT

Useful.

EQUIPMENT EXTRAS

Gelpi self-retaining retractors; hand-held Langenbeck and Hohmann retractors.

SURGICAL TECHNIQUE

The greater trochanter is identified and its proximodistal height estimated by palpation; this distance will be the central third of the incision. The skin incision begins dorsally, courses over the cranial aspect of the greater trochanter and extends distally, towards the patella. Loose fascia and fat is dissected and Gelpi retractors applied to reveal the fascia lata and the biceps femoris muscle. The superficial fascia lata is incised along the cranial border of the biceps femoris muscle (Figure 22.36a). Further loose fascia is dissected to reveal the deep layer of the fascia lata, which is incised along the junction between the tensor fasciae latae and the superficial gluteal muscles; this incision is extended distally along the caudal border of the tensor fasciae latae muscle for the full length of the skin incision. The superficial and middle gluteal muscles can then be retracted dorsally and the tensor fasciae latae cranially, using Langenbeck retractors. The deep gluteal tendon of insertion is then identified as it attaches on the greater trochanter; this has a characteristic silver appearance. This is separated from the underlying joint capsule using a periosteal elevator. If necessary, additional exposure can be obtained by making an inverted L-shaped incision in the tendon before it is retracted cranially (Figure 22.36b). Sufficient tissue should be left at the insertion on the proximal femur to allow sutures to be

→ **OPERATIVE TECHNIQUE 22.1 CONTINUED**

placed to repair the tenotomy. If this additional tenotomy is not performed, the tendon is retracted dorsally using the Langenbeck retractor. The femoral head and neck is then identified by palpation, and using a sharp blade, a longitudinal incision is made from the acetabulum extending laterally across the femoral head and down on to the base of the femoral neck. In most cases, the incision is extended laterally into the origin of the vastus medialis and intermedius; these muscles can then be retracted distally to expose the femoral neck.

If necessary, the hip is luxated by firm external rotation of the femur. The ligament of the femoral head can be cut most easily using a Hatt spoon; alternatively, a disarticulator or curved Mayo scissors can be used. Ensuring adequate external rotation of the femur and placement of Hohmann retractors under the femoral head and neck can assist with exposure at this stage (Figure 22.36c).

WARNING
Avoid excessive dissection caudally under the biceps femoris muscle; this would take the approach directly on to the sciatic nerve

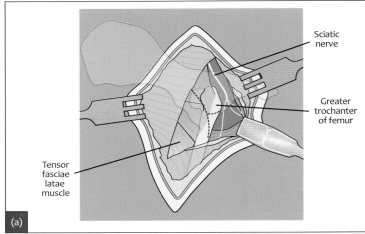

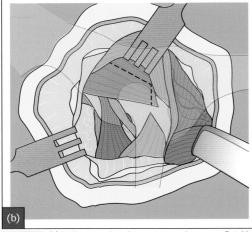

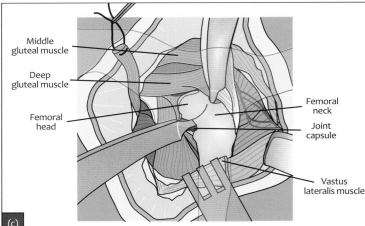

22.36 (a) Following the skin incision, the superficial layer of the fascia lata is incised along the cranial border of the biceps femoris muscle which is retracted caudally. The deep layer of the fascia lata is then incised along the junction between the tensor fasciae latae and the superficial gluteal muscles; this incision is extended distally, caudal to the tensor fasciae latae (dotted line). (b) The superficial and middle gluteal muscles are retracted dorsally to reveal the deep gluteal tendon. To improve exposure, this can be incised using an inverse 'L' shaped incision if necessary (dotted line). (c) The joint capsule is incised parallel to the femoral neck. External rotation of the femur and placement of Hohmann retractors allows exposure of the femoral head and neck.

Closure

The joint capsule and origin of the vastus muscles are sutured using cruciate mattress sutures. The deep gluteal tenotomy is repaired using a suitable tendon suture pattern, most commonly a locking loop pattern. The deep and superficial layers of the fascia lata are then closed using continuous sutures before routine closure of the superficial layers and skin.

POSTOPERATIVE CARE

Depends on underlying condition and surgical procedure performed.

COMPLICATIONS

Depends on underlying condition and surgical procedure performed.

OPERATIVE TECHNIQUE 22.2

Dorsal approach to the hip

INDICATIONS

Open reduction of dorsal hip luxation; complex fractures of the femoral head; central and caudal fractures of the acetabulum.

POSITIONING

Lateral recumbency with the affected limb uppermost, as in Operative Technique 22.1.

ASSISTANT

Useful.

EQUIPMENT EXTRAS

Gelpi self-retaining retractors; hand-held Langenbeck and Hohmann retractors; oscillating saw or sharp osteotome and mallet; Kirschner wires and orthopaedic wire; drill.

SURGICAL TECHNIQUE

The initial approach is identical to Operative Technique 22.1. Following incision of the deep layer of the tensor fasciae latae, the biceps femoris muscle is retracted caudally and the superficial gluteal tendon sectioned close to its insertion on the third trochanter, leaving sufficient tissue to allow closure. The origin of the vastus lateralis muscle is incised and retracted distally.

The greater trochanter is then exposed and blunt dissection continued caudally, taking care to avoid the sciatic nerve. A straight haemostat is then passed from caudal to cranial, medial to the greater trochanter and deep to the insertion of the middle and deep gluteal tendons (Figure 22.37a). The base of the greater trochanter is then identified and the greater trochanter osteotomy performed in a distolateral to proximomedial direction, aiming towards the pre-placed haemostat (Figure 22.37b). Further soft tissue attachments are then cut and the greater trochanteric fragment retracted dorsally (Figure 22.37c). If necessary, the internal obturator tendon can be cut and retracted caudodorsally; this allows atraumatic retraction of the sciatic nerve and improves exposure of the caudal aspect of the acetabulum. An incision can now be made into the joint capsule if necessary.

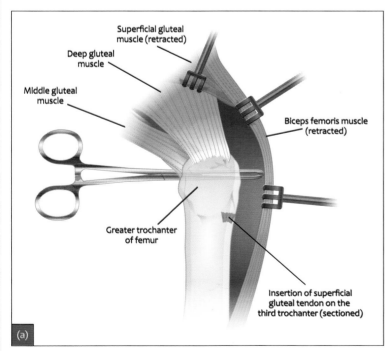

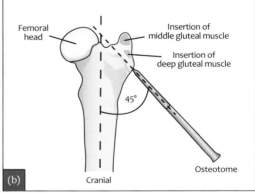

22.37 Osteotomy of the greater trochanter.
(a) Following retraction of the biceps femoris and superficial gluteal muscles, an instrument is placed medial to the greater trochanter deep to the insertions of the middle and deep gluteal tendons. (b) A 45-degree osteotomy of the greater trochanter is performed, starting at the base of the trochanter and aiming proximomedially. (continues) ▶

➡

→ **OPERATIVE TECHNIQUE 22.2 CONTINUED**

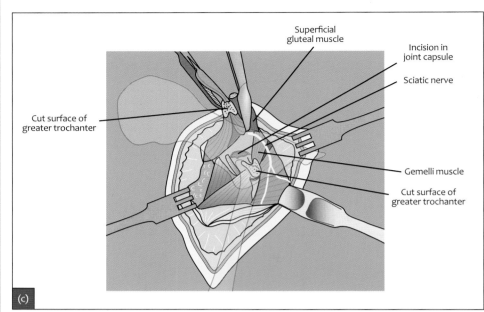

Superficial gluteal muscle

Incision in joint capsule

Sciatic nerve

Cut surface of greater trochanter

Gemelli muscle

Cut surface of greater trochanter

(c)

22.37 (continued) Osteotomy of the greater trochanter. (c) The greater trochanter can then be retracted proximally.

Alternative technique

In young animals with open proximal femoral physes, tenotomy of the gluteal tendons at their insertion on the greater trochanter can allow adequate exposure and an osteotomy can be avoided. Exposure using this technique is inferior to that achieved using an osteotomy.

> **WARNING**
>
> Great care must be taken to avoid damaging the sciatic nerve during dissection or retraction

Closure

The joint capsule is repaired using cruciate mattress sutures, and the external hip rotator tendons using a suitable tendon holding pattern such as a locking loop.

The greater trochanteric osteotomy is stabilized using pins and tension-band wire. The fragment is held in position either manually or using pointed forceps. Two K-wires are then driven into the fragment at an angle of approximately 45 degrees to the long axis of the bone; the wires should engage the medial cortex of the femur in the region of the lesser trochanter. Following a longitudinal incision in the vastus lateralis and soft tissue retraction, a transverse bone tunnel is drilled from cranial to caudal through the femoral diaphysis. The distance between the K-wires and the distal extent of the osteotomy is measured; using the distal extent of the osteotomy as a reference, the bone tunnel should be located at least the same distance distally. A length of orthopaedic wire is placed through the bone tunnel and around the K-wires in a figure-of-eight pattern. The tension-band is tightened using two twist knots. The twist knots and the K-wires are then bent over and cut short.

The superficial gluteal tendon is reattached using a tendon holding pattern. The deep and superficial layers of the fascia lata and superficial tissues are closed in layers.

POSTOPERATIVE CARE

Depends on underlying condition and surgical procedure performed.

COMPLICATIONS

Depends on underlying condition and surgical procedure performed.

OPERATIVE TECHNIQUE 22.3

Ventral approach to the hip

INDICATIONS

Open reduction of ventral luxation of the hip.

POSITIONING

Dorsal recumbancy with the hindlimbs in a 'frog-legged' position. The affected limb should be four-quarter draped with the paw covered in a sterile shroud to allow manipulation during surgery; the contralateral limb can be loosely secured using tape or rope ties. The hair should be clipped well beyond the ventral midline.

ASSISTANT

Useful.

EQUIPMENT EXTRAS

Gelpi self-retaining retractors; hand-held Langenbeck retractors.

SURGICAL TECHNIQUE

A longitudinal incision is made over the pectineus muscle, starting just lateral to the ventral midline and extending distally. The pectineus tendon can be sectioned at its insertion on the pubis, if necessary, to improve exposure. Blunt dissection through loose fascia allows exposure of the joint capsule. The joint capsule is incised in a craniocaudal direction.

WARNING

Great care is needed to avoid multiple branches of the femoral artery and vein, the proximal circumflex femoral vessels, and the femoral and obturator nerves

Closure

The joint capsule is closed with cruciate mattress sutures. The pectineus tendon is left unsutured. The superficial layers are closed routinely. Intradermal sutures are preferred to avoid the challenges associated with removal of skin sutures in this region.

POSTOPERATIVE CARE

Depends on underlying condition and surgical procedure performed.

COMPLICATIONS

Depends on underlying condition and surgical procedure performed.

OPERATIVE TECHNIQUE 22.4

Hip toggle

INDICATIONS

Open reduction and stabilization of dorsal or ventral coxofemoral luxation.

POSITIONING AND APPROACH

Lateral recumbency with the affected limb uppermost; craniolateral approach as described in Operative Technique 22.1. It is easier to perform the approach if the luxation is first reduced, although this is not possible in every case. It is usually unnecessary to perform a deep gluteal tenotomy. An additional longitudinal incision is made on the vastus lateralis muscle to expose the lateral aspect of the femur immediately distal to the greater trochanter.

ASSISTANT

Useful.

EQUIPMENT EXTRAS

Gelpi self-retaining retractors; hand-held Langenbeck and Hohmann retractors; drill and drill bits; drill aiming device; hip toggle.

SURGICAL TECHNIQUE

Following the initial approach, the first step is to create a bone tunnel through the femoral head and neck. On the lateral aspect of the femur, the site for starting the bone tunnel is identified immediately distal to the distal extent of the greater trochanter. A small drill bit is used to mark the bone at this site with a mono-cortical hole. The femur is then externally rotated through 90 degrees and Hohmann retractors placed to expose the femoral head. The fovea capitis is identified and the remnants of the ligament of the femoral head removed. The femoral head is marked at this point with a mono-cortical hole using a small drill bit. The tip of an aiming device is then placed into the hole in the femoral head, and the femur rotated internally to allow exposure of the lateral entry point. Using the aiming device a hole is then drilled through the femoral head and neck in a lateral to medial direction (Figure 22.38).

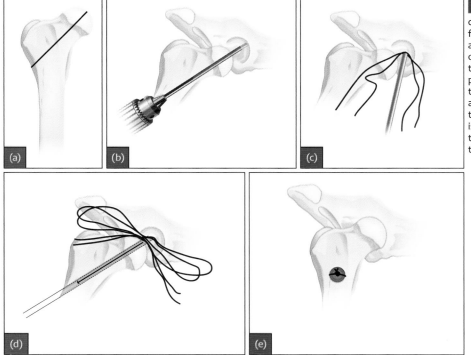

22.38 Toggle stabilization for hip luxation. (a) A bone tunnel is drilled along the femoral neck, running from the base of the greater trochanter and exiting the bone at the fovea capitis of the femoral head. (b) A hole is drilled in the acetabular fossa. (c) The toggle rod is placed through the acetabular hole into the pelvic canal. Pulling on the sutures allows the rod to be positioned against the medial acetabular wall. (d) The suture is passed through the femoral bone tunnel. (e) Following reduction of the hip, the suture is secured laterally to a button.

→ **OPERATIVE TECHNIQUE 22.4 CONTINUED**

> **PRACTICAL TIP**
>
> It is usually easier to use a small drill bit initially, and then to over-drill the hole using the appropriate slightly larger drill bit. The final size of the bone tunnel ranges from 1.8 mm to 2.7 mm depending on the size of the patient

The femur is then retracted caudodorsally to expose the acetabulum, and the remnants of the ligament of the femoral head are removed to expose the trochanteric fossa. A hole is drilled into the pelvic canal through the fossa, taking to care to avoid damaging the underlying pelvic viscera.

The toggle suture is then placed on to the toggle pin, which is pushed through the drill hole in the acetabular fossa. Gentle pulling on the suture allows the toggle pin to rotate and engage on the medial aspect of the medial acetabular wall. The toggle suture is then pulled through the femoral bone tunnel using a straight needle, twisted piece of wire or a piece of stiff suture material. The femoral head is relocated in the acetabulum and maintained by application of lateral to medial pressure. The ends of the toggle suture are secured on the lateral aspect of the femur using another toggle pin or a polyethylene button.

> **PRACTICAL TIP**
>
> Although the toggle pin can be made from a twisted K-wire, a commercially available toggle rod is easier to use

> **PRACTICAL TIP**
>
> In most cases, a strong, large gauge, non-absorbable suture material is used. Monofilament leader line is popular but can lead to osteolysis of the femoral neck; braided materials such as polyester or polyethylene are also suitable, but great care is needed to maintain asepsis when using these materials

Closure

A secure capsular closure can add significantly to the stability of the hip, although in some cases capsular trauma will preclude this. If possible, the capsule is closed using a cruciate mattress pattern. The deep gluteal tendon is repaired using a suitable tendon holding suture pattern. The superficial layers are closed routinely.

POSTOPERATIVE CARE

Radiographs are obtained to document appropriate placement of the toggle and reduction of the hip. Strict rest is recommended to allow healing of the joint capsule, although short lead walks can be allowed. Exercise is gradually increased after 6 weeks, provided clinical progress is satisfactory.

COMPLICATIONS

The most common complication is re-luxation of the hip, which is seen in around 10–15% of cases. This generally necessitates revision surgery, either to restabilize the hip or to perform a salvage procedure. Other complications are less common but can include sciatic nerve damage or infection. Infection appears to be more common if permanent braided suture materials are used.

OPERATIVE TECHNIQUE 22.5

Iliofemoral suture

INDICATIONS

Open reduction and stabilization of dorsal coxofemoral luxation.

POSITIONING AND APPROACH

Lateral recumbency with the affected limb uppermost; craniolateral approach as described in Operative Technique 22.1. It is usually not necessary to perform a deep gluteal tenotomy.

ASSISTANT

Useful.

EQUIPMENT EXTRAS

Gelpi self-retaining retractors; hand-held Langenbeck and Hohmann retractors; drill and drill bits; ± screws and washers; ± suture anchor.

SURGICAL TECHNIQUE

Following exposure of the hip, the remnants of the ligament of the femoral head are removed from the femoral head and the acetabulum. The hip is then reduced. Reduction is maintained using medial pressure on the greater trochanter. The joint capsule is sutured, if possible.

The site for placement of the iliofemoral suture on the ilium is identified, immediately dorsal to the origin of the rectus femoris muscle on the iliopubic eminence. There are various options for securing the suture.

- A bone tunnel can be drilled through the ventral aspect of the ilium in a dorsolateral to ventromedial direction to allow passage of the suture material. This can give a secure anchor point, but it can be difficult to retrieve the suture end after passage through the tunnel.
- A screw and washer or suture anchor can be placed immediately dorsal to the origin of the rectus femoris muscle. This is relatively straightforward, although most suture anchors or cortical screws have a tendency to cut through the suture material. This might be avoided by use of a 4.0 mm partially threaded cancellous screw and washer; the suture is attached around the smooth part of the screw.
- A single bone tunnel can be drilled in a direct lateral to medial direction and a hip toggle placed in a similar fashion to that described in Operative Technique 22.4.
- Using a curved needle, the suture can be placed through the origin of the rectus femoris muscle, immediately adjacent to the bone.

To attach the suture to the greater trochanter, two small drill tunnels, 1.5–2.0 mm, can be drilled through the base of the trochanter; the femur is internally rotated and drilled in a caudal to cranial direction to avoid traumatizing the sciatic nerve. The suture can be placed from caudal to cranial through one tunnel, attached to the ilial anchor point, and then passed cranial to caudal through the second tunnel (Figure 22.39). Alternative techniques include placement of the suture through a single tunnel with the second end of the suture passed lateral to the trochanter, or passage of the suture medial to the trochanter with the second end passed laterally. Whichever method is selected, it is easiest if the knot between the two suture ends is positioned caudal to the trochanter rather than between the trochanter and the ilium.

The femur is then internally rotated with the hip reduced, and held by an assistant while the suture is tightened and knotted.

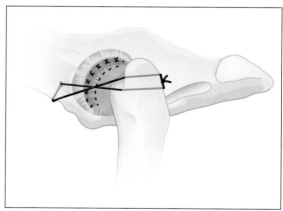

22.39 Iliofemoral suture. The suture is placed from the greater trochanter to the pelvis in the region of the origin of the rectus femoris muscle. Tightening the suture with internal rotation of the femur maintains reduction of the hip.

→ **OPERATIVE TECHNIQUE 22.5 CONTINUED**

PRACTICAL TIP

In most cases, a strong, large gauge, non-absorbable suture material is used. Monofilament leader line is popular but can lead to osteolysis if placed through bone tunnels; braided materials such as polyester or polyethylene are also suitable, but great care is needed to maintain asepsis when using these. Use of absorbable materials such as polydioxanone or polyglactin 910 has been described, but early breakage of these materials may lead to recurrence of the luxation

---

Closure

The deep gluteal tendon is repaired using a suitable tendon holding pattern. Routine closure of the fascia lata and superficial layers is then performed.

POSTOPERATIVE CARE

Radiographs are obtained to document reduction of the hip. Strict rest is recommended for around 6 weeks to allow healing of the joint capsule, although short lead walks can be allowed. The pelvic limb is held internally rotated for a few weeks following surgery, but then a more normal posture is regained, presumably as the suture stretches or breaks. Exercise is gradually increased after 6 weeks provided clinical progress is satisfactory.

COMPLICATIONS

The most common complication is re-luxation of the hip, which is seen in around 10–15% of cases. This generally necessitates revision surgery, either to restabilize the hip or to perform a salvage procedure. Other complications are less common but can include sciatic nerve damage or infection. Infection appears to be more common if permanent braided suture materials are used.

OPERATIVE TECHNIQUE 22.6

Transarticular pin

INDICATIONS

Open reduction and stabilization of dorsal or ventral coxofemoral luxation.

POSITIONING AND APPROACH

Lateral recumbency with the affected limb uppermost; craniolateral approach as described in Operative Technique 22.1. It is usually unnecessary to perform a deep gluteal tenotomy. An additional longitudinal incision is made on the vastus lateralis muscle to expose the lateral aspect of the femur immediately distal to the greater trochanter.

ASSISTANT

Useful.

EQUIPMENT EXTRAS

Gelpi self-retaining retractors; hand-held Langenbeck and Hohmann retractors; drill and drill bits; drill aiming device; Steinmann pins.

SURGICAL TECHNIQUE

Following the initial approach, the first step is to create a bone tunnel through the femoral head and neck. On the lateral aspect of the femur, the site for starting the bone tunnel is identified immediately distal to the base of the greater trochanter. A small drill bit is used the mark the bone at this site with a mono-cortical hole. The femur is then externally rotated through 90 degrees and Hohmann retractors placed to expose the femoral head. The fovea ➡

→ **OPERATIVE TECHNIQUE 22.6 CONTINUED**

capitis is identified and the remnants of the ligament of the femoral head removed. The femoral head is marked at this point with a mono-cortical hole using a small drill bit. The tip of an aiming device is then placed into the hole in the femoral head, and the femur rotated internally to allow exposure of the lateral entry point. Using the aiming device, a hole is then drilled through the femoral head and neck in a lateral to medial direction. The appropriate pin is then selected and is driven from lateral to medial through the tunnel until the tip is just present at the articular surface.

PRACTICAL TIP

Pin size can range from 1.6 mm in small cats up to 3.5 mm in larger dogs

PRACTICAL TIP

It is usually easier to use a small drill bit initially, and then to over-drill the hole using the appropriate slightly larger drill bit. The final size of the bone tunnel should be slightly smaller than the diameter of the pin which will be used

The femur is then retracted caudodorsally to expose the acetabulum, and the remnants of the ligament of the femoral head are removed to expose the trochanteric fossa. The hip is reduced; reduction is maintained by application of medial pressure to the greater trochanter. With the limb held in slight internal rotation and abduction, the pin is driven across the joint space and through the medial acetabular wall. The end of the pin is then bent over, taking care not to move the pin in or out of the femur, and the pin cut short; it can be left relatively proud so that identification for removal several weeks later is easy (Figure 21.40).

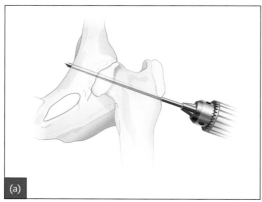
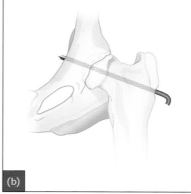

22.40 Transarticular pin. The pin is driven through a pilot hole drilled along the femoral neck. The entry point for the pin is the base of the greater trochanter; the exit point is the fovea capitis. (a) Following reduction of the hip, the pin is driven just through the medial acetabular wall. (b) The end of the pin is then bent over to prevent migration into the pelvis.

PRACTICAL TIP

The distance between the femoral head and the medial acetabular wall can be estimated from preoperative radiographs of the contralateral intact hip. The tip of the pin should penetrate into the pelvic canal by a few millimetres. If there is any doubt regarding the length of the pin, an unscrubbed assistant can perform a gloved digital rectal examination to check the pin is not too long

Closure

A secure capsular closure can add significantly to the stability of the hip, although in some cases capsular trauma will preclude this. If possible, the capsule is closed using a cruciate mattress pattern. The deep gluteal tendon is repaired using a suitable tendon holding suture pattern. The superficial layers are closed routinely.

POSTOPERATIVE CARE

Radiographs are obtained to document appropriate placement of the pin and reduction of the hip. Strict rest is recommended postoperatively. The pin is removed via a limited lateral approach after around 4 weeks. Exercise is gradually increased thereafter, provided clinical progress is satisfactory.

COMPLICATIONS

Re-luxation of the hip can occur if pin breakage or retrograde migration occurs. This generally necessitates revision surgery, either to re-stablize the hip or to perform a salvage procedure. Antegrade pin migration could cause devastating damage to pelvic viscera, but is avoided by bending over the pin end. Other complications are less common but can include sciatic nerve damage or infection.

OPERATIVE TECHNIQUE 22.7

Dorsal capsular sling

INDICATIONS

Open reduction and stabilization of dorsal coxofemoral luxation.

POSITIONING AND APPROACH

Lateral recumbency with the affected limb uppermost; a dorsal approach (see Operative Technique 22.2) is usually made. It is possible to perform the procedure via a craniolateral approach (see Operative Technique 22.1) but this can be more challenging.

ASSISTANT

Useful.

EQUIPMENT EXTRAS

Gelpi self-retaining retractors; hand-held Langenbeck and Hohmann retractors; drill and drill bits; K-wires; orthopaedic wire; ± screws and washers; ± suture anchors.

SURGICAL TECHNIQUE

Following exposure of the hip, the remnants of the ligament of the femoral head are cleared from the femoral head and the acetabulum. The hip is reduced. The sites for attachment of the dorsal capsular sutures are then identified on the dorsal acetabular bone at the ten and two o'clock positions. Various options exist for attachment of the sutures.

- Screws and washers – These are simple to place, although the threads of the cortical screws can cut through the sutures; this problem can be reduced by the use of partially threaded cancellous screws and washers.
- Suture anchors – These are simple to apply, although most suture anchors have relatively sharp edges which can cut through the sutures.

> **PRACTICAL TIP**
>
> Check the range of motion of the hip after placement of each screw or suture anchor to make sure the joint has not been compromised. If necessary, the hip can be probed using a blunt instrument

Bone tunnels are drilled from cranial to caudal through the dorsal aspect of the femoral neck for attachment of the sutures on the femur. Reduction of the hip is checked and the joint capsule repaired, if possible. The dorsal sutures are placed between the pelvic anchor points and the bone tunnels in the femoral neck (see Figure 22.25). The limb should be held in slight abduction as the knots are tightened.

> **PRACTICAL TIP**
>
> Heavy gauge, long-acting or non-absorbable suture material is used. If braided non-absorbable material is used great care is needed to maintain asepsis as these materials are associated with a higher risk of postoperative infection

The trochanteric osteotomy is then stabilized using pins and a tension-band wire as described in Operative Technique 22.2. In larger dogs, it is possible to reattach the greater trochanter in a slightly more caudal and distal location (Figure 22.41); this increases tension in the gluteal tendons, internally rotating the hip and improving stability.

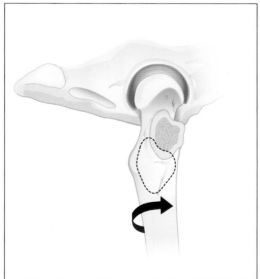

22.41 Following a dorsolateral approach to the hip, the greater trochanter can be reattached in a slightly caudal and distal location in larger dogs. This increases tension in the gluteal tendons, internally rotating the hip and improving stability.

→ **OPERATIVE TECHNIQUE 22.7 CONTINUED**

Closure

Routine closure of the superficial layers.

POSTOPERATIVE CARE

Radiographs are obtained to document appropriate placement of the implants and reduction of the hip. Strict rest is recommended for 6 weeks postoperatively. Exercise is gradually increased thereafter, provided clinical progress is satisfactory.

COMPLICATIONS

Re-luxation is the most common complication, seen in around 10–15% of cases. This can lead to rapid erosion of the femoral head which impinges on the acetabular screws and necessitates revision surgery, either to restabilize the hip or to perform a salvage procedure. Other complications are less common but can include sciatic nerve damage, infection, or failure of fixation of the trochanteric osteotomy. Radiographically, a degree of osteolysis of the greater trochanter is common but is rarely associated with any clinical signs.

OPERATIVE TECHNIQUE 22.8

Femoral head and neck excision

INDICATIONS

Salvage of any painful condition of the hip that cannot be managed by alternative means, excluding locally invasive neoplasia. Femoral head and neck excision gives a less predictable outcome than total hip replacement, regardless of patient size. While the procedure is technically much more straightforward, strict attention to detail, in particular with regard to the position and orientation of the line of osteotomy, is vital.

POSITIONING AND APPROACH

Lateral recumbency with the affected limb uppermost; craniolateral approach as described in Operative Technique 22.1. It is helpful to perform a deep gluteal tenotomy in most cases.

ASSISTANT

Useful but not essential.

EQUIPMENT EXTRAS

Gelpi self-retaining retractors; hand-held Langenbeck and Hohmann retractors; oscillating saw or osteotome and mallet.

SURGICAL TECHNIQUE

The hip is luxated and the femur externally rotated by 90 degrees. It is extremely important that the femur is maintained in this orientation throughout the procedure, to avoid the osteotomy being performed at an inappropriate angle. Exposure is assisted by placement of two or three Hohmann retractors under the femoral head and neck (see Figure 22.36c). It is important to expose the femoral neck as well as the femoral head. The capsular incision is continued along the cranial aspect of the femoral neck immediately distal to the small ridge of bone marking the origin of the vastus medialis and intermedius, ending at the craniolateral aspect of the femur. The joint capsule and vastus muscles should be elevated from the femoral neck and retracted distally. It is helpful to palpate the lesser trochanter on the medial aspect of the bone; this marks the distal extent of the osteotomy.

The site for the osteotomy is then identified, beginning at the proximal aspect of the femoral neck immediately medial to the greater trochanter, and extending distomedially towards the proximal aspect of the lesser trochanter (Figure 22.42).

With the femur held externally rotated by 90 degrees with the patella uppermost, the osteotomy is made aiming directly at the floor. If the patient is positioned securely in true lateral recumbency and the femur is held

→ **OPERATIVE TECHNIQUE 22.8 CONTINUED**

appropriately, this should be in the true craniocaudal plane. Any anteversion of the femoral neck should be ignored. An oscillating saw is preferred, but if this is unavailable a sharp osteotome and mallet can be used. If an osteotome is used it should be aimed in a craniocaudal direction with respect to the femur, never proximodistally as this can lead to a spiral fracture of the femur. Use of a Gigli wire is not advisable as the wire tends to slip medially and proximally and therefore the femoral neck is not resected adequately. Once the osteotomy is complete, the femoral head can be grasped with pointed forceps, any remaining capsular attachments cut using curved Mayo scissors or a sharp blade, and the fragment removed.

The osteotomy should be carefully checked and palpated. It should exit the bone distally immediately proximal to the lesser trochanter, and there should be no sharp spikes of bone caudally. If any unwanted bone remains it can be removed at this stage using an oscillating saw, rongeurs or a rasp. The femur is then returned to a normal weight-bearing position and the hip checked for range of motion and any evidence of impingement or crepitus.

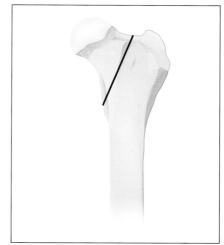

22.42 Femoral head and neck excision. It is very important that the femur is externally rotated by 90 degrees and oriented so the stifle is pointing at the ceiling of the room. The osteotomy is made along a line starting medial to the greater trochanter and ending immediately proximal to the lesser trochanter.

> **PRACTICAL TIP**
>
> The lesser trochanter should not be mistaken for a remaining spike of bone at the base of the femoral neck. These can be differentiated by identifying the iliopsoas muscle that inserts on the lesser trochanter

> **PRACTICAL TIP**
>
> Techniques have been described to interpose soft tissues between the femur and the pelvis, such as biceps femoris muscle flaps. These techniques will increase surgical time, morbidity and complications and are not recommended

Closure

As described for Operative Technique 22.1.

POSTOPERATIVE CARE

Postoperative radiographs are usually obtained to check the orientation of the osteotomy. Early controlled use of the operated limb is encouraged by allowing slow lead walks. Aggressive analgesia is provided for the first 2–3 weeks; longer term analgesia using NSAIDs is continued for 2–3 months. Physiotherapy techniques such as passive range of motion and hydrotherapy can be extremely useful; professional advice from a chartered physiotherapist may be helpful.

> **PRACTICAL TIP**
>
> Postoperative analgesia should be continued for 2–3 months; this is especially important in larger patients

COMPLICATIONS

Limb use generally steadily improves over the course of several weeks. In some patients poor limb use can persist; this is more commonly encountered in animals that have inadequate postoperative analgesia or physiotherapy. Owners should be warned that in the long term, limb function is unlikely to be normal and mild lameness is common. Outcome is less predictable in larger patients, especially if postoperative physiotherapy is neglected. Other complications are less common but could include sciatic nerve damage, femoral fracture and infection.

Chapter 23

The stifle

Mike Farrell

Clinical anatomy

The stifle joint is a complex hinge joint consisting of distinct femorotibial and femoropatellar articulations. A large femoropatellar joint cavity communicates with a smaller femorotibial joint cavity. The joint capsule is divided into inner synovial and outer fibrous layers that are separated distal to the patella by the infrapatellar fat pad. Ligamentous support of the stifle joint is provided by the medial and lateral collateral ligaments and the cranial and caudal cruciate ligaments (Figure 23.1). The medial collateral ligament (MCL) originates on the medial femoral epicondyle and blends with the joint capsule and medial meniscus before inserting over a large rectangular area on the caudoproximal aspect of the tibia. The lateral collateral ligament originates on the lateral femoral epicondyle immediately proximal to the origin of the popliteal muscle and passes caudodistally to insert on the fibular head. The collateral ligaments are primarily responsible for limiting valgus and varus stifle motion especially when the stifle joint is extended. Functional anatomy of the cranial and caudal cruciate ligaments is described below.

The major blood supply to the stifle joint is derived from branches of the middle genicular artery, which arises from a direct branch of the femoral artery called the popliteal artery. The middle genicular artery penetrates the joint capsule caudally and passes through the intercondylar notch between the cruciate ligaments. The infrapatellar fat pad also contributes to the vascular supply of the cruciate ligaments.

The periarticular tissues of the stifle are innervated by branches of the saphenous, tibial and common peroneal nerves. The synovial tissue covering the cruciate ligaments, the ligaments themselves, and the menisci are richly innervated with sensory and mechanical nerve endings.

Examination

Lameness examination

Lameness is an abnormality of gait and/or posture. Postural abnormalities including abnormal sitting and stationary lameness are sometimes described in the clinical history. If the dog or cat is allowed to walk around the consulting room, postural abnormalities are frequently displayed. Canine gait examination is usually performed outdoors. Examination of cats is more challenging because nervous cats typically adopt a stealthy crouching gait or hide in a corner. Examination can be more rewarding when cats are left alone in a closed room and observed through a window or video captured. The reader is referred to Chapter 2 for further details.

- **Limping** can be defined as visible asymmetry in load transfer of one limb compared with the contralateral limb. There is no particular gait abnormality that allows definitive localization to the stifle joint. For example, although skipping lameness is often attributed to patellar luxation, it is also seen with lameness localized to other areas including the foot, hip and lumbosacral spine. Limping can be difficult to detect in small dogs with rapid limb movement; video capture and slow motion playback can be useful in these cases.

23.1 Flexed canine stifle joint with the patella luxated medially. 1a = caudolateral band of the cranial cruciate ligament; 1b = craniomedial band of the cranial cruciate ligament 2 = caudal cruciate ligament; 3 = medial meniscus; 4 = lateral meniscus; 5 = long digital extensor tendon; 6 = medial humeral condyle; 7 = tibial tuberosity.

- **Bilateral pelvic limb lameness.** Several conditions affecting the stifle joint can present bilaterally. Limping is only seen when one limb transfers significantly more load than the other. Otherwise, more subtle lameness may be present, including a pottery, shuffling gait, difficulty on rising and abnormal sitting. Mechanical lameness can be seen with severe bilateral medial patellar luxation (MPL) with genu varum and an inability to extend the stifle joints.
- **Abnormal sit.** Dogs with stifle pain, such as seen with cranial cruciate ligament (CCL) disease, are often reluctant to sit with the stifle fully flexed. The affected limb is preferentially extended and is usually the lowermost limb when dogs display an asymmetrical sit (Figure 23.2).

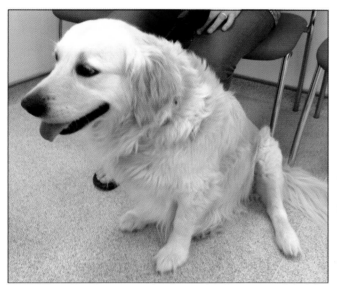

23.2 Positive sit test. Note the abnormal sitting posture of the left hind limb.
(Courtesy of Rob Pettitt)

Orthopaedic examination

Examination of the stifle joint of small dogs is best performed with the dog on a table. An assistant's hand can be placed under the abdomen to prevent the dog from sitting down. Large dogs are examined on the floor. They can be prevented from sitting by positioning a knee under the pelvis during the examination (Figure 23.3).

The stifle should be gently palpated without manipulation to determine abnormalities in the position of anatomical landmarks (e.g. patellar luxation) and to assess for the presence of joint effusion; the latter is a fluid swelling either side of the patellar tendon that makes its borders palpably indistinct. Normal range of motion is tested, with concurrent assessment of pain response, crepitus and patellar tracking. Pain on full extension is common in dogs with partial tears of the cranial cruciate ligament. Specific tests for cranial cruciate ligament insufficiency include the cranial draw and the tibial compression tests (Figures 23.4 and 23.5).

Integrity of the collateral ligaments is tested by application of valgus stress to test the medial collateral ligament, and varus stress to test the lateral collateral ligament; for this, the stifle joint is held in full extension. Landmarks are the medial and lateral femoral condyles for the upper hand and the fibular head and opposing proximal tibia for the lower hand. The fingers and thumbs of each hand are

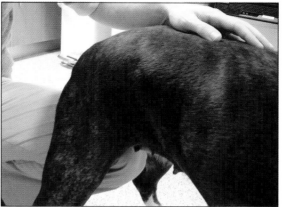

23.3 Placement of the clinician's knee beneath the pelvic floor frees both hands for examination of a standing dog.

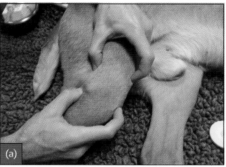

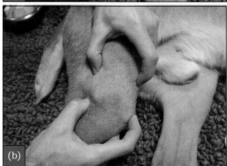

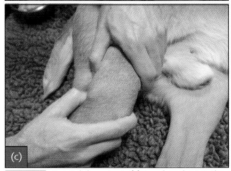

23.4 Cranial draw test. (a) Landmarks are the patella and lateral fabella for the finger and thumb of the upper hand and the tibial tuberosity and fibular head for the finger and thumb of the lower hand. A cranial force is applied to the tibia with the joint in a neutral position and in 30–60 degrees of flexion to aid in the detection of partial cranial crucial ligament (CCL) ruptures. (b) Cranial draw of 5–10 mm is common after complete CCL rupture in large-breed dogs. The caudolateral band of the CCL is taut when the stifle is in a neutral position but not when the stifle is flexed. Therefore a small amount of draw (<3 mm) with the stifle in flexion is consistent with partial CCL rupture of the craniomedial band. (c) Inappropriate technique frequently results in false-positive cranial draw. The tips of the fingers and thumb must be directly in contact with the bony landmarks. If the fingertips wrap around the landmarks as shown, they tend to apply cranial draw to skin and subcutaneous tissues. These structures displace easily in normal patients.

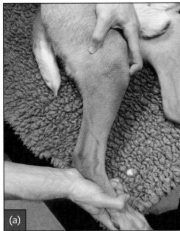

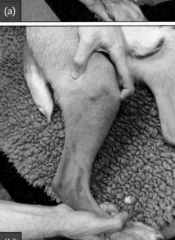

23.5 Tibial compression (cranial tibial thrust) test. (a) The stifle is held in a neutral position by all the fingers of the upper hand except the index finger, which is used to press caudally on the tibial tuberosity. The hock is flexed with the lower hand while the upper hand maintains the same stifle flexion angle. (b) The test mimics the loading conditions that generate tibial thrust. If the tibia thrusts cranially during testing, this is a positive tibial compression test and is diagnostic of cranial cruciate ligament (CCL) insufficiency. The tibial compression test is more difficult to perform correctly than the cranial draw test but is sometimes better tolerated in the conscious patient. It is also useful for distinguishing cranial from caudal ligament ruptures.

positioned directly over these periarticular landmarks because there is less potential for false-positives caused by stifle joint flexion or rotation which can occur if the femur and tibia are manipulated from their mid-diaphyses. The collateral ligaments should prevent all varus or valgus deviation in the extended stifle joint.

Diagnostic imaging

Specific details on appropriate imaging techniques for the stifle are provided in the imaging section at the end of this chapter. For more general information on imaging techniques and their application, see Chapter 3.

Radiography

Patient positioning:

- **Mediolateral view** – The patient should be positioned in lateral recumbency with the affected limb on the table (Figure 23.6a). Excessive or insufficient retraction of the contralateral limb results in external or internal rotation of the affected stifle, respectively. Internal stifle rotation is also caused by insufficient elevation of the proximal limb to the level of the film cassette. These errors result in a lack of superimposition of the femoral condyles. Accurate superimposition of the condyles and inclusion of the hock joint are critical for accurate measurement of the tibial plateau angle. Stifle flexion angle is important for pre-surgical planning: for tibial tuberosity advancement surgery, the recommended angle is 135-degree extension; whereas for tibial

plateau levelling osteotomy (TPLO) surgery, a 90-degree stifle angle is used. The X-ray beam should always be centred on the stifle. It should be noted that use of a 10 cm magnification marker allows appropriate calibration for surgical templating.

- **Caudocranial view** – The caudocranial view (Figure 23.6b) allows easier acquisition of correctly positioned radiographs than the craniocaudal view. External rotation is avoided by elevation of the contralateral limb. The tail can be tucked under the contralateral stifle. If the patient tips towards the affected limb, sandbags can be tucked under the ipsilateral groin. Cotton wool positioned directly under the stifle prevents slipping on the surface of the cassette. Symmetrical positioning of the femoral condyles, fabellae and patella is critical for assessment of angular and rotational limb deformities.

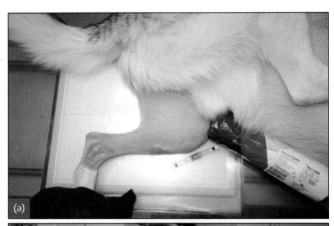

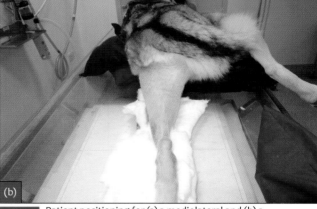

23.6 Patient positioning for (a) a mediolateral and (b) a caudocranial view of the stifle.

Radiographic views: The radiographic views required vary according to the suspected clinical problem. Bilateral radiographs should always be obtained due to the high incidence of bilateral stifle pathology.

- **Cranial cruciate ligament disease** – Diagnosis has usually already been confirmed with a positive cranial draw or tibial compression test. Mediolateral and caudocranial radiographs allow evaluation of secondary changes such as synovial effusion and periarticular osteophytes, and the exclusion of joint neoplasia (Figure 23.7). Radiographic measurements are used for surgical planning, particularly when tibial osteotomy surgery is being considered.

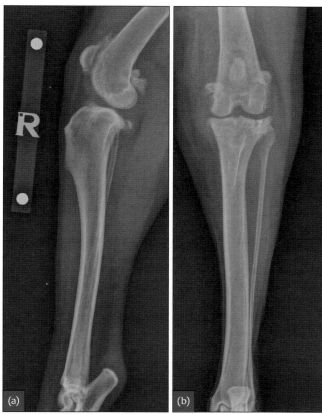

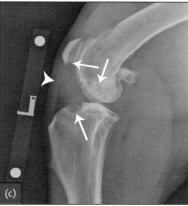

23.7 (a) Mediolateral and (b) caudocranial radiographs showing periarticular osteophyte and enthesiophyte formation. Note the reduction in the infrapatellar fat pad size consistent with joint effusion. Periarticular osteophytosis should not be used as a predictor of the degree of cartilage pathology, particularly in dogs with cranial cruciate ligament (CCL) disease in which osteophytes can indicate a response to instability rather than acting as an indicator of the severity of osteoarthritis. (c) An intra-articular tumour (synovial sarcoma) causes impingement of the infrapatellar fat pad (arrowhead) as well as osteolysis of the femur, tibia and patella (arrowed). Ultrasonography can be used to differentiate soft tissue masses from synovial effusion.

- **Patellar luxation** – Radiographs are assessed for the presence of angular and/or torsional limb deformities. Femoral radiographs used to assess distal femoral varus require precise X-ray beam orientation perpendicular to the bone. Precise radiographic positioning is necessary to correctly assess the degree of femoral varus (Dudley *et al.*, 2006) and identify the optimum site for osteotomy if distal femoral corrective osteotomy is intended. Bisection of the fabellae by the femoral cortices is commonly used as a repeatable reference point (Kowaleski, 2006; Roch and Gemmill, 2008).

Synovial fluid analysis

The canine stifle joint is one of the easiest joints to aspirate. Synovial fluid analysis is usually undertaken when there is a high index of suspicion of septic arthritis or immune-mediated polyarthritis. For further details, the reader is referred to Chapter 4.

Canine cranial cruciate ligament disease

Canine CCL disease is the most common cause of pelvic limb lameness in dogs. In contrast, rupture of the CCL is uncommon in cats. The term 'disease' is used to cover a spectrum of pathology that ranges from stretching to partial or complete rupture. Stifle joint instability resulting from CCL disease results in pain, lameness and progressive osteoarthritis.

Anatomy and function

The CCL originates on the axial aspect of the lateral femoral condyle and crosses the joint diagonally to insert on the cranial intercondylar region of the tibial plateau (Figure 23.8). The CCL is narrowest in its mid-section and it fans out proximally and distally. It is covered by synovial membrane so that it is intra-articular but extrasynovial. The CCL is composed of numerous bundles of collagen fibres separated by thin membranous sheets containing blood vessels and nerves. Vascularization is from the overlying synovial vessels emanating from the infrapatellar fat pad and caudal soft tissues. The central core of the mid-section of the CCL is relatively poorly vascularized. Mechanoreceptors in the ligament detect increased strain and initiate neural reflex arcs resulting in contraction of the caudal thigh muscles and simultaneous relaxation of the quadriceps muscles. This is a protective mechanism that contributes to joint stability.

The CCL is composed of two functional components: the narrow craniomedial band and the broad caudolateral band. The craniomedial band remains taut in all positions, in contrast to the caudolateral band which is only taut when the stifle joint is extended. The CCL functions as an important stabilizer to cranial displacement of the tibia and also prevents hyperextension of the stifle joint. In conjunction with the caudal cruciate ligament and collateral ligaments it has a secondary role of preventing excessive internal rotation of the tibia. It also prevents excessive varus or valgus movement when the stifle is flexed.

Aetiopathogenesis

There is considerable controversy regarding the aetiopathogenesis of CCL disease and there have been important recent advances in our understanding of the genetic, biological and mechanical influences on the integrity of the canine CCL.

Genetics of CCL disease

A high incidence of bilateral CCL disease and a predisposition of certain breeds are suggestive of a genetic predisposition to CCL disease. Approximately 50% of Labrador Retrievers will rupture the contralateral CCL within 5.5 months of the initial rupture (Buote *et al.*, 2009).

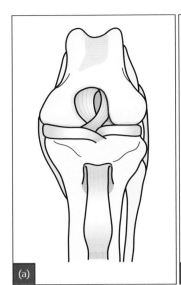
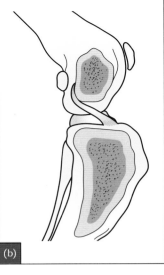
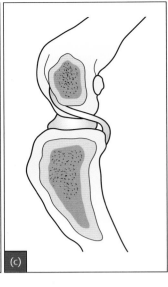

23.8 Anatomy of the cruciate ligaments. (a) The cranial cruciate ligament dominates the cranial view. (b) The cranial cruciate ligament arises in the medial aspect of the lateral condyle and inserts in the intercondylar region. (c) The caudal cruciate ligament arises from the lateral aspect of the medial condyle and inserts on the caudal aspect of the tibia.

A genetic basis for CCL disease has been identified in Newfoundlands, with a heritability of 0.27 and a possible recessive mode of inheritance (Wilke *et al.*, 2006). It is unknown whether the genetic defect causes structural alteration of the CCL, or an altered mechanical or biological environment predisposes to premature CCL degeneration.

Mechanical hypotheses

Conformational variations including stifle joint hyper-extension, narrow intercondylar notch, steep tibial plateau slope and MPL have all been hypothesized as causes of abnormal stress and micro-injury of the CCL resulting in progressive ligament rupture (Aiken *et al.*, 1995; Comerford *et al.*, 2006; Duerr *et al.*, 2007).

Intercondylar notch stenosis: A stenotic intercondylar notch causes impingement of the CCL. This can result in ligament micro-injury (Dienst *et al.*, 2007) and has been proposed as a potential risk factor for CCL disease in pre-disposed breeds such as the Labrador Retriever (Comerford *et al.*, 2006; Lewis *et al.*, 2008).

Steep tibial plateau: The stifle is subjected to external ground reaction forces applied to the limb during weight-bearing and internal forces generated by muscle contrac-tion (Figure 23.9). These forces generate a cranially oriented shear force of the tibia, termed 'cranial tibial thrust' (Slocum and Devine, 1984). Higher tibial plateau angles result in increased tibial thrust (Warzee *et al.*, 2001). Cranial tibial thrust is opposed passively by the CCL and actively by the hamstring and biceps femoris muscles.

There have been numerous studies evaluating the association of tibial plateau angle and CCL rupture but there is no clear answer. Pathological increases in tibial plateau angle (>55 degrees) have uncommonly been corre-lated with CCL rupture (Read and Robins, 1982; Macias *et al.*, 2002). Other studies have shown that the tibial plateau angle is not significantly different in Labrador Retrievers with and without CCL disease (Reif and Probst, 2003), or between Greyhounds (which rarely suffer CCL disease) and Labrador Retrievers (Wilke *et al.*, 2002).

Medial patellar luxation: Rates of clinical CCL disease of up to 25% have been reported in dogs with MPL (Campbell *et al.*, 2010). It has been theorized that increased internal

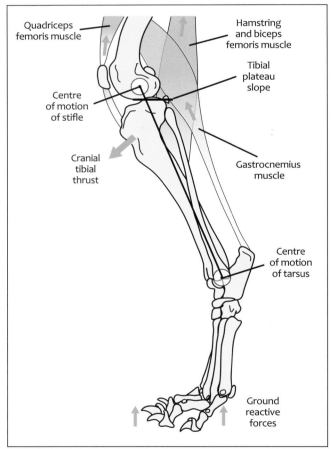

23.9 Stifle joint forces and cranial tibial thrust.

tibial rotation attributable to MPL may contribute to increased strain on the CCL and eventual rupture. Other theories for an increased risk of developing CCL disease include malalignment of the extensor mechanism and absence of a caudally directed vector force of the patello-femoral joint in dogs with grade IV MPL. An association has yet to be proven between MPL grades ≤III and CCL disease, although the association between grade IV patellar luxation and CCL rupture is statistically significant (Campbell *et al.*, 2010).

Biological hypotheses

Development of CCL rupture usually involves gradual degeneration of the ligament, generalized stifle joint inflammation, initial partial CCL rupture and gradual progression to complete rupture. Initially, slight CCL insufficiency may not cause visible lameness but can produce mild joint instability and progressive osteoarthritis. Dogs with incipient CCL disease can have a palpably stable joint but present with lameness, stifle effusion, and synovitis. Recent research suggests that the stifle synovitis precedes the development of CCL rupture rather than being a consequence of instability. Activation of immune responses within the stifle appear important to the development of synovitis and subsequent CCL degeneration (Muir *et al.*, 2007). The precise biological mechanisms responsible for this synovitis and its contribution to the development of CCL disease are the subject of ongoing research.

Meniscal anatomy and pathology

The medial and lateral menisci are semilunar fibrocartilaginous structures interposed between the articular surfaces of the femur and tibia (Figure 23.10). They are wedge-shaped in cross-section with the thicker peripheral border attached to the joint capsule. The menisci play an important role in stabilization and function of the stifle joint. They aid in load transmission, shock absorption, joint stability, lubrication and proprioception. Only the thick peripheral 15% of the meniscus has a vascular supply and the thin avascular inner portion heals poorly. The medial and lateral menisci both have tibial ligamentous attachments; the caudal horn of the lateral meniscus also attaches to the femur via the meniscofemoral ligament but the medial meniscus does not. The meniscofemoral ligament maintains the position of the caudal horn of the lateral meniscus relative to the lateral femoral condyle; this in turn prevents crushing or tearing of the caudal horn by the lateral femoral condyle during craniocaudal femur–tibia translation in the CCL deficient stifle. In contrast, the medial meniscus is firmly attached to the tibial plateau by the joint capsule, MCL and menisco-tibial ligaments. During abnormal craniocaudal translation, the medial meniscus becomes the primary restraint against cranial tibial thrust and is prone to injury (Figure 23.11).

The prevalence of reported meniscal injuries in dogs with CCL injuries is 10 to 70% and these injuries are almost exclusively confined to the medial meniscus.

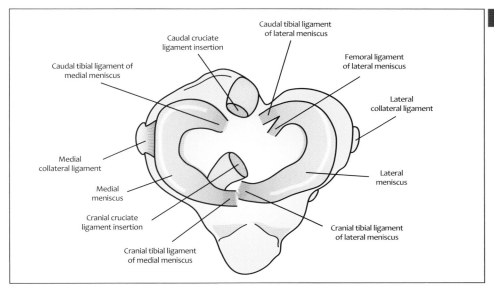

23.10 Anatomy of the medial and lateral menisci.

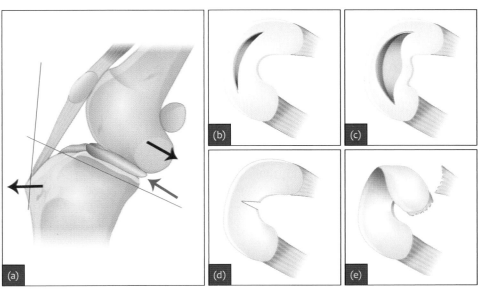

23.11 (a) In a cranial cruciate ligament (CCL) deficient stifle, the medial meniscus becomes the primary restraint against cranial tibial thrust and is prone to injury, particularly in the caudal horn. The blue arrows denote the relative movement of the tibia and femoral condyle; the red arrow indicates the medial meniscus. (b–e) Common medial meniscal injuries: (b) longitudinal tear; (c) bucket-handle tear; (d) transverse tear; and (e) caudal pole avulsion (folding injury).

Meniscal injuries most commonly involve the caudal horn and are frequently a longitudinal tear known as a bucket-handle tear (Figure 23.11c). Risk factors for meniscal injury in association with CCL rupture include complete rupture (12.9 times higher odds with complete *versus* partial CCL rupture), delayed surgery, high bodyweight (1.4% increase for every additional kilogram of body-weight) and breed predisposition (Golden Retrievers and Rottweilers have a higher risk and West Highland White Terriers have a lower risk compared with Labrador Retrievers) (Hayes *et al.*, 2010).

Diagnosis
Signalment
Any breed of dog may be presented with CCL disease but the breeds at highest risk for CCL rupture are medium, large and giant breeds including Newfoundlands, Mastiffs, Rottweilers, retrievers, Bulldogs and Boxers. Peak incidence is reported between 2 and 10 years of age (Whitehair *et al.*, 1993; Duval *et al.*, 1999; Witsberger *et al.*, 2008), with dogs less than 4 years of age being signifi-cantly less likely to be diagnosed with CCL rupture com-pared with dogs over 4 years of age (Witsberger *et al.*, 2008). Over the last four decades, the reported preva-lence of CCL disease has increased, and it has become relatively common for large and giant-breed dogs to be presented with bilateral cranial cruciate ligament disease under 2 years of age. Neutered dogs have significantly increased odds for having CCL rupture compared with intact dogs of both genders (Witsberger *et al.*, 2008). In addition, early neutering (before 6 months of age) was reported to be a significant risk factor for development of excessive tibial plateau angles in large-breed dogs with CCL rupture (Duerr *et al.*, 2007).

History
Onset of lameness can be acute or insidious. Acute-onset severe pelvic limb lameness may occur in dogs with com-plete rupture of a degenerated CCL. The main differential diagnosis when there is sudden worsening of lameness in a dog with previously mild or intermittent lameness is menis-cal injury. An audible click is sometimes reported in dogs with concurrent meniscal injury, but absence of a click should not be used as an indicator of normal meniscal integrity. One study reported audible or palpable clicks in only 28% of dogs with confirmed meniscal injuries (Case *et al.*, 2008).

Clinical examination
Gait examination: Lameness grade is variable and depends on whether or not the CCL injury is acute or chronic, the completeness of CCL rupture and whether or not there are concurrent injuries (e.g. meniscal injury). If lameness is bilateral, dogs will often lean forward to unload the pelvic limbs. Dogs with unilateral lameness may externally rotate the affected limb.

Orthopaedic examination: Palpation of the medial aspect of the stifle will often reveal a firm thickening, indicative of periarticular fibrosis, that is commonly termed 'medial but-tress'. This pathological change almost always indicates CCL disease. Deep palpation of the caudomedial aspect of the tibial plateau may be especially painful in dogs affected by injuries to the caudal horn of the medial men-iscus (Figure 23.12). Detection of stifle instability and

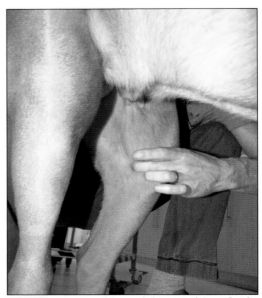

23.12 Palpation of the medial aspect of the stifle often reveals a firm thickening, indicative of periarticular fibrosis, that is commonly termed 'medial buttress'. Deep palpation using a single digit pressed into the caudomedial aspect of the stifle joint often causes a pain response in dogs with injuries to the caudal horn of the medial meniscus.

cranial translation of the tibia relative to the femur provides definitive confirmation of complete or partial CCL rupture (see Figures 23.3 and 23.4). In immature dogs, cranial translation of the tibia relative to the femur of a few milli-metres is normal due to slight laxity in the ligament; the small amount of tibiofemoral translation will come to an abrupt stop. In contrast, in dogs with CCL rupture, the tibiofemoral translation will end in a soft or spongy stop.

Treatment
Non-surgical management
Paatsama originally reported that complete severance of the canine CCL invariably resulted in osteoarthritis and that the associated lameness never totally resolved (Paatsama, 1952). Subsequently, only two clinical studies have specifically evaluated the long-term outcome after non-surgical management of canine CCL injury (Pond and Campbell, 1972; Vasseur, 1984). A conclusion of both studies was that non-surgical management can return small-breed dogs to 'normal', but recovery rates were poor for large-breed dogs. Small-breed dogs were arbitrarily defined as <15kg. Non-surgical management was defined as restriction to lead walks for 3–8 weeks, weight loss (if indicated) and strategic analgesic medication. On the basis of these studies, it has become widely accepted that non-surgical management is a good option for small-breed dogs; thus, it is important that the available data are thoroughly evaluated (Figure 23.13).

Despite several important study limitations, it is appro-priate to deduce that small-breed dogs have a better chance of improvement after non-surgical management of CCL insufficiency than large-breed dogs. In one of the aforementioned studies, only 19% of large-breed dogs returned to 'normal' in the long term (Vasseur, 1984). Potential reasons for a better outcome in small-breed dogs include:

* Lower mechanical demands placed upon the unstable articulation due to lower bodyweight

Feature	Pond and Campbell, 1972	Vasseur, 1984
Number of small-breed dogs	32	28
Study design	Retrospective	Retrospective
Outcome measures	Subjective owner assessment ('Is there lameness?')	Owner and veterinary assessment (Subjective: 'normal' or 'improved')
Pre-operative lameness grade and duration	Not stated	Not stated
Pre-operative degree of CCL injury (partial or complete)	Not stated	Not stated
Incidence of bilateral CCL insufficiency	Incidence not stated for small dogs	Not stated
Frequency of reassessment	Two assessments (3 months short-term assessment; duration of long-term follow-up not stated)	One reassessment 2–7 years (mean 3 years) after treatment
Success rate	90% 'normal'	75% 'normal', 11% improved
Long-term activity level	Not defined	Poorly defined
Time to recover completely	Not stated	Estimated by owners as 4 months (range 2.5–5 months)
Surgical control group	Yes – variable techniques	No

23.13 Data defining outcome following non-surgical management of cranial cruciate ligament (CCL) injury in small-breed dogs. Although these data are frequently used to support non-surgical management in small-breed dogs, they must be interpreted in light of several important limitations, including poorly defined pre-treatment status, subjective outcome measures, and absence of short- and medium-term follow-up.

- Lower mechanical demands due to lifestyle. Small-breed dogs typically develop clinical CCL disease later in life than large-breed dogs (Vasseur, 1984)
- Differing owner expectations of what constitutes normal function in young large-breed dogs and old small-breed dogs
- Challenges in evaluating lameness in small-breed dogs due to their rapid limb movement (Off and Matis, 2010).

In contrast to non-surgical treatment, surgical management produces rapid and predictable functional improvement, with the potential to return dogs to a status that is objectively indistinguishable from that of a normal dog in the long term (Gordon-Evans et al., 2013; Nelson et al., 2013). Thus, regardless of animal size, non-surgical management should be reserved for patients with mild, intermittent lameness that are poor anaesthesia candidates and those that suffer significant comorbidities or whose owners lack the financial means for surgical intervention or the ability to accept the risks associated with surgery. When non-surgical management is chosen for overweight dogs, function is optimized by the use of an effective weight-loss programme (Wucherer et al., 2013). See Chapter 6 for details of medical management of degenerative joint disease.

Stifle orthoses

Stifle orthoses (braces) are available as an alternative to surgical intervention or as a means of augmenting extracapsular CCL repair (Figure 23.14). A custom orthosis is made-to-order based on a fibreglass impression provided by the primary care practitioner. Fibreglass cast material is applied to the limb of the standing dog. The negative impression of the limb is used to fabricate a positive impression that is used as a template to build the orthosis. An open access video describes the recommended technique for making the fibreglass impression and correctly fitting the completed orthotic (www.orthopets.com). Tolerance of the orthotic depends in part on the temperament of the dog, with stoical dogs taking 1–2 weeks to become accustomed to the device. The manufacturers recommend that stifle orthoses should be

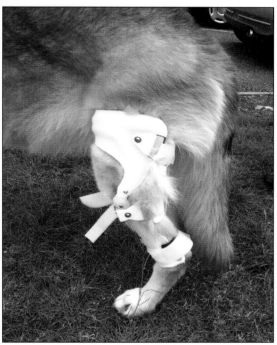

23.14 A custom hinged stifle orthosis.
(Reproduced with permission from OrthoPets Europe)

maintained for all waking hours (i.e. they should only be removed at night) for the rest of the animal's life. One study reported the outcome and complications for dogs treated for CCL injury with either orthoses or TPLO (Hart, et al, 2015). The study did not report the duration of follow up or the total duration of external support. Data were available for 203 dogs treated with orthoses. Although rates of owner satisfaction were high for both non-surgically and surgically managed dogs, the proportion of owners who reported that their dogs had mild or no lameness and rated the intervention as excellent, very good or good was significantly greater for the TPLO group. In addition, complications related to the orthoses were common, with skin lesions in 46%, treatment failure and subsequent surgery in 11% and intolerance of the device in 7%. Contraindications include:

- Aggressive temperament
- Body conformation that does not allow at least 50% of the femur to be enclosed within the orthosis (e.g. dogs with short femurs, heavily muscled proximal limbs and/or pendulous abdomens)
- Excessive skin folds (e.g. Shar Peis, Chow Chows and Bulldogs)
- Uncontrolled skin disease (e.g. atopy) or endocrinopathies that cause skin fragility (e.g. hyperadrenocorticism)
- Suspected meniscal injury – this represents a challenging problem because meniscal injury is difficult to diagnose by clinical examination.

Surgical options

Surgical treatment options for CCL disease are broadly divided into those that provide either passive or dynamic stifle stability. Extracapsular and intracapsular stabilization techniques confer passive stability to the joint. In contrast, tibial osteotomy techniques provide dynamic stability while the joint is loaded. Techniques differ in concept, technical difficulty, invasiveness, potential risks, equipment, rate of recovery, completeness of recovery and cost. Treatment should be recommended based on the best possible evidence, particularly in an age when owners are increasingly well informed. Information available on the Internet with respect to canine CCL disease is of highly variable quality and can be misleading (Taggart et al., 2010). Until recently, clinical studies had failed to establish a clear advantage of one surgical technique above another, although one study showed a significantly worse outcome after intracapsular stabilization (Conzemius et al., 2005). Two recent studies applied random allocation of dogs into groups treated either by TPLO or lateral fabellotibial suture (LFS) and a third study compared the outcome of TPLO, tibial tuberosity advancement (TTA) and LFS without random allocation of dogs to each treatment group. Dogs were reassessed in the short, medium and long term using owner evaluation and force plate analysis (Gordon-Evans et al., 2013; Nelson et al., 2013; Krotscheck et al., 2016). All surgical procedures induced improvements in limb function with comparable improvement in clinical outcomes such as goniometry and thigh circumference, but dogs treated by TPLO had better ground reaction forces and higher owner satisfaction than those treated via LFS.

Intra-articular inspection: Examination of the stifle joint can be performed via arthroscopy or arthrotomy. Arthrotomy is more invasive but less costly than the more technically demanding arthroscopic procedure. Surgical technique for canine stifle arthroscopy has been described (Gemmill and Farrell, 2009). Compared with arthrotomy, stifle arthroscopy provides increased visibility of the joint, and results in faster recovery times and increased mobility in the first 8 weeks postoperatively (Hoelzler et al., 2004). Although stifle joint inspection should be considered mandatory in patients presenting with CCL disease, there has been recent controversy regarding the necessity for arthrotomy. The evidence supporting intra-articular inspection of stifle joints affected by CCL disease is compelling:

- Advantages of stifle joint inspection:
  - Meniscal injury is a very common cause of significant morbidity: in one study, dogs with concurrent meniscal injury were found to be more lame based on force plate analysis than those without meniscal injury (Wustefeld-Janssens et al., 2014)

- Reported incidence rate of meniscal injury is 10–70% (Hayes et al., 2010)
  - Clinically unimportant meniscal injuries have not been reported either in dogs or humans. Human meniscal damage causes discomfort and progression of degenerative joint disease (Rath and Richmond, 2000)
  - Meniscal injuries are often the cause of a poor response to non-surgical management. In one study, 73% of large-breed dogs and 100% of small-breed dogs that did not improve after non-surgical management had meniscal injuries (Vasseur, 1984)
  - Failure to improve after CCL repair is frequently attributed to lack of identification of meniscal tears at the time of surgery (Thieman et al., 2006)
  - Visual confirmation of CCL injuries can be made prior to performing potentially invasive surgery
- Disadvantages of stifle joint inspection:
  - Although meniscal injuries can occur with partial CCL rupture, they are uncommon in dogs with mild lameness and minimal instability
  - In one study, the overall complication rate after TPLO was significantly higher in dogs that had a full arthrotomy than those that had no arthrotomy (Stauffer et al., 2006); however, there were some important flaws in this study that make meaningful interpretation challenging. For example, the differences could be a consequence of relatively limited surgeon experience in the dogs treated by arthrotomy.

The indications and technique for meniscal inspection, partial meniscectomy and medial meniscal release are described in Operative Technique 23.5.

Resection of the CCL remnant: Removal of frayed ends of a (partially) ruptured CCL is recommended if the frayed ends prevent proper inspection of the medial meniscus. However, removal of grossly normal CCL is not recommended. Conserved CCL remains functional, providing stability to the joint (craniocaudal, varus–valgus, rotational) resulting in improved centring of the femoral condyles within the confines of the menisci. The effect of conserved CCL after debridement of small partial tears is a significant reduction in the incidence of subsequent (late) meniscal injury and articular cartilage damage (Hulse et al., 2010).

Stabilization surgery: An algorithmic approach can be applied to the decision-making process for CCL stabilization surgery, whereby each patient is assessed according to the unique mechanical, biological and clinical factors that influence the healing process (Figure 23.15). A numerical score from 1 to 10 is assigned to the mechanical, biological and clinical factors that influence the healing environment after CCL repair. Low mechanical and clinical scores imply a suboptimal mechanical environment during the first few weeks of recovery. This should prompt the selection of a robust and durable repair that is not reliant on good patient compliance for an optimal outcome. Tibial osteotomy has an advantage over extracapsular repair in this instance. Low biological scores imply a greater chance of relatively slow and potentially incomplete recovery. Surgery that relies on a benign intra-articular environment (intra-articular repair) or periarticular fibrosis for stabilization of the joint (extracapsular repair) carries a higher risk in patients with low biological scores. The decision process is also strongly influenced by the incidence and nature of intraoperative and postoperative complications (see Figure 23.19).

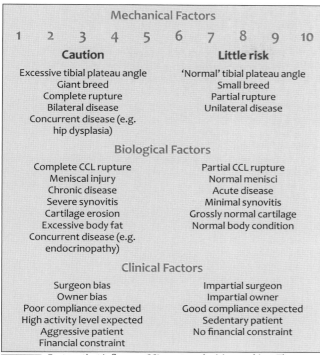

Mechanical Factors	
1 2 3 4 5 6 7 8 9 10	
Caution	**Little risk**
Excessive tibial plateau angle	'Normal' tibial plateau angle
Giant breed	Small breed
Complete rupture	Partial rupture
Bilateral disease	Unilateral disease
Concurrent disease (e.g. hip dysplasia)	
Biological Factors	
Complete CCL rupture	Partial CCL rupture
Meniscal injury	Normal menisci
Chronic disease	Acute disease
Severe synovitis	Minimal synovitis
Cartilage erosion	Grossly normal cartilage
Excessive body fat	Normal body condition
Concurrent disease (e.g. endocrinopathy)	
Clinical Factors	
Surgeon bias	Impartial surgeon
Owner bias	Impartial owner
Poor compliance expected	Good compliance expected
High activity level expected	Sedentary patient
Aggressive patient	No financial constraint
Financial constraint	

23.15 Factors that influence CCL surgery decision-making. These risks must be carefully considered when selecting the most appropriate surgical technique. In some cases, a particular risk may drive a decision towards or away from a specific surgical technique. For example, in dogs with very steep tibial plateau angles (>34 degrees), it is often impossible to create an appropriate patellar tendon angle using TTA surgery. If this is the case, alternative techniques should be considered in preference to TTA. In other circumstances, a particular risk should be considered and discussed with an owner, although it might not exert an influence on the chosen surgical technique. CCL = cranial cruciate ligament; TTA = tibial tuberosity advancement.

Intra-articular stabilization: The damaged CCL is replaced with a ligament prosthesis intended to replicate the original CCL. Many graft tissues have been used including fascia lata, patellar tendon, hamstring fascia and skin. Intra-articular CCL stabilization has fallen out of favour due to a relatively slow, inferior recovery and a high incidence of complications compared with other techniques (Conzemius *et al.*, 2005). Experimental dogs treated using hamstring grafts remained significantly lame 12 weeks postoperatively and often took up to 52 weeks for lameness to resolve (Lopez *et al.*, 2003).

Extracapsular stabilization: Although there are many variations in surgical technique, the commonest method employed for femorotibial joint stabilization is LFS. Stability is conferred by passing non-absorbable suture material medial and cranial to the lateral fabella within the gastrocnemius muscle origin, i.e. the femorofabellar ligament, and through one or more bone tunnels in the tibial tuberosity. The suture position is intended to mimic the orientation of the CCL, thus limiting cranial draw and internal tibial rotation. Concurrent imbrication of the lateral fascia may help to further stabilize the stifle joint. Monofilament materials used for LFS include nylon, polypropylene and stainless steel. Multifilament materials include polyblend (Fiberwire® or TightRope®, Arthrex) and polyethylene (LigaFiba, Veterinary Instrumentation). Braided materials have improved handling properties and superior biomechanics compared with monofilament materials but carry a significantly increased risk of infection and sinus formation (see below). The LFS technique relies on periarticular fibrosis for permanent stabilization of the joint.

Extracapsular stabilization mitigates cranial draw but residual postoperative cranial draw is common. Most surgeons aim to reduce cranial draw to <2 mm but not to eliminate it entirely. Extracapsular sutures cannot precisely mimic the functions of the CCL because it is impossible to achieve isometric anchorage points. Consequently, overtensioning of a LFS causes reduced stifle range of motion, pathologically increased joint compressive forces, and excessive external tibial rotation (Chailleux *et al.*, 2007; Tonks *et al.*, 2010). This may predispose to early failure due to suture creep, breakage or failure of the fabellar anchorage site (Hill *et al.*, 1999; Figure 23.16). Conversely, undertensioning leads to persistent stifle instability that can cause ongoing pain, loss of function and meniscal injury. In the long term, significant ongoing cranial draw has been recognized in approximately half of dogs treated by extracapsular stabilization (Moore and Read, 1995); however, the relationship between recurrent cranial draw and lameness is complex because the presence of cranial draw 6 weeks postoperatively does not relate to lameness (Hill *et al.*, 1999). As ≤2 mm postoperative cranial draw is expected, extracapsular stabilization is most appropriate when >2 mm of preoperative cranial draw is present. In animals with early partial CCL rupture in which cranial draw is subtle, tibial osteotomy is a more suitable alternative.

Tibial plateau levelling osteotomy: Slocum originally hypothesized that levelling the tibial plateau would provide functional femorotibial stability during weight-bearing by reducing cranial tibial thrust (Slocum and Devine, 1983). He proposed two surgical procedures to reduce the tibial plateau slope angle and thus, cranial tibial thrust. The initial technique involved a proximal cranial tibial wedge osteotomy (Slocum and Devine, 1984). Subsequently, radial osteotomy TPLO was developed and patented using a

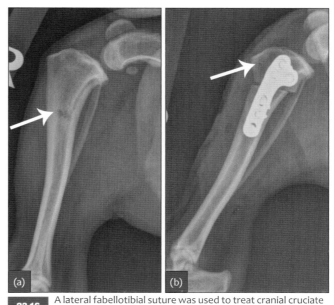

23.16 A lateral fabellotibial suture was used to treat cranial cruciate ligament (CCL) insufficiency in a 6-year-old mixed-breed dog. Lameness did not improve postoperatively. (a) Note the very distal position of the tibial bone tunnel (arrowed). Tension applied to the fabellotibial suture causes non-physiological stifle joint flexion, tibial external rotation and compression of the lateral joint compartment. There was a subsequent meniscal injury diagnosed 4 months postoperatively. (b) Revision surgery involved caudal pole hemimeniscectomy and cranial closing wedge tibial plateau levelling osteotomy (TPLO). Note the correct position of the tibial bone tunnel (arrowed). A fabellotibial suture was used due to overt stifle instability (1.5 cm draw).

technique involving creation of a crescent-shaped osteotomy caudal to the insertion of the patellar tendon. With either technique the tibial plateau angle is reduced to approximately 6 degrees rather than 0 degrees. Over-rotation of the tibial plateau (<6 degrees) has the potential to produce caudal tibial thrust and damage the caudal cruciate ligament. The decision on whether to perform cranial closing wedge TPLO or radial osteotomy TPLO is usually based on personal preference. Cranial closing wedge TPLO is often performed in small dogs with very steep tibial plateau angles (>34 degrees) where tibial plateau rotation after radial osteotomy would result in an exposed tibial tuberosity segment that is vulnerable to avulsion fracture. In comparison to radial osteotomy TPLO, cranial closing wedge TPLO results in a smaller surface area of compression (theoretically resulting in reduced stability), and allows less precise control of final tibial plateau angle. A higher incidence of complications that required surgical revision was reported for cranial closing wedge TPLO in one study (Corr and Brown, 2007); however, another study demonstrated no significant differences in major complication rates, re-operation rates or final tibial plateau angles between TPLO and a modified cranial closing wedge technique (Oxley et al., 2013).

Tibial tuberosity advancement: TTA was developed at the University of Zurich in the late 1990s according to principles derived from biomechanical models of joint forces in the human knee. The premise of these models is that the tibiofemoral compressive force is approximately the same magnitude, and oriented in the same direction, as the patellar tendon force. The relative directions of the

tibiofemoral and patellar tendon forces vary according to the stifle flexion angle. When the patellar tendon angle (PTA) is >90 degrees, there is a resultant tibiofemoral shear force that is directed cranially. In CCL deficient stifles, this results in cranial tibial thrust during normal weight-bearing. When the PTA is <90 degrees, the direction of the shear force is reversed, and the CCL is unloaded while the caudal cruciate ligament is loaded. The principle of TTA is to advance the tibial tuberosity sufficiently far cranially to maintain a PTA ≤90 degrees in order to obtain a neutral or caudally directed tibiofemoral shear force during ambulation. The effect of advancing the tibial tuberosity has been validated in an *in vitro* experimental study (Apelt *et al.*, 2007). The surgical technique of TTA has been described in detail (Lafaver *et al.*, 2007). The relative advantages and disadvantages of TTA and TPLO have been discussed in detail (Boudrieau, 2009). TTA is widely and erroneously considered to be less technically demanding than TPLO. For this reason, several variants on the original TTA procedure are now available in an attempt to make TTA surgery more accessible (Figure 23.17).

Explaining surgical options to owners: The principles of CCL repair are complex. Tibial osteotomy surgery, in particular, can appear counter-intuitive to laypeople. This produces a challenge for veterinary surgeons tasked with explaining the available surgical options. Video animations have been demonstrated to significantly improve owners' understanding of CCL injuries and the surgical options available to treat them (Clements *et al.*, 2013). These animations are available as an open access online resource (Figure 23.18).

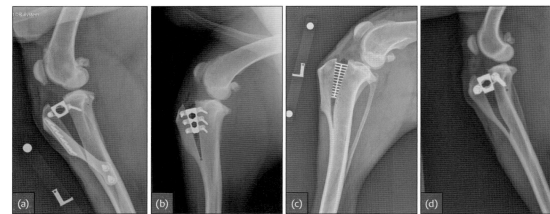

23.17 Multiple variations of tibial tuberosity advancement (TTA) are commercially available. The proposed advantage of these modifications is reduced technical demand compared with standard TTA. In the author's opinion, creation and advancement of an incomplete osteotomy as shown is technically demanding. This requires meticulous precision in locating the distal extremity of the osteotomy and very patient advancement (this can take >5 minutes). The consequence of suboptimal osteotomy or advancement technique is iatrogenic fracture of the hinge of distal bone.
(a) Standard TTA. (b) TTA rapid. (c) TTA2. (d) Modified Maquet Technique using a standard TTA cage. (e) Modified Maquet procedure.
(b, Courtesy of Toby Gemmill; e, Courtesy of Orthomed UK)

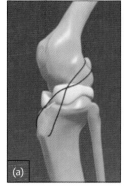
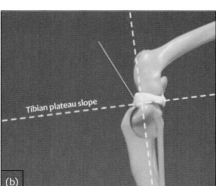
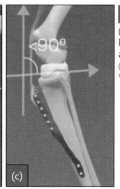

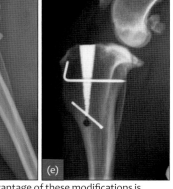

23.18 Video animation stills showing the principles and technique for (a) extra-capsular stabilization, (b) tibial plateau levelling osteotomy and (c) tibial tuberosity advancement.
(Courtesy of the University of Edinburgh, available from http://www.ed.ac.uk/vet/services/cclr

Postoperative rehabilitation

Postoperative rehabilitation after CCL repair surgery has benefits including decreased muscle spasm, improved tissue healing, increased range of motion and increased muscle strength and endurance. The goal is to return the patient to normal function as quickly as possible while minimizing the possibility of postoperative complications. Protocols should be tailored to the individual. Further details can be found in the *BSAVA Manual of Canine and Feline Rehabilitation, Supportive and Palliative Care*.

Lead walking: The simplest postoperative physical therapy protocol involves a recommendation for slow lead walking for at least 6 weeks postoperatively. Stairs and slippery surfaces should be avoided and an abdominal sling can provide additional support in the first 2–3 weeks. This is the most commonly recommended protocol and has been associated with good results in the medium term in several studies involving various surgical techniques.

Hydrotherapy: Hydrotherapy has a proven benefit in terms of recovery rate after extracapsular stabilization (Marsolais *et al.*, 2002). Swimming protocols typically involve 1-minute bursts with 1-minute rest over a total session of 10 minutes. Underwater treadmill walking can be performed for longer sessions, with the water level usually fixed at the level of the hip joint.

Passive range of motion exercises: Passive range of motion exercises can improve stifle range of motion after surgical treatment of CCL rupture (Monk *et al.*, 2006).

Transcutaneous electrical nerve stimulation, neuromuscular electrical stimulation and extracorporeal shock wave therapy: These techniques have all been recommended for rehabilitation after CCL stabilization surgery but there is no evidence that shows a better outcome for the dog with such therapy.

Complications

Postoperative complications are broadly divided into mechanical and biological categories. Mechanical complications include implant failure, subsequent (late) meniscal injury, tibial or fibular fracture, patellar luxation and patellar tendinitis. Biological complications include periprosthetic infection, septic arthritis and delayed osseous healing. The complications associated with osteotomy procedures can have potentially severe consequences (Figure 23.19). For example, patellar luxation, septic arthritis and diaphyseal tibial fracture (Figure 23.20) are all uncommon complications that require major surgical

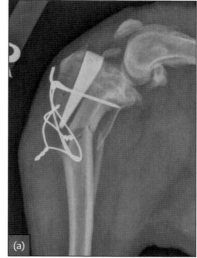
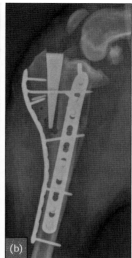
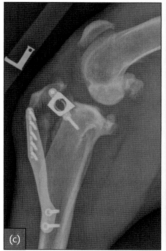
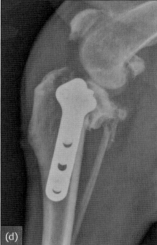

23.20 Mechanical complications after tibial osteotomy surgeries. (a) This diaphyseal tibial fracture occurred 1 month after a modified Maquet procedure. The fracture propagated from the drill hole at the distal limit of the advancement. (b) Surgical repair using orthogonal locking plate fixation. (c) Tibial tuberosity avulsion fracture diagnosed 4 weeks after tibial tuberosity advancement (TTA). (d) Fibular fracture and 'rock-back' of the tibial plateau segment diagnosed 6 weeks after tibial plateau levelling osteotomy (TPLO).

intervention or long-term medical management to treat successfully. Tibial osteotomies are advanced orthopaedic procedures that should be undertaken only by surgeons with sufficient training and experience.

If recurrent lameness occurs after CCL repair, there are several potential causes but the two most frequent complications following CCL surgery are septic arthritis

Procedure	Overall complication rate	Re-operation rate	Meniscal injury	Incisional complications	Other complications
LFS	17.4–21%	7.2–21%	1.9–19%	8.8%	Common peroneal nerve entrapment, ongoing instability, patellar luxation, periprosthetic infection, septic arthritis
TPLO	14.8–28%	5–9%	0–10.5%	2–16%	Popliteal artery laceration, tibial tuberosity fracture, fibular fracture, implant failure, patellar tendinitis, patellar luxation, delayed osseous healing, periprosthetic infection, septic arthritis
TTA	19–59%	6.2–11.3%	3.4–21.7%	6.6–21%	Tibial tuberosity fracture, diaphyseal tibial fracture, implant failure, patellar tendinitis, patellar luxation, delayed osseous healing, periprosthetic infection, septic arthritis

23.19 Complications following cranial cruciate ligament stabilization surgery. LFS = lateral fabellotibial suture; TPLO = tibial plateau levelling osteotomy; TTA = tibial tuberosity advancement.

and late medial meniscal injury. Implant failure and tibial or fibular fracture can be ruled out by clinical and radiographic assessment. Septic arthritis is ruled out by synovial fluid analysis. After these differential diagnoses have been ruled out in dogs with recurrent lameness, joint effusion and stifle pain, the most likely diagnosis is meniscal injury. Confirmation of meniscal injury can be made using ultrasonography, MRI, arthroscopy or exploratory arthrotomy.

Postoperative infection:

Extracapsular stabilization: Postoperative surgical site infection rate after extracapsular suture was as high as 18–21% when multifilament suture material was used for extracapsular stabilization (Dulisch, 1981ab). Infection rate with monofilament suture material is less than 5% (Casale and McCarthy, 2009). Nevertheless, due to mechanical concerns related to monofilament suture materials, there has been a recent resurgence of multifilament suture for extracapsular stabilization. As there are currently no long-term studies assessing complication rates for these recent variations in extracapsular implants, it remains to be seen whether the previous problems of chronic periprosthetic infection will resurface. When periprosthetic infection or septic arthritis occurs after extracapsular stabilization, resolution of infection usually requires removal of the non-absorbable suture (Marchevsky and Read, 1999). The diagnosis and management options for acute septic arthritis are discussed in Chapter 6.

Tibial plateau levelling osteotomy: Postoperative infection after TPLO manifests as superficial wound infection, septic arthritis or osteomyelitis. The reported infection rates of 0–7% (Pacchiana et al., 2003; Priddy et al., 2003; Stauffer et al., 2006; Fitzpatrick and Solano, 2010) are higher than the 1.5–2.6% reported for clean surgical procedures (Rosin et al., 1993; Lipowitz, 1996). Radiographs should always be acquired in the event of sudden onset lameness after any osteotomy surgery because of the close relationship between mechanical instability (related to bone/implant failure) and infection. Treatment of deep periprosthetic infection and septic arthritis after TPLO requires a long duration of oral antibiotic therapy (e.g. 2 months) and, in one-third to two-thirds of cases, implant removal after the bone has healed (Fitzpatrick and Solano, 2010; Nicoll et al., 2014).

Tibial tuberosity advancement: A postoperative TTA incisional infection rate of 6.6% has been reported (Wolf et al., 2012). Although this is in a similar range to the overall infection rate after TPLO, rates of deep periprosthetic infection and septic arthritis are as low as 0–1% (Hoffmann et al., 2006; Lafaver et al., 2007; Stein and Schmoekel, 2008; Wolf et al., 2012). If recalcitrant deep infection does occur and implant removal is required to resolve the infection, this can be technically demanding. Standard TTA cages and forks can be removed, but cages typically have sufficient osseous ingrowth that they can only be explanted after removing the adjacent bone using an oscillating saw or osteotome. Removal of OrthoFoam MMP implants is particularly challenging. An additional important problem occurs because advancement cannot be maintained after removal of the titanium wedge. Revision therefore requires replacement of the tibial tuberosity in its original anatomical position with pin and tension-band wire fixation of the tuberosity fragment, or revision to stan-dard TTA with insertion of an antibiotic impregnated collagen sponge.

Terrier skipping syndrome

Intermittent skipping is common in terrier breeds. After ruling out MPL, CCL insufficiency and hip dysplasia, it is common practice to attribute this lameness to habitual behaviour. However, these dogs should be carefully screened for evidence of stifle pain and effusion, because CCL disease without palpable instability (termed 'stable CCL disease') is a common finding. In many affected terriers, there is an excessive tibial plateau slope (>34 degrees). In these dogs, it is likely that the cause of the skipping is recurrent low-grade CCL sprain injury.

Feline cruciate ligament rupture

Feline CCL injuries can be divided into two distinct groups: those with atraumatic isolated CCL rupture and those with traumatic CCL rupture that is often part of a complex of multi-ligamentous stifle injuries but can occur as an isolated injury. Cats with atraumatic CCL disease are typically older and heavier than the general population and often suffer from bilateral pathology (Harasen, 2005). The pathogenesis of atraumatic feline CCL rupture is thought to parallel the degenerative CCL ruptures seen in overweight small-breed dogs (Harasen, 2005) but evidence is limited. Degenerative CCL disease may be less common in cats than in dogs because the CCL in dogs is smaller than the caudal cruciate ligament, whereas the reverse is true in cats. Also, the genetic inheritance of CCL rupture documented in the dog may be absent or less likely in the more heterozygous feline population (Harasen, 2007). A possible link has been proposed between hyperthyroidism and feline CCL disease (Harasen, 2005).

Although one study documented favourable results after non-surgical management of degenerative feline CCL rupture (Scavelli and Schrader, 1987), it can take up to 3 months of confinement to achieve the required improvement. Published results of feline extracapsular stabilization (Figure 23.21) indicate that results are at least as good as those achieved with non-surgical treatment, and that surgery provides quicker and more reliable return to function (Harasen, 2005). TTA in the cat has also been reported (Perry and Fitzpatrick, 2010).

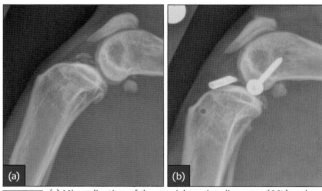

23.21 (a) Mineralization of the cranial cruciate ligament (CCL) and menisci is common in cats with degenerative CCL disease but can also be seen in clinically normal cats. (b) In the author's experience, the feline femorofabellar ligament is weaker than the equivalent ligament in dogs, which creates a higher risk of fabellar avulsion after lateral fabellotibial suture placement. A screw and washer have been used in this case to create a femoral anchor point.

Traumatic CCL rupture and multi-ligamentous injuries

Traumatic isolated CCL rupture occurs rarely. It is thought to occur as a result of stifle joint hyperextension and/or internal rotation, usually after trapping the affected limb and attempting to forcefully withdraw it. Currently, there is no objective evidence to support one technique of stifle stabilization above another after traumatic CCL rupture; however, if translational femorotibial instability is severe, the most appropriate surgical technique is probably intracapsular or extracapsular stabilization. In most cases of traumatic CCL rupture, especially those occurring after high-rise injuries or vehicular trauma, injuries to other ligaments and tendons (i.e. the caudal cruciate ligament, collateral ligaments, patellar tendon and long digital extensor tendons), articular cartilage and the menisci are common.

The collateral ligaments are major stabilizers of the stifle joint, counteracting valgus/varus, rotational and translational instabilities. If there is a suspicion of collateral ligament injury, the joint should be subjected to varus and valgus stress testing under deep sedation or general anaesthesia. Caudocranial radiographs can also be taken with stress applied to document valgus or varus instability after collateral ligament injury.

Management

Isolated low-grade collateral ligament sprains (see Chapter 9) may be amenable to non-surgical therapy, consisting of strict rest, non-steroidal anti-inflammatory drugs and a structured physical therapy programme. High-grade sprains causing palpable collateral ligament instability should be managed surgically. The goal of surgical treatment is to re-establish the functional length of the ligament and attain adequate joint stability and function through healing with fibrous tissue formation. This goal can be accomplished by various means:

- Ligament imbrication
- Primary suture repair
- Synthetic ligament replacement using screws or tissue anchors and suture
- Reattachment of avulsed fragments using screws and spiked washers or pins and tension-band wires.

Regardless of the method used for repair, external ancillary support is required for 4–6 weeks postoperatively. The stifle joint is very difficult to immobilize effectively using splint coaptation, so transarticular external skeletal fixation (see Figure 23.31b) is recommended in most cases (Higgins et al., 2010).

If trauma to the stifle is sufficiently severe to cause multiplanar instability or complete luxation, complete patient assessment (including complete blood counts, serum biochemistry and thoracic and abdominal radiography) should be performed to rule out important comorbidities. An important combination of injuries associated with stifle luxation is CCL rupture, MCL insufficiency and joint capsule tears. Avulsion of the caudal horn of the medial meniscus from the torn joint capsule is another common concurrent injury. Surgical exploration can be performed via a long medial or lateral parapatellar approach to allow inspection of the medial and lateral compartments. Each damaged structure must be addressed in turn. Avulsed menisci can theoretically be reattached to the joint capsule using fine absorbable mattress sutures, but crushing or tearing injuries require partial or complete meniscectomy. If both cruciate ligaments are torn, the stifle joint should be temporarily fixed in a normal weight-bearing position using an intraoperative transarticular pin (1.1–2.0 mm Kirschner wire) (Keely et al., 2007). It is vital that a normal femorotibial articulation is restored before soft tissue reconstructive surgery is performed. Avulsed cruciate ligaments can be reattached using screws or Kirschner wires, while mid-substance tears are treated by debridement and intra-articular or extracapsular repair. Joint capsule tears are either primarily repaired or allowed to heal by second intention. Once the intraoperative transarticular pin is removed, stifle joint stability and range of motion are tested before closure. Transarticular external skeletal fixation is recommended for 4–6 weeks postoperatively. Hinged transarticular skeletal fixation systems are commercially available and have an advantage of allowing increased stifle joint range of motion while providing adequate postoperative stability (Aron et al., 1997).

Multi-ligamentous stifle injuries are more common in cats than in dogs. In cats with complete stifle luxation, irreparable meniscal injuries are common. Stifle arthrodesis or hinged total knee replacement are both associated with good long-term function in cats and small dogs (see below).

Prognosis

With appropriate surgical treatment and physical rehabilitation, the prognosis for functional limb use is good. Obvious reduction of stifle range of motion is common immediately after removal of transarticular skeletal fixators, but this rapidly improves over the ensuing 2–3 weeks. Mild intermittent lameness is inevitable in a proportion of cases due to the severity of post-traumatic osteoarthritis. Athletic and working dogs are unlikely to return to pre-injury levels of performance.

Caudal cruciate ligament rupture

The caudal cruciate ligament arises within the intercondylar fossa from the lateral aspect of the medial femoral condyle and extends caudodistally to the lateral edge of the popliteal notch of the tibia (see Figure 23.8). The caudal cruciate ligament prevents caudal translation of the tibia relative to the femur and helps limit internal rotation of the tibia during joint flexion by twisting together with the CCL. It is a secondary restraint to hyperextension and helps limit valgus and varus movement when the stifle is flexed.

Caudal cruciate ligament injuries most commonly occur as a component of multi-ligamentous injuries of the stifle. There is also a theoretical risk of caudal cruciate ligament rupture after TPLO surgery if the plateau has been inadvertently over-rotated. Traumatic isolated rupture of the caudal cruciate ligament is very rare. When it does occur, it is usually in young large-breed dogs that have sustained severe trauma. Avulsion of the femoral origin of the ligament is the commonest mode of failure. Diagnosis is made from the presence of caudal draw. If differentiation of caudal draw from cranial draw is difficult, a tibial compression test should be performed. This test is positive in CCL rupture but negative in caudal cruciate ligament rupture. Radiographs show obvious caudal tibial subluxation (Figure 23.22).

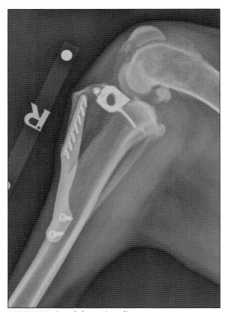

23.22 Caudal cruciate ligament rupture occurred secondary to septic arthritis as a late complication after tibial tuberosity advancement (TTA) surgery to treat complete CCL rupture. Note the caudal displacement of the tibial eminences relative to the femoral condyles.

Conservative management is justified in most cases because normal function was reported after non-surgical management of caudal cruciate ligament transection in experimental dogs (Harari *et al.*, 1987). If caudal cruciate ligament rupture results from over-rotation of the tibial plateau during TPLO, surgery should be revised to restore an appropriate tibial plateau angle (~6 degrees) and the caudal cruciate ligament should be replaced via intra-articular or extracapsular repair.

Septic arthritis

Septic arthritis (see Chapter 6) is a debilitating disease that presents most commonly as a severe acute lameness, although a chronic form exists which causes a milder weight-bearing lameness. Previous reports have found stifle surgery or haematological spread to account for most cases of septic arthritis (Marchevsky and Read, 1999; Clements *et al.*, 2005). Other rare sources of infection include foreign body penetration of the joint or local spread from adjacent tissues. The most common bacteria isolated in septic arthritis are skin commensals including *Staphylococcus pseudintermedius*, *S. aureus*, and β-haemolytic *Streptococcus* spp. Unlike horses and farm animals, which can be affected by a septic polyarthropathy caused by haematogenous spread from a septic focus, canine bacterial septic arthritis is almost always a monoarthropathy.

Medial patellar luxation in dogs
Signalment and history

MPL is most commonly recognized in toy and miniature breeds, especially Miniature Poodles and Yorkshire Terriers. This condition occurs less frequently in large and giant-breed dogs but when it does occur, certain breeds

are predisposed. These include English and Staffordshire Bull Terriers, English Bulldogs, Labrador Retrievers and Mastiffs. Many dogs are presented before reaching skeletal maturity; however, in some cases lameness may only become a feature later in life or secondary to stifle effusion and instability caused by CCL rupture. Unilateral MPL often presents as an intermittent 'skipping' lameness. In dogs with low-grade MPL, the patella may spontaneously relocate resulting in immediate lameness resolution. Lameness may become continuous in dogs with high-grade luxation (see below), if retropatellar chondromalacia develops, or in dogs affected by concurrent CCL injury. Anatomical deformities causing intermittent luxation may progress over time, potentially resulting in permanent luxation later in life. Although MPL is sometimes the result of severe trauma, most cases are considered developmental because they occur at an early age and there is no history of trauma. Deformities such as medial displacement of the quadriceps muscle group, lateral torsion or bowing of the distal femur, femoral epiphyseal dysplasia, internal tibial torsion and rotational instability of the stifle joint present either in isolation or in combination in dogs affected by MPL.

Clinical findings

The clinical signs of MPL vary according to the degree of deformity, chronicity of the condition and whether or not one or both stifles are affected. A 'bow-legged' conformation (genu varum) is a feature in some dogs. Patellar tracking and the angle of the femorotibial joint when the patella luxates should be determined. Integrity of the cruciate ligaments, evidence of femoropatellar crepitus and pain, and any reduced range of stifle extension should be noted.

Grading patellar luxations is useful for monitoring progression of the condition and response to surgery. The following clinical grades have been proposed:

- **Grade I** – The patella can be manually luxated but returns to a normal position when released
- **Grade II** – The patella may luxate during stifle flexion or manual manipulation and remains luxated until stifle extension or manual replacement occurs. This grade covers a broad spectrum of disease severity in that the patella may luxate infrequently or frequently
- **Grade III** – The patella is permanently luxated but can be manually replaced. It reluxates spontaneously when manual pressure is removed
- **Grade IV** – The patella is permanently luxated and cannot be replaced.

The dog should be examined initially in a normal standing position without manipulating either pelvic limb. If periarticular soft tissue thickening makes identification of the patella difficult, the tibial tuberosity should be palpated first and the fingers should follow the patellar tendon proximally towards the femoral trochlear groove. If the finger identifies the trochlear groove, the patella is luxated. Cranial draw testing should always be performed because concurrent CCL disease has been documented in up to 42% of dogs presenting for MPL repair (Brower *et al.*, 2017).

Radiography

Radiographs are assessed for the presence of angular and/or torsional limb deformities (see above). If possible (grades I and II), radiographs should be acquired with the patella reduced because patellar luxation exaggerates the appearance of osseous deformities. Tangential ('sky-line') views of the flexed stifle are of limited value because depth of the femoral trochlear sulcus is best assessed surgically. Computed tomography (CT) is particularly useful for preoperative planning before femoral corrective osteotomy (Figure 23.23).

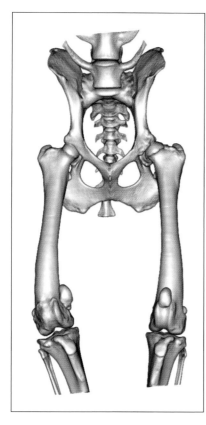

23.23 CT scan showing deformities in a 22-month-old Akita with grade III medial patellar luxation of the right hindlimb (left on the image). Note the distal femoral varus, the medial luxated position of the patella and the internal rotation of the tibia and tibial tuberosity. The left hindlimb (right on the image) has mild distal femoral varus.
(Courtesy of Gareth Arthurs)

Surgical management

MPL presents either as an important clinical problem causing intermittent or constant lameness, or as an incidental finding during routine physical examination. There is no evidence to support 'prophylactic' surgery in clinically occult cases of MPL because the progression of osteoarthritis is not influenced by whether or not surgery is performed (Willauer and Vasseur, 1987; Roy et al., 1992). Thus, in skeletally mature dogs, the decision to operate is usually made based on the frequency of lameness episodes; for example, limping once every month might be managed non-surgically while daily lameness would be managed surgically. Decision making is more controversial in puppies because clinically mild MPL can develop into severe MPL as a consequence of progressive limb deformity. Skeletal deformities progress secondary to abnormal forces exerted on the distal femoral and proximal tibial physes as a result of displacement of the quadriceps muscle during the growth phase. Reduced femoropatellar pressure secondary to MPL leads to underdevelopment of the femoral trochlear sulcus. Progression of these deformities can be mitigated by early restoration of normal patellar tracking.

Surgical treatments of patellar luxation may be subdivided into those that improve alignment of the quadriceps mechanism, those that deepen the femoral trochlear sulcus, and soft tissue reconstructive procedures that influence medial or lateral patellar support. With the exception of puppies with the potential for improved limb alignment and femoropatellar congruity, over-reliance on soft tissue reconstructive procedures should be avoided. Failure to correct tibial and/or femoral misalignment is a common cause of MPL recurrence following surgical repair (Arthurs and Langley-Hobbs, 2006; Roch and Gemmill, 2008).

Tibial tuberosity transposition

With the exception of skeletally immature puppies, realignment of the quadriceps muscle should always be performed via tibial tuberosity transposition. Tibial tuberosity transposition (see Operative technique 23.7) results in a lower incidence of major complications including clinically important patellar re-luxation (Arthurs and Langley-Hobbs, 2006). Meticulous attention to detail is required to ensure that the extensor mechanism has been adequately realigned and stabilized using a pin and tension-band wire technique.

Deepening the femoral trochlear sulcus (sulcoplasty)

Many techniques have been described for deepening the femoral trochlea. Trochleoplasty (block and wedge recession) and trochlear chondroplasty (preserves intact hyaline cartilage in young puppies) have been associated with good success in numerous studies. Nevertheless, all sulcoplasty procedures cause some degree of hyaline cartilage morbidity. Damaged hyaline cartilage is permanently replaced with fibrocartilage that is weaker and less suited to articulation than the hyaline cartilage it replaces. Even minor cartilage damage can trigger an inflammatory cascade that contributes to the progression of osteoarthritis. Radiographic osteophytosis has been shown to progress significantly faster in dogs treated for MPL with trochleoplasty compared to dogs treated surgically but without trochleoplasty (Yoon, 2014). Thus, trochleoplasty should only be performed if there is an obviously shallow groove. In one study of 91 dogs in which MPL surgery was performed without trochleoplasty, there was a patellar re-luxation rate of 20% and a revision surgery (major complication) rate of 6.6% (Linney et al., 2011). These complication rates are similar to previously reported rates of 5–6% patellar re-luxation, 6–11% major complications and 0–11% revision surgery when trochleoplasty was not performed (Arthurs and Langley-Hobbs, 2006; Gibbons et al., 2006). However, when an obviously shallow groove is present, there is a clear indication for trochleoplasty. Another study reported a 5-fold reduction of patellar re-luxation when trochleoplasty was performed in addition to tibial tuberosity transposition (Cashmore et al., 2014).

Block recession sulcoplasty: Block recession sulcoplasty (see Operative Technique 23.8) utilizes a rectangular osteochondral autograft that is harvested from the trochlea and replaced into the deepened recipient bed (Talcott et al., 2000). Compared with wedge recession sulcoplasty, block recession resulted in improved patellar recession in the extended cadaveric canine stifle and reduced re-luxation during internal torsion of the tibia (Johnson et al., 2001).

Wedge recession sulcoplasty: Wedge recession sulcoplasty (see Operative Technique 23.8) is frequently performed in preference to block recession sulcoplasty because it is perceived to be an easier procedure.

However, there are several important disadvantages of wedge recession. Firstly, the osteotomies must be created at an acute angle to the cartilage surface. Consequently, it is common for the saw blade to slip and excoriate the articular cartilage of the wedge. Secondly, if the osteotomies are not sufficiently convergent, they can drift towards the intercondylar notch and damage the origin of the caudal cruciate ligament. Finally, the tapering proximal end of the wedge may prevent adequate recession of the proximal trochlea so that the patella remains vulnerable to reluxation when the stifle is extended.

Medial trochlear buttress: At the time of writing, a system that employs a polyethylene buttress to increase the height of the medial trochlear ridge has recently become available (RidgeStop™, Orthomed; Figure 23.24). Various sizes of implant can be applied to multiple sizes of dogs. The main advantages of this technique in comparison to trochleoplasty are that prosthetic trochlear ridge height is maximized proximally and there is no hyaline cartilage morbidity. Despite these important advantages, it is vital to recognize that this implant should only be considered an alternative to trochleoplasty. It should not be employed as the sole corrective procedure without adequate correction of quadriceps mechanism malalignment. At the time of writing, the potential complications and long-term outcome after medial trochlear buttress surgery are unknown.

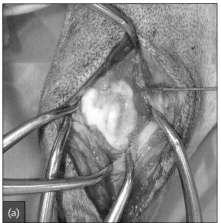

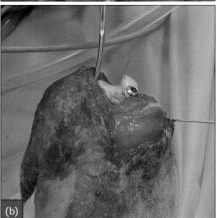

23.24 (a) Diffuse full-thickness cartilage erosion is present on the medial trochlear ridge of this 2-year-old French Bulldog with grade III medial patellar luxation (MPL) (medial is to the right of the image). (b) A RidgeStop™ implant was used to cover the cartilage defect and increase the height of the medial trochlear ridge. Quadriceps realignment was also performed via tibial tuberosity transposition.

Lateral soft tissue tightening

The lateral joint capsule and fascia lata may be tightened after reduction of the patella. Care should be taken to avoid excessive tightening, which can cause lateral patellar luxation. Occasionally it is necessary to place a non-absorbable suture or strip of fascia lata from the lateral fabella to the patella to augment other stabilizing procedures, especially in dogs with increased internal rotational laxity. Tightening is achieved by resection of an elliptical piece of joint capsule and fascia lata or via capsular/fascial overlap or a combination of both.

Medial soft tissue release

The surgical approach to the stifle joint for MPL repair usually involves a lateral parapatellar arthrotomy. Concurrent medial parapatellar arthrotomy can also be performed to release taut or fibrotic medial retinacular tissues. The proximal extent of the release varies according to the amount of soft tissue fibrosis. Medial soft tissue release should only be performed if it is otherwise impossible to relocate the patella and realign the quadriceps mechanism because a higher frequency of major complications has been reported after release (Arthurs and Langley-Hobbs, 2006).

Corrective osteotomy

The majority of cases of MPL can be successfully managed using tibial tuberosity transposition, trochleoplasty and soft tissue reconstructive procedures. Corrective distal femoral osteotomy (Figure 23.25) is advocated as a component of MPL repair when osseous deformities include excessive femoral varus. The selection criteria are poorly defined, but angles >12 degrees have been used

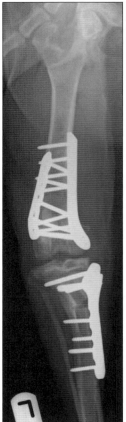

23.25 Distal femoral and proximal tibial osteotomies have been performed to treat excessive distal femoral and proximal tibial varus and torsion.

because this is outside the reported reference ranges (Dudley *et al.*, 2006). The two most common indications for distal femoral osteotomy are grade III and IV MPL in large-breed dogs (Swiderski and Palmer, 2007) and for revision of patellar re-luxation in any dog with significant distal femoral varus (Roch and Gemmill, 2008). Patellar re-luxation following traditional surgical treatment is more frequent in large-breed dogs than in small-breed dogs (Arthurs and Langley-Hobbs, 2006). This has led to speculation that untreated excessive femoral varus may play a role in postoperative patellar re-luxation following traditional MPL treatment in large-breed dogs (Swiderski and Palmer, 2007). Distal femoral osteotomy surgery is associated with high success rates (Brower *et al.*, 2017) but requires meticulous attention to detail in the preoperative planning, especially the radiographic assessment of the required degree of correction. The surgical technique itself is also more demanding than traditional MPL repair.

Trochlear sulcus replacement

In dogs with severe irreversible pathology to the trochlear ridges or sulcus, the entire trochlea can be replaced by a prosthesis. Diamond-like-coated titanium implants are commercially available for this purpose (Kyon, Switzerland; Figure 23.26). Early clinical results of a patellar groove replacement system are encouraging, but there are no long-term outcome studies available at the time of writing.

Concomitant patellar luxation and CCL rupture

Anecdotally, correction of femoropatellar instability has been considered more important than management of the CCL rupture. Affected stifles often have significant osteoarthritis and the associated periarticular fibrosis reduces femorotibial instability. When significant cranial draw is present in dogs with low scores in the CCL decision-making algorithm, a LFS may provide adequate stability. The Kirschner wires stabilizing the tibial tuberosity transposition may be used as the distal anchor. Arthrotomy to allow meniscal inspection is mandatory. Tibial plateau

levelling techniques may be used to manage MPL and concurrent CCL rupture. With the TPLO procedure, the craniodistal fragment, including the tibial tuberosity, can be externally rotated in order to effect modest quadriceps mechanism realignment (Langenbach and Marcellin-Little, 2010). In cases requiring substantial quadriceps mechanism re-alignment, TPLO can be combined with tibial tuberosity transposition (Leonard *et al.*, 2016). TTA has also been successfully modified to incorporate lateral and distal tibial tuberosity transposition for the treatment of MPL and concomitant CCL disease in large-breed dogs (Yeadon *et al.*, 2011).

Prognosis

The prognosis following MPL surgery is generally good, although postoperative complications are reported in 18–29% of operated stifles (Arthurs and Langley-Hobbs, 2006; Gibbons *et al.*, 2006). An increased risk for postoperative complications has been identified in heavier dogs, higher grades of MPL and after failure to address the underlying conformational abnormalities using tibial tuberosity transposition and recession trochleoplasty. In small-breed dogs with grade IV MPL complicated by severe anatomical deformities, stifle arthrodesis offers a reasonable salvage option.

Lateral patellar luxation in dogs

Although the accepted dogma is that, typically, MPL affects small-breed dogs and lateral patellar luxation (LPL) affects large-breed dogs, MPL is more frequently recognized in dogs of all sizes (Hayes *et al.*, 1994). Compared with MPL, LPL is rare; when it is seen, it more often affects large and giant-breed dogs. LPL is typically associated with a distinct complex of severe limb deformities including hip dysplasia, increased anteversion of the femoral neck, increased angle of inclination (*coxa valga*), medial bowing of the distal femur, shallow trochlea, lateral displacement of the tibial tuberosity, lateral bowing of the tibia and external rotation of the paw.

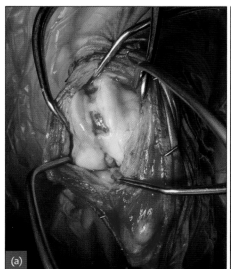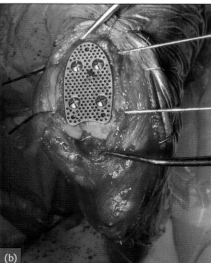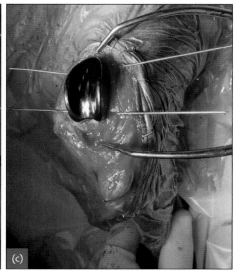

23.26 (a) A block recession sulcoplasty had been performed but there was recurrent patellar luxation and almost complete necrosis of the cartilage surface of the osteochondral graft. (b) The trochlea has been resected (K-wires were used for soft tissue retraction) and the base-plate has been screwed into place. (c) The patellar groove prosthesis *in situ*.

Due to the complexity of the anatomical deformities associated with LPL, surgical outcome is often described as being worse than the outcome after surgical correction of MPL. Complication rates after LPL surgery are high, with one study reporting an overall complication rate of 51%, with 38% major complications. Of these, patellar re-luxation was the commonest problem. The principles of surgical correction of MPL should also be applied to LPL; most importantly, failure to appreciate the underlying skeletal deformities and apply appropriate corrective surgery is likely to result in a suboptimal outcome (Kalff *et al.*, 2014).

Patellar luxation in cats

In cats, MPL is more common than LPL, and Devon Rex and Abyssinian breeds appear to be predisposed as a result of developmental hypoplasia of the medial femoral condyle. Affected cats are also frequently affected by hip dysplasia. Patellar luxation is often an incidental finding, since the majority of cats with patellar luxation are not lame. The normal feline patella has a relatively higher range of medial-to-lateral mobility within the trochlear groove than the canine patella; thus, feline patellar 'subluxation' is considered a normal finding. When lameness does occur, it is often described by owners as a 'collapsing' or 'buckling' of the affected limb or a crouched stance rather than the skipping lameness that is typical of canine patellar luxation.

Treatment

Skeletal deformity is generally less severe than in dogs. When patellar luxation results in lameness, surgical correction is indicated. Tibial tuberosity transposition, with or without a recession trochleoplasty technique, is often necessary. In general, the surgical techniques used to correct canine patellar luxation can be successfully performed in cats; however, the reported complication rate of 26% (Rutherford *et al.*, 2014) is higher than the complication rate reported after similar procedures in dogs. The most common complications reported after feline patellar luxation repair were implant-related problems after tibial tuberosity transposition. The feline proximal tibia is thinner in the sagittal plane than the canine proximal tibia; consequently, the tibial tuberosity fragment is often small and may be more prone to fracture after fixation with a pin and tension-band wire construct, especially if the pins are oversized. In addition, tibial tuberosity transposition appears to be less effective at preventing patellar re-luxation than it is in dogs (Arthurs and Langley-Hobbs, 2006; Rutherford *et al.*, 2014).

Partial parasagittal patellectomy

The feline stifle is unusual because the patella is wider in a mediolateral direction relative to the femoral trochlear sulcus (Rutherford and Arthurs, 2014). This shape hinders stable tracking of the patella even after recession sulcoplasty (Rutherford and Arthurs, 2014). Parasagittal patellectomy can be performed in order to match the mediolateral width of the patella to the dimensions of the trochlear sulcus. This involves lateral partial patellar ostectomy using an oscillating saw. At the time of writing, successful partial parasagittal patellectomy has only been reported in four cats (Rutherford and Arthurs, 2014) and the long-term outcome is unknown.

Osteochondrosis

Osteochondrosis (OC) is a developmental cartilage disorder most commonly affecting young, rapidly growing, large or giant-breed dogs. The disease is characterized by disruption of the normal process of endochondral ossification and focal osteonecrosis. When cartilage fails to mature into bone, it becomes thickened and the deeper chondrocytes become necrotic due to lack of diffusion of nutrients. Unlike normal articular cartilage, thickened cartilage has a poor resistance to shear forces. When the shear resistance is exceeded, fissures form in the deeper zones. If these fissures propagate into a dissecting flap, the condition is termed osteochondritis dissecans. The ultimate cause of OC is unknown, but commonly cited aetiological factors include genetic predisposition, rapid growth, anatomical conformation and nutritional imbalances. Some of the postulated causes of OC may be interrelated. For example, inherited factors have been closely associated with rapid growth rate or joint conformations that predispose to OC (Ytrehus *et al.*, 2007). Phenotypic expression in predisposed individuals can be influenced by environmental factors including calcium supplementation, which has been implicated in the development of OC in Great Dane puppies (Goedegebuure and Hazewinkel, 1986).

OC of the stifle joint is an uncommon cause of lameness in dogs, occurring less frequently than OC of the shoulder, elbow or hock joints (Montgomery *et al.*, 1994). The axial weight-bearing portion of the lateral condyle is most frequently affected, although the medial condyle can be involved either concurrently or in isolation. In one case series, the medial condyle was more commonly affected than the lateral condyle (Bertrand *et al.*, 1997). Patellar OC has also been described in humans, horses, pigs and dogs and was implicated as a cause of pathological bilateral patellar fractures in a cat (Palierne *et al.*, 2010). The concept that atraumatic feline patellar fractures can be caused by OC might help explain their unpredictable healing characteristics (Langley-Hobbs, 2009) (see the *BSAVA Manual of Canine and Feline Fracture Repair and Management*).

Presentation

Predisposed breeds include Great Danes, Labrador Retrievers, Golden Retrievers, Newfoundlands, Mastiffs and German Shepherd Dogs. Age at presentation typically ranges from 5–12 months; however, late diagnosis is common, particularly when radiographs are not obtained as part of the initial database. Affected dogs usually present with insidious onset lameness affecting one or both pelvic limbs. Bilateral lesions are recognized in approximately one-quarter of affected dogs (Bertrand *et al.*, 1997; Cook *et al.*, 2008). The degree of lameness varies from subtle to non-weight-bearing, and is often exacerbated by vigorous exercise. Joint effusion can be overt, but stifle pain varies. When typical clinical signs are recognized, the principal differential diagnoses are CCL disease and septic arthritis. Imaging is required to achieve a definitive diagnosis of stifle OC.

Radiographic assessment

Standard caudocranial and mediolateral radiographs (Figure 23.27) of both stifles are acquired (see above) due to the possibility of bilateral pathology. The radiographic findings associated with stifle OC include:

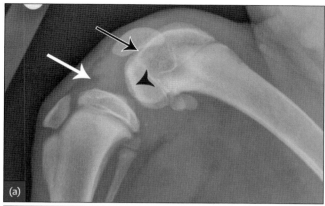

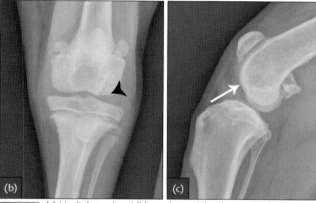

23.27 (a) Mediolateral and (b) caudocranial radiographs showing osteochondrosis of the lateral femoral condyle in a 5-month-old Hungarian Vizsla. Note that marked stifle effusion causes compression of the fat pad (white arrow) as well as the fascial plane caudal to the stifle joint. Flattening of the lateral femoral condyle can be seen on both views (arrowheads) and sclerosis can be seen in the adjacent subchondral bone on the mediolateral view. The black arrow shows the typical location of the extensor fossa that appears as an indentation in the contour of the lateral femoral trochlear ridge and should not be mistaken for an OC lesion. (c) The normal extensor fossa (arrowed) in this 1.5-year-old Newfoundland affected by a partial cranial cruciate ligament (CCL) rupture is very obvious. This appearance is common in giant-breed dogs.

- Joint effusion (recognized as compression of the infrapatellar fat pad)
- Radiolucent defects of the subchondral bone of one or both femoral condyles
- Sclerosis associated with the defect and adjacent femoral condyle
- Calcified free bodies ('joint mice')
- Periarticular osteophytes (in chronic cases).

Advanced imaging and arthroscopic assessment are rarely necessary to achieve a definitive diagnosis but are useful for preoperative planning when resurfacing procedures are being considered (see below).

Treatment

Non-surgical management

Non-surgical management consists of short-term exercise restriction and non-steroidal anti-inflammatory medications. Non-surgical management is appropriate in stifle joints in which OC is an incidental finding with no associated clinical signs; for example, after screening a contralateral stifle joint in a dog with unilateral clinical signs. Clinical and radiographic reassessment is recommended after 4–6 weeks to ensure that there is no evidence of disease progression that might warrant surgical intervention.

Surgical debridement

Palliative surgical treatment is recommended in cases showing persistent lameness. This involves removal of pathological cartilage and bone with subsequent curettage, forage or micro-picking of subchondral bone to stimulate bleeding that, in turn, induces fibrocartilage proliferation within the defect. Inspection of, and access to, the OC lesion can be accomplished via a lateral or medial para-patellar approach, depending on lesion location. Based on the limited current evidence, a guarded to poor prognosis for high-level, pain-free function is expected after palliative debridement of stifle OC lesions. Outcome is likely to depend on the size and location of the lesion, with smaller, axial lesions carrying a more favourable prognosis. Early intervention and arthroscopic treatment may optimize surgical outcome, with one report suggesting that arthroscopic treatment resulted in subjectively better short-term outcomes when compared with cases treated by arthrotomy (Bertrand *et al.*, 1997). Suboptimal outcomes for canine stifle OC have been attributed to extensive loss of weight-bearing articular cartilage and subchondral bone, joint incongruity, inferior biomechanics of reparative tissue and/or pre-existing or subsequent secondary osteoarthritis in this high-demand and complex joint (Cook *et al.*, 2008).

Osteochondral grafting

Stifle OC defects can be resurfaced using either auto-genous tissue or synthetic graft substitutes. Based on encouraging results in humans, the Osteochondral Autograft Transfer System (OATS®, Arthrex) was applied to 12 stifle joints in 10 dogs affected by OC of the lateral femoral condyle (Cook *et al.*, 2008). Specific equipment used to harvest and transfer the osteochondral graft can be obtained as either a single-use disposable kit or as a reusable kit. Articular cartilage is harvested from the non-weight-bearing distal femoral trochlea at the sulcus terminalis (Figure 23.28). Large defects can be resurfaced using multiple osteochondral grafts arranged in an overlapping mosaic pattern. Autografts are integrated into the subjacent subchondral bone. Second-look arthroscopic follow-up showed maintenance of articular cartilage composition and architecture, and restoration of articular surface contour and congruity (Cook *et al.*, 2008). Although this procedure is low risk (the only reported complication was transient periarticular swelling) and all dogs sustained significant long-term clinical improvements, only 2/10 dogs were completely free from pain or lameness in the long term.

Synthetic resurfacing

Synthetic resurfacing of femoral condylar OC lesions is possible using a commercial polyurethane titanium-backed plug (SynaCart®, Arthrex; Figure 23.29). There are three potential advantages of this system:

- Donor site morbidity is avoided
- The synthetic graft can be contoured *in situ* to produce a congruent surface
- Implants are available in multiple diameters.

These implants show a great deal of potential, with good results being demonstrated in an experimental canine stifle model (Cook *et al.*, 2014); however, although they are commercially available at the time of writing, they are still undergoing clinical evaluation.

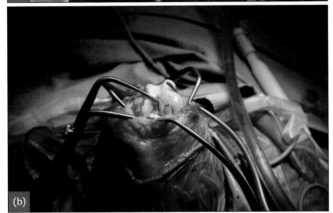

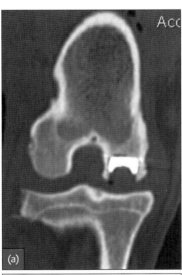

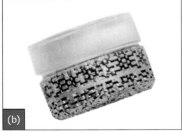

23.28 Osteochondral autograft transfer in a 7-month-old Labrador Retriever with osteochondrosis. Note (a) the harvest site in the non-weight-bearing sulcus terminalis of the femoral trochlea and (b) the transposed graft *in situ*, which should have a surface contour that is continuous with the surrounding cartilage.

23.29 (a) Computed tomographic and (b) photographic images of a SynaCart® implant used for resurfacing a medial condylar osteochondrosis lesion.
(Courtesy of Noel Fitzpatrick)

Patellar tendon injuries

The names patellar tendon and patellar ligament are used interchangeably. Conditions affecting the patellar tendon are unusual in dogs and rare in cats.

Patellar tendon rupture

Traumatic injuries of the patellar tendon are rare. At the time of writing, there have been a total of 14 reported cases, including 13 dogs and one cat (Ries and Harris, 1982; Gilmore, 1983; Bloomberg and Parker, 1984; Culvenor, 1988; Aron et al., 1997; Smith et al., 2000; Gemmill and Carmichael, 2003; Shipov et al., 2008; Archer et al., 2010; Farrell and Fitzpatrick, 2013). The most common injury is direct penetrating trauma. Indirect trauma can cause rupture via forceful contraction of the quadriceps muscle against a flexed and immobile stifle joint. Patellar tendon injury could also occur as a consequence of tibial tuberosity surgery, e.g. tibial tuberosity transposition (Figure 23.30), or stabilization of a tibial tuberosity fracture. It may be associated with placement of K-wire and tension band constructs that 'cheese-wire' through the patellar tendon. For this reason, when it is necessary to place K-wires relatively proximally in the patellar tendon insertion, it may be prudent to place these wires in series so that the tension-band wire only engages the proximal wire.

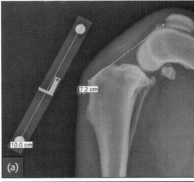

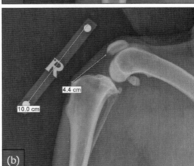

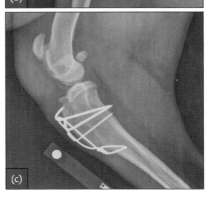

23.30 (a) Mediolateral radiograph showing left patellar tendon rupture in a 4-year-old Rhodesian Ridgeback. A penetrating injury had been sustained 10 days previously. Note the patella alta caused by lengthening of the patellar tendon mechanism. (b) The normal stifle joint is shown for comparison. (c) Patellar tendon rupture can be seen in this 1-year-old Labrador Retriever. This mediolateral radiograph was taken 6 weeks after tibial tuberosity transposition.

Diagnosis

Any age or breed of animal with a suggestive history or penetrating trauma can be affected. Clinical diagnosis of patellar tendon insufficiency relies on identification of patella alta (i.e. proximal displacement of the patella) and a reduced or absent patellar reflex. Plain radiography can be used to confirm a diagnosis of complete tendon rupture by documentation of patella alta. If patella alta is not radiographically demonstrable, ultrasonography is the first choice imaging modality (see Figure 23.41). CT and MRI are usually reserved for cases of chronic patellar tendinitis.

Treatment

Surgical intervention is indicated if a patellar tendon injury is sufficiently severe that patella alta is identifiable. Acute ruptures in dogs can be repaired primarily, with good clinical results. Mid-tendon ruptures are repaired using a paired locking loop or 3-loop pulley suture pattern with 3 metric (2/0 USP) polydioxanone (PDS). Insertional avulsions can be repaired using suture and bone tunnels. Regardless of the technique, augmentation and protection of the repair are essential because tensile forces transmitted through the patellar tendon during normal ambulation (including slow walking) significantly exceed the tensile strength of the tenorrhaphy. Techniques used to augment the repair include:

- A loop of suture (nylon or stainless steel) passed through bone tunnels in the patella and tibial tuberosity or through the quadriceps tendon immediately proximal to the patella and a bone tunnel in the tibial tuberosity
- Fascial or tendon allograft (Veterinary Transplant Services, Kent, WA, USA)
- Autogenous fascia lata or hamstring graft (Figure 23.31a; Farrell and Fitzpatrick, 2013)
- A transarticular external skeletal fixator (ESF) can be used to protect the internal repair. Where possible, the ESF (Figure 23.31b) should be maintained for a minimum of 4 weeks. Maintenance for >6 weeks is challenging because of a tendency for pins to loosen causing significant morbidity.

Chronic patellar tendon ruptures typically result from delayed diagnosis or unsuccessful surgical intervention. Under these circumstances, post-traumatic tendon degeneration can result in a significant defect that necessitates partial or complete patellar tendon replacement. Allograft or autogenous graft tissues can be used to repair defects and augmentation can be applied as described above. When patellar tendon injuries involve non-reconstructable local soft tissue loss, stifle arthrodesis may be indicated.

Postoperative care includes strict exercise restriction for a minimum of 6 weeks, regular clinical and radiographic reassessment and physical rehabilitation after removal of any external protection. The prognosis for return to full athletic function depends on the severity of the injury and is guarded when complete tendon replacement is required.

Patellar tendinitis

Low-grade patellar tendon strains usually occur secondary to surgery that isolates the tibial tuberosity or changes stifle biomechanics and thereby alters tendon loading (i.e. TPLO, TTA and tibial tuberosity transposition). Patellar tendon thickening after TPLO is common and has also been reported after TTA (Pettitt *et al.*, 2014). Multiple risk

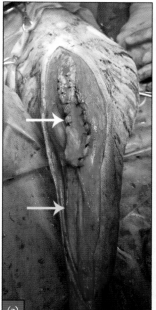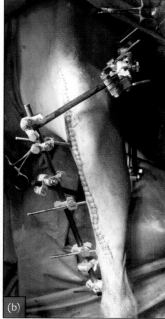

23.31 Surgical reconstruction of the patellar tendon (left is medial). (a) The patellar defect was reconstructed and the primary repair has been internally augmented using a hamstring graft. Note the defect in the donor bed along the medial aspect of the tibia (yellow arrow), and the transposed graft sutured to the abaxial borders of the patellar tendon (white arrow). (b) A transarticular external skeletal fixator has been used to protect an internal patellar tendon reconstruction. The four pins transfixing the femur are placed from lateral to medial and the four tibial pins are placed from medial to lateral to maximize the use of safe corridors.

factors have been identified including an excessively cranial tibial osteotomy, a partially intact CCL in conjunction with a cranial osteotomy and postoperative tibial tuberosity fracture (Carey *et al.*, 2005). Affected dogs typically have a lameness that is more obvious when they are stationary than when they are walking or trotting. Lameness grade is variable and depends on the severity of strain injury. The tendon is usually most affected at its distal insertion where it is palpably thickened, and can be painful and crepitant in some dogs. A presumptive diagnosis can be made based on radiographic patellar tendon thickening (Figure 23.32). Ultrasonography can be used to assess changes to the architecture of the tendon. In most dogs, post-surgical patellar tendinitis spontaneously resolves after rest and non-steroidal anti-inflammatory

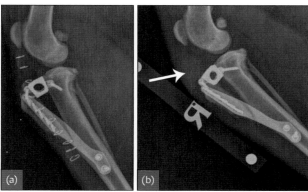

23.32 Mediolateral radiographs of the stifle joint of a 6-year-old Springer Spaniel taken (a) immediately and (b) 6 weeks postoperatively following TTA surgery. Note the severe insertional thickening of the patellar tendon (arrowed).

medication, but recovery can take several months. In humans, recovery times after patellar tendinitis can be shortened using acupuncture or extracorporeal shockwave therapy. These techniques are equally applicable in affected dogs.

Tibial tuberosity apophysitis

Osgood–Schlatter disease is a traction injury affecting the patellar tendon–tibial tuberosity complex of young active adolescent humans. The condition causes pain and swelling that is localized to the insertion of the patellar tendon, and is bilateral in 20–30% of affected individuals (von Pfeil et al., 2009). Dogs are affected by a similar condition although it is rare; one study reported an incidence of 0.08% of referral hospital admissions (Ehrenborg and Olsson, 1962). The pathogenesis of tibial tuberosity apophysitis is not completely understood, although there is thought to be a traumatic component. In humans with Osgood–Schlatter disease, forceful contraction of the quadriceps muscle in young individuals exceeds the tensile strength of the patellar tendon insertion, resulting in avulsion of small pieces of cartilage or bone from the tibial tuberosity. A similar pathogenesis is likely in dogs; however, a genetic predisposition has also been suggested (Skelly et al., 1997). In the United Kingdom, Staffordshire Bull Terriers are most commonly affected.

In dogs with apophysitis without avulsion of the apophysis, lameness can resolve spontaneously with strict rest and non-steroidal anti-inflammatory drugs, but complete resolution of lameness can take several weeks. Surgery involves the application of a pin and tension-band wire construct. Surgery is indicated in dogs with intractable pain and lameness, if radiographs show moderate to significant displacement of the tibial tuberosity or if radiographic fusion of the apophysis is not apparent after 4–6 weeks of non-surgical management.

Long digital extensor tendon injuries

The long digital extensor (LDE) tendon originates in the extensor fossa of the lateral femoral epicondyle. Nearly the entire tendon is intra-articular. The muscle belly passes through the extensor groove on the craniolateral aspect of the tibia, and inserts on digits 2–5. Its primary functions include flexion of the tarsus and extension of the digits (Smith, 1999).

Long digital extensor tendon avulsion

Avulsion of the LDE tendon is an uncommon injury seen in young large and giant-breed dogs. Most affected dogs are less than 6 months old when the injury occurs and have a history of mild trauma (e.g. jumping or falling). There is a variable amount of stifle joint effusion, pain and soft tissue thickening lateral to the joint. Insufficiency of the LDE can be confirmed by simultaneously fully flexing the stifle, extending the hock and attempting to flex the digits. The digits will flex without tension if the LDE mechanism is not intact. In the acute stage, avulsion fragments can be detected radiographically near the extensor fossa. Radiographic changes observed with chronic avulsion include mineralization of the LDE tendon and an osseous defect at the extensor fossa. CT, MRI, exploratory arthroscopy and arthrotomy can all be used to confirm the diagnosis.

The treatment of choice for LDE tendon avulsion is surgical reattachment of the tendon origin. This can be accomplished via:

- Screw or divergent K-wire fixation of an avulsed bone fragment
- Resection of the bone fragment then screw and spiked washer reattachment of the avulsed tendon.

If reattachment to the femur cannot be achieved, tenodesis to the proximal tibia should be performed using a screw and spiked washer or staple fixation.

The repair should be protected by strict exercise restriction and prevention of stifle flexion using a soft padded bandage, splint or cast for 2–3 weeks. Physical rehabilitation should be employed over the following 4–6 weeks to optimize healing and function. To date, all reported cases have returned to a sound gait (Pond, 1973; Lammerding et al., 1976; Bardet and Piermattei, 1983; Stramel, 1997).

Long digital extensor tendon luxation

Luxation of the LDE tendon has been reported as a complication after TPLO surgery in four dogs (Haaland and Sjostrom, 2007). Luxation was thought to have been a consequence of iatrogenic injury to the retinaculum that normally secures the LDE within the extensor fossa. Lameness occurred suddenly 1–12 months postoperatively and LDE luxation was easily palpated. Treatment involved securing the LDE tendon in its normal position, or transection and tenodesis. Lameness resolved in all four cases.

Gastrocnemius muscle avulsion

The gastrocnemius muscle is divided proximally into medial and lateral bellies that originate on the medial and lateral femoral supracondylar tuberosities. Each head contains a sesamoid bone, i.e. the fabella. The two muscle bellies merge distally to comprise the major component of the common calcaneal tendon that inserts on the mid to lateral aspect of the proximal calcaneus. The gastrocnemius muscle acts to flex the stifle and extend the hock. Avulsion injuries can affect the lateral or medial heads or both. This unusual injury is assumed to occur as a result of low-grade trauma although there is often no witnessed event. Athletic large-breed dogs are most commonly affected but it can occur in cats (Figure 23.33). Clinical presentation is of weight-bearing lameness with varying degrees of hyperflexion of the hock (plantigrade stance). Localized swelling and pain may be present. Radiographs reveal distal displacement of one or both fabellae with associated soft tissue swelling. Pathological displacement of a fabella must be distinguished from normal fabellar asymmetry that occurs commonly in terriers, in particular West Highland White Terriers (Figure 23.33c).

The treatment of choice for gastrocnemius avulsion is surgical reattachment of the muscle at its natural origin. This can be achieved via:

- A screw and spiked washer
- Direct suturing to the adjacent periosteum
- Suture reattachment to bone tunnels or suture anchors.

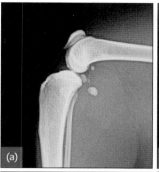
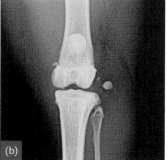
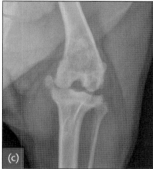

23.33 (a) Mediolateral and (b) caudocranial radiographs of the stifle of a 2-year-old Domestic Shorthaired cat presenting after unknown trauma with a moderate weight-bearing lameness and plantigrade stance affecting the right pelvic limb. Note the distolateral displacement of the lateral fabella and small fragments of bone. This is pathognomic for lateral gastrocnemius avulsion. (c) Normal fabellar asymmetry in a 10-year-old West Highland White Terrier.
(a, b Courtesy of Alex Belch)

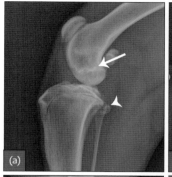
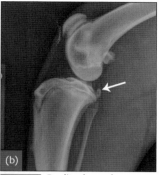
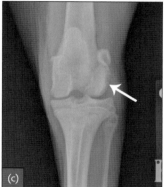

23.34 Popliteal muscle avulsion in a 10-month-old Saluki with moderate weight-bearing lameness of the right pelvic limb. (a) Note the lucency distal to a sclerotic line that demarcates the proximal margin of the origin of the popliteal tendon (arrowed). There is also distal displacement of the popliteal sesamoid bone (arrowhead); compare with the (b) normal contralateral limb (arrowed). (c) The caudocranial radiograph shows a lucent defect (arrowed).

Purchase of the tendon suture can be improved by passing the suture around the displaced fabella. Significant avulsion forces acting on the repair can be mitigated by the application of a transarticular ESF across the hock joint to prevent hock flexion. This should be maintained for 3 weeks prior to the instigation of a physical rehabilitation programme. Lead walking should be maintained for a minimum of 6 weeks. The prognosis for a return to normal long-term function is very good.

Popliteal tendon avulsion

The popliteal tendon originates on the lateral femoral epicondyle medial to the lateral collateral ligament, and contains a sesamoid bone. The tendon continues caudally to the muscle belly on the caudal aspect of the stifle joint. The popliteus muscle acts to flex the stifle joint and rotate the tibia internally. Avulsion of the tendon is a very unusual injury that can occur in skeletally immature large-breed dogs. Clinical signs include weight-bearing lameness, local swelling and pain. Radiographs may show an avulsion fragment adjacent to the tendon origin, although avulsion can occur without discrete fragmentation. An osseous defect may be visible at the same site (Figure 23.34) and there is distal displacement of the popliteal sesamoid bone. Popliteal sesamoid bone displacement is also present in some cases of CCL rupture but cranial draw is the defining clinical feature in affected dogs.

Treatment of choice is surgical exploration and reattachment of the avulsed tendon. Reattachment can be achieved via:

- A screw and spiked washer
- Direct suturing to the adjacent periosteum
- Suture reattachment to bone tunnels or suture anchors.

Purchase of the tendon suture can be improved by passing the suture around the displaced sesamoid bone. The repair should be protected postoperatively by

strict exercise restriction and use of a splinted bandage for 2–3 weeks. Physical rehabilitation should be employed over the following 4–6 weeks. The prognosis for a return to normal long-term function is very good. Non-surgical management can result in a gradual return to normal function.

Stifle salvage options

Total knee replacement

Total knee replacement (TKR) is indicated for end-stage stifle joint osteoarthritis (Figure 23.35). It may be contraindicated if there is collateral ligament damage (system dependent), septic arthritis or periarticular infection. If infection is present, either the infection must be resolved prior to consideration of TKR, or stifle arthrodesis should be considered instead. A modular TKR system (Canine Total Knee, Biomedtrix; see Figure 23.35a) has been commercially available since 2005. At the time of writing, over 300 dogs have been treated using this system. The surgical technique has been described in detail (Liska and Doyle, 2009) and is well illustrated by an open access video clip (http://www.biomedtrix.com/total-knee-replacement) that can be shown to owners. The implant system uses a metal-on-plastic condylar design (a cobalt-chrome femoral component and an ultra-high molecular weight polyethylene tibial component) that mimics the geometry of the articulating surfaces of the normal canine femur and tibia. Canine TKR produces rapid improvements in function that are maintained in the medium term (Allen et al., 2009; Liska and Doyle, 2009). Clinical studies are underway to establish whether canine TKR is capable of producing full restoration of high-level function in the long term. Reported complications in human TKR include aseptic loosening, infection and implant wear.

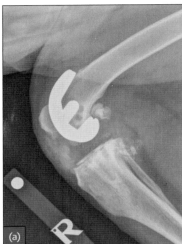

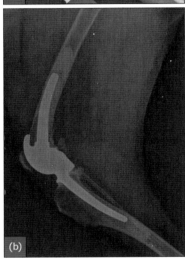

23.35 (a) The Biomedtrix canine total knee replacement (TKR) is only suitable when the collateral ligaments are intact. (b) This custom-made hinged TKR was used to treat end-stage osteoarthritis secondary to multi-ligamentous instability.
(Courtesy of Noel Fitzpatrick)

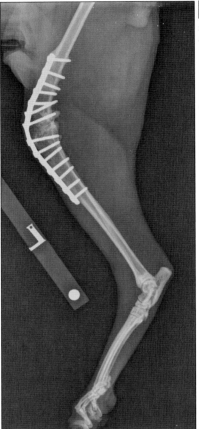

23.36 Mediolateral radiograph showing complete stifle arthrodesis 1.5 years postoperatively in an 8-year-old Domestic Shorthaired cat that had previous unsuccessful surgical reconstruction of a traumatic multi-ligamentous injury. The radiograph shows the cranial plate position and a 120-degree flexion angle.

Stifle arthrodesis

Stifle arthrodesis is a salvage procedure for animals suffering from severe irreparable compromise to the stifle joint, usually secondary to ligament damage, osteoarthritis, articular fractures or septic arthritis. Other reasons for stifle arthrodesis include congenital limb malformation, intractable patellar luxation, shearing injury, joint luxation, patellar tendon rupture or as a treatment for selected peripheral nerve injuries. The aim of stifle arthrodesis is to provide acceptable joint function and relieve pain when amputation or TKR are not options. Although lameness as a result of pain should be ameliorated by stifle arthrodesis, mechanical lameness persists. The impact of mechanical lameness probably varies according to animal size. Small dogs and cats are the primary candidates for stifle arthrodesis.

Arthrodesis at the correct stifle angle is essential in order to optimize surgical outcome. The best guide for selection of the appropriate arthrodesis angle involves measurement of the standing angle of the contralateral limb (if it is normal). In dogs, the published arthrodesis angle is 135–140 degrees and recommended angles in cats range from 110–125 degrees. Resection of the menisci and articular cartilage is typically performed by en bloc ostectomy to produce flat surfaces that can be compressed together using lag screws and/or compression plates. Rigid internal fixation (Figure 23.36) is recommended because times to achieve complete fusion are

often longer than it is possible to maintain an ESF. Surgical technique and aftercare are well described (Bonath and Vannini, 2005).

Complications are relatively common with stifle arthrodesis. These include iatrogenic trauma to the popliteal artery, failure of fusion, infection, implant loosening and fracture occurring at the stress riser at either end of the plate and screws.

References and further reading

Aiken SW, Kass PH and Toombs JP (1995) Intercondylar notch width in dogs with and without cranial cruciate ligament injuries. *Veterinary and Comparative Orthopaedics and Traumatology* **8**, 128–132

Allen MJ, Leone KA, Lamonte K, Townsend KL and Mann KA. (2009) Cemented total knee replacement in 24 dogs: surgical technique, clinical results, and complications. *Veterinary Surgery* **38**, 555–567

Apelt A, Kowaleski MP and Boudrieau RJ (2007) Effect of tibial tuberosity advancement on cranial tibial subluxation in canine cranial cruciate-deficient stifle joints: an *in vitro* experimental study. *Veterinary Surgery* **36**, 170–177

Archer RM, Sissener TR and Spotswood TC (2010) What is your diagnosis? Patellar tendon rupture. *Journal of the American Veterinary Medicine Association* **237**, 273–274

Aron DN, Selcer BA and Smith JD (1997) Autogenous tensor fascia lata graft replacement of the patellar ligament in a dog. *Veterinary and Comparative Orthopaedics and Traumatology* **10**, 141–145

Arthurs GI and Langley-Hobbs SJ (2006) Complications associated with corrective surgery for patellar luxation in 109 dogs. *Veterinary Surgery* **35**, 559–566

Bardet J and Piermattei D (1983) Long digital extensor and popliteal tendon avulsion associated with lateral patellar luxation in a dog. *Journal of the American Veterinary Medicine Association* **183**, 465–466

Barrett E, Barr F, Owen M *et al.* (2009) A retrospective study of the MRI findings in 18 dogs with stifle injuries. *Journal of Small Animal Practice* **50**, 448–455

Bertrand SG, Lewis DD, Madison JB *et al.* (1997) Arthroscopic examination and treatment of osteochondritis dissecans of the femoral condyle of six dogs. *Journal of the American Animal Hospital Association* **33**, 451–455

Bloomberg MS and Parker RB (1984) Chronic lameness in the dog due to delayed diagnosis of disruption of the patellar ligament. *Journal of the American Animal Hospital Association* **20**, 899–904

Boettcher P, Bruehschwein A, Winkels P *et al.* (2010) Value of low-field magnetic resonance imaging in diagnosing meniscal tears in the canine stifle: A prospective study evaluating sensitivity and specificity in naturally occurring cranial cruciate ligament deficiency with arthroscopy as the gold standard. *Veterinary Surgery* **39**, 296–305

Bonath KH and Vannini R (2005) Arthrodesis of the stifle. In: *AO Principles of Fracture Management in the Dog and Cat*, pp. 459–463. AO Publishing, Davos, Switzerland

Boudrieau RJ (2009) Tibial plateau leveling osteotomy or tibial tuberosity advancement? *Veterinary Surgery* **38**, 1–22

Brower BE, Kowaleski MP, Peruski AM *et al.* (2017) Distal femoral lateral closing wedge osteotomy as a component of comprehensive treatment of medial patellar luxation and distal femoral varus in dogs. *Veterinary and Comparative Orthopaedics and Traumatology* **30**, 20–27

Buote N, Fusco J and Radasch R (2009) Age, tibial plateau angle, sex, and weight as risk factors for contralateral rupture of the cranial cruciate ligament in Labradors. *Veterinary Surgery* **38**, 481–489

Campbell CA, Horstman CL, Mason DR and Evans RB (2010) Severity of patellar luxation and frequency of concomitant cranial cruciate ligament rupture in dogs: 162 cases (2004–2007). *Journal of the American Veterinary Medical Association* **236**, 887–891

Carey K, Aiken SW, DiResta GR, Herr LG and Monette S (2005) Radiographic and clinical changes of the patellar tendon after tibial plateau leveling osteotomy: 94 cases (2001–2003). *Veterinary and Comparative Orthopaedics and Traumatology* **18**, 235–242

Casale SA and McCarthy RJ (2009) Complications associated with lateral fabellotibial suture surgery for cranial cruciate ligament injury in dogs: 363 cases (1997–2005) *Journal of the American Veterinary Medical Association* **234**, 229–235

Case JB, Hulse D, Kerwin SC and Peycke LE (2008) Meniscal injury following initial cranial cruciate ligament stabilization surgery in 26 dogs (29 stifles). *Veterinary and Comparative Orthopaedics and Traumatology* **21**, 365–367

Cashmore RG, Havlicek M, Perkins NR *et al.* (2014) Major complications and risk factors associated with surgical correction of medial patellar luxation in 124 dogs. *Veterinary and Comparative Orthopaedics and Traumatology* **27**, 263–270

Chailleux N, Lussier B, De Guise J, Chevalier Y and Hagemeister N (2007) In vitro 3-dimensional kinematic evaluation of 2 corrective operations for cranial cruciate ligament-deficient stifle. *Canadian Journal of Veterinary Research* **71**, 175–180

Clements DN, Broadhurst H, Clarke SP *et al.* (2013) The effectiveness of 3D animations to enhance understanding of cranial cruciate ligament rupture. *Journal of Veterinary Medical Education* **40**, 29–34

Clements DN, Owen MR, Mosley JR *et al.* (2005) Retrospective study of bacterial infective arthritis in 31 dogs. *Journal of Small Animal Practice* **46**, 171–176

Comerford EJ, Tarlton JF, Avery NC, Bailey AJ and Innes JF (2006) Distal femoral intercondylar notch dimensions and their relationship to composition and metabolism of the canine anterior cruciate ligament. *Osteoarthritis and Cartilage* **14**, 273–278

Conzemius MG, Evans RB, Faulkner Besancon M *et al.* (2005) Effect of surgical technique on limb function after surgery for rupture of the cranial cruciate ligament in dogs. *Journal of the American Veterinary Medical Association* **226**, 232–236

Cook JL, Hudson CC, Kuroki K (2008) Autogenous osteochondral grafting for treatment of stifle osteochondrosis in dogs. *Veterinary surgery* **37**, 311–321

Cook JL, Kuroki K, Bozynski CC *et al.* (2014) Evaluation of synthetic osteochondral implants. *The Journal of Knee Surgery* **27**, 295–302

Corr SA and Brown C (2007) A comparison of outcomes following tibial plateau levelling osteotomy and cranial tibial wedge osteotomy procedures. *Veterinary and Comparative Orthopaedics and Traumatology* **20**, 312–319

Culvenor JA (1988) Fascia lata flap to reinforce repair of patella ligament injuries in the dog and cat. *Journal of Small Animal Practice* **29**, 559–563

Dienst M, Schneider G, Altmeyer K *et al.* (2007) Correlation of intercondylar notch cross sections to the ACL size: a high resolution MR tomographic *in vivo* analysis. *Archives of Orthopaedic and Trauma Surgery* **127**, 253–260

Dudley RM, Kowaleski MP, Drost WT and Dyce J (2006) Radiographic and computed tomographic determination of femoral varus and torsion in the dog. *Veterinary Radiology and Ultrasound* **47**, 546–552

Duerr FM, Duncan CG, Savicky RS *et al.* (2007) Risk factors for excessive tibial plateau angle in large-breed dogs with cranial cruciate ligament disease. *Journal of the American Veterinary Medical Association* **231**, 1688–1691

Dulisch ML (1981a) Suture reaction following extra-articular stifle stabilization in the dog. Part I: A retrospective study of 161 stifles. *Journal of the American Animal Hospital Association* **17**, 569–571

Dulisch ML (1981b) Suture reaction following extra-articular stabilization in the dog. Part II: A prospective study of 66 stifles. *Journal of the American Animal Hospital Association* **17**, 572–574

Duval JM, Budsberg SC, Flo GL and Sammarco JL (1999) Breed, sex and bodyweight as risk factors for rupture of the cranial cruciate ligament in young dogs. *Journal of the American Veterinary Medical Association* **215**, 811–814

Ehrenborg G and Olsson SE (1962) Avulsion of the tibial tuberosity in the dog. A comparative roentgenologic study with special reference to the Osgood-Schlatter lesion in man. *Acta Chirurgica Scandinavica* **123**, 28–37

Farrell M and Fitzpatrick N (2013) Patellar ligament-bone autograft for reconstruction of a distal patellar ligament defect in a dog. *Journal of Small Animal Practice* **54**, 269–274

Fitzpatrick N and Solano MA (2010) Predictive variables for complications after TPLO with stifle inspection by arthrotomy in 1000 consecutive dogs. *Veterinary Surgery* **39**, 460–474

Gemmill TJ and Carmichael S (2003) Complete patellar ligament replacement using a fascia lata autograft in a dog. *Journal of Small Animal Practice* **44**, 456–459

Gemmill T and Clements D (2016) *BSAVA Manual of Canine and Feline Fracture Repair and Management, 2nd edn.* BSAVA Publications, Gloucester

Gemmill TJ and Farrell M (2009) Evaluation of a joint distractor to facilitate arthroscopy of the canine stifle. *Veterinary Surgery* **38**, 588–594

Gibbons SE, Macias C, Tonzing MA, Pinchbeck GL and McKee WM (2006) Patellar luxation in 70 large breed dogs. *Journal of Small Animal Practice* **47**, 3–9

Gilmore DR (1983) Patellar ligament rupture in a dog. *Journal of the American Veterinary Medical Association* **183**, 228–229

Goedegebuure SA and Hazewinkel HAW (1986) Morphological findings in young dogs chronically fed a diet containing excess calcium. *Veterinary Pathology Online* **23**, 594–605

Gordon-Evans WJ, Griffon DJ, Bubb C *et al.* (2013) Comparison of lateral fabellar suture and tibial plateau leveling osteotomy techniques for treatment of dogs with cranial cruciate ligament disease. *Journal of the American Veterinary Medical Association* **243**, 675–680.

Haaland PJ, Sjöström L (2007) Luxation of the long digital extensor tendon as a complication to Tibial Plateau Levelling Osteotomy. *Veterinary and Comparative Orthopaedics and Traumatology* **20**, 224–226

Harari J, Johnson L, Stein LE, Kneller SK, Pijanowski G (1987) Evaluation of experimental transection and partial excision of the caudal cruciate ligament in dogs. *Veterinary Surgery* **16**, 151–154

Harasen G (2005) Feline cranial cruciate rupture: 17 cases and a review of the literature. *Veterinary and Comparative Orthopaedics and Traumatology* **18**, 254–257

Harasen G (2007) Feline cruciate rupture. *The Canadian Veterinary Journal* **48**, 639–640

Hart JL, May KD, Kieves NR *et al.* (2015) Comparison of owner satisfaction between stifle joint orthoses and tibial plateau leveling osteotomy for the management of cranial cruciate ligament disease in dogs. *Journal of the American Veterinary Medical Association* **249**, 391-398

Hayes AG, Boudrieau RJ and Hungerford LL (1994) Frequency and distribution of medial and lateral patellar luxation in dogs: 124 cases (1982–1992). *Journal of the American Veterinary Medical Association* **205**, 716–720

Hayes AG, Boudrieau RJ and Hungerford F (1994) Frequency and distribution of medial and lateral patellar luxation in dogs: 124 cases (1982–1992). *Journal of the American Veterinary Medical Association* **205**, 716–720

Hayes GM, Langley-Hobbs SJ and Jeffery ND (2010) Risk factors for medial meniscal injury in association with cranial cruciate ligament rupture. *Journal of Small Animal Practice* **51**, 630–634

Higgins B, Coughlan A, Pettitt R *et al.* (2010) The use of transarticular external skeletal fixation in the management of failed tibial tuberosity transposition in five dogs. *Veterinary and Comparative Orthopaedics and Traumatology* **23**, 109–113

Hill CM, Conzemius MG, Smith GK, McManus PM and Maloney D (1999) Bacterial culture of the canine stifle joint following surgical repair of ruptured cranial cruciate ligament. *Veterinary and Comparative Orthopaedics and Traumatology* **12**, 1–5

Hoelzler MG, Millis DL, Francis DA and Weigel JP (2004) Results of arthroscopic versus open arthrotomy for surgical management of cranial cruciate ligament deficiency in dogs. *Veterinary Surgery* **33**, 146–153

Hoffmann DE, Miller JM, Ober CP *et al.* (2006) Tibial tuberosity advancement in 65 canine stifles. *Veterinary and Comparative Orthopaedics and Traumatology* **19**, 219–227

Hofmeister EH, Watson V, Snyder LB and Love EJ (2008) Validity and client use of information from the World Wide Web regarding veterinary anesthesia in dogs. *Journal of the American Veterinary Medical Association* **233**, 1860–1864

Hulse D, Beale B and Kerwin S (2010) Second look arthroscopic findings after tibial plateau leveling osteotomy. *Veterinary Surgery* **39**, 350–354

Johnson AL, Probst CW, Decamp CE *et al.* (2001) Comparison of trochlear block recession and trochlear wedge recession for canine patellar luxation using a cadaver model. *Veterinary Surgery* **30**, 140–150

Johnson KA (1994) Osteomyelitis in dogs and cats. *Journal of the American Veterinary Medical Association* **205**, 1882–1887

Kalff S, Butterworth SJ, Miller A *et al.* (2014) Lateral patellar luxation in dogs: a retrospective study of 65 cases. *Veterinary and Comparative Orthopaedics and Traumatology* **2**, 130–134

Keely B, Glyde M, Guerin S and Doyle R (2007) Stifle joint luxation in the dog and cat: The use of temporary intraoperative transarticular pinning to facilitate joint reconstruction. *Veterinary and Comparative Orthopaedics and Traumatology* **20**, 198–203

Kowaleski MP (2006) Patellar luxation – preoperative evaluation and surgical planning for femoral corrective osteotomy. *13th Conference of the European Society of Veterinary Orthopaedics and Traumatology, September 7 to 10, 2006, Munich, Germany*, 87–90

Krotscheck U, Nelson SA, Todhunter RJ, Stone M and Zhang Z (2016) Long term functional outcome of tibial tuberosity advancement *versus* tibial plateau leveling osteotomy and extracapsular repair in a heterogeneous population of dogs. *Veterinary Surgery* **45**, 261–268

Lafaver S, Miller NA, Stubbs WP, Taylor RA and Boudrieau RJ (2007) Tibial tuberosity advancement for stabilization of the canine cranial cruciate ligament-deficient stifle joint: surgical technique, early results, and complications in 101 dogs. *Veterinary Surgery* **36**, 573–586

Lammerding JJ, Noser GA, Brinker WO and Carrig CB (1976) Avulsion fracture of the origin of the extensor digitorum longus muscle in 3 dogs. *Journal of the American Animal Hospital Association* **12**, 764–767

Langenbach A and Marcellin-Little DJ (2010) Management of concurrent patellar luxation and cranial cruciate ligament rupture using modified tibial plateau levelling. *Journal of Small Animal Practice* **51**, 97–103

Langley-Hobbs SJ (2009) Survey of 52 fractures of the patella in 34 cats. *Veterinary Record* **164**, 80–86

Leonard KC, Kowaleski MP, Saunders WB, McCarthy RJ and Boudrieau RJ (2016) Combined tibial plateau levelling osteotomy and tibial tuberosity transposition for treatment of cranial cruciate ligament insufficiency with concomitant medial patellar luxation. *Veterinary and Comparative Orthopaedics and Traumatology* **29**, 536-540.

Lewis BA, Allen DA, Henrikson TD and Lehenbauer TW (2008) Computed tomographic evaluation of the canine intercondylar notch in normal and cruciate deficient stifles. *Veterinary and Comparative Orthopaedics and Traumatology* **21**, 119–124

Lindley S and Watson P (2010) *BSAVA Manual of Canine and Feline Rehabilitation, Supportive and Palliative Care.* BSAVA Publications, Gloucester

Linney WR, Hammer DL and Shott S (2011) Surgical treatment of medial patellar luxation without femoral trochlear groove deepening procedures in dogs: 91 cases (1998–2009). *Journal of the American Veterinary Medical Association* **238**, 1168–1172

Lipowitz AJ (1996) Surgical wounds. In: *Complications in Small Animal Surgery: Diagnosis, Management, Prevention*, ed. DD Caywood and CD Newton, pp. 1–6. Williams and Wilkins, Philadelphia

Liska WD and Doyle ND (2009) Canine total knee replacement: surgical technique and one-year outcome. *Veterinary Surgery* **38**, 568–582

Lopez MJ, Markel MD, Kalscheur V, Lu Y and Manley PA (2003) Hamstring graft technique for stabilization of canine cranial cruciate ligament deficient stifles. *Veterinary Surgery* **32**, 390–401

Luther JK, Cook CR and Cook JL (2009) Meniscal release in cruciate ligament intact stifles causes lameness and medial compartment cartilage pathology in dogs 12 weeks postoperatively. *Veterinary Surgery* **38**, 520–529

Macias C, McKee WM and May C (2002) Caudal proximal tibial deformity and cranial cruciate ligament rupture in small breed dogs. *Journal of Small Animal Practice* **43**, 433–438

Mahn MM, Cook JL and Balke MT (2005) Arthroscopic verification of ultrasonographic diagnosis of meniscal pathology in dogs. *Veterinary Surgery* **34**, 318–323

Marchevsky AM and Read RA (1999) Bacterial septic arthritis in 19 dogs. *Australian Veterinary Journal* **77**, 233–237

Marsolais GS, Dvorak G and Conzemius M (2002) Effects of postoperative rehabilitation on limb function after cranial cruciate ligament repair in dogs. *Journal of the American Veterinary Medical Association* **220**, 1325–2330

Monk ML, Preston CA and McGowan CM (2006) Effects of early intensive postoperative physiotherapy on limb function after tibial plateau leveling osteotomy in dogs with deficiency of the cranial cruciate ligament. *American Journal of Veterinary Research* **67**, 529–536

Montgomery RD, Hathcock JT, Milton JL and Fitch RB (1994) Osteochondritis dissecans of the canine tarsal joint. *Compendium on Continuing Education for the Practicing Veterinarian* **16**, 835–845

Moore KW and Read RA (1995) Cranial cruciate ligament rupture in the dog – a retrospective study comparing surgical techniques. *Australian Veterinary Journal* **72**, 281–285

Muir P, Schaefer SL, Manley PA *et al.* (2007) Expression of immune response genes in the stifle joint of dogs with oligoarthritis and degenerative cranial cruciate ligament rupture. *Veterinary Immunology and Immunopathology* **119**, 214–221

Nelson SA, Krotscheck U, Rawlinson J *et al.* (2013) Long-term functional outcome of tibial plateau leveling osteotomy versus extracapsular repair in a heterogeneous population of dogs. *Veterinary Surgery* **42**, 38–50

Nicoll C, Singh A and Weese JS (2014) Economic impact of tibial plateau leveling osteotomy surgical site infection in dogs. *Veterinary Surgery* **43**, 899–902

Off W and Matis U (2010) Excision arthroplasty of the hip joint in dogs and cats. *Veterinary and Comparative Orthopaedics and Traumatology* **23**, 297–305

Oxley B, Gemmill TJ, Renwick AR, Clements DN and McKee WM (2013) Comparison of complication rates and clinical outcome between tibial plateau leveling osteotomy and a modified cranial closing wedge osteotomy for treatment of cranial cruciate ligament disease in dogs. *Veterinary Surgery* **42**, 739–750

Paatsama S (1952) *Ligamentous injuries in the canine stifle joint* [Thesis]. Helsinki: Royal Veterinary College

Pacchiana PD, Morris E, Gillings SL, Jessen CR and Lipowitz AJ (2003) Surgical and postoperative complications associated with tibial plateau leveling osteotomy in dogs with cranial cruciate ligament rupture: 397 cases (1998–2001). *Journal of the American Veterinary Medical Association* **222**, 184–193

Palierne S, Palissier F, Raymond-Letron I and Autefage A (2010) A case of bilateral patellar osteochondrosis and fracture in a cat. *Veterinary and Comparative Orthopaedics and Traumatology* **21**, 427–433

Perry K and Fitzpatrick N (2010) Tibial tuberosity advancement in two cats with cranial cruciate ligament deficiency. *Veterinary and Comparative Orthopaedics and Traumatology* **23**, 196–202

Pettitt R, Cripps S, Baker M *et al.* (2014) Radiographic and ultrasonographic changes of the patellar ligament following tibial tuberosity advancement in 25 dogs. *Veterinary and Comparative Orthopaedics and Traumatology* **27**, 216–221

Pond MJ (1973) Avulsion of the extensor digitorum longus muscle in the dog: a report of four cases. *Journal of Small Animal Practice* **14**, 785–796

Pond MJ and Campbell JR (1972) The canine stifle joint I. Rupture of the anterior cruciate ligament. *Journal of Small Animal Practice* **13**, 1–10

Priddy NH, Tomlinson JL, Dodam JR and Hornbostel JE (2003) Complications with and owner assessment of the outcome of tibial plateau leveling osteotomy for treatment of cranial cruciate ligament rupture of dogs: 193 cases (1997–2001). *Journal of the American Veterinary Medical* **222**, 1726–1732

Rath E and Richmond JC (2000) The menisci: basic science and advances in treatment. *British Journal of Sports Medicine* **34**, 252–257

Read RA and Robins GM (1982) Deformity of the proximal tibia in dogs. *Veterinary Record* **111**, 295–298

Reif U and Probst CW (2003) Comparison of tibial plateau angles in normal and cranial cruciate deficient stifles of Labrador Retrievers. *Veterinary Surgery* **32**, 385–389

Ries RL and Harris LR (1982) Patellar ligament avulsion in a dog. *Modern Veterinary Practice* **63**, 969–971

Roch SP and Gemmill TJ (2008) Treatment of medial patellar luxation by femoral closing wedge osteotomy using a distal femoral plate in four dogs. *Journal of Small Animal Practice* **49**, 152–158

Rosin E, Dow S, Daly W, Peterson SW and Penwick RC (1993) Surgical wound infection and use of antibiotics. In: *Textbook of Small Animal Surgery, Vol. 1, 2nd edn*, ed. DH Slatter, pp. 94–95. WB Saunders, Philadelphia

Roy RG, Wallace LJ, Johnston GR and Wickstrom SL (1992) A retrospective evaluation of stifle osteoarthritis in dogs with bilateral medial patellar luxation and unilateral surgical repair. *Veterinary Surgery* **21**, 475–479

Rutherford L and Arthurs GI (2014) Partial parasagittal patellectomy: a novel method for augmenting surgical correction of patellar luxation in four cats. *Journal of Feline Medicine and Surgery* **16**, 689–694

Rutherford L, Langley-Hobbs S, Whitelock RJ and Arthurs GI (2014) Complications associated with corrective surgery for patellar luxation in 85 feline surgical cases. *Journal of Feline Medicine and Surgery* **16**, 1–6

Samii VF, Dyce J, Pozzi A *et al.* (2009) Computed tomographic arthrography of the stifle for detection of cranial and caudal cruciate ligament and meniscal tears in dogs. *Veterinary Radiology and Ultrasound* **50**, 144–150

Scavelli TD and Schrader SC (1987) Nonsurgical management of rupture of the cranial cruciate ligament in 18 cats. *Journal of the American Animal Hospital Association* **23**, 337–340

Shipov A, Shahar R, Joseph R and Milgram J (2008) Successful management of bilateral patellar tendon rupture in a dog. *Veterinary and Comparative Orthopaedics and Traumatology* **21**, 181–184

Skelly CM, McAllister H and Donnelly WJC (1997) Avulsion of the tibial tuberosity in a litter of greyhound puppies. *Journal of Small Animal Practice* **38**, 445–449

Slocum B and Devine T (1983) Cranial tibial thrust: a primary force in the canine stifle. *Journal of the American Veterinary Medical Association* **183**, 456–459

Slocum B and Devine T (1984) Cranial tibial wedge osteotomy: a technique for eliminating cranial tibial thrust in cranial cruciate ligament repair. *Journal of the American Veterinary Medical Association* **84**, 564-569

Smith BJ (1999) Muscles of the pelvic limb. In: *Canine Anatomy*, ed. BJ Smith, pp. 524–542. Philadelphia: Lippincott, Williams and Wilkins

Smith MEH, de Haan JJ, Peck J and Madden SN (2000) Augmented primary repair of patellar ligament rupture in three dogs. *Veterinary and Comparative Orthopaedics and Traumatology* **13**, 154–157

Stauffer KD, Tuttle TA, Elkins AD, Wehrenberg AP and Character BJ (2006) Complications associated with 696 tibial plateau leveling osteotomies (2001–2003). *Journal of the American Animal Hospital Association* **42**, 44–50

Stein S and Schmoekel H (2008) Short-term and eight to 12 months results of a tibial tuberosity advancement as treatment of canine cranial cruciate ligament damage. *Journal of Small Animal Practice* **49**, 398–404

Stramel D (1997) Avulsion of the long digital extensor tendon. *Canine Practice* **22**, 16–17

Swiderski JK and Palmer RH (2007) Long-term outcome of distal femoral osteotomy for treatment of combined distal femoral varus and medial patellar luxation: 12 cases (1999–2004). *Journal of the American Veterinary Medical Association* **231**, 1070–1075.

Taggart R, Wardlaw J, Horstman CL *et al.* (2010) An analysis of the quality of canine cranial cruciate ligament disease information available on the internet. *Veterinary Surgery* **39**, 278–283

Talcott KW, Goring RL and De Haan JJ (2000) Rectangular recession trochleoplasty for treatment of patellar luxation in dogs and cats. *Veterinary and Comparative Orthopaedics and Traumatology* **13**, 39–43

Taylor-Brown F, Lamb CR, Tivers MS *et al.* (2014) Magnetic resonance imaging for detection of late meniscal tears in dogs following tibial tuberosity advancement for treatment of cranial cruciate ligament injury. *Veterinary and Comparative Orthopaedics and Traumatology* **27**, 141–146

Thieman KM, Tomlinson JL, Fox DB, Cook C and Cook JL (2006) Effect of meniscal release on rate of subsequent meniscal tears and owner-assessed outcome in dogs with cruciate disease treated with tibial plateau leveling osteotomy. *Veterinary Surgery* **35**, 705–710

Tivers MS, Mahoney PN, Baines EA *et al.* (2009) Diagnostic accuracy of positive contrast computed tomography arthrography for the detection of injuries to the medial meniscus in dogs with naturally occurring cranial cruciate ligament insufficiency. *Journal of Small Animal Practice* **50**, 324–332

Tonks CA, Pozzi A, Ling HY and Lewis DD (2010) The effects of extra-articular suture tension on contact mechanics of the lateral compartment of cadaveric stifles treated with the TightRope CCL® or lateral suture technique. *Veterinary Surgery* **39**, 343–349

Vasseur PB (1984) Clinical results following nonoperative management for rupture of the cranial cruciate ligament in dogs. *Veterinary Surgery* **13**, 243–246

Von Pfeil DJ, DeCamp CE and Abood SK (2009) The epiphyseal plate: nutritional and hormonal influences; hereditary and other disorders. *Compendium on Continuing Education for the Practicing Veterinarian* **31**, E1–E4

Warzee CC, Dejardin LM, Arnoczky SP and Perry RL (2001) Effect of tibial plateau leveling on cranial and caudal tibial thrusts in canine cranial cruciate–deficient stifles: An *in vitro* experimental study. *Veterinary Surgery* **30**, 278–286

Whitehair JG, Vasseur PB and Willits NH (1993) Epidemiology of cranial cruciate ligament rupture in dogs. *Journal of the American Veterinary Medical Association* **203**, 1016–1019

Wilke VL, Conzemius MG, Besancon MF, Evans RB and Ritter M (2002) Comparison of tibial plateau angle between clinically normal Greyhounds and Labrador Retrievers with and without rupture of the cranial cruciate ligament. *Journal of the American Veterinary Medical Association* **221**, 1426–1429

Wilke VL, Conzemius MG, Kinghorn BP *et al.* (2006) Inheritance of rupture of the cranial cruciate ligament in Newfoundlands. *Journal of the American Veterinary Medical Association* **228**, 61–64

Willauer CC and Vasseur PB (1987) Clinical results of surgical correction of medial luxation of the patella in dogs. *Veterinary Surgery* **16**, 31–36

Witsberger TH, Villamil JA, Schultz LG, Hahn AW and Cook JL (2008) Prevalence of and risk factors for hip dysplasia and cranial cruciate ligament deficiency in dogs. *Journal of the American Veterinary Medical Association* **232**, 1818–1824

Wolf RE, Scavelli TD, Hoelzler MG, Fulcher RP and Bastian RP (2012) Surgical and postoperative complications associated with tibial tuberosity advancement for cranial cruciate ligament rupture in dogs: 458 cases (2007–2009). *Journal of the American Veterinary Medical Association* **240**, 1481–1487

Wucherer KL, Conzemius MG, Evans R and Wilke VL (2013) Short-term and long-term outcomes for overweight dogs with cranial cruciate ligament rupture treated surgically or nonsurgically. *Journal of the American Veterinary Medical Association* **242**, 1364–1372

Wustefeld-Janssens BG, Pettitt RA, Cowderoy EC *et al.* (2016) Peak vertical force and vertical impulse in dogs with cranial cruciate ligament rupture and meniscal injury. *Veterinary Surgery* **45(1)**, 60–65

Yeadon R, Fitzpatrick N and Kowaleski MP (2011) Tibial tuberosity transposition-advancement for treatment of medial patellar luxation and concomitant cranial cruciate ligament disease in the dog. Surgical technique, radiographic and clinical outcomes. *Veterinary and Comparative Orthopaedics and Traumatology* **24**, 18–26

Yoon D (2014) Degenerative joint disease after medial patellar luxation repair in dogs with or without trochleoplasty. *Journal of Veterinary Clinics* **32(1)**, 22

Ytrehus B, Carlson CS and Ekman S (2007) Etiology and pathogenesis of osteochondrosis. *Veterinary Pathology Online* **44**, 429–448

IMAGING TECHNIQUES

Thomas W. Maddox

A combination of soft tissue and osseous conditions affect the stifle joint. Many of these can be assessed by radiography, and the specific anatomy of the stifle (see Chapter 3) does allow for better evaluation of soft tissue lesions than is possible for most other joints. Nevertheless, the use of modalities other than radiography is increasing.

RADIOGRAPHY

Standard views

The standard orthogonal views are the mediolateral and caudocranial views. The depth of the stifle means that a radiographic grid should not be required.

Mediolateral view

This view is essential for assessment of joint effusion, tibial translation and osteophyte formation.

- The patient is placed in lateral recumbency with the target limb dependent against the cassette/plate and the contralateral limb retracted craniodorsally; superimposition of the prepuce in male dogs should be avoided (Figure 23.37).
- The stifle should be in a neutral position and the distal limb supported with a foam wedge to alleviate stifle rotation.
- The primary beam is centred distal to the medial femoral condyle and caudal to the patellar ligament.
- Collimate to include the cranial skin margins and approximately one-third of the femur and tibia.

This view can be adapted for surgical planning of TTA by extending the stifle joint to 135 degrees; this is confirmed using a goniometer.

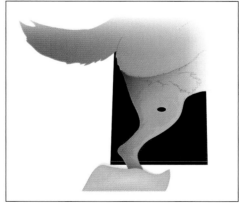

23.37 Patient positioning for a mediolateral view of the stifle.

→ **IMAGING TECHNIQUES CONTINUED**

Caudocranial view

- The patient is placed in sternal recumbency (stabilization with a positioning trough, sandbags or wedges may be required) and the pelvic limb drawn caudally (Figure 23.38).
- The stifle of the target limb should be extended and slightly internally rotated, with elevation of the contralateral limb using sponges.
- The primary beam is centred on the midline just distal to the femoral condyles.
- Collimate to include the medial and lateral skin margins and approximately one-third of the femur and tibia.

Special views

Special views are not commonly acquired of the stifle, but the most important are listed below.

Stressed views

Stressed views are useful for assessment of the collateral ligaments. The limb proximal to the stifle is stabilized with ties and an opposing shearing force is applied distal to the stifle. Caudocranial or craniocaudal radiographs are obtained as described above (Figure 23.39). As with all stressed views, radiographs of the contralateral limb are advised for the purpose of comparison.

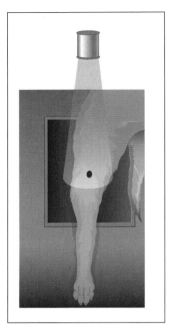
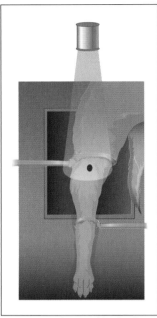

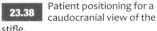 **23.38** Patient positioning for a caudocranial view of the stifle.

23.39 Patient positioning for a stressed caudocranial view of the stifle. Placing ties as shown will stress the lateral aspect of the joint.

Horizontal beam radiographs

Horizontal beam radiographs are theoretically helpful but are rarely obtained because of the radiation safety issues associated with horizontal beams. Examples of such views include the caudocranial view of the stifle, and the craniodistal–cranioproximal view of the patella for the assessment of patellar luxation and patellar fractures.

Tibial osteotomy view

This view is required for surgical planning of techniques such as tibial plateau levelling osteotomy or closing wedge osteotomy. It is advised that specific texts are consulted to achieve the views required for the different techniques.

COMPUTED TOMOGRAPHY

CT allows much better identification of the osseous and soft tissue structures of the stifle compared with radiography. Articular fractures, luxations, avulsions, OC lesions, femoral trochlear depth, trochlear ridge height and changes associated with degenerative conditions affecting the stifle are much better appreciated with CT than with radiography. Contrast CT arthrography is required to fully assess some of the intra-articular soft tissue structures such as the cruciate ligaments and menisci.

Standard technique

- Sternal recumbency is generally used (dorsal recumbency is also suitable) with extension of the pelvic limbs.
- Both stifles can be scanned concurrently.
- The scan margins should extend from proximal to the patella to include the proximal one-quarter of the tibia.
- Once acquired, separate images of both stifles should be reconstructed with as small a field of view as feasible.
- Reconstruction using bone and soft tissue algorithms is advisable.

CT arthrography

This technique is required to demonstrate the cruciate ligaments and menisci. A low concentration of contrast medium is required (non-ionic, low osmolar contrast medium diluted to 50–150 mg iodine/ml) and approximately 3–6 ml is injected into the stifle following aseptic preparation.

Dorsal and sagittal reformatting is generally required for interpretation of these images, but cruciate ruptures and meniscal injuries can be identified (Figure 23.40), with meniscal damage appearing as distortions of the normal wedge-like meniscal shape or occasionally as contrast extending into the body of the meniscus (Samii et al., 2009; Tivers et al., 2009).

→ IMAGING TECHNIQUES CONTINUED

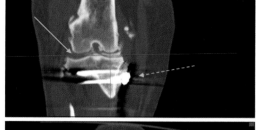

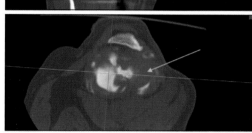

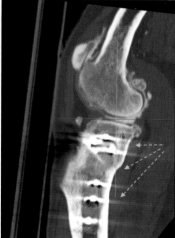

23.40 Multiplanar reconstruction (MPR) CT positive contrast arthrograms of the right stifle of a 10-year-old female Labrador Retriever with late (medial) meniscal injury post tibial plateau levelling osteotomy (TPLO) surgery. Contrast medium is seen filling the region normally occupied by the medial meniscus (crosshairs) and contrasts with the normal lateral meniscal filling defect (solid arrows). Note the metal streak artefacts as a result of the TPLO implants (dashed arrows).

MAGNETIC RESONANCE IMAGING

The multiple soft tissue pathologies that can affect the stifle joint mean that MRI has a role to play in the imaging of stifle disease. Cranial cruciate ligament rupture and meniscal damage in dogs can be identified. While ligament rupture and even degeneration can be readily assessed, more variable results have been reported for meniscal injuries, particularly with low field systems (Barrett *et al.*, 2009; Boettcher *et al.*, 2010).

A standardized protocol has not been developed, but images are generally acquired with the patient in lateral recumbency with the stifle mildly flexed, using small flexible coils. T2- and proton density-weighted sequences are the minimum required, with sagittal and dorsal plane images appearing more useful than images of the transverse plane. Cruciate ligament disease may be apparent as increased signal intensity or discontinuity of the ligament fibres, or sometimes as complete absence of the ligament with irregular, heterogeneous soft tissue at its approximate location. Normal menisci generally have low signal intensity and so mixed (increased) signal intensity within the meniscus is suggestive of meniscal pathology, especially if it extends to the meniscal margins (Barrett *et al.*, 2009). Linear hyperintensities extending into the meniscus, as well as shape changes and flattening of the meniscus are also seen (Taylor-Brown *et al.*, 2014).

ULTRASONOGRAPHY

The superficial soft tissue structures of the stifle are amenable to ultrasound examination. A high frequency linear ultrasound probe is preferred. Moderate to severe joint effusions can be seen as a dilatation of the suprapatellar recess proximal to the patella, and compression of the infrapatellar fat pad can sometimes be identified. The medial and lateral menisci can be clearly seen on the abaxial aspects of the stifle; medial meniscal pathology can be seen as medial bulging of the border, sometimes with displacement, and a heterogeneous echogenicity of the meniscus (Mahn *et al.*, 2005).

On the cranial aspect of the joint the patella tendon can easily be observed, with tendinopathy and tendon ruptures being readily identified (Figure 23.41).

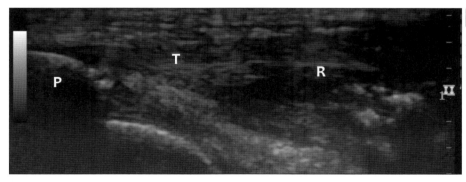

23.41 Ultrasonogram of the stifle of a dog. The patella (P) can be seen proximally with some normal patellar tendon (T); more distally near the insertion there is hypoechoic tissue and loss of normal tendon fibre pattern (R), indicating severe pathology (rupture/partial rupture) of the distal part of the tendon.

OPERATIVE TECHNIQUE 23.1

Patient preparation for stifle surgery

POSITIONING

Limb alignment is best assessed with the patient in dorsal or dorsolateral recumbency with the affected side tipped towards the table. Tibial osteotomies require instrumentation from medial to the tibia. If sandbags are used to support the thorax, it is easy to roll the patient into lateral recumbency after draping has been completed so that the affected limb is positioned flat against the operating table. A loose tie is applied to the contralateral limb to prevent it from rolling towards the surgical field. Extra-capsular repair is usually performed with the patient in lateral recumbency with the affected limb uppermost (Figure 23.42a).

DRAPING

Inclusion of the hock joint within the surgical field facilitates limb alignment assessment. The foot is covered with unsterile Vetrap and is suspended from a ceiling-mounted or stand-mounted clip (Figure 23.42b). The surgeon uses a small piece of sterile drape to hold the foot while the theatre assistant removes the clip. The drape is covered with a layer of sterile Vetrap that can be secured to the skin using a towel clip (Figure 23.42c).

Final draping

A waterproof drape is useful as a final drape during stifle surgery due to the copious amount of irrigation fluid that would otherwise strike through cotton drapes (Figure 23.42d).

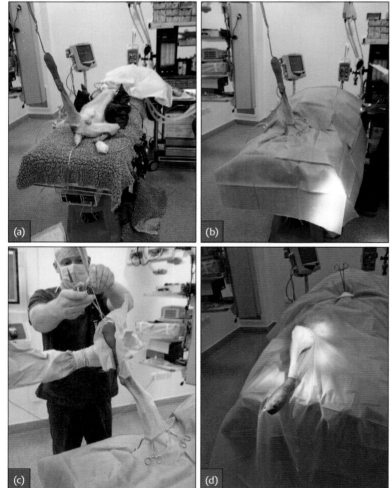

23.42 Patient preparation for stifle surgery. (a) Dorsal recumbency allows the best appreciation of limb alignment and facilitates the medial approach to the stifle. (b) Four sterile drapes have been placed (use of adhesive drapes, as in this case, is optional). (c) A piece of sterile drape material, or a sterile glove, can be used to grasp the unsterile foot dressing. This is secured with sterile cohesive bondage material (e.g. Vetrap). (d) A large waterproof drape can be fenestrated and passed over the limb. This is especially useful in operations involving significant surgical site irrigation.

OPERATIVE TECHNIQUE 23.2

Lateral parapatellar approach

POSITIONING

Lateral or dorsolateral recumbency, with the affected limb uppermost.

ASSISTANT

No.

EQUIPMENT EXTRAS

See Operative Technique 23.4.

SURGICAL TECHNIQUE

The skin incision is made on the craniolateral aspect of the stifle from the distal third of the femur to the tibial tuberosity. The fascia lata and lateral fascia of the stifle are exposed. Another incision is made along the cranial border of the biceps femoris muscle. This is continued distally a few millimetres lateral and parallel to the patella and patellar tendon (Figure 23.43). The biceps femoris muscle is retracted caudally. The joint capsule is incised using a stab incision that is extended using Mayo (blunt-tipped) scissors from the level of the tibial plateau to the level of the proximal extremity of the lateral trochlear ridge. With the stifle joint extended, the patella is luxated medially. Flexion of the joint exposes the intra-articular structures (see Operative Technique 23.4).

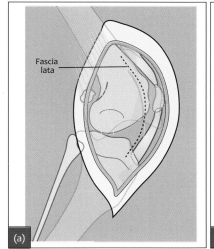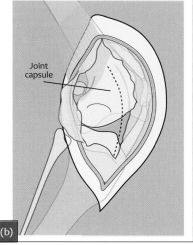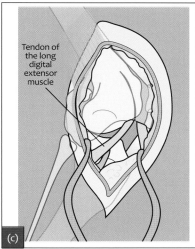

23.43 Lateral parapatellar approach. (a) Incision along the cranial border of the biceps femoris muscle. (b) The biceps femoris muscle and fascia lata are retracted. (c) Retraction of the infrapatellar fat pad exposes the intra-articular structures.

Closure

The joint capsule and fascia lata are closed in separate layers using absorbable sutures in a continuous or interrupted pattern. The remaining wound closure is routine.

POSTOPERATIVE CARE

See appropriate Operative Technique.

COMPLICATIONS

Medial patellar luxation if wound dehiscence occurs.

OPERATIVE TECHNIQUE 23.3

Medial parapatellar approach

POSITIONING

See Operative Technique 23.1.

ASSISTANT

No.

EQUIPMENT EXTRAS

See Operative Technique 23.4.

SURGICAL TECHNIQUE

The skin incision is made on the craniomedial aspect of the stifle starting at the distal third of the femur. The distal limit of the incision depends on the surgery being performed (e.g. TPLO, tibial tuberosity transposition). The medial parapatellar fascial incision is extended proximally into the cranial sartorius and vastus medialis muscles (Figure 23.44). The joint capsule is incised using a stab incision that is extended using Mayo (blunt-tipped) scissors from the level of the tibial plateau to the level of the proximal extremity of the medial trochlear ridge. With the stifle joint extended, the patella is luxated laterally. Flexion of the joint exposes the intra-articular structures (see Operative Technique 23.4). A limited medial approach uses a shorter craniomedial skin incision extending from the distal pole of the patella to the tibial tuberosity (Figure 23.45).

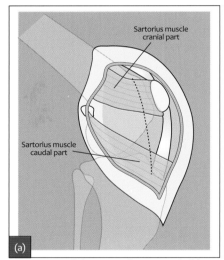
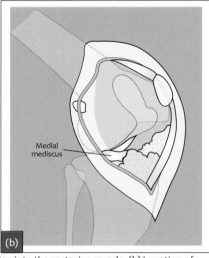
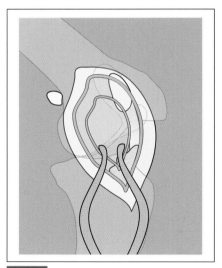

23.44 Medial parapatellar approach. (a) Incision into the sartorius muscle. (b) Luxation of the patella and stifle flexion exposes the intra-articular structures.

23.45 Limited medial approach.

Closure

The joint capsule and fascia lata are closed in separate layers using absorbable sutures in a continuous or interrupted pattern. The remaining wound closure is routine.

POSTOPERATIVE CARE

See appropriate Operative Technique.

COMPLICATIONS

Lateral patellar luxation if wound dehiscence occurs after a full medial parapatellar approach.

OPERATIVE TECHNIQUE 23.4

Intra-articular stifle joint inspection

POSITIONING

Dorsal recumbency and as described in Operative Techniques 23.1 and 23.2.

ASSISTANT

Helpful to hold the limb still and in the correct position to maximize intra-articular exposure.

EQUIPMENT EXTRAS

- **Focal light source** – if the operating room lights do not provide sufficient light to clearly assess the caudal compartment of the stifle joint, a head-mounted LED light source can be very useful.
- **Meniscal probe** – a Dandy nerve hook (Veterinary Instrumentation) is available in two sizes. This hook is essential for assessing the integrity of the menisci.
- **Beaver blade** – Beaver-type scalpel blades (Veterinary Instrumentation) have a fine handle and disposable blades with a cutting surface on the tip. These blades are particularly useful for meniscal surgery.
- **Suction unit** – suction is very useful to evacuate haemorrhage and irrigation fluid.

SURGICAL TECHNIQUE

Two sizes of stifle distractors are available (Veterinary Instrumentation) for large and small-breed dogs, although the large size (Figure 23.46a) can be introduced into the stifle joint of small-breed dogs if the CCL is ruptured.

1 One or two Gelpi retractors are introduced into the joint to expose the femoral trochlear groove and intercondylar notch. The stifle distractors are introduced into the intercondylar fossa from cranial to caudal; they must be fully closed and should be introduced with the tips pointing medially and laterally to minimize the chance of iatrogenic trauma to the cartilage surfaces. The tips should be positioned as caudally as possible to improve distraction of the caudal compartment of the joint (Figure 23.46b).

2 The stifle distractors are rotated through 90 degrees and slowly ratcheted open. Positioning the upper tip more caudally in the intercondylar fossa than the lower tip on the tibial plateau induces cranial translation of the tibia and improves access to the caudal compartment.

3 If access to the caudal compartment of the stifle is suboptimal, a second stifle distractor can be inserted with the jaws positioned deep to the jaws of the first distractor. This provides even distraction of the joint and can significantly improve access for inspection of the caudal poles of the menisci. Alternatively, applying rotational force to the stifle distractors can improve exposure of the caudal joint compartment.

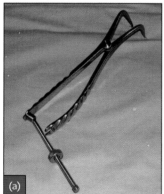
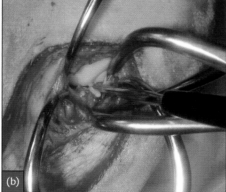

23.46 Correct use of Gelpi retractors and stifle distractors. (a) Two sizes of stifle distractors are available (Veterinary Instrumentation) for large- and small-breed dogs, although the large size (a) can be introduced into the stifle joint of small-breed dogs, if the cranial cruciate ligament (CCL) is ruptured. (b) One or two Gelpi retractors are introduced into the joint to expose the femoral trochlear groove and intercondylar notch. The stifle distractors are introduced into the intercondylar fossa from cranial to caudal; they must be fully closed and should be introduced with the tips pointing medially and laterally to minimize the chance of iatrogenic trauma to the cartilage surfaces. The tips should be positioned as caudally as possible to improve distraction of the caudal compartment of the joint. The stifle distractors are rotated through 90 degrees and slowly ratcheted open. Positioning the upper tip more caudally in the intercondylar fossa than the lower tip on the tibial plateau induces cranial translation of the tibia and improves access to the caudal compartment. If access to the caudal compartment of the stifle is suboptimal, a second stifle distractor can be inserted with the jaws positioned deep to the jaws of the first distractor. This provides even distraction of the joint and can significantly improve access for inspection of the caudal poles of the menisci (see Equipment Extras above).

OPERATIVE TECHNIQUE 23.5

Meniscal inspection, partial meniscectomy and medial meniscal release

POSITIONING

See Operative Technique 23.1.

ASSISTANT

Very helpful to hold the limb still and in the correct position to maximize exposure of the menisci.

EQUIPMENT EXTRAS

See Operative Technique 23.4.

SURGICAL APPROACH

A limited medial approach can be extended to a full medial arthrotomy (see Operative Technique 23.3) if exposure of the caudal compartment of the stifle joint is suboptimal. A full lateral parapatellar approach (see Operative Technique 23.2) is used if concomitant intra-articular or extra-capsular stabilization is planned.

SURGICAL TECHNIQUE

Observation of the caudal horns of the menisci can be challenging but can be improved using good surgical technique (see Operative Technique 23.4).

Partial meniscectomy

Observation of the menisci without palpation is insufficient because injuries may be present that can only be detected by probing. A Dandy nerve hook or similar instrument is inserted below the caudal horn of the medial meniscus and rotated so that the hook is pointing towards the meniscus. If a bucket-handle tear is present, the tip of the probe will hook the axial portion and reveal the tear as the hook is drawn towards the arthrotomy. Removal of the torn portion requires two incisions with a Beaver or No. 11/15 scalpel blade. Firstly, the caudal attachment is sectioned taking care to avoid the caudal cruciate ligament. Secondly, a radial cut is made at the cranial extent of the injured section of meniscus (Figure 23.47). Small mosquito or meniscal forceps are used to remove the damaged portion of the meniscus from the joint. After removal of an axial tear (bucket-handle), the remaining meniscus should be probed to check for the presence of multiple bucket-handle tears.

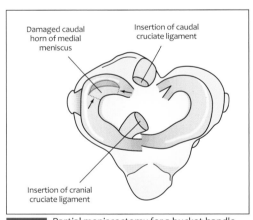

23.47 Partial meniscectomy for a bucket-handle tear. After the caudal attachment is sectioned, a radial cut is made at the cranial extent of the injured section.

Medial meniscal release – axial (caudal) meniscal release

Routine meniscal release is not recommended because meniscal function is compromised after meniscal release. Indications for meniscal release include cases where an axial partial meniscectomy has been performed and the remaining abaxial portion of the meniscus is thought to be at a high risk for subsequent meniscal injury, or where there is abnormal mobility of the caudal horn of the medial meniscus without a tear being identified after thorough probing. Release of the caudal horn of the medial meniscus (axial meniscal release) is performed after inspection of the joint through a medial or lateral parapatellar arthrotomy. 'Blind' mid-body (abaxial) meniscal release, whereby a radial incision is created across the mid-body of the medial meniscus via a stab incision caudal to the medial collateral ligament, is not recommended. The stifle joint should be routinely inspected and normal menisci should not be damaged.

COMPLICATIONS

Although clinically important complications after meniscal release are rarely reported, the procedure has been shown to cause articular cartilage loss, further meniscal pathology, degenerative joint disease and lameness in experimental dogs (Luther *et al.*, 2009).

OPERATIVE TECHNIQUE 23.6

Crimped lateral fabellotibial suture

PLANNING

Ensure that extracapsular stabilization is appropriate (see Figure 23.15).

POSITIONING

See Operative Technique 23.1.

ASSISTANT

Very helpful to enable simultaneous holding of the limb, tensioning of the suture and crimping of the suture.

EQUIPMENT EXTRAS

Hohmann retractors; small graft passer; heavy-gauge semicircular needles; monofilament nylon leader line (dogs <15 kg – single strand of 50 lb (22.7 kg) nylon leader line; dogs 15–30 kg – single strand of 80 lb (36 kg) nylon leader line; dogs 30–40 kg – double strand of 80 lb (36 kg) or single strand of 100 lb (45.4 kg) nylon leader line); drill and drill bits; 16 G hypodermic needle.

SURGICAL TECHNIQUE

For approach, see Operative Technique 23.2. The extra-articular suture is placed once the joint capsule has been closed following joint inspection to attend to any meniscal injury and excise redundant cranial cruciate ligament remnants.

Fabellar anchor point

The tip of a Hohmann retractor is placed caudal to the lateral fabella to retract the biceps femoris muscle. Most suture prostheses are available with swaged-on needles that can be passed around the lateral fabella. The needle tip should be passed around the lateral fabella from cranioproximal to caudodistal. Ideal positioning is around the femorofabellar ligament, just cranial to the fabella. The loop of suture material is elevated and tensioned to ensure that the fabella is properly engaged. If the suture is positioned too caudally, the gastrocnemius muscle will be distracted by the suture loop. Alternatively, a small graft passer can be used to pass the suture material, again in a cranioproximal to caudodistal direction around the femorofabellar ligament. A correctly positioned strand should be robustly anchored.

SUTURE PASSAGE

On the medial aspect of the stifle, a stab incision is created immediately caudal to the insertion of the patellar tendon though the extra-articular bursa that is located here. A pair of mosquito forceps is inserted from medial to lateral through the stab incision. The swaged needle is cut off the suture material and the resulting suture end is grasped in the mosquito forceps and retracted through the stab incision.

Tibial anchor point

Fascia is dissected from the insertion of the patellar tendon until the distinct line where the fibres terminate is identified (Figure 23.48). A 2–2.5 mm drill hole is created from medial to lateral 5–8 mm caudal to this point. The cranial tibial muscle is sharply dissected from cranial to caudal to expose the lateral exit of the tibial bone tunnel. The free end of the suture is passed from medial to lateral through the tibial tunnel.

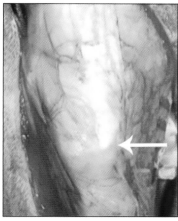

23.48 A 2–2.5 mm drill hole is created from medial to lateral starting 5–8 mm caudal to the point of insertion of the patellar tendon (arrowed). The cranial tibial muscle is sharply dissected from cranial to caudal to expose the lateral exit of the tibial bone tunnel. The free end of the suture is passed from medial to lateral through the tibial tunnel.

→ **OPERATIVE TECHNIQUE 23.6 CONTINUED**

Suture crimping and tensioning

Joint capsule closure should be performed prior to tensioning the extracapsular suture. The free ends of the nylon leader line are passed in opposing directions through the crimp tube. Tension may be applied using instrumentation (Tensioning clamps, Veterinary Instrumentation) or by hand. If tension is applied by hand, the crimping tool is used to crimp with moderate tension across the centre of the wide edge of the oval crimping tube. The suture ends are tensioned until the crimp tube is pulled flat against the joint capsule (Figure 23.49). If insufficient force is applied to the crimping tool, the suture will slide through and tension will be lost. If excessive force is applied, it will not be possible to tension the suture. If the applied force is ideal, the crimp will hold the tensioned suture allowing cranial draw to be tested. Cranial draw should be <2 mm and there should be a normal stifle range of motion. The crimping device is used to crimp the tube with maximum force (both hands can be used) in the centre of the crimp tube and at both ends (not within 1 mm of the extremities of the crimp tube) to make three crimps in total.

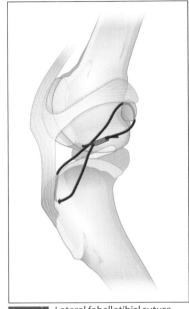

 Lateral fabellotibial suture with a crimped configuration.

OPERATIVE TECHNIQUE 23.7

Tibial tuberosity transposition

PLANNING

The position of the tibial tuberosity should be assessed relative to the quadriceps muscle group and femoral trochlea during weight-bearing with the patella reduced. The position of the tibial osteotomy should be pre-planned using the tibial tuberosity as a landmark (see Operative Technique 23.6 and Figure 23.48).

POSITIONING

See Operative Technique 23.1.

ASSISTANT

No.

EQUIPMENT EXTRAS

Periosteal elevator; microsagittal oscillating saw with multiple blades or hacksaw; drill; Kirschner wires; orthopaedic wire; wire benders; wire cutters.

SURGICAL APPROACH

See Operative Technique 23.3.

SURGICAL TECHNIQUE

A craniomedial approach to the stifle and proximal tibia is made, with elevation and caudal retraction of the aponeurotic insertion of the sartorius muscle. The tibial crest should be completely exposed. A medial arthrotomy is performed for joint inspection. An oscillating saw is used to create the tibial osteotomy starting proximally at a

→ **OPERATIVE TECHNIQUE 23.7 CONTINUED**

point that is at least 3–4 mm cranial to the cranial extremity of the tibial plateau (Figure 23.50a). If an oscillating saw is not available, the cranial tibial muscle is reflected from the craniolateral aspect of the proximal tibia and the tuberosity is separated using a hacksaw. In some cases, a distal periosteal attachment can be maintained, although in severe cases it is frequently necessary to detach the tuberosity completely. If necessary, cortical bone on the caudolateral aspect of the osteotomy site may be removed to expose cancellous bone and provide a level bed for the transposed tuberosity. The tibial tuberosity is rotated laterally and stabilized with one or two Kirschner wires and a tension-band wire (Figure 23.50b). Femoropatellar stability is assessed by flexing and extending the stifle while internally rotating the distal limb. In cases of patella alta (where the patella is located proximally with luxation when the stifle is extended) the tuberosity may be transposed distally in addition to laterally.

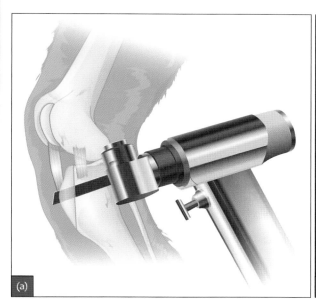 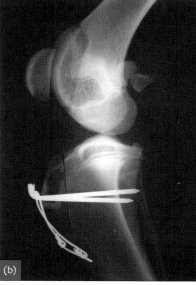

23.50 (a) An oscillating saw is used to separate the tibial tuberosity. (b) Tibial tuberosity transposition stabilized with two Kirschner wires and a tension-band wire in a 2.5-year-old Labrador Retriever. There is evidence of a rectangular recession trochleoplasty.

Closure

See Operative Technique 23.3.

POSTOPERATIVE CARE

Controlled lead walking is recommended until follow-up radiographs are obtained 4–6 weeks postoperatively.

COMPLICATIONS

If a hacksaw is used, care must be taken to ensure that the back edge of the saw does not contact the patellar tendon because this can result in laceration of the tendon. The risk of injury to the patellar tendon is minimized by holding the stifle joint in full extension while the osteotomy is performed. The tuberosity should be transposed until there is normal alignment of the quadriceps mechanism. Excessive lateralization can result in lateral patellar luxation while insufficient lateralization can cause recurrent medial luxation. Other mechanical complications include implant failure and iatrogenic injury to the patellar tendon due to suboptimal implant positioning (see main text).

OPERATIVE TECHNIQUE 23.8

Recession trochleoplasty

The location of the patella relative to the femoral trochlea when it luxates should be determined by palpation. The decision as to whether or not to deepen the trochlea is based on intraoperative findings (see text).

POSITIONING

See Operative Technique 23.1.

ASSISTANT

Helpful to help hold and stabilize the limb.

EQUIPMENT EXTRAS

Fine-toothed saw (e.g. X-ACTO saw, Veterinary Instrumentation) (Figure 23.51); modular osteotome with handle (available from 2 mm wide, Veterinary Instrumentation; see Chapter 14) or a fine oscillating microsagittal saw; a motorized burr (useful but not essential); various sizes of sharp chisels or osteotomes; mallet.

SURGICAL APPROACH

- Medial patellar luxation: lateral parapatellar approach (see Operative Technique 23.2).
- Lateral patellar luxation: medial parapatellar approach (see Operative Technique 23.3).

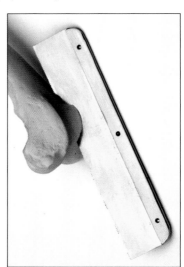

23.51 A fine-toothed hard-backed saw blade. This is similar to the X-ACTO saw but is stiffer, resulting in improved handling during recession sulcoplasty.
(Courtesy of Veterinary Instrumentation)

SURGICAL TECHNIQUE

Wedge recession sulcoplasty

Marks are made on the medial and lateral trochlear ridges with a scalpel blade to define the borders of the wedge. A fine-toothed saw is used to create a wedge-shaped segment. Saline irrigation of the blade helps prevent sticking. The wedge segment is carefully stored and a second cut is made parallel to the first on the side opposite the direction of the patellar luxation (Figure 23.52a). The osteotomy must be made so that the two oblique planes of the cuts intersect proximally at the proximal edge of the trochlear articular cartilage and distally at the intercondylar notch. The wedge is replaced in the recessed defect (Figures 23.52b and 23.53). Removal of a sliver of bone along the apex of the wedge can reduce the tendency for the wedge to rock from side to side. Occasionally, the wedge fits better if it is rotated through 180 degrees.

Block recession sulcoplasty

Parallel incisions are made on the medial and lateral trochlear ridges with a scalpel blade to define the margins of the block. The width

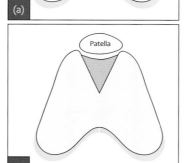

23.52 Wedge recession trochleoplasty. (a) Following removal of a wedge-shaped section, a parallel cut is made in the opposite side to the direction of patellar luxation. (b) After removal of the second section, the original wedge is replaced. The caudal ridge has been removed to secure a tight fit.

23.53 Intraoperative view of a wedge recession trochleoplasty.

→ **OPERATIVE TECHNIQUE 23.8 CONTINUED**

of the cut should be sufficient to accept the patella, and the trochlear ridges should be maintained. Each cut is angled approximately 10 degrees axially towards the sagittal plane of the femur (Figure 23.54a) to ensure subsequent compression between the autograft and recipient bed. The cuts extend from the proximal transtrochlear margin to the intercondylar fossa. The rectangular block is separated using a fine osteotome, Beaver blade or oscillating saw, working towards the centre of the block from the proximal and distal extremities. Care is taken to avoid fracturing the osteochondral segment. The block segment is carefully stored and the defect bed is deepened using an osteotome, oscillating saw or motorized burr. The block is replaced into the defect bed (Figures 23.54b and 23.55) and the patella is reduced so that tracking can be examined. Occasionally, the block fits better if it is rotated through 180 degrees.

POSTOPERATIVE CARE

Controlled lead only exercise is recommended for 4–6 weeks postoperatively.

COMPLICATIONS

Complications include recession of the medial or lateral trochlear ridges due to the wedge being too wide, fracture of the osteochondral block or necrosis of the osteochondral fragment. Migration of the osteochondral fragment is very rare.

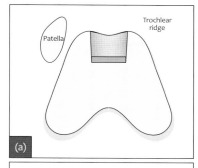

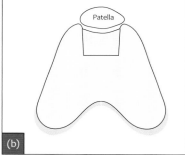

23.54 Block recession trochleoplasty. (a) Parallel incisions in the trochlear ridges, angled at approximately 10 degrees axially. (b) Following resection of cancellous bone, the osteochondral block is replaced.

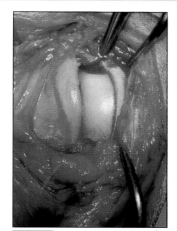

23.55 Intraoperative view of a block recession trochleoplasty.

OPERATIVE TECHNIQUE 23.9

Tibial osteotomy procedures – Editor's guide

Gareth Arthurs

Multiple tibial osteotomy procedures have been described for the treatment of canine and feline CCL insufficiency (see text). Regardless of the selected technique, meticulous attention to detail is required in preoperative planning and surgical implementation. Surgeons should be aware that the initial learning curve for these procedures can be steep and minor technical errors can result in severe complications. It is recommended that surgeons planning to perform tibial osteotomy surgeries are proficient in general orthopaedic surgery and, in particular, have an understanding of fracture biomechanics and fixation techniques. All surgeons should attend a training course relevant to that procedure, and be confident and have significant experience of internal fixation to deal with complications, should they occur. A very simple explanation is provided here to give a basic understanding of how these procedures may be performed.

CRANIAL WEDGE OSTECTOMY–TIBIAL PLATEAU LEVELLING OSTEOTOMY (CWO–TPLO)

Templating

1 The tibial plateau angle (TPA) is calculated from the preoperative radiograph (Figure 23.56).

2 The size and position of the wedge to be removed is carefully calculated and templated on the radiograph.

Surgery

3 A (mini) medial arthrotomy is performed and the cruciate ligaments and menisci are inspected. Damaged tissue is resected as appropriate.

4 The medial aspect of the proximal tibia is exposed by elevation of the soft tissues.

5 The planned wedge ostectomy is transferred from the radiograph to the bone, using pre-planned measurements to ensure that the ostectomy is made in the correct position.

6 Holes may be pre-drilled for placement of K-wires or tension-bands to facilitate reduction post-ostectomy.

7 The ostectomy is made using an oscillating saw, flush and suction, and the wedge of bone is removed.

8 The ostectomy site is reduced and stabilized using implants or reduction forceps.

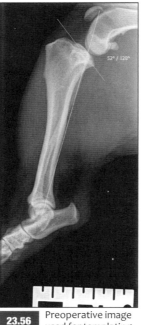

23.56 Preoperative image used for templating of CWO-TPLO surgery; lines to measure the TPA are shown.

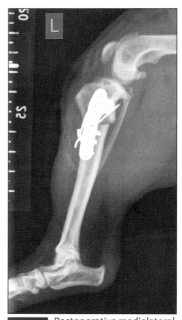

23.57 Postoperative mediolateral radiograph showing the ostectomy site reduced and compressed with implants *in situ*. Locking implants are used for greater stability. The adjusted TPA can also be calculated from this image.

9 A plate is applied to the medial aspect of the tibia to stabilize and compress the osteotomy; use of a locking plate gives greater construct stability. Care must be taken to ensure that the screws do not penetrate the joint.

10 Orthogonal radiographs are taken postoperatively to confirm appropriate implant position, osteotomy position and reduction, limb alignment and postoperative TPA (Figure 23.57)

TIBIAL PLATEAU LEVELLING OSTEOTOMY

Templating

1 The TPA is calculated from the preoperative radiograph (Figure 23.58).

2 The size and position of the curved osteotomy is carefully calculated and templated on the radiograph.

→ **OPERATIVE TECHNIQUE 23.9 CONTINUED**

Surgery

3 A (mini) medial arthrotomy is performed and the cruciate ligaments and menisci are inspected. Damaged tissue is resected as appropriate.

4 The medial aspect of the proximal tibia is exposed by elevation of the soft tissues.

5 The planned radial osteotomy is transferred from the radiograph to the bone, using pre-planned measurements to ensure that the osteotomy is made in the correct position.

6 The osteotomy is made (with or without the use of a procedure specific jig) using an oscillating bi-radial TPLO saw, flush and suction. After the cut has been made in the *cis*-cortex only, the predetermined amount of rotation is marked on the tibia adjacent to the radial osteotomy before completion of the osteotomy.

7 A pin is driven into the tibial plateau segment to rotate this segment of bone, and the plateau is rotated by the pre-calculated amount until the markers on the bone lie adjacent to each other.

8 The tibial plateau is stabilized to the tibial shaft in this new position using K-wires, bone forceps or a combination of both.

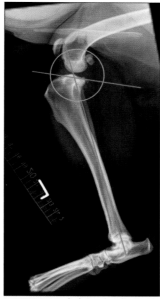
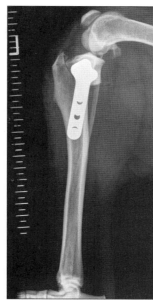

23.58 Mediolateral radiograph of the tibia used to measure TPA and template the radial TPLO.

23.59 Postoperative mediolateral radiograph showing the tibial osteotomy reduced and compressed with implants *in situ*. The adjusted TPA can be calculated from this image.

9 A plate is applied to the medial aspect of the tibia to stabilize and compress the osteotomy; ideally a locking plate is used. Care must be taken to ensure that the screws do not penetrate the joint.

10 Orthogonal radiographs are taken postoperatively to confirm appropriate implant position, osteotomy position and reduction, limb alignment and postoperative TPA (Figure 23.59).

TIBIAL TUBEROSITY ADVANCEMENT

Templating

1 The amount of tibial advancement is calculated from the preoperative radiograph.

2 The position of the osteotomy is carefully calculated and measured from the preoperative radiograph.

3 The size of the implants to be applied to the tibial tuberosity and diaphysis are carefully measured from the radiograph using dedicated templates (Figure 23.60).

Surgery

4 A (mini) medial arthrotomy is performed and the cruciate ligaments and menisci are inspected. Damaged tissue is resected as appropriate.

5 The craniomedial aspect of the proximal tibia is exposed by elevation of the soft tissues.

6 The planned tibial advancement osteotomy is carefully measured and executed using an oscillating saw, flush and suction.

7 Depending on the TTA system being used, some implants (original Kyon TTA plate with forks) may need to be applied to the tibial tuberosity before the osteotomy is complete (Figure 23.61). With other systems the osteotomy can be completed, although it may be desirable to leave a distal bridge of bone and periosteum intact, and the implants may be applied later.

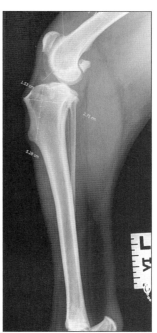

23.60 Mediolateral preoperative radiograph for calculation of tibial tuberosity advancement and planning of implant size and position.

→ **OPERATIVE TECHNIQUE 23.9 CONTINUED**

8 The tibial tuberosity is advanced cranially and a cage of the appropriate size is placed at the proximal aspect of the osteotomy.

9 The size and position of all the implants relative to the tibial diaphysis and the tibial metaphysis are carefully assessed.

10 The implants are applied to the bone; the cage and plate are secured to the tibia using screws.

11 Bone graft may be applied to the gap created by the tibial advancement.

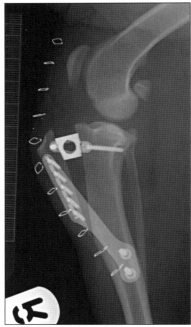

23.61 Mediolateral postoperative radiograph showing implant positioning and osteotomy location following a forked Kyon TTA technique.

PRACTICAL TIP

The original Kyon TTA procedure used a cage with two screws, and a plate with forks securing it to the tibial tuberosity proximally and two screws distally to the tibial diaphysis. There are now many different types of TTA procedures available that are an evolution of the original Kyon TTA procedure. These include the Orthomed MMP, the Leibinger TTA Rapid and the Fusion TTA; each has a very different and specific surgical technique that is learnt at the training course for that procedure

Chapter 24

The tarsus

Rob Pettitt, Gareth Arthurs, Brian Beale and Don Hulse

Surgical anatomy

The tarsus (hock) is a composite joint consisting of seven tarsal bones that articulate in in a complex fashion. It has four major joints: from proximal to distal these are the tarsocrural (tibiotarsal), proximal intertarsal, distal intertarsal and tarsometatarsal joints (Figure 24.1).

The tarsus primarily moves in flexion and extension with more than 95% of the range of motion occurring at the tarsocrural joint. The tarsocrural joint is formed by the articulation of the cochlea of the tibia and the distal fibula with the paired trochlear ridges of the talus. The talar ridges are semicircular and are angled approximately 25 degrees laterally. This allows for clearance of the hind paws past the forepaws during running. The normal tarsus will flex to an angle of around 20–30 degrees and extend to an angle of around 180–190 degrees.

Mediolateral stability is provided principally by the collateral ligaments (Figure 24.2), both of which have long and short components in the dog. Both ligaments originate on the respective malleoli. The short component of the medial collateral ligament (MCL) courses caudally and inserts on the medial aspect of the plantar end of the medial ridge of

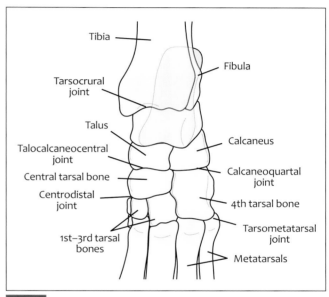

24.1 The bones and joints of the canine tarsus.

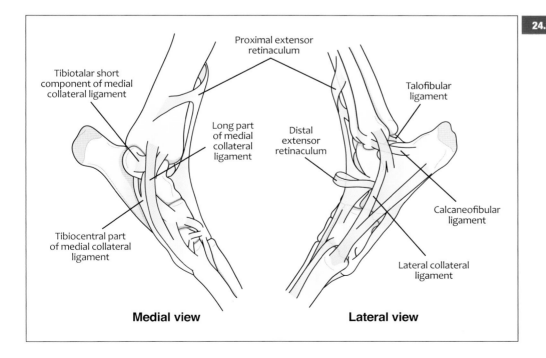

24.2 The ligaments of the canine tarsus.

the talus, while the long component courses distally and has an attachment to the talus before finally inserting on the first tarsal bone. The short component of the lateral collateral ligament (LCL) again courses caudally and inserts on the calcaneus. The long component passes over and attaches to the calcaneus and fourth tarsal bone and finally inserts on the head of the fifth metatarsal bone. The long components of the collateral ligament are taut in extension and relaxed in flexion. The short component is most taut in flexion and less taut in extension.

In the cat there are no long components of the ligament. On the lateral aspect there are the fibulotalar and fibulocalcaneal ligaments and the fibularis brevis tendon. On the medial aspect there are the tibiotalar (craniodistal and caudoproximal parts) and tibiocentral ligaments and the tibialis caudalis tendon. A number of tendons cross the tarsocrural joint to provide active and passive joint support and the joint capsule is also a significant stabilizer of the joint in the domestic cat (Young *et al.*, 1993; Nicholson *et al.*, 2012).

The Achilles (common calcaneal) tendon inserts on the tuber calcaneus and plays an important role in maintaining support and proper angulation of the tarsus. It comprises the tendon of insertion of the gastrocnemius and the combined tendon of the gracilis, biceps femoris and semitendinosus muscles. The superficial digital flexor tendon is associated with, but functionally discrete from, the Achilles tendon proximal to the calcaneus; it passes over the tuber calcaneus and continues distally over the caudal aspect of the calcaneus, plantar ligament and metatarsal bones to insert on the flexor processes of the second phalanges of each of the four digits.

The proximal intertarsal joint includes:

- The talocalcaneocentral joint, comprising proximally and laterally the articulation between the plantar surface of the talus and the sustentaculum tali of the calcaneus, and distally and medially the articulation between the head of the talus, distal calcaneus and proximal central tarsal bone
- The calcaneoquartal joint, comprising the articulation between the calcaneus proximally and fourth tarsal bone distally.

The joint is supported on the plantar aspect by ligaments which span the joint from the calcaneus to the fourth and central tarsal bones, before passing distally to contribute to the plantar tarsal fibrocartilage. Mediolateral support is provided by the long components of the collateral ligaments. There are also dorsal intertarsal ligaments, but these are of little clinical significance.

The distal intertarsal or centrodistal joint is present only on the medial aspect and includes the articulation between the central tarsal bone and the tarsal bones 1, 2 and 3. It is spanned laterally by tarsal bone 4, which helps to protect the distal intertarsal joint from injury.

The tarsometatarsal joint consists of the articulations between the tarsal bones 1, 2, 3 and 4 and the base of the metatarsal bones. It is supported by distal extensions of the collateral and plantar ligaments and the plantar fibrocartilage.

Examination of the tarsus

Signs of tarsal lameness

Dogs and cats with pathology localized to the tarsus may show some or all of the following signs:

- Postural abnormality, e.g. hyperextension in osteochondritis dissecans (OCD) or hyperflexion following Achilles tendon injury or intertarsal subluxation (Figure 24.3)
- Periarticular swelling, usually visible upon inspection
- Altered range of motion, e.g. reduction in flexion of the tarsocrural joint with OCD, or increased flexion with disruption of the Achilles tendon
- Joint instability, e.g. hyperextension of the proximal intertarsal joint, or collateral ligament injury causing varus or valgus tarsal instability
- Pain or crepitus upon palpation.

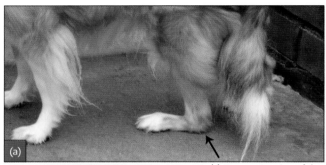

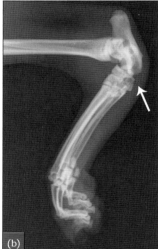

24.3 (a) Hyperextension of the proximal intertarsal joint in the left hindlimb of a Shetland Sheepdog. Note the abnormal dropped posture of the hock, the mid-tarsal angulation and the absence of a visible calcaneus projecting caudally (arrowed). (b) A mediolateral radiograph of a tarsus showing the same pathology. Note the severe subluxation with loss of plantar support at the proximal intertarsal joint (arrowed).
(Courtesy of Gareth Arthurs)

Physical examination of the tarsus

Physical examination of the tarsus is facilitated by the minimal soft tissues surrounding the joint and should include assessment of the following features:

- Palpation for tarsocrural joint swelling (Figure 24.4). Fluctuant swelling is common with acute disease and firm swelling is more common with chronic conditions
- Palpation of the talar ridges is particularly important when surgically approaching the joint for treatment of OCD. The plantar aspects of the medial and lateral trochlear ridges can usually be palpated during full flexion of the tarsocrural joint. The dorsal aspects of the medial and lateral trochlear ridges can usually be palpated during full extension of the tarsocrural joint. Palpation of these landmarks is often limited if the joint is thickened or an effusion is present
- Palpation of the Achilles tendon. This should normally be well defined and should be taut during weight-bearing (Figure 24.5). Abnormal thickening and pain upon palpation may indicate Achilles tendinopathy.

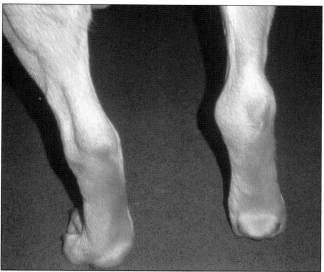

24.4 Swelling of the caudomedial aspect of the right tarsocrural joint in a dog with osteochondritis dissecans (OCD) of the medial ridge of the talus.

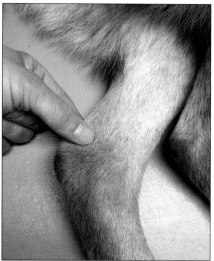

24.5 Palpation of the distal Achilles tendon. The tendon should be examined for thickness, tautness and any pain on palpation. This is best done during weight-bearing.

Partial tears of the insertion of the gastrocnemius tendon are common and may appear as a thickening of the distal aspect of the Achilles tendon. Pain, lack of tension upon weight-bearing or forced flexion against an extended stifle may indicate Achilles tendon rupture or avulsion

• Examination for joint instability. Tarsal instability should be assessed in the frontal and sagittal planes. This should include mediolateral angulation of the tarsocrural and tarsometatarsal joints (frontal plane) and dorsoplantar angulation of the proximal intertarsal and tarsometatarsal joints especially (sagittal plane). The cause of mediolateral angulation should be differentiated between ligamentous instability (MCL injury) and bony deformity (e.g. pes varus). In the dog the medial and lateral collateral ligaments have long straight and short oblique components. Disruption of the long straight component leads to valgus (MCL) or varus (LCL) instability when the tarsus is extended or held in a weight-bearing position. Rotational instability and subtle subluxation of the tibiotarsal joint can occur with an isolated tear of the short oblique component of the collateral ligament when assessing collateral instability with the tarsus flexed. In the cat, it is more complex.

Disruption to the tibiocentral ligament, craniodistal part of the tibiotalar ligament and tendon of the tibialis caudalis muscle will lead to instability in extension. Conversely, damage to the caudoproximal structures will lead to instability in flexion (Nicholson *et al.*, 2012)

• Examination for pain. Pain in tarsal lameness may be elicited by full flexion (e.g. OCD), during examination for joint instability, or by direct palpation (e.g. tarsal bone fractures). Intertarsal rotation of the tarsus with the joint in full extension may elicit pain in cases of centrodistal lameness (Guilliard, 2005).

> **PRACTICAL TIP**
>
> Clinical findings that indicate a tarsal problem include firm or fluctuant joint swelling, instability, loss of range of motion, abnormal angulation and pain

Diagnostic tools

Radiography

The anatomy of the tarsus is complex and the reader should be familiar with the radiographic appearance of this region to allow adequate interpretation. The use of an equivalent view of the contralateral limb or radiology textbooks is recommended (see Imaging Techniques). Standard views should include mediolateral and extended dorsoplantar (or plantarodorsal) views (Figure 24.6). Oblique views and flexed dorsoplantar (skyline) views can be useful to evaluate regions of the trochlea that are difficult to view due to superimposition of adjacent structures (Figure 24.7). Stressed radiographs can be helpful in documenting joint

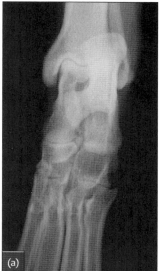

24.6 (a) Dorsoplantar radiograph of the normal canine tarsus. Note the uniformly narrow tarsocrural joint space and the superimposition of the calcaneus over the lateral tarsocrural joint space. (b) Mediolateral radiograph of the normal canine tarsus. Note the limits of the calcaneoquartal joint (arrowed).

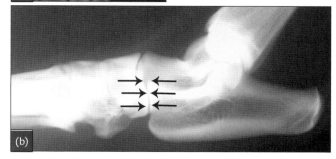

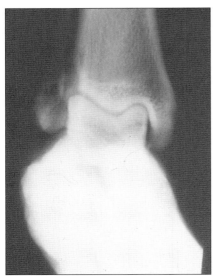

24.7 Flexed dorsoplantar radiograph of the normal canine tarsus. Note the increased visibility of the lateral aspect of the tarsocrural joint space.

instability and determining the level of instability. The tarsus should be stressed by applying a valgus (lateral) force distally to assess MCL stability on a dorsoplantar view. Conversely, application of a varus (medial) force distally is used to assess LCL stability. Similarly, hyperextension and hyperflexion mediolateral stressed views are used to assess dorsal or plantar instability.

Computed tomography

Computed tomography (CT) can be invaluable to assess bony abnormalities of the tarsus and has been shown to be much more sensitive than radiography when identifying fractures (Hercock *et al.*, 2011). It is often the imaging technique of choice when assessing bony abnormalities of the tarsus. The extent and location of OCD lesions can be clearly identified, assisting the surgeon's choice of surgical approach. CT is also a valuable tool to assess articular fractures and deformities of the tarsus (Figure 24.8).

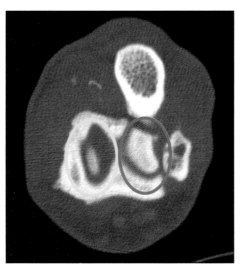

24.8 Dorsal plane CT image of the hock at the level of the trochlear ridges of the talus. The lateral trochlear ridge (red circle) is normal but the medial trochlear ridge (yellow circle) is almost completely missing secondary to osteochondrosis. This is much easier to appreciate on a CT image than it would be on the equivalent radiographs.
(Courtesy of Gareth Arthurs)

Synovial fluid analysis

Synovial fluid analysis is useful to differentiate inflammatory arthritis from osteoarthritis and trauma. Marked elevation of neutrophils is consistent with immune-mediated arthritis and septic arthritis. Mild elevation of mononuclear cells may be seen with traumatic injury and osteoarthritis. Sampling techniques are discussed in Chapter 4, and joint inflammation is covered in Chapter 6.

Surgical approaches

Arthrotomy

A number of surgical approaches to the tarsocrural joint have been described. Exposure is limited by the mortise nature of the trochlear joint and collateral ligamentous stability. Maximum exposure is offered by medial malleolar osteotomy (Sinibaldi, 1979) or collateral desmotomy. However, such techniques have been associated with complications such as prolonged morbidity, failure of orthopaedic implants, joint instability, inaccurate articular reconstruction, iatrogenic cartilage trauma and subsequent osteoarthritis (Smith and Vasseur, 1985; Beale *et al.*, 1991). Approaches that do not involve an osteotomy or desmotomy are preferred, but access is limited (Beale and Goring, 1990; Goring and Beale, 1990); therefore, accurate localization of lesions is essential before surgery is undertaken.

Osteochondrosis of the medial or lateral trochlear ridges of the talus is the most common indication for tarsocrural arthrotomy. Plantaromedial, dorsomedial, plantarolateral and dorsolateral approaches, all of which conserve the collateral ligaments, have been described in detail (Beale and Goring, 1990; Goring and Beale, 1990). Dorsal and plantar approaches may be combined via a single incision. Conservation of the collateral ligaments reduces postoperative morbidity, and while exposure of the trochlear ridges (particularly the medial ridge) is limited, these approaches are usually adequate for recovery of osteochondral fragments. Tenotomy of the lateral head of the deep digital flexor tendon to give improved plantar access has also been described (Dew and Martin, 1993). Surgical approaches to the bones and other joints of the tarsus are simple and direct as there is little intervening soft tissue. Tendinous and neurovascular structures are retracted as appropriate.

Arthroscopy of the tarsus

The tarsal joint is small and tight and, therefore, difficult to investigate arthroscopically, even for the experienced surgeon. For this reason, the surgeon must be prepared to convert the arthroscopic procedure into an open arthrotomy. Early arthroscopic intervention is recommended because intra-articular observation becomes more difficult as joint capsule fibrosis and synovial proliferation advance with articular disease. Although infrequently used in the majority of practices currently, arthroscopy of the tarsus is likely to become more common as future applications, expertise and experience are gained. The indications for arthroscopy of the tarsus include:

- Diagnosis and treatment of OCD of the medial or lateral trochlear ridges of the talus
- Synovial biopsy
- Treatment of infective arthritis.

When evaluating the tarsus arthroscopically, the arthroscope portal can be placed directly over the anatomical area of interest or it can be introduced on the opposite side of the joint to help prevent inadvertent withdrawal of the arthroscope. Once a lesion is localized to a specific region of the tarsus, the surgical approach or arthroscopic portal that gives best access to the area of interest can be selected. If the dorsal aspect of the joint is to be approached, the dog is positioned in dorsal recumbency with the pelvic limbs extended. If the plantar aspect of the joint is to be approached, the patient can be best assessed in sternal recumbency, again with the pelvic limbs extended.

The tarsocrural joint is the only site where arthroscopy is possible within the tarsus (Figure 24.9). When evaluating the tarsus arthroscopically, it is often useful to utilize multiple portals to allow thorough examination of the joint. Hyperflexion and hyperextension may improve inspection of the articular surfaces, by separating the joint surfaces and increasing the amount of articular surface visible from each portal.

Viewing the dorsal aspect of the tarsocrural joint

The tarsus should be positioned in extension. While maintaining the position of the camera head, the light post is rotated to the side to view other regions of the trochlear ridges, the trochlear sulcus, synovial membrane and collateral ligaments. The articulation of the tibia, fibula and talus is also visible. As the light post is rotated to the 6 o'clock (distal) position, the articular surface of the distal tibia can be seen.

Viewing the plantar aspect of the tarsocrural joint

The tarsus should be positioned in flexion. While maintaining the position of the camera head, the light post is rotated to the side to view other regions of the trochlear ridges, trochlear sulcus, flexor hallucis longus tendon, synovial membrane and collateral ligaments. The articulation of the tibia, fibula and talus is also visible. As the light post is rotated to the 6 o'clock (distal) position, the articular surface of the distal tibia can be seen. The medial and lateral collateral ligaments are also visible.

The number of portals used varies depending on the objective of the procedure. If joint exploration is the goal of the surgery, an arthroscope portal and egress portal are all that are required. If tissue biopsy or treatment is

required, the egress portal is converted to an instrument portal. Ancillary instrument portal sites can be triangulated to a region as needed. The most commonly used portal sites are the plantarolateral (Figure 24.10) and plantaromedial (Figure 24.11) The surgeon should be familiar with all of the arthroscopic portals of the tarsus because complete inspection and access to the joint may require use of multiple portals. The surgeon should not hesitate to change to a new portal if the field of view is inadequate or if the scope is difficult to maintain in an intra-articular position.

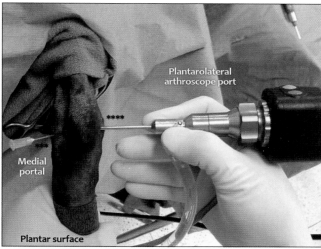

24.10 Positioning of the plantarolateral portal for arthroscopy of the tarsus.

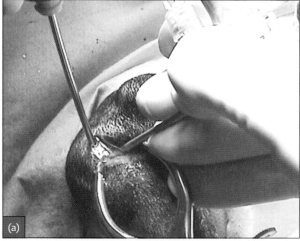

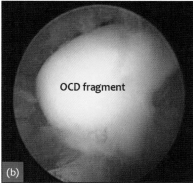

24.11 (a) Performing an arthroscopic mini-arthrotomy through a plantaromedial approach to remove (b) an osteochondritis dissecans (OCD) fragment of the medial ridge of the talus.

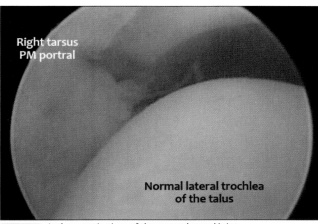

24.9 Arthroscopic view of the normal tarsal joint. PM = plantaromedial.

Congenital conditions of the tarsus

Congenital anomaly of the central tarsal bone

This is an uncommon finding that occurs in large and giant breeds of dog. It consists of medial osseous 'spurs' of variable size that project beyond the proximal and distal extremities of the bone. This anomaly is usually an incidental radiographic finding and does not appear to be associated with lameness (Figure 24.12).

Torsion of the tarsus

Large and giant dog breeds may exhibit abnormal external rotation of the limb distal to the tarsus. This rotation appears to originate within the tarsal region at the level of the proximal intertarsal joint and can result in significant external rotation (up to 80 degrees) of the foot (Petazzoni *et al.*, 2009). Metatarsal dysplasia may also be present. Lameness is a common sign associated with this abnormality.

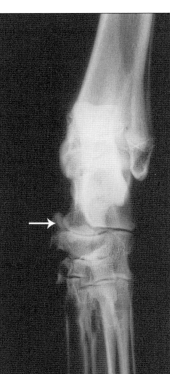

24.12 Dorsoplantar radiograph of a Newfoundland with congenital medial 'spur' formation affecting the central tarsal bone (arrowed). There is also marked rotation of the tarsus and metatarsus in relation to the distal tibia and fibula. There was no lameness related to these abnormalities.

Developmental conditions of the tarsus

Hyperextension of the tarsus

The tarsus is occasionally seen to 'pop' forwards into over-extension, usually at rest. The condition is typically not painful and does not appear to be a cause of lameness. This condition is poorly understood, but it can be associated with more significant abnormalities more proximally, e.g. hip dysplasia and cranial cruciate ligament

problems. It is more common in young large-breed dogs. Specific treatment is usually unnecessary and many dogs improve spontaneously as they mature. Bandaging and splinting techniques are not thought to be helpful. Correction of hip or stifle problems may improve this condition in some patients.

Angular deformity of the distal tibia/fibula

Angular deformities of the distal crus occur far less commonly than in the distal antebrachium. While they may occur as a result of trauma to the physes, they are usually developmental as a result of asymmetrical growth or premature closure of the distal physes. Lateral angulation (pes valgus) may be seen in Collies, Shetland Sheepdogs (McCarthy, 1998) and large breeds (Figure 24.13), and medial angulation (pes varus) has been described in Dachshunds (Johnson *et al.*, 1989). Diagnosis should be straightforward upon inspection and easy to confirm radiographically. Treatment is by corrective osteotomy if the degree of angulation is severe enough to cause lameness.

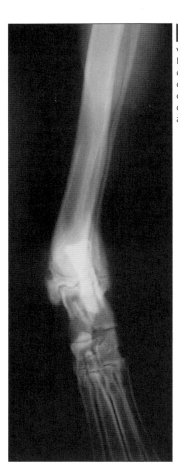

24.13 Valgus deviation of the tarsus and foot (pes valgus) in a juvenile Newfoundland. This deviation was causing lameness and was corrected by a medially based closing wedge osteotomy. The opposite limb was less severely affected.

Osteochondritis dissecans of the medial ridge of the talus

OCD of the tarsus most commonly involves the plantaromedial ridge of the talus, with Labrador Retrievers, Rottweilers and Bull Terriers most commonly affected. Most dogs are presented at 5–9 months of age, although later presentation for chronic mild lameness can occur. Clinical signs may be bilateral, which can complicate diagnosis. Affected animals may have a hyperextended tarsal posture and careful inspection or palpation will reveal swelling of the caudomedial tarsocrural joint. Flexion can be significantly restricted, especially in more chronic cases, and pain is a common finding.

A diagnosis of OCD of the medial ridge of the talus can usually be confirmed radiographically but subtle changes may not be visible. On a mediolateral view, flattening of the trochlear ridge can be seen and there will often be marginal osteophyte formation at the caudal aspect of the distal tibia, as secondary osteoarthritis tends to develop early and progresses rapidly (Figure 24.14a). A mineralized fragment may be seen caudal to the talus if the OCD lesion has detached. On the plantarodorsal view, there is flattening of the medial trochlear ridge, with an increase in medial tarsocrural joint space (Figure 24.14b). A mineralized fragment may be seen proximal to the trochlear ridge and there will usually be osteophyte formation along the medial aspect of the talus. In some cases the lesion cannot be seen radiographically as it sits more plantar on the talar ridge and the hock cannot be extended far enough to skyline the lesion. If there is doubt, the diagnosis can be confirmed by CT scan, arthroscopy or arthrotomy (Figure 24.15).

Although most affected dogs appear to benefit from surgical removal of the OCD lesion via a plantaromedial arthrotomy or arthroscopy, the outcome for this disease remains guarded (van der Peijl et al., 2012). Postoperative

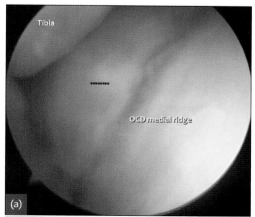

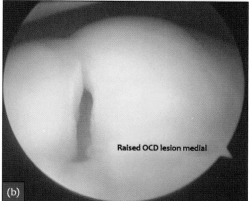

24.15 Arthroscopic diagnosis of OCD of the tarsus. (a) OCD of the medial ridge of the talus. (b) Raised OCD lesion of the medial ridge of the talus. OCD = osteochondritis dissecans.

osteophyte size, degree of swelling and range of motion seem to be the main prognostic indicators.

The majority of tarsal OCD lesions are located at the plantaromedial aspect of the trochlea and the location of the lesion should guide the surgeon's approach. For example, the most common arthroscopic portal is the plantarolateral one.

A soft support bandage is applied for 4–5 days postoperatively and exercise is restricted to short walks on a lead only for 4 weeks, with a phased increase in the lengths of walks after that period.

Most owners feel that their pet's comfort, exercise tolerance and quality of life are improved by surgery. The hyperextended joint posture and periarticular thickening may persist and osteoarthritis progresses despite surgery. Many dogs may remain lame despite removal of the OCD lesion, or lameness may recur in the future (Miller and Beale, 2008). If significant lameness cannot be controlled by conservative means, pantarsal arthrodesis is available as a salvage procedure.

Osteochondritis dissecans of the lateral ridge of the talus

OCD occasionally affects the lateral trochlear ridge of the talus (Robins et al., 1983). Physical signs are similar to lesions of the medial ridge, although periarticular swelling is more evident laterally. The lesion may be located caudally, plantarly or more cranio-dorsally on the trochlear ridge. The radiographic signs are the same as in medial ridge lesions, although diagnosis is more difficult due to superimposition of the calcaneus and lateral trochlear

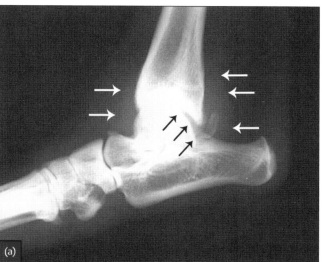

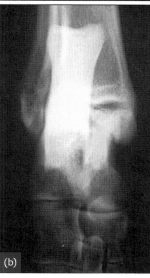

24.14 (a) Mediolateral radiograph of OCD of the hock. There is periarticular soft tissue swelling (white arrows) and the tarsocrural joint space is widened caudally. Flattening of the trochlear ridge is evident (black arrows) and the caudal edge of the distal tibia appears extended by marginal osteophyte formation. There is a free mineralized body (the OCD lesion) caudal to the trochlear ridge. (b) Plantarodorsal radiograph of OCD of the medial trochlear ridge. The medial joint space is abnormally widened (compare with Figure 24.6a). OCD = osteochondritis dissecans.

ridge on the plantarodorsal view. Oblique views or a flexed dorsoplantar view may be more helpful. CT is ideal for evaluation of hock OCD lesions.

Treatment options are similar to those for medial ridge OCD, although a craniolateral and/or dorsolateral surgical approach can be advantageous for treatment of more cranially positioned lesions due to better access.

Acquired conditions of the tarsus

Fractures

Fractures involving the tarsus are covered in detail within the *BSAVA Manual of Canine and Feline Fracture Repair and Management*. Most commonly, they involve the calcaneus, the talus, the central tarsal and the numbered tarsal bones. They are generally closed, comminuted and due to indirect trauma. They are most frequently seen in racing and working dogs, although calcaneal fractures can also occur in the pet animal, usually as a result of direct trauma.

Collateral ligament injury

Injuries to the tarsal collateral ligaments are usually associated with acute trauma, either closed (e.g. a fall or twisting injury) or in association with open or shearing injuries (e.g. road traffic accident). Diagnosis is easy in shearing injuries and can usually be made by palpation or by the use of stress radiography in closed injuries. Radiography is used to identify avulsion fractures of ligamentous attachment points.

Tarsocrural collateral ligament injury

Most cases of tarsocrural collateral ligament injury involve complete injury to the medial and/or lateral collateral ligament complex, although isolated injury to the short component of the lateral collateral has been described as a cause of lameness (Sjöstrom and Hakanson, 1994).

Shearing injuries can affect the medial or lateral aspect of the joint. In addition to loss of collateral support there will be loss of varying amounts of bone and overlying soft tissues. These injuries are best managed initially using transarticular external skeletal fixation and appropriate open wound management. Soft tissue defects can be allowed to heal by secondary intention or treated by delayed primary closure or skin grafting techniques. Where there is instability due to loss of collateral ligament support, primary repair using ligament prostheses or temporary stabilization with a transarticular external skeletal fixator (TESF) to allow periarticular fibrosis is recommended (Kulendra *et al.*, 2011; Kulendra and Arthurs, 2014). If there has been significant loss of bone beyond the axial margin of the malleolus, or joint stability cannot be restored, pantarsal arthrodesis should be considered.

Simple malleolar avulsion fractures are best treated by open reduction and internal fixation using pin(s) and a tension-band wire. Comminuted malleolar fractures are difficult to manage. If primary repair is not possible then indirect stabilization using a TESF or pantarsal arthrodesis are alternative options.

When planning prosthetic replacement of the tarsocrural collateral ligaments, it is essential to mimic as closely as possible the normal anatomy so that the joint can be stabilized throughout its full range of movement

(Aron and Purinton, 1985). In the dog two prosthetic ligaments need to be inserted, with a single anchor point proximally but two distinct points distally (Figure 24.16). The proximal anchor point is usually a bone screw with a washer. The distal anchor points may also be small screws with washers, although the insertion of the short component of the medial collateral is on the abaxial aspect of the medial trochlear ridge of the talus but a protruding screw head at this point may impinge on the medial malleolus when the joint extends. Therefore a suture anchor (see Chapter 14) recessed beneath the bone surface is probably more appropriate in this location. In a recent study (Beever *et al.*, 2016) prosthetic ligament replacement was associated with a high risk of complication in dogs with tarsocrural injury. The recommendation for cats is to place a series of four prosthetic ligaments through bone tunnels, two tight in flexion and two tight in extension (Nicholson *et al.*, 2012).

> **PRACTICAL TIP**
>
> Consider the use of suture anchors for prosthetic ligament replacement: this avoids interference with joint motion and facilitates wound closure

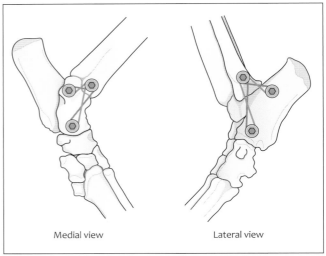

Medial view   Lateral view

24.16 Positioning of anchorage points for prosthetic tarsocrural collateral ligaments.

Depending upon the size of the patient, braided non-absorbable material or monofilament nylon leader line are suitable materials for the ligament prosthesis. Leader line tends to result in a bulkier knot so a crimp is preferable. The long component should be tightened with the joint extended and the short component with the joint flexed to recreate the correct combination of joint stability without interfering with normal mobility. Unfortunately, there are no good guidelines in use on which to base selection of implant size.

> **PRACTICAL TIP**
>
> In cats, imbrication of the local soft tissues (if present) or periarticular fibrosis associated with open wound healing in shearing injuries managed with a TESF usually seems to provide sufficient long-term stability without the need for prosthetic ligaments

Following surgery to manage instability without use of a TESF, the tarsus should be supported in a splint or cast for 6–8 weeks, followed by a further 4–6 weeks of restricted exercise. Most dogs seem to have a favourable result, although some degree of joint stiffness, lameness or osteoarthritis may result.

Intertarsal and tarsometatarsal collateral ligament injury

Loss of collateral support at the intertarsal or tarsometatarsal joints can be seen in isolation or as part of a more complex soft tissue injury. In either event, partial (intertarsal and/or tarsometatarsal) arthrodesis usually represents the best treatment. This is typically best performed using a plate and screws located medially or laterally (Dyce *et al.*, 1998), depending upon the joint involved and the location of the major soft tissue injury. The lateral surface is usually preferred as it is flatter, much less plate contouring is required, and it allows placement of a screw in the large fourth tarsal bone. Standard compression plates, purpose-made hybrid intertarsal arthrodesis plates or sections of cuttable plate can be used, depending upon patient size (Figure 24.17). Alternatively, in cats, fine pins may be introduced into the distal metatarsal bones via dorsal cortical slots and driven across the tarsometatarsal joint into the tarsal bones, although the outcome with this technique is not as well understood.

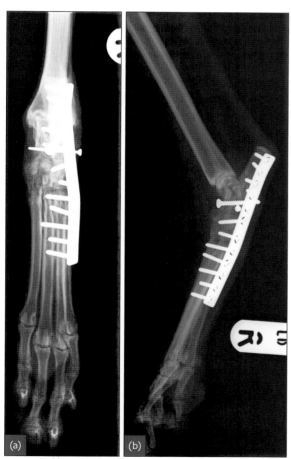

24.17 (a) Dorsoplantar and (b) mediolateral radiographs of a partial tarsal arthrodesis performed in a dog 6 months previously using a contoured 2.7 mm dynamic compression plate on the lateral aspect of the tarsus. Note that only the 'ghost' outline of the proximal and distal rows of intertarsal joints are visible, consistent with progressive arthrodesis.
(Courtesy of Gareth Arthurs)

Whatever technique is used, standard principles of arthrodesis, i.e. removal of articular cartilage, insertion of a cancellous bone graft and consideration of additional external support following surgery, should always be adhered to. Intertarsal and tarsometatarsal fusions usually provide good results.

Closure of the surgical wounds, especially in smaller dogs and cats, may be challenging due to the relatively little soft tissue in that area. Careful pre-incision planning is needed to avoid the incision lying over the implant. In some cases, multiple tension-releasing incisions may be required in order to facilitate a tension-free closure.

Plantar ligament degeneration

Idiopathic degeneration of the plantar supporting structures of the proximal intertarsal joint is seen uncommonly, with middle-aged Shetland Sheepdogs over-represented. Affected individuals are typically overweight and usually have a sedentary lifestyle. Progressive ligament degeneration allows hyperextension of the proximal intertarsal (calcaneoquartal and talocentral) joints, causing a plantigrade posture and lameness. Such changes may be bilateral; if not, soft tissue swelling can often be detected on the plantar surface of the contralateral proximal intertarsal joint and this frequently indicates incipient plantar ligament degeneration.

Affected dogs may be lame if there is unilateral hyperextension, or exercise intolerant if affected bilaterally. The affected tarsus (tarsi) will be dropped and the calcaneus will be rotated proximally by the pull of the Achilles tendon. There is usually palpable instability (hyperextension) of the proximal intertarsal joint but manipulation appears to cause little discomfort.

Mediolateral and dorsoplantar non-stressed radiographs of the affected tarsus (tarsi) will confirm the diagnosis, and are used for surgical planning. Stressed films, with hyperextension of the proximal intertarsal joint, will accentuate the abnormality if there is doubt (Figure 24.18). Specifically, new bone formation/enthesopathy, indicating chronic pathology, is usually seen on the plantar aspect of the distal calcaneus, and this can also be seen as a sign of impending plantar ligament failure in the contralateral limb (Figure 24.19).

As opposed to ligamentous degeneration, any breed of dog can suffer traumatic injury to the plantar ligamentous support, usually with obvious local swelling and visible or palpable instability. The treatment in either case is selective arthrodesis of the calcaneoquartal joint (Allen *et al.*,

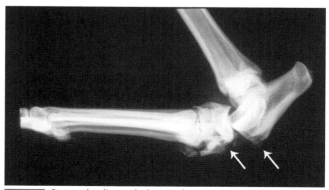

24.18 Stressed radiograph showing hyperextension of the proximal intertarsal joint due to plantar ligament degeneration in a Shetland Sheepdog. There is enthesophyte formation on the plantar aspect of the calcaneoquartal joint (arrowed) and new bone formation dorsal to the centrodistal joint.

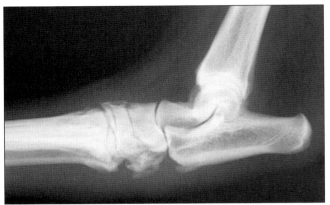

24.19 Mediolateral radiograph of the contralateral, apparently normal, limb of a dog with subluxation of the proximal intertarsal joint. There is periarticular soft tissue swelling and plantar enthesophyte formation adjacent to the calcaneoquartal joint. These changes signify ongoing degenerative changes that may lead to failure of plantar ligament support.

1993). Several techniques have been described to achieve this and the most popular are a pin and plantar tension-band, a lag screw (± plantar tension-band) or a compression plate applied laterally. The lateral plate has been shown to be associated with fewer complications than either lag screw or pin combined with tension-band wire (Barnes *et al.*, 2013). In each case articular cartilage should be completely removed from the joint surfaces and a cancellous bone graft should be used. External support can be applied for 6–8 weeks, or until signs of osseous fusion are visible radiographically, although the need for this is unproven and dressing-associated complications are common (Meeson *et al.*, 2011). Recent evidence for pancarpal arthrodesis is that a cast is not needed (Ramirez and Macias, 2016); therefore, it is reasonable to believe the same is true for partial tarsal arthrodesis where the plate is edge loaded and so mechanically stronger and less prone to premature cyclic fatigue. In bilateral cases, surgeries should be staged if possible, with an interval of 6–8 weeks between operations.

If a successful arthrodesis can be achieved, the vast majority of dogs will return to a good level of function. The most common complication is failure to achieve arthrodesis and subsequent fixation failure, especially in dogs affected bilaterally. Prolonged external support prior to surgery seems to be associated with a greater risk of postoperative complications, so surgery should normally be undertaken as soon as possible after diagnosis.

Dorsal ligament rupture

Rupture of dorsal intertarsal ligaments occurs sporadically, usually following traumatic hyperflexion of the intertarsal or tarsometatarsal joint. Instability can be detected by palpation and stressed radiography (Figure 24.20).

Isolated dorsal ligament rupture can be managed non-surgically using external support for 4–6 weeks, as weight-bearing automatically holds the affected joint in reduction. If there is gross instability, imbricating the ruptured dorsal soft tissues using polydioxanone can be helpful. Arthrodesis should be required only in extremely unstable joints.

Achilles tendon injuries

The common calcaneal tendon (CCT) consists of the gastrocnemius as well as the common tendon of the gracilis,

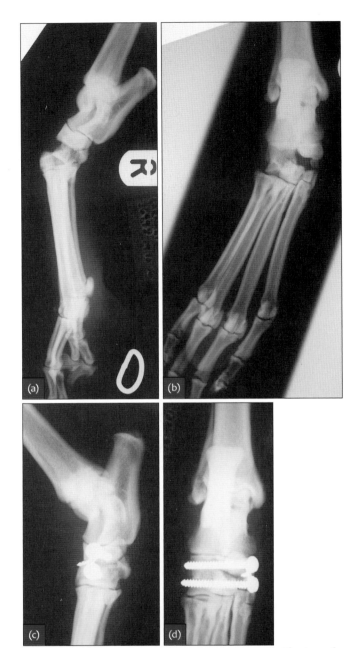

24.20 (a–b) Stressed views of the tarsus demonstrating fracture of the first tarsal bone with resulting medial and dorsal instabilities originating at the centrodistal joint. (c–d) Selective stabilization of the affected centrodistal joint using two screws, washers and a figure-of-eight wire. Management in this case was successful. (Courtesy of Gareth Arthurs)

biceps femoris and semitendinosus muscles, and inserts on the tuber calcaneus. The superficial digital flexor tendon is closely associated with the CCT proximal to the calcaneus but does not insert on the tuber calcaneus. Instead it passes over the tuber calcaneus with a bursa interposed between the tuber calcaneus and the tendon. Injury to the Achilles mechanism encompasses complete ruptures, partial ruptures and avulsion/enthesopathy at the point of insertion on the calcaneus. Injury can be due to acute trauma, e.g. a penetrating wound or sharp laceration, or can be more chronic, e.g. tendinopathy. Achilles tendon injuries have been classified into three main types by Meustege (1993). Physical signs vary depending upon the severity of injury and may be bilateral in chronic cases.

- **Complete rupture** results in a plantigrade tarsal posture or severely dropped tarsus (Figure 24.21). The tarsus can be manually hyperflexed while the stifle is fixed in extension (which should be mechanically impossible). There may be a palpable defect in the substance of the tendon in acute rupture but there may be no palpable defect in chronic injuries.
- **Partial rupture** (e.g. injury to the gastrocnemius tendon in isolation) may result in a partially dropped tarsus with hyperflexion ('clenching') of the digits during weight-bearing or manual flexion of the tarsus (Figure 24.22). The appearance of the digits is due to the superficial digital flexor tendon remaining intact and being tensioned as the tarsus hyperflexes. This appearance is most commonly recognized in middle-aged Dobermanns affected by gastrocnemius enthesopathy (Bonneau *et al.*, 1982; Butterworth, 1995). In these cases there is usually palpable swelling of the tendon insertion on the calcaneus and pain upon digital pressure.
- **Tendinosis/peritendinitis** may cause palpable thickening of the Achilles mechanism but with no rupture and without any alteration in joint posture.

Radiography (mediolateral view) will reveal soft tissue swelling. Cases of chronic gastrocnemius avulsion/enthesopathy may show small islands of mineralization proximal to the insertion of the tendon and new bone formation ('capping') around the free end of the calcaneus. Ultrasonography is a useful modality for scanning the tendon in order to assess fibre alignment and disruption to the tendon (Figures 24.23 and 24.24). Treatment of Achilles tendon ruptures may be conservative or surgical, depending upon presentation. There are no clear guidelines for decision-making but as a general guide:

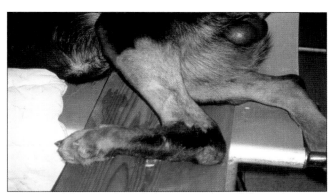

24.21 Adult Rottweiler with chronic complete Achilles tendon rupture. There is a pressure sore on the plantar aspect of the calcaneus and thickening of the distal Achilles tendon. The hock is hyperflexed.

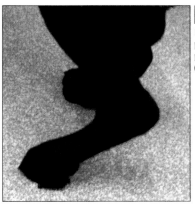

24.22 Gastrocnemius avulsion in a Labrador Retriever. Note the partially 'dropped' hock posture with hyperflexion ('clenching') of the digits.

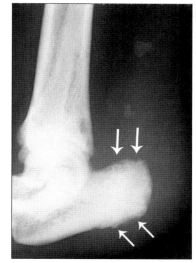

24.23 Mediolateral radiograph of gastrocnemius avulsion. Note the small areas of mineralization proximal to the calcaneus and the 'capping' of the tip of calcaneus by new bone formation (arrowed).

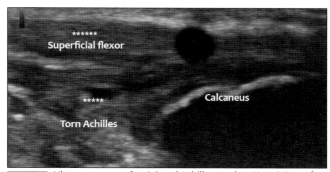

24.24 Ultrasonogram of an injured Achilles tendon. Note injury of the gastrocnemius insertion at the calcaneus. The superficial flexor tendon is intact.

- Dogs with normal joint and digital posture and mild lameness may be suitable for non-surgical management. Restriction to leash exercise for 6–8 weeks and use of non-steroidal anti-inflammatory drugs, if required, may allow resolution of lameness
- If not, or if progressive postural changes develop, surgery is indicated including exploration, debridement and suturing of the tendon and/or placement of a transarticular external skeletal fixator to hold the hock in extension and thereby allow the tendinopathy to consolidate (see Operative Technique 24.5). The prognosis is somewhat variable depending on the level, extent and nature of the injury, and multiple complications are possible
- As a salvage procedure, pantarsal arthrodesis is possible (see Operative Technique 24.4). This is considered by some surgeons as the technique of first choice in chronic degenerative tendinosis/insertionopathy cases because of the complications and variable outcomes associated with tendon repair surgical techniques.

Superficial digital flexor tendon luxation

Lateral luxation of the superficial digital flexor tendon from the calcaneus as a result of rupture of its medial retinacular attachment occurs most commonly in Shetland Sheepdogs and racing Greyhounds (Vaughan, 1987), but can occur in many different breeds. The luxation can be palpated as a slipping of the tendon on and off its normal location in acute cases, although it may become more fixed laterally in time, in which case there will only be local swelling. Medial luxation following failure of the lateral retinaculum occurs much less commonly.

Surgical repair of the torn retinaculum via a plantaromedial (or if necessary, plantarolateral) incision is best. The torn or stretched retinaculum is sutured directly or overlapped using polydioxanone mattress sutures. In chronic cases, or if primary repair fails, revision surgery using polypropylene mesh to reinforce the repair has been described (Houlton and Dyce, 1993). Suture anchors can also be used as an interference post to prevent lateral displacement of the tendon and as an anchor to secure the torn retinaculum. The sulcus at the proximal aspect of the calcaneus can also be deepened in a similar fashion to trochlear block recession of the femoral trochlear for treatment of patellar luxation.

Acknowledgement

The authors would like to acknowledge the contribution of Andy Miller to the chapter in the first edition of this manual.

References and further reading

Allen MJ, Dyce J and Houlton JEF (1993) Calcaneoquartal arthrodesis in the dog. *Journal of Small Animal Practice* **34**, 205–210

Aron DA and Purinton PT (1985) Replacement of the collateral ligaments of the canine tarsocrural joint – a proposed technique. *Veterinary Surgery* **14**, 178–184

Baltzer WI and Rist P (2009) Achilles tendon repair in dogs using the semitendinosus muscle: surgical technique and short-term outcome in five dogs. *Veterinary Surgery* **38**, 770–779

Barnes DC, Knudsen CS, Gosling M et al. (2013) Complications of lateral plate fixation compared with tension band wiring and pin or lag screw fixation for calcaneoquartal arthrodesis. Treatment of proximal intertarsal subluxation occurring secondary to non-traumatic plantar tarsal ligament disruption in dogs. *Veterinary and Comparative Orthopaedics and Traumatology* **26**, 445–452

Beale BS and Goring RL (1990) Exposure of the medial and lateral trochlear ridges of the talus in the dog. Part I. Dorsomedial and plantaromedial surgical approaches to the medial trochlear ridge. *Journal of the American Animal Hospital Association* **26**, 13–18

Beale BS, Goring RL, Herrington J et al. (1991) A prospective evaluation of four surgical approaches to the talus of the dog used in the treatment of osteochondritis dissecans. *Journal of the American Animal Hospital Association* **27**, 221–229

Beale BS, Hulse DA, Schulz K and Whitney WO (2003) *Small Animal Arthroscopy*. Saunders, Philadelphia

Beever LJ, Kulendra ER and Meeson RL (2016) Short and long-term outcome following surgical stabilization of tarsocrural instability in dogs. *Veterinary and Comparative Orthopaedics and Traumatology* **29**, 142–148

Benlooch-Gonzalez M, Grapperon-Mathis M and Boury B (2014) Computed tomography assisted determination of optimal insertion points and bone corridors for transverse implant placement in the feline tarsus and metatarsus. *Veterinary and Comparative Orthopaedics and Traumatology* **27(6)**, 441–446

Bonneau NH, Olivieri M and Breton L (1982) Avulsion of the gastrocnemius tendon in the dog causing flexion of the hock and digits. *Journal of the American Animal Hospital Association* **19**, 717–722

Braden TD (1976) Fascia lata transplant for repair of chronic Achilles tendon defects. *Journal of the American Animal Hospital Association* **12**, 800–805

Butterworth SJ (1995) Gastrocnemius enthesopathy. *Veterinary Practice* **1**, 8

Caine A, Agthe P, Posch B et al. (2009) Sonography of the soft tissue structures of the canine tarsus. *Veterinary Radiology and Ultrasound* **50(3)**, 304–308

Deruddere K, Milne M, Wilson K et al. (2014) Magnetic resonance imaging, computed tomography, and gross anatomy of the canine tarsus. *Veterinary Surgery* **43**, 912–919

Dew TL and Martin RA (1993) A caudal approach to the tibiotarsal joint. *Journal of the American Animal Hospital Association* **29**, 117–121

Diserens KA and Venzin C (2015) Chronic Achilles tendon rupture augmented by transposition of the fibularis brevis and fibularis longus muscles. *Schweizer Archiv fur Tierheilkunde* **157**, 519–524

Dyce J, Whitelock RG, Robinson KV, Forsythe F and Houlton JEF (1998) Arthrodesis of the tarsometatarsal joint using a laterally applied plate in 10 dogs. *Journal of Small Animal Practice* **39**, 19–22

Fitzpatrick N, Sajik D and Farrell M (2013) Feline pantarsal arthrodesis using pre-contoured dorsal plates applied according to the principles of percutaneous plate arthrodesis. *Veterinary and Comparative Orthopaedics and Traumatology* **26**, 399–407

Gemmill T and Clements D (2016) *BSAVA Manual of Canine and Feline Fracture Repair and Management, 2nd edn*. BSAVA Publications, Gloucester

Gielen I, van Ryssen B and van Bree H (2005) Computerized tomography compared with radiography in the diagnosis of lateral trochlear ridge talar osteochondritis dissecans in dogs. *Veterinary and Comparative Orthopaedics and Traumatology* **18(2)**, 77–82

Goring RL and Beale BS (1990) Exposure of the medial and lateral trochlear ridges of the talus in the dog. Part II. Dorsolateral and plantarolateral surgical approaches to the lateral trochlear ridge. *Journal of the American Animal Hospital Association* **26**, 19–24

Guilliard MJ (2005) Centrodistal joint lameness in dogs. *Journal of Small Animal Practice* **46**, 199–202

Hercock CA, Innes JF, McConnell F et al. (2011) Observer variation in the evaluation and classification of severe central tarsal bone fractures in racing Greyhounds. *Veterinary and Comparative Orthopaedics and Traumatology* **24** 215–222

Houlton JEF and Dyce J (1993) The use of polypropylene mesh for revision of failed repair of superficial flexor tendon luxation in three dogs. *Veterinary and Comparative Orthopaedics and Traumatology* **6**, 129–130

Jenkins DHR, Forster IW, McKibbin B and Ralis ZA (1977) Induction of tendon and ligament formation by carbon implants. *Journal of Bone and Joint Surgery* **59B**, 53–57

Johnson SG, Hulse DA, Vangundy TE and Green RW (1989) Corrective osteotomy for pes varus in the dachshund. *Veterinary Surgery* **18**, 373–379

Katayama M (2016) Augmented repair of an Achilles tendon rupture using the flexor digitorum lateralis tendon in a Toy Poodle. *Veterinary Surgery* **45**, 1083–1086

Kornmayer M, Amort K, Failing K and Kramer M (2014) Medullary cavity diameter of metacarpal and metatarsal bones in cats. A cadaveric radiographic and computed tomographic analysis. *Veterinary and Comparative Orthopaedics and Traumatology* **27(6)**, 447–452

Kulendra E and Arthurs GI (2014) Management and treatment of feline tarsal injuries. *In Practice* **36**, 119–132

Kulendra E, Grierson J, Okushima S, Cariou M and House A (2011) Evaluation of the transarticular ESF for the treatment of tarsocrural instability in 32 cats. *Veterinary and Comparative Orthopaedics and Traumatology* **24**, 320–325

McCarthy PE (1998) Bilateral pes valgus deformity in a Shetland Sheepdog. *Veterinary and Comparative Orthopaedics and Traumatology* **11**, 197–199

Meeson RL, Davidson C and Arthurs GI (2011) Soft-tissue injuries associated with cast application for distal limb orthopaedic conditions. A retrospective study of sixty dogs and cats. *Veterinary and Comparative Orthopaedics and Traumatology* **24**, 126–131

Meustege FJ (1993) The classification of canine Achilles tendon lesions. *Veterinary and Comparative Orthopaedics and Traumatology* **6**, 53–55

Miller J and Beale B (2008) Tibiotarsal arthroscopy. Applications and long-term outcome in dogs. *Veterinary and Comparative Orthopaedics and Traumatology* **21**, 159–165

Moores AP, Owen MR and Tarlton JF (2004) The three-loop pulley suture versus two locking-loop sutures for the repair of canine Achilles tendons. *Veterinary Surgery* **33**, 131–137

Morton MA, Thomson DG, Rayward RM, Jimenez-Peleaz M and Whitelock RG (2015) Repair of chronic rupture of the insertion of the gastrocnemius tendon in the dog using a polyethylene terephthalate implant. Early clinical experience and outcome. *Veterinary and Comparative Orthopaedics and Traumatology* **28**, 282–287

Nicholson I, Langley-Hobbs S, Sutcliffe M, Jeffrey N and Radke H (2012) Feline talocrural luxation: A cadaveric study of repair using ligament prostheses. *Veterinary and Comparative Orthopaedics and Traumatology* **2**, 116–123

Petazzoni M, Piras A, Jaeger GH and Marioni C (2009) Correction of rotational deformity of the pes with external fixation in four dogs. *Veterinary Surgery* **38**, 506–514

Ramirez JM and Macias C (2016) Pancarpal arthrodesis without rigid coaptation using the hybrid dynamic compression plate in dogs. *Veterinary Surgery* **45**, 303–308

Robins GM, Read RA, Carlisle CH and Webb SM (1983) Osteochondritis dissecans of the lateral ridge of the trochlea of the tibial tarsal bone in the dog. *Journal of Small Animal Practice* **24**, 675–685

Roch SP, Clements DN, Mitchell RA et al. (2008) Complications following tarsal arthrodesis using bone plate fixation in dogs. *Journal of Small Animal Practice* **49**, 117–126

Sinibaldi KR (1979) Medial approach to the tarsus. *Journal of the American Animal Hospital Association* **15**, 77

Sjöstrom L and Hakanson N (1994) Traumatic injuries associated with the short lateral collateral ligaments of the tarsocrural joint of the dog. *Journal of Small Animal Practice* **35**, 163–168

Smith MM and Vasseur PB (1985) Clinical evaluation of dogs after surgical and non surgical management of osteochondritis dissecans of the talus. *Journal of the American Veterinary Medical Association* **187**, 31–35

van der Peijl GJ, Scaeffer IG, Theyse LF et al. (2012) Osteochondrosis dissecans of the tarsus in Labrador Retrievers: clinical signs, radiological data and force plate gait evaluation after surgical treatment. *Veterinary and Comparative Orthopaedics and Traumatology* **25**, 126–134

Vaughan LC (1987) Disorders of the tarsus in the dog parts 1 and 2. *British Veterinary Journal* **143**, 388–498

Young RP, Scott SH and Loeb GE (1993) The distal hindlimb musculature of the cat: multiaxis moment arms of the ankle joint. *Experimental Brain Research* **96** 141–151

IMAGING TECHNIQUES

Thomas W. Maddox

The tarsus is a complex joint and there is considerable superimposition of the component bones seen on radiography. This can result in changes that are difficult to interpret and even detect on conventional radiographs, especially in cases of traumatic injury. As a consequence of this, computed tomographic examination of the joint is being used more frequently.

RADIOGRAPHY

Standard views

Standard views of the tarsus are the mediolateral and plantarodorsal or dorsoplantar views. The small size of the limb at this level means that radiographic grids are not required and a high detail system should be used if available.

Mediolateral view

Superimposition of the tarsal bones and joints on this view is not quite as problematic as for the same view of the carpus, but pathology involving the small tarsal bones is still difficult to evaluate. Dorsoplantar subluxation can be well assessed, and although there is some superimposition of the medial and lateral parts of the tarsocrural joint, these can still be evaluated.

- The patient is placed in lateral recumbency with the target limb dependent against the cassette/plate and the contralateral limb retracted cranially (Figure 24.25).
- The tarsus should be in a neutral position.
- Primary beam is centred just distal to the medial and lateral malleoli.
- Collimate to include one-third of the distal crus and most of the metatarsals.

Plantarodorsal view

This view is useful for assessment of the medial and lateral aspects of the tarsus, and the medial part of the tarsocrural joint is well seen as there is no superimposition of additional structures to the talus and distal tibia.

- The patient is placed in sternal recumbency with the target limb extended; radiographic positioning aids can be placed under the contralateral limb to rotate the animal slightly to the side of interest (Figure 24.26).
- Primary beam is centred just on the midline distal to the medial and lateral malleoli.
- Collimate to include one-third of the distal crus and most of the metatarsals.

Special views

The complex anatomy of the tarsus sometimes necessitates the use of oblique views to allow accurate assessment of fractures and some osteochondrosis lesions. Full evaluation of the tarsocrural articulation requires a flexed dorsoplantar view. Stressed views of the joint can be obtained in both orthogonal planes. As with all stressed views, radiographs of the contralateral limb are advised for comparative purposes. Interpretation of these views can be problematic due to the complex anatomy and superimposition inherent to the tarsus.

Palmarolateral–dorsomedial oblique view

- The animal is positioned as for the plantarodorsal view and the distal limb rotated by approximately 45 degrees to bring the plantar surface of the tarsus medially; rotation of the thorax/abdomen away from the target limb can sometimes help achieve this.
- Positioning, centring and collimation are otherwise as the standard plantarodorsal view.

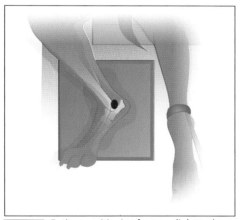

24.25 Patient positioning for a mediolateral view of the tarsus.

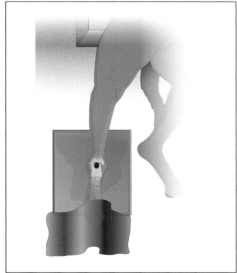

24.26 Patient positioning for a plantardorsal view of the tarsus.

→ **IMAGING TECHNIQUES CONTINUED**

Palmaromedial–dorsolateral oblique view

- The animal is positioned as for the plantarodorsal view and the distal limb rotated by approximately 45 degrees to bring the plantar surface of the tarsus laterally; rotation of the thorax/abdomen towards the target limb can sometimes help achieve this.
- Positioning, centring and collimation are otherwise as the standard plantarodorsal view.

Flexed dorsoplantar view

The calcaneus is superimposed over the lateral trochlear ridge of the talus and lateral part of the tarsocrural joint on the standard plantarodorsal view, and the two parts of the joint cannot be easily differentiated on the mediolateral view. The flexed dorsoplantar view eliminates the superimposition of the calcaneus over the articuation of the distal tibia with the talus.

- The animal is placed in dorsal recumbency (stabilized with a positioning trough).
- The target limb is elevated and placed on a block to flex the stifle to approximately 90 degrees (Figure 24.27).
- A cassette/plate is placed under the caudal aspect of the distal crus and the tarsus is flexed 15 degrees off perpendicular to this.
- Primary beam is centred on the tarsocrural joint.
- Collimate to include one-third of the distal crus.

Stressed extended view

This view has limited applications but has been used to assess the dorsodistal parts of the trochlear ridges of the talus (although they are superimposed) or to evaluate the integrity of the dorsal intertarsal ligaments:

- The animal is positioned as for a mediolateral view
- Cranially secured (proximally) and plantarly secured (distally) tapes or ties are used to maintain the tarsus in maximal extension (Figure 24.28)
- Positioning, centring and collimation are otherwise as the standard mediolateral view.

Flexed mediolateral view

This view is useful for assessing injuries of the plantar supporting tissues.

- The animal is positioned as for a mediolateral view.
- Tapes or ties across the angle of the joint are used to maintain the tarsus in maximal flexion (Figure 24.29).
- Positioning, centring and collimation are otherwise as the standard mediolateral view.

Medially and laterally stressed plantarodorsal views

These views are useful to demonstrate insufficiency of the collateral ligaments. The proximal part is stabilized with ties and an opposing shearing force is applied distal to the tarsus (Figure 24.30). Standard plantarodorsal radiographs are obtained.

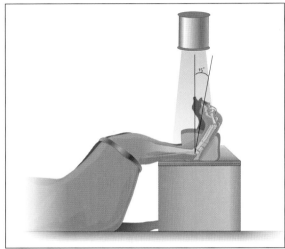

24.27 Patient positioning for a flexed dorsoplantar view of the tarsus.

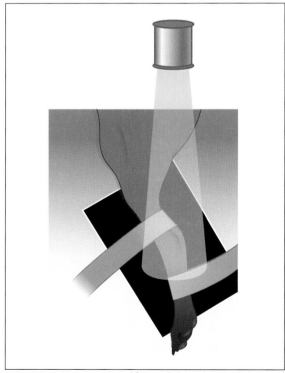

24.28 Patient positioned for mediolateral extended view of the canine tarsus. Adhesive tape is used to stabilize the hock in the extended position.

→ IMAGING TECHNIQUES CONTINUED

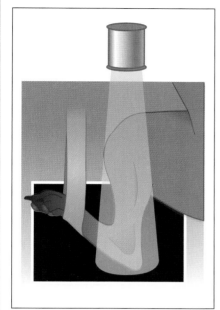

24.29 Patient positioning for a mediolateral flexed view of the canine hock. Adhesive tape is used to hold the tarsocrural joint in a fully flexed position.

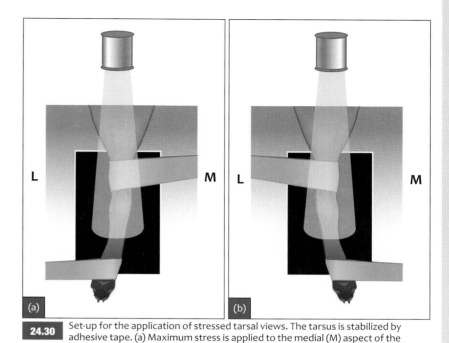

24.30 Set-up for the application of stressed tarsal views. The tarsus is stabilized by adhesive tape. (a) Maximum stress is applied to the medial (M) aspect of the tarsus. (b) Maximum stress is applied to the lateral (L) aspect of the tarsus.

COMPUTED TOMOGRAPHY

CT is an excellent modality for the evaluation of conditions affecting the tarsus; the tarsal bones can be individually examined without any superimposition, and the morphology of complex lesions can be more simply assessed. Lesions of the medial and lateral trochlear ridges of the talus such as osteochondrosis can be equally easily evaluated, with no requirement for special positioning (Gielen *et al.* 2005). Complex fractures can be more readily assessed on CT images than on multiple radiographic views (including oblique views), with the images also less challenging to obtain.

Standard technique

The animal should be placed in sternal or dorsal recumbency with the pelvic limbs fully extended.

* The scan margins should extend from the distal one-quarter of the crus to include the metatarsals.
* Once acquired, separate images of both tarsi must be reconstructed with as small a field of view as feasible.
* Reconstruction using bone and soft tissue algorithms is advisable.

Arthrography of the tarsus is technically difficult and largely unnecessary. Systemic contrast can allow enhanced visualization of the soft tissues of the tarsus, but is rarely required.

MAGNETIC RESONANCE IMAGING

MRI has not been extensively used for imaging of the tarsus, although it offers similar advantages to CT. The small size of the tarsus can create some problems in acquiring sufficient signal to generate useful images, but careful selection of imaging parameters will result in the production of acceptable studies.

ULTRASONOGRAPHY

Most of the tarsus presents a limited opportunity for ultrasonography. However, lesions of the calcaneal tendon are well-suited to ultrasound examination. The main components of the tendon, gastrocnemius, superficial digital flexor and common calcaneal (biceps femoris, semitendinosus, gracilis), can all be identified.

A high frequency, linear ultrasound probe is used to examine the tendon with the tarsocrural joint slightly in flexion. Partial and complete ruptures and degenerative tendinopathy can be identified, with varying degrees of heterogeneity of the tendon and mineralization in chronic cases. Irregularity on the proximal aspect of the calcaneus representing enthesopathy can also be recognized (Caine *et al.*, 2009).

OPERATIVE TECHNIQUE 24.1

Medial malleolar osteotomy and repair

> **WARNING**
>
> Osteotomy of the medial malleolus is not a low morbidity procedure and it should be avoided unless extensive exposure of the joint is necessary. Medial malleolar osteotomy is a difficult procedure that creates an intra-articular osteotomy. It can be difficult to achieve anatomical reduction and stable fixation which can lead to osteoarthritis, joint instability and possibly non-union

POSITIONING

Lateral recumbency on the affected side with the unaffected limb abducted and drawn cranially. The affected limb is suspended to allow free limb draping.

ASSISTANT

Not essential.

EQUIPMENT EXTRAS

Powered sagittal or reciprocating saw, or osteotome and mallet if preferred; standard and small Gelpi self-retaining retractors; pointed reduction forceps; powered drill and range of arthrodesis pins; pin benders and cutters; orthopaedic wire and twisters.

Care must be taken with the osteotome and mallet: note that the direction of the osteotomy is poorly controlled and/or fissuring of the bone may occur; use a thin and sharp osteotome to minimize the chance of this occurring.

SURGICAL APPROACH

A medial skin incision is made over the malleolus, extending proximally to the distal third of the tibia and distally to the level of the tarsometatarsal joint. The malleolus, collateral ligaments and caudal tendons (tibialis caudalis and deep digital flexor) are identified.

SURGICAL TECHNIQUE

1   The tendons are retracted caudally and the malleolus isolated, either by marking with fine hypodermic needles, or by making small arthrotomies cranial and caudal to the collateral ligament complex (Figure 24.31).

2   Holes slightly smaller than the fixation pins to be used in repair of the malleolar osteotomy can be pre-drilled at this stage. Pre-drilling should facilitate optimal reduction at the completion of the procedure. The drill holes should start distally and be angled sufficiently proximally to avoid entering the joint; joint mobility should be checked with the drill bit in place as each hole is drilled to verify this. A preoperative craniocaudal radiograph should be used to assist calculation of appropriate angulation of the drill position and direction.

3   The osteotomy should be angled sufficiently to produce a large enough fragment for repair but not so angled that the cut violates the weight-bearing articular surface of the distal tibia. Preoperative images are used to plan the osteotomy position and direction. The cut portion of the malleolus is retracted distally and the arthrotomy is extended transversely as far as necessary to complete the exposure.

4   The osteotomy is reduced in a perfect position using pointed reduction forceps and repaired using two K-wires inserted into the holes previously pre-drilled. The K-wire ends are bent over to prevent migration and a tension-band wire is secured around them and through a transverse bone tunnel drilled proximally in the tibia.

5   Following placement of each K-wire, the tarsocrural joint should be tested for pin impingement on the joint by manipulating the joint through a full range of flexion and extension and checking for crepitus or limited range of movement.

→ **OPERATIVE TECHNIQUE 24.1 CONTINUED**

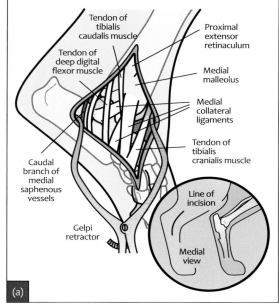

(a)

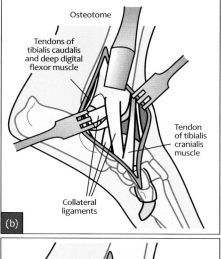

(b)

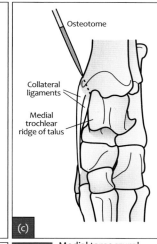

(c)

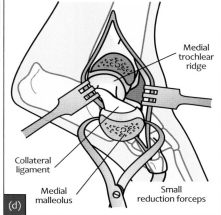

(d)

24.31 Medial tarsocrural arthrotomy by osteotomy of the medial malleolus. (a) Exposure of the medial aspect of the tarsus. (b) Retraction of caudal tendons prior to osteotomy. (c) Position of osteotomy. (d) Distal reflection of medial malleolus to expose the medial trochlear ridge.

Alternative technique

- The pins used to repair the osteotomy may be inserted directly through the malleolus at the time of repair rather than using pre-drilled tunnels (if a small enough drill bit is not available).
- Arthrodesis pins are superior to K-wires in this event, as they have a cutting trocar tip at each end.

PRACTICAL TIP

When drilling fine K-wires into bone it is important that only a short portion of the K-wire protrudes from the chuck, otherwise the wire will be too flexible and it will bend. To accomplish this, several pauses to adjust pin length while drilling are likely to be necessary

Closure

The arthrotomy incisions are closed using a fine synthetic absorbable material of the surgeon's preference, e.g. 2 metric (3/0 USP) polydioxanone (PDS). The remainder of the closure is routine.

POSTOPERATIVE CARE

A postoperative radiograph should be taken to assess reduction of the osteotomy and implant positioning. A padded support bandage should be applied for 2 weeks and activity restricted to short walks on a lead only for 4 weeks after that. Analgesia should be provided for as long as necessary. Follow-up radiographs should be taken after 6 weeks to assess healing of the osteotomy and check for any implant migration. Implants are not removed routinely.

OPERATIVE TECHNIQUE 24.2

Medial arthrotomy for osteochondritis dissecans of the medial ridge of the talus

POSITIONING

Lateral recumbency with the affected side down but the affected limb suspended to allow free limb draping. The unaffected limb is uppermost, abducted and drawn cranially out of the way.

ASSISTANT

Not essential but very useful to hold the hock in the correct position to facilitate surgical exposure.

EQUIPMENT EXTRAS

Small Gelpi self-retaining retractors; small grasping forceps; small elevator (Freer); small curette; electrocautery is very helpful if available.

SURGICAL APPROACH

A medial skin incision is made caudal to the malleolus, extending proximally to the tibial metaphysis and distally to the level of the talocentral joint. The incision is centred over the palpable plantaromedial trochlear ridge. The arthrotomy is made while holding the tibiotarsal joint in flexion. The tendons lying caudally (tibialis caudalis and deep digital flexor) should be identified and retracted caudally. This can be difficult due to periarticular swelling and fibrosis in cases of OCD.

SURGICAL TECHNIQUE

A vertical arthrotomy is made between the collateral complex and the retracted caudal tendons (Figure 24.32). Commonly this corresponds with the area of greatest swelling. The arthrotomy is opened using small Gelpi retractors and the medial ridge of the talus can then be seen. The caudal end of an OCD lesion is usually easy to see but full flexion of the tarsus is necessary for a more cranial exposure. The OCD flap is elevated, grasped and removed. The edges of the defect are inspected and remaining loose osteochondral fragments are removed by gentle curettage. More vigorous curettage should be avoided as this only increases what may already be substantial loss of the medial ridge of the talus and could contribute to joint instability. The joint should be lavaged using sterile lactated Ringer's solution or saline prior to closure.

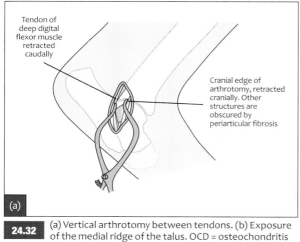

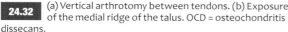

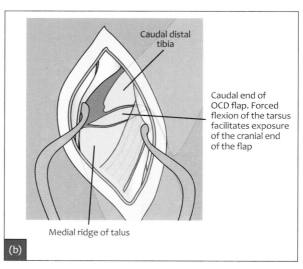

24.32 (a) Vertical arthrotomy between tendons. (b) Exposure of the medial ridge of the talus. OCD = osteochondritis dissecans.

→ **OPERATIVE TECHNIQUE 24.2 CONTINUED**

PRACTICAL TIP

Haemorrhage from periarticular tissues can reduce visibility, and electrocautery, if available, is very helpful. Full flexion of the tarsus is necessary for inspecting the cranial end of the lesion so a tourniquet cannot be used

Alternative technique

Attempts at reattaching large osteochondral fragments in OCD have been reported. For this, or in other situations where a more extensive exposure is required, osteotomy of the medial malleolus (see Operative Technique 24.1) is necessary.

Closure

The arthrotomy is closed using a fine synthetic absorbable material of the surgeon's preference. The remainder of the closure is routine.

POSTOPERATIVE CARE

A padded bandage should be applied for 4 or 5 days and analgesics used for as long as necessary. Exercise is restricted to short (10–15 minute) bouts of lead walking for 4 weeks with a phased increase in the level of activity after that.

OPERATIVE TECHNIQUE 24.3

Partial tarsal arthrodesis

PLANNING

The most common indications for partial arthrodesis are tarsal fractures, plantar ligament degeneration, intertarsal or tarsometatarsal instability or osteoarthritis. Instability commonly involves the calcaneoquartal and tarsometatarsal joints following acute or repetitive trauma. Chronic instability may be associated with considerable periarticular fibrosis. Intraoperative haemorrhage may hamper visibility and diathermy is very useful to limit this. Alternatively, a tourniquet can be used to control haemorrhage (see Chapter 13). Reference should be made on preoperative radiographs to the amount of new bone formation on the plantar surface of the intertarsal and tarsometatarsal joints. Excision of excessive bone or fibrous tissue formation may facilitate placement of the implant used for partial arthrodesis. A donor site for harvesting cancellous bone graft should be prepared if using autogenous bone graft. This can be the ipsilateral tuber coxae, proximal lateral humeral metaphysis (recommended) or, if preferred, the contralateral proximal medial tibial metaphysis.

POSITIONING

Lateral recumbency with the affected limb uppermost and suspended for free limb draping. If the ipsilateral proximal humerus is to be the source of cancellous bone for grafting it is helpful to have this limb drawn caudally.

ASSISTANT

Very helpful but not essential.

EQUIPMENT EXTRAS

Standard and small Gelpi self-retaining retractors; appropriately sized drill bit and spoon curette for harvesting cancellous bone; small curette or high-speed burrs for removal of articular cartilage; small rongeurs; appropriately sized drills, depth gauge, tap etc. for insertion of bone screws and/or plate; orthopaedic wire and instrumentation for its insertion (if desired).

→

→ **OPERATIVE TECHNIQUE 24.3 CONTINUED**

SURGICAL APPROACH

A skin incision is made along the plantarolateral edge of the calcaneus and extended proximally 2–3 cm beyond the tip of the calcaneus and distally 2–6 cm beyond the tarsometatarsal joint, depending upon the size of patient and the technique selected. The superficial digital flexor is reflected medially from the calcaneoquartal joint and calcaneus.

PRACTICAL TIP

Make the skin incision plantar to the intended position of the plate in order that at the end of the surgery, the skin incision is not closed directly over the plate

SURGICAL TECHNIQUE

For all techniques, reactive soft tissue and new bone formation are removed as required from the plantar aspect of the calcaneoquartal joint to allow inspection of the articular surfaces. The joint is forcibly hyperextended and articular cartilage is removed from the joint surfaces, ideally using a high-speed burr, although a sharp curette can be used. Articular cartilage should be removed from the tarsal and metatarsal bones if instability is present at these joint levels.

Lateral bone plate

1 The lateral prominence of the proximal end of the fifth metatarsal bone can be removed using rongeurs or a high-speed burr; this is recommended as it facilitates positioning of the plate on the lateral aspect and this means less plate contouring is required.

2 Cancellous bone is packed into the joint spaces and the calcaneoquartal joint is reduced and held in position. A temporary transarticular pin can be placed to assist in stabilizing the proximal intertarsal joint and, if wished, this can be used to form a plate–rod combination.

3 An appropriately sized plate is contoured to fit the lateral aspect. Intertarsal plates, dynamic compression plates, hybrid pancarpal arthrodesis plates or veterinary cuttable plates suit this location well. Usually three screws are placed in the calcaneus, one in the fourth tarsal bone, and three or four in the proximal metatarsal bones. The proximal two metatarsal screws should engage as many metatarsal bones as possible (Figure 24.33). More distal screws should only engage one or two metatarsal bones. The proximal calcaneal screws and the distal metatarsal screws are used to generate axial compression against the fixed middle screw in the fourth tarsal bone. Locking plates and screws can be useful to reduce the chance of screw loosening, although they should be used in combination with compression. Plate contouring should be performed in order to prevent problems with soft tissue closure due to a proud plate.

Lag screw and tension-band

1 A gliding hole is drilled in a retrograde direction from the calcaneal articular surface proximally, to exit the proximal tuber calcaneus immediately dorsal to the insertion site of the common calcaneal tendon.

2 An insert guide is placed into the proximal end of this drill hole and cancellous bone graft is packed into the intertarsal and tarsometatarsal joints.

3 The joint is then forcibly hyperflexed to ensure proper alignment of the calcaneoquartal articular surfaces.

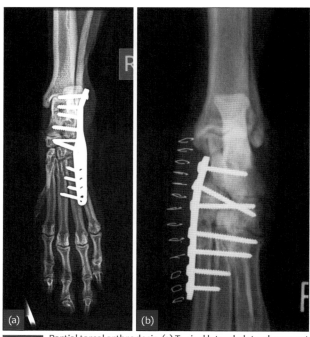

24.33 Partial tarsal arthrodesis. (a) Typical lateral plate placement (see also Figure 24.17). The twist in the plate is usually necessary in order to apply it flush to the bone, to ensure that the screws engage the metatarsal bones correctly and to avoid causing a rotational deformity of the metatarsal bones relative to the proximal tarsus. (b) Contoured medial bone plate placement. The use of a medial plate is unusual as much more contouring is required and it is difficult to place the plate as proximal on the talus as is possible on the calcaneus when the plate is placed laterally.
(a, Courtesy of Gareth Arthurs)

→ **OPERATIVE TECHNIQUE 24.3 CONTINUED**

4 A pilot hole is drilled through the insert guide into the fourth tarsal bone and proximal metatarsus. The drill hole is measured and tapped and an appropriately sized bone screw, 2 mm shorter than the measured depth, is inserted and tightened to produce compression of the joint space. Alternatively, a large pin can be placed instead of a screw.

5 An orthopaedic tension-band wire should be placed in order to secure the repair. This is placed as a figure-of-eight pattern through bone tunnels in the calcaneus and proximal end of the fifth metatarsal bone. The wire protects the screw from bending. Further cancellous bone graft is then packed into the plantar aspect of the joint.

WARNING

Outcome with the screw and tension-band technique is associated with a higher failure and re-operation rate compared with the lateral plate technique (Barnes *et al.*, 2013)

WARNING

A common mistake is to fail to identify the distal articular surface of the calcaneus properly and start the gliding hole too far plantar. This directs the pilot hole and consequently the lag screw into the fibrocartilage plantar to the fourth tarsal bone rather than into its proper location within the bone

Closure

The superficial digital flexor tendon is apposed to the lateral periarticular soft tissues using fine polydioxanone sutures to help in retaining the ventral cancellous bone graft. The remainder of the closure is routine.

POSTOPERATIVE CARE

- Postoperative radiographs should be taken to assess alignment and implant positioning.
- External support can be applied postoperatively if desired and this may be a cast, splint or orthotic brace, depending upon patient size and compliance. It is not necessary to immobilize the tarsocrural joint. External support may be used for 1–6 weeks depending on mechanical, biological and patient or owner factors.
- Follow-up radiographs should be taken after 6 or 8 weeks. Assuming there is sufficient evidence of healing, external support can usually be discontinued. Return to normal activity should be accomplished gradually over a 4-week period following radiographic union of the arthrodesis.

OPERATIVE TECHNIQUE 24.4

Pantarsal arthrodesis

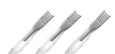

PLANNING

Pantarsal arthrodesis is an advanced, technically demanding procedure and should never be undertaken lightly. The standing angle of the hock can be measured from the unaffected limb but a range of standard pantarsal plates are widely available to choose from that set the standing angle of the hock and minimize the need for plate contouring. Locking plates and screws can be helpful to reduce the chance of screw loosening but, as mentioned previously for partial tarsal arthrodesis, they should be combined with compression. Depending upon surgeon preference, the plate can be positioned, dorsally, medially (the authors, RP and GA's preference) or laterally. Consideration must also be given to harvesting cancellous bone for grafting. For a medial approach the contralateral proximal humeral metaphysis is advised.

POSITIONING (FOR MEDIAL APPROACH)

Lateral recumbency with the affected limb down but suspended to allow free limb draping. The unaffected limb is uppermost, abducted and drawn cranially. The cancellous bone graft donor site selected should be readily accessible.

ASSISTANT

Essential.

→ **OPERATIVE TECHNIQUE 24.4 CONTINUED**

EQUIPMENT EXTRAS

Pantarsal arthrodesis hybrid compression plate; appropriate bone plate and screw instrumentation, i.e. drills, depth gauges, taps, screwdrivers etc.; plate-bending instruments; appropriately sized drill bit and curette for harvesting cancellous bone; Gelpi self-retaining retractors (standard and small); rongeurs; powered bone saw, or (if preferred) osteotome/bone chisel and mallet; high-speed burr or small curette for removal of articular cartilage. Tourniquets are useful but electrocautery is essential for these surgeries.

SURGICAL APPROACH

An angled skin incision is made medially from the mid tibia to the level of the second metatarsophalangeal joint.

> **PRACTICAL TIP**
>
> Make the skin incision away from/plantar to the intended position of the plate in order that at the end of the surgery, the skin incision is not closed directly over the plate

SURGICAL TECHNIQUE

1 A suitable volume of cancellous bone for grafting is harvested, or allograft (demineralized bone matrix or similar) may be used.

2 A modified osteotomy of the medial malleolus is performed in such a way that the osteotomy site, distal tibia and tarsal/metatarsal bones are flush.

3 The osteotomized malleolus can be morsalized and used as bone graft.

4 The articular surfaces of the tarsocrural joint are thoroughly debrided of articular cartilage.

5 The talocentral, centrodistal and medial tarsometatarsal joints are opened and the articular cartilage and dense subchondral bone plate are removed using a drill or (ideally) a high-speed burr.

Note: It has been suggested that care should be taken when debriding the tarsometatarsal joints to preserve the perforating metatarsal artery as not to do so has been linked with plantar necrosis (Roch *et al.*, 2008); however, this is speculative, no direct link has been proven, and it is likely that other factors such as general vascular compromise and postoperative dressing application contribute to the complication.

6 Preserving the normal contour of the tarsocrural joint facilitates reduction and stabilization.

7 The proximal metatarsal prominence is removed using rongeurs. The exposed joint spaces are lavaged using sterile lactated Ringer's solution or saline, and cancellous bone is packed into the joint spaces. The tarsus is positioned at the appropriate angle and the plate is contoured to fit the limb perfectly. The first screw to be placed is inserted into the talus; this is a neutral screw. Load screws are then placed into the distal tibia and proximal metatarsus. Subsequent screws are inserted sequentially proximally and distally. In the proximal metatarsus, two screws should engage three or four metatarsal bones. The distal plate screws should engage several metatarsal bones.

8 Once the plate has been applied, a calcaneotibial position screw can be placed to protect the plate from bending in the sagittal plane.

Alternative techniques

- The tarsocrural articular surfaces can also be removed using a saw. This involves a transverse cut across the distal tibia and an appropriately angled cut across the talus. Calculating the angle of the talar cut is challenging but this method does produce a substantial area of cancellous bone-to-bone contact at the arthrodesis site.
- A pantarsal arthrodesis plate may also be applied laterally, although the plate and screws can be more awkward to seat satisfactorily on that side.
- Dorsal application of a contoured straight plate or a dorsal pre-contoured pantarsal arthrodesis plate is also possible and has been described (Fitzpatrick *et al.*, 2013).
- Arthrodesis of the tarsocrural joint alone has been reported using multiple screw techniques but is not advised due to a significant failure rate.

Closure

Routine in most cases, although tension-relieving incisions may be needed if the closure is overly taut.

→ **OPERATIVE TECHNIQUE 24.4 CONTINUED**

POSTOPERATIVE CARE

- Postoperative radiographs should be taken to assess reduction and alignment of the arthrodesis as well as implant positioning (Figure 24.34).
- External support for around 6 weeks with a cast can be employed although, as mentioned in the main text, its necessity is questionable and it should be used with caution.
- Many surgeons prefer to apply a padded support bandage for the first week after surgery to allow postoperative swelling to subside, either prior to cast application or regardless of cast application.
- Analgesia should be provided for as long as necessary.
- Follow-up radiographs should be taken 8 weeks postoperatively; typically, some progression of arthrodesis fusion should be seen at that time and if so, external support can be discarded and a phased increase in lead exercise allowed. Off-lead exercise should not be permitted for 6 weeks after cast removal.

Pantarsal arthrodesis, if well executed, should give good results in the majority of cases, although angular or rotational deformities can be created by surgery and some dogs will be lame despite successful arthrodesis.

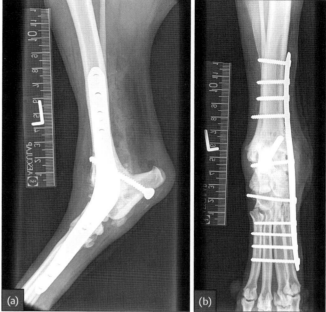

24.34 (a) Mediolateral and (b) dorsoplantar views immediately postoperatively following pantarsal arthrodesis surgery in a 40 kg Labrador Retriever. A minimally contoured 3.5/2.7 mm hybrid pantarsal arthrodesis plate (Veterinary Instrumentation) has been placed on the medial aspect of the tibia and a 4.5 mm calcaneotibial positional screw has been placed to augment the strength of the repair.
(Courtesy of Gareth Arthurs)

OPERATIVE TECHNIQUE 24.5

Repair of Achilles tendon rupture

PLANNING

Treatment of Achilles tendon ruptures may be conservative or surgical, depending upon presentation. Surgery is indicated in dogs with abnormal joint and digital posture and/or obvious lameness. A tourniquet should not be used as it might compromise manipulation of the tarsus during surgery.

POSITIONING

Sternal recumbency with the affected limb extended caudally and suspended for free limb draping.

ASSISTANT

Helpful but not essential.

EQUIPMENT EXTRAS

Standard Gelpi self-retaining retractors; appropriately sized drill, depth gauge, tap etc. for insertion of positional calcaneotibial bone screw; appropriately sized drill for creation of bone tunnel in calcaneus (if necessary). →

→ **OPERATIVE TECHNIQUE 24.5 CONTINUED**

SURGICAL APPROACH

The calcaneus is exposed via a plantarolateral approach. The superficial digital flexor tendon is reflected medially after sectioning its lateral retinaculum and the tarsus is maximally extended using pointed reduction forceps applied to the tip of the calcaneus and the cranial tibia. This permits fixation of the tarsus in extension using an appropriately sized calcaneotibial screw. It is essential to measure the approximate screw length from preoperative radiographs and ensure that a screw of adequate diameter and length is available. Bi-cortical purchase in the distal tibia is essential.

SURGICAL TECHNIQUE

Positional calcaneotibial screw

The tarsus is fixed in extension using an appropriately sized calcaneotibial screw (e.g. 4.5 mm diameter screw in a Dobermann or large Labrador Retriever).

With the joint fully extended and held in position with pointed reduction forceps, a pilot hole is drilled in a plantarolateral to dorsomedial direction through the proximal aspect of the calcaneus to emerge at the cranial aspect of the tibia. The length of the entire drill hole is measured and the calcaneal and tibial holes are tapped. An appropriately sized bone screw, 3–4 mm longer than the measured depth, is inserted and tightened. The screw should be inserted as a position screw, **not as a lag screw** (Figure 24.35).

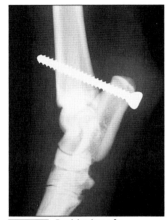

PRACTICAL TIP

Fixing the tarsus in extension with a pair of pointed reduction forceps during the entire procedure will simplify lining up the bone tunnel in the calcaneus with the one in the tibia

WARNING

The screw tip should extend 3–4 mm beyond the cranial cortex of the tibia so that, if it breaks postoperatively, both ends can be removed if required

24.35 Positioning of a calcaneotibial screw. The screw tip should protrude sufficiently from the cranial cortex of the tibia so that each part can be removed if the screw breaks.

Repair of the tendon rupture/injury

Acute laceration injuries

In acute, complete injuries it should be easy to identify the transected ends of the gastrocnemius and superficial digital flexor components. These should be repaired separately using polydioxanone or non-absorbable monofilament nylon. A modified Kessler locking loop or a three-loop pulley suture pattern (Moores *et al.*, 2004) is recommended.

Chronic laceration injuries

Muscle contracture may create difficulties in re-apposing the tendon ends. Lateral digital flexor tendon (Katayama, 2016), fibularis brevis and longus (Diserens and Venzin, 2015), polyethylene terephthalate implant (Morton *et al.*, 2015) and semitendinosus muscle (Baltzer and Rist, 2009) have all been described to fill the defect. Older descriptions include using carbon fibre or polyester (Jenkins *et al.*, 1977) or fascia lata grafts (Braden, 1976) to fill the defect.

Repair of gastrocnemius tendon avulsion

Gastrocnemius tendon avulsions should be reattached via one or two bone tunnels drilled transversely across the tip of the calcaneus to act as distal anchorage points for locking loop or similar sutures.

Mechanical protection of the surgical repair

This can be achieved by:

- Placement of a calcaneotibial positional screw, in turn protected against failure by a padded splint or cast. The screw is removed after 6 weeks
- Placement of a trans-articular ESF with the hock in extension; the ESF is removed after 6 weeks
- When the screw or ESF is removed, a padded splint, cast or brace should be placed to further protect the repair for another 3–6 weeks.

→ **OPERATIVE TECHNIQUE 24.5 CONTINUED**

Closure

The lateral retinaculum of the superficial digital flexor should be repaired using polydioxanone sutures. The remainder of the closure is routine.

POSTOPERATIVE CARE

* Postoperative radiographs should be taken to assess alignment and implant positioning.
* Postoperative external skeletal fixator care.
* Postoperative dressing care.

PRACTICAL TIP

If primary treatment of Achilles mechanism injuries fails, pantarsal arthrodesis (see Operative Technique 24.4) can be considered as a salvage procedure. This may also be a valid consideration from the outset in chronic tendon avulsions but it is usually preferable to attempt to save tendon and joint function rather than to opt immediately for pantarsal arthrodesis

Chapter 25

The temporomandibular joint

Andy Moores

Clinical and surgical anatomy

The temporomandibular joint (TMJ) is a synovial condylar (hinge) joint formed between the condyloid process of the mandible and the mandibular fossa of the temporal bone. The retroarticular process is a caudoventral protrusion of the temporal bone which limits the potential for caudal luxation of the condyloid process. A joint capsule provides support for the joint and is thickened laterally to form the lateral ligament. A thin fibrocartilaginous articular disc sits between the articular surfaces and improves congruency. It is attached to the joint capsule at its periphery thus separating the joint into dorsal and ventral compartments.

Laterally the joint is covered by the masseter muscle, which must be reflected ventrally away from the caudal part of the zygomatic arch to access the TMJ. The palpebral and dorsal buccal branches of the facial nerve run superficially just dorsal and ventral to the zygomatic arch respectively and must be avoided during surgery. The maxillary artery lies ventromedial to the mandibular condyle.

Clinical examination

A history of facial trauma warrants careful examination of the cranial nerves and assessment of jaw movement and occlusion. While the patient is conscious, careful attention is paid to assessing for lateral deviation of the mandible and whether the patient can fully close the mouth. An oral examination is performed under sedation or anaesthesia to assess for wounds inside the mouth and to palpate and manipulate the mandible. Occlusion and the ability to close and fully open the mouth should be evaluated.

Diagnostic imaging

Specific details on appropriate imaging techniques for the TMJ are provided in the imaging section at the end of this chapter. For more general information on imaging techniques and their application, see Chapter 3.

Temporomandibular joint conditions

Luxation of the TMJ

Luxation of the TMJ is most commonly seen in cats and is associated with trauma to the head, most often caused by a road traffic accident. TMJ luxation is rarely seen in dogs. Most luxations are rostrodorsal and unilateral and the mandible will be deviated to the unaffected side. Occasionally bilateral luxations may be seen in which case the mandible will be symmetrical but deviated rostrally. Caudal luxation is unusual but is possible in association with fracture of the retroarticular process of the temporal bone. Luxation of the TMJ results in an inability to close the mouth fully due to malocclusion of the teeth. Care should be taken to distinguish TMJ luxation from fractures of the mandible, although both can occur concurrently.

Imaging is required to confirm the diagnosis. With rostral luxation a widened joint space is visible on a dorsoventral radiograph (Figure 25.1). If computed tomography (CT) is available then this is preferred to identify additional osseous injuries which may not be apparent on radiographs (Figure 25.2) (Bar-Am et al., 2008).

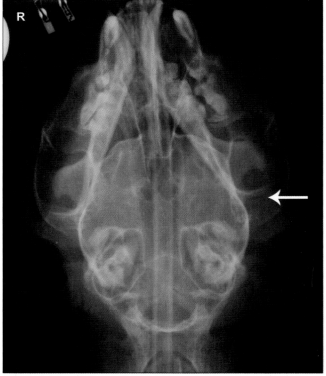

25.1 Dorsoventral radiograph of a cat with a unilateral (left) temporomandibular joint (TMJ) luxation (arrowed).

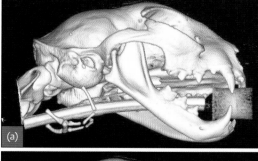

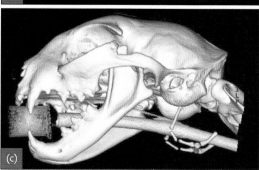

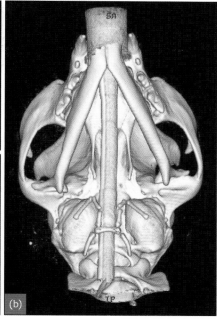

25.2 CT 3D reconstructions from a cat with a left rostrodorsal temporomandibular joint (TMJ) luxation. (a) Oblique lateral view of the normal right side. (b) Ventrodorsal and (c) oblique lateral views of the luxated left side.

Recent rostral luxations can usually be reduced closed by manipulation under anaesthesia. A rod (5–10 mm diameter) is placed horizontally across the mouth as caudal as possible, to act as a fulcrum. A wooden pencil is ideal for this since it is soft enough to protect the teeth, and the teeth are unlikely to slip on the pencil. With the pencil in place between the maxillary and mandibular dental arcades, the rostral jaw is closed to lever the caudal mandible ventrally (Figure 25.3). At the same time a caudal force is applied to the affected side to reduce the condyloid process. A return of normal dental occlusion and jaw movement signifies a successful reduction. In order for this technique to be successful the ipsilateral mandible does of course need to be intact; if this is not the case, open reduction is likely to be required.

Rarely, luxation of the TMJ may be associated with impingement of the coronoid process of the mandible on the zygomatic arch or even displacement of the coronoid process lateral to the arch (Figure 25.4). These cases will present with a mouth that is locked open or unable to fully close. Closed reduction is unlikely to be successful in which case open reduction is indicated.

Following open or closed reduction additional support is usually not necessary. If additional support is required then an open mouth maxillomandibular fixation technique

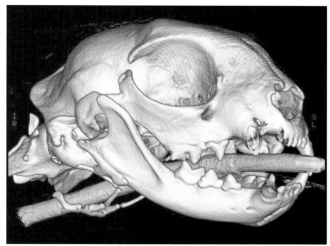

25.4 CT 3D reconstruction from a cat with a laterally displaced coronoid process associated with a traumatic lateral temporomandibular joint (TMJ) subluxation.

is considered for a short period of time (see below). Soft food is fed for 10–14 days post reduction regardless of the method of reduction.

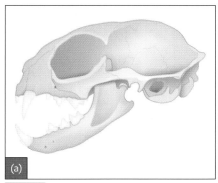

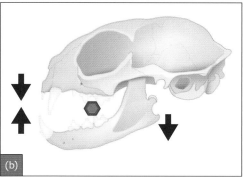

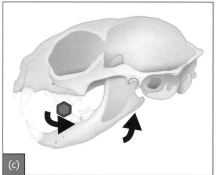

25.3 Diagrams showing technique for the closed reduction of a temporomandibular joint (TMJ) luxation.

Fractures involving the TMJ

Similarly to luxations of the TMJ, fractures of the condyloid process and pericondylar fractures are most often seen in cats and there may be concurrent TMJ luxation or subluxation. CT is invaluable in identifying and understanding the fracture (Figure 25.5). Decision-making will depend on the presence of other mandibular or skull fractures. In cats and all but the largest dogs, articular fracture fragments are too small to be stabilized by internal fixation; therefore, the normal rules of articular fracture repair which dictate accurate anatomical reduction and rigid internal fixation cannot be followed. If the fracture is minimally displaced and jaw alignment and dental occlusion are unaffected, the fracture is managed conservatively, with a 4 to 6 week restriction to soft food. Bone healing may be by osseous union or via a functional fibrous union. If the mandible is displaced than it will need to be maintained in a reduced position for the duration of healing. In mesaticephalic and dolichocephalic dogs a tape muzzle (Figure 25.6) may be sufficient to achieve this. These muzzles are difficult to maintain in cats and brachycephalic dogs. A subcutaneous suture which encircles the rostral jaw performs a similar role to a tape muzzle and may be more applicable to short-nosed animals (Nicholson *et al.*, 2010).

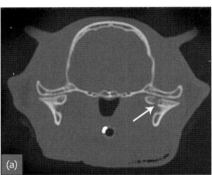

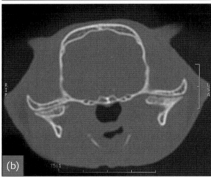

25.5 Transverse CT images of a cat with a left condyloid process fracture (arrowed). (a) Preoperative and (b) after 4 weeks of maxillomandibular fixation with an external skeletal fixator, showing bone healing.
(Reproduced from Moores, 2011 with permission from *The Journal of Small Animal Practice*)

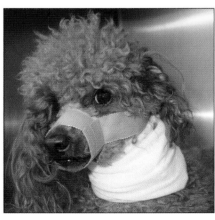

25.6 A tape muzzle fashioned from strips of inelastic adhesive tape.

Tape muzzles and encircling sutures may not provide adequate stability, particularly in the lateral plane. More rigid immobilization of the TMJ can be provided by maxillomandibular fixation. Closed mouth and open mouth techniques are described (Lantz, 1981; Bennett *et al.*, 1994). Open mouth techniques are preferred since they allow oral feeding, there is less risk of respiratory obstruction (nasal airflow is often compromised in head trauma patients), and there is less risk from vomiting. To allow full access to the oral cavity and assessment of dental occlusion, the endotracheal tube is diverted via a pharyngotomy incision during surgical fixation. An oesophagostomy tube may also be placed to provide nutrition in the early post-fixation period, although most patients are able to lap a semi-liquid diet within a day or two. The jaw is immobilized with the crowns of the canine teeth overlapping by 30–50%. In cats, this equates to a 10–12 mm gap between the maxillary and mandibular incisors. It is important that the mouth is not fixed too open since this will prevent the patient from being able to swallow.

Pharyngotomy intubation

The patient is anaesthetized and intubated in a standard manner. It is important that every part of the endotracheal tube, including the cuff inflation mechanism, will fit through a small stab incision. For a right-handed surgeon it is easiest to perform the pharyngotomy intubation on the left side. The left side of the head is clipped and aseptically prepared. The surgeon places a gloved finger in the oral cavity to identify the space between the ramus of the mandible and the hyoid apparatus; this is where the intubation is performed. A stab incision is made in the skin using the finger in the oral cavity as a landmark, ensuring the neurovascular structures have been identified and are away from the incision site (Figure 25.7a). Blunt dissection with a pair of forceps creates a tunnel into the pharynx (Figure 25.7b). The forceps are passed into the pharynx and out of the mouth. The end of the endotracheal tube's cuff is grasped in the jaws of the forceps, and pulled through the pharyngotomy incision. The forceps are returned through the incision and, after disconnecting the tube from its connector, the tube itself is grasped and pulled through the incision (Figure 25.7c). The circuit is reconnected and the endotracheal tube is secured to the skin with a finger-trap suture (Figure 25.7d). At the end of the procedure the incision is left to heal by second intention

Open mouth maxillomandibular fixation can be achieved by interdental composite bonding of the canine teeth (Bennett *et al.*, 1994). This requires access to and familiarity with dental acrylic techniques, and four intact canine teeth for optimal fixation. Fixation failure is a recognized complication and repeat bondings may be required. Maxillomandibular external skeletal fixation is an alternative technique that can be performed without intact canine teeth (Moores, 2011). For this, one to two Kirschner wires are placed extraorally across both the maxilla and the mandible, taking great care to avoid tooth roots and the mandibular canal. With dental occlusion restored, the wires are bent over and joined with epoxy putty (Veterinary Instrumentation) (Figure 25.8).

With any maxillomandibular fixation technique, tools (such as wire cutters for external skeletal fixation) must be kept close to the patient in the immediate postoperative period in case of emergencies that require removal of the fixation and re-intubation.

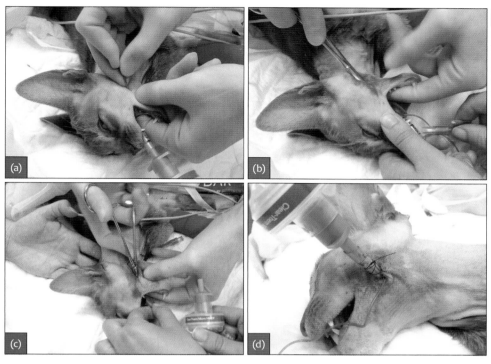

25.7 Pharyngotomy endotracheal intubation. (a) A stab incision is made caudal to the mandible using a finger in the pharynx as a guide. (b) Forceps are used to create a tunnel into the pharynx and to retrieve the cuff tube. (c) The endotracheal tube is disconnected and retrieved in the same way as the cuff tube. (d) The tube is secured with a finger-trap suture.

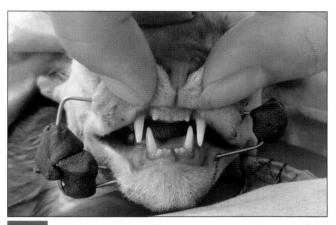

25.8 Cat with a maxillomandibular external skeletal fixator in place.

The duration of fixation will depend on the age of the patient and the nature of the injuries present, but will typically be around 3–4 weeks. This should allow time for clinical union, if not osseous union, to occur. A soft diet is continued for 4 weeks after removal of the fixator. Imaging of these patients prior to implant removal can often be unsatisfactory due to the overlying osseous structures and presence of metalwork and putty. Careful assessment of mandibular stability post frame removal is essential while the animal remains sedated and, if necessary, further stabilization may need to be considered.

Given that the majority of fractures are managed by conservative means or by indirect reduction, inevitably a degree of malunion and joint incongruity will result with the associated development of varying degrees of degenerative joint disease. The clinical significance of post-traumatic TMJ osteoarthritis is unknown but in one study (Arzi *et al.*, 2013) osteoarthritis (OA) was the most frequent finding in dogs undergoing CT evaluation for investigation of suspected TMJ disorders. In those cases where OA was the only significant abnormality detected in the TMJ, it was judged to be asymptomatic in 11/15 (73%) individuals.

TMJ ankylosis

Ankylosis is the consolidation of a joint resulting in immobility. Immobility of the TMJ may be due to 'true' ankylosis where there is intracapsular pathology that has resulted in fibrosis and restriction. This may occur secondary to traumatic injuries. 'False' ankylosis is caused by pathology in the tissues around the TMJ that limits joint movement; causes may include fibrous tissue or callus formation secondary to fractures, neoplasia or infection. Occasionally craniomandibular osteopathy (see Chapter 7) may result in extracapsular TMJ ankylosis. Masticatory muscle myopathy is a differential diagnosis for inability to open the mouth but this is often associated with more severe muscle atrophy than cases of ankylosis.

In advanced cases of TMJ ankylosis, it may not be possible to open the mouth more than a few millimetres and weight loss will be marked. Endotracheal intubation for anaesthesia will be problematic. If it is known that the pathology is unilateral then mandibular symphysiotomy can be performed with a mallet and osteotome via a small rostral incision. This will allow intubation by opening one half of the mouth. The symphysiotomy is repaired with orthopaedic wire once the ankylosis has been corrected. Alternatively, if the mouth can be opened sufficiently, an endotracheal tube can be pre-placed over a small flexible endoscope and intubation can be performed by endoscopic observation of the larynx and trachea. The endotracheal tube can then be advanced over the endoscope into the trachea. In all situations, a tracheotomy kit should be available in case these methods fail and an urgent restoration of the airway is required.

The conservative management of TMJ ankylosis by repeated forced opening of the jaw under anaesthesia is unlikely to be successful. Surgical management of the ankylosis will be dependent on the pathology present and this is ideally determined by CT imaging. If the pathology is extracapsular then all involved tissue will need to be removed and this may require resection of the zygomatic arch as well as part of the mandible (Figure 25.9).

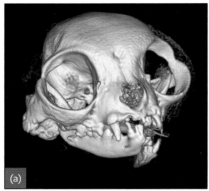
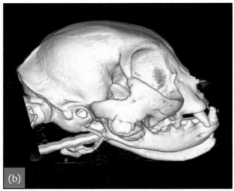
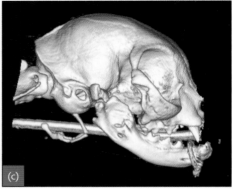

25.9 CT 3D reconstructions from a cat with a right zygomatic arch osteoma causing complete extracapsular ankylosis of the right TMJ. Mandibular symphysiotomy was performed to allow endotracheal intubation. (a–b) Preoperative scans. (c) Postoperative scan demonstrating complete resection of the zygomatic arch and the coronoid process of the mandible.

Intracapsular ankylosis is managed by condylectomy (excision arthroplasty) (see Operative Technique 25.1). Preservation of the articular disc may reduce postoperative adhesions between the temporal bone and the osteotomy site. Unilateral condylectomy is well tolerated and malocclusion is not expected. Malocclusion is more likely following bilateral condylectomy. If this is persistent, crown reduction or extraction of canine teeth may be required.

The prognosis following the management of ankylosis for non-malignant disease is generally good as long as all of the affected tissue is removed (Maas and Theyse, 2007).

TMJ dysplasia/locking jaw syndrome

Locking jaw syndrome is the intermittent locking of the jaw in an open position when the mouth is opened fully, for example while yawning (Figure 25.10). The coronoid process of the mandible deviates laterally and impinges on the ventral aspect of the zygomatic arch, thus creating the 'lock'. The lock may occur on one side only or on either side. The locked open jaw may only last for a few seconds or may persist until the jaw can be manually reduced. Locking jaw syndrome has been reported in cats and dogs. Since developmental factors are often involved, most patients are young adults at first presentation (Lantz, 2012).

TMJ dysplasia has been described as excessive mediolateral laxity in one or both TMJs and this has been proposed as a mechanism for jaw locking. The author has also seen jaw locking in dogs with skull deformities such as mandibular prognathism (overshot jaw, i.e. excessively long mandible). In cats, the predisposition of Persians suggests skull conformation plays a role in jaw locking.

When the jaw is locked the rostral mandible will be slightly deviated towards the side of the impingement. It may be possible to palpate the lateralized coronoid process ventral to the zygomatic arch on the affected side. It is often possible to reduce the lock in the conscious patient by opening the mouth further, applying a medial pressure to the displaced coronoid process and pushing the rostral mandible to the opposite side.

Condylectomy and partial coronoidectomy have been described to manage locking jaw syndrome but partial zygomatic arch resection is less invasive, does not compromise joint function and in the author's experience is a very successful technique for these cases (see Operative Techniques 25.1 and 25.2). Since the area of impingement will not be the same for every patient, the area to be resected is ideally determined on the basis of imaging with the jaw in a locked position to ensure the correct part of the zygomatic arch is resected. CT 3D reconstructions are ideal for this purpose (Figure 25.11). If CT is not available it may be possible to determine the area to be resected at the time of surgery, although it is not always straightforward to recreate the 'lock' at surgery. If the lock cannot be induced at surgery, wide resection of the zygomatic arch could be considered but at the expense of greater surgical trauma, particularly if the ventral border of the orbit is resected. Even if the history is of a unilateral locking, while the patient is anaesthetized the jaw should be manipulated to try to recreate the locking on both sides in case there is bilateral impingement. As well as opening the mouth fully and moving the rostral jaw to one side, lateral pressure on the medial aspect of the coronoid process (from within the oral cavity) may help to recreate the lock.

Zygomatic arch resection is very well tolerated and as long as the correct area is resected, the prognosis following either unilateral or bilateral surgery is very good.

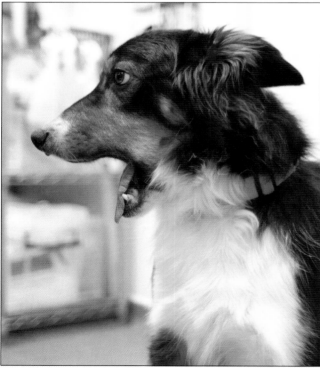

25.10 A dog with a locked open jaw due to coronoid process–zygomatic arch impingement.

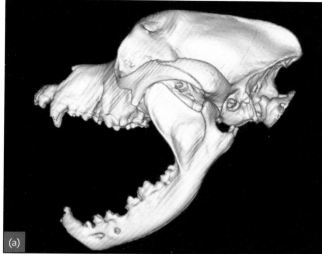

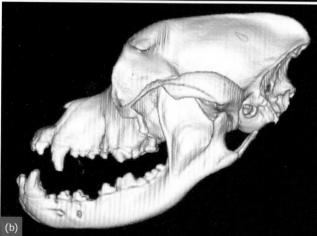

25.11 CT 3D reconstructions from a Boxer with a locked jaw. (a) Preoperative scan with the jaw in a locked position. (b) Postoperative scan showing partial resection of the zygomatic arch. The locking was bilateral and a similar resection was performed on the right side.

Neoplasia

To the author's knowledge, neoplasia of the TMJ itself has not been reported in cats or dogs, although in humans there are sporadic reports of primary TMJ tumours. Tumours of the tissues surrounding the TMJ may have an effect on TMJ function and treatment will of course be dictated by the location and nature of the primary lesion. The reader is referred to the *BSAVA Manual of Canine and Feline Head, Neck and Thoracic Surgery* and the *BSAVA Manual of Canine and Feline Oncology* for further information.

References and further reading

Arzi B, Cissell D, Verstraete F *et al.* (2013) Computed tomographic findings in dogs and cats with temporomandibular joint disorders – 58 cases (2006–2011). *Journal of the American Veterinary Medical Association* **242**, 69–75

Bar-Am Y, Pollard RE, Kass PH and Verstraete FJM (2008) The diagnostic yield of conventional radiographs and computed tomography in dogs and cats with maxillofacial trauma. *Veterinary Surgery* **37**, 294–299

Bennett JW, Kapatkin AS and Marretta SM (1994) Dental composite for the fixation of mandibular fractures and luxations in 11 cats and 6 dogs. *Veterinary Surgery* **23**, 190–194

Dobson J and Lascelles D (2011) *BSAVA Manual of Canine and Feline Oncology, 3rd edn.* BSAVA Publications, Gloucester

Holt D, Haar G and Brockman D (2018) *BSAVA Manual of Canine and Feline Head, Neck and Thoracic Surgery, 2nd edn.* BSAVA Publications, Gloucester

Lantz GC (1981) Interarcade wiring as a method of fixation for selected mandibular injuries. *Journal of the American Animal Hospital Association* **17**, 599–603

Lantz GC (2012) Temporomandibular joint dysplasia. In: *Oral and Maxillofacial Surgery in Dogs and Cats*, ed. FJM Verstraete, MJ Lommer and AJ Bezuidenhout, pp. 531–537. Saunders, Edinburgh.

Maas C and Theyse L (2007) Temporomandibular joint ankylosis in cats and dogs. A report of 10 cases. *Veterinary and Comparative Orthopaedics and Traumatology* **20**, 192–197

Macready DM, Hecht S, Craig LE *et al.* (2010) Magnetic resonance imaging features of the temporomandibular joint in normal dogs. *Veterinary Radiology and Ultrasound* **51**, 436–440

Moores AP (2011) Maxillomandibular external skeletal fixation in five cats with caudal jaw trauma. *Journal of Small Animal Practice* **52**, 38–41

Nicholson I, Wyatt J, Radke H and Langley-Hobbs SJ (2010) Treatment of caudal mandibular fracture and temporomandibular joint fracture-luxation using a bi-gnathic encircling and retaining device. *Veterinary and Comparative Orthopaedics and Traumatology* **23**, 102–108

Schwarz T, Weller R, Dickie AM *et al.* (2002) Imaging of the canine and feline temporomandibular joint: A review. *Veterinary Radiology and Ultrasound* **43**, 85–97

IMAGING TECHNIQUES

Thomas W. Maddox

Due to its small size and location at the base of the skull, the TMJ is difficult to image with radiography. Aside from the dorsoventral and lateral (where the two joints are superimposed), all views that visualize the TMJ are some form of oblique view and will inevitably result in a degree of distortion of the anatomy. For this reason, CT is a technically easier and more rewarding modality for imaging of the TMJ (Schwarz *et al.*, 2002).

RADIOGRAPHY

Standard views

The standard lateral view of the skull is of little use for imaging the TMJ and so will not be described here. The use of a radiographic grid is not required, except for very large dogs.

Dorsoventral view

This view allows good visualization of both TMJs simultaneously and is useful for assessment of subluxation and some articular fractures. Exact congruence of the joint can be difficult to assess.

- The animal is positioned in sternal recumbency with the head extended and the hard palate approximately parallel with the cassette/plate (Figure 25.12).
- Larger dogs may require elevation of the head on a foam pad/block.
- The primary beam is centred on the midline at the level of the orbits.
- As mandibular symmetry often forms part of the assessment, collimate rostrally to the nose and caudally to the back of the skull.

Special views

The normal lateral oblique view (left/right 30-degree dorsal–right/left ventral oblique; obtained by axially rotating the skull from a lateral position) allows observation of the TMJs separately, but generally results in an overly oblique view of the joint. However, sagittal oblique views provide a more accurate representation of joint morphology.

Sagittal oblique view

- The animal is positioned in lateral recumbency with the target joint dependent against the cassette/plate (Figure 25.13).
- From this the nose is tilted up by 5–25 degrees from the true lateral position.
- The primary beam is centred on the TMJ by direct palpation of the joint.
- Collimate tightly to include the caudal angle of the mandible and dorsally to the zygomatic arch.

With the right TMJ closest to the cassette, the resulting radiograph is properly termed a left rostral–right caudal oblique. Brachycephalic dogs require a greater angle of elevation compared with dolichocephalic breeds. Occasionally slight axial rotation of the skull will assist in avoiding superimposition of the TMJ with the base of the skull. The view can be obtained with the mouth open or closed.

This is a view for which comparison with the contralateral joint is often beneficial, and both joints should be radiographed. Care should be taken to replicate the view as closely as possible in terms of positioning, in order to allow direct comparison to be made more easily.

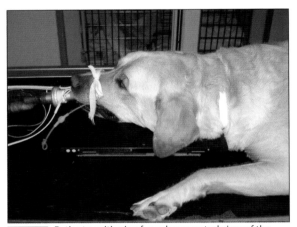

25.12 Patient positioning for a dorsoventral view of the skull including the temporomandibular joints.

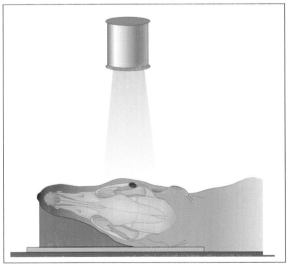

25.13 Patient positioning for a sagittal oblique view of the temporomandibular joint. The joint projected rostrally is the dependent one (i.e. the one nearest the cassette).

→ **IMAGING TECHNIQUES CONTINUED**

COMPUTED TOMOGRAPHY

The TMJs are very well visualized on CT examination, with no special positioning required, and even small, minimally displaced articular fractures can be well imaged (Arzi *et al.*, 2013). Multiplanar reconstruction is also very useful in appreciating conditions affecting the morphology of the joints (Figure 25.14). However, assessment of the soft tissue components, such as the fibrocartilagenous meniscus, is limited. Despite this, the other advantages mean that CT, if available, should be considered the modality of choice for imaging of TMJ disease.

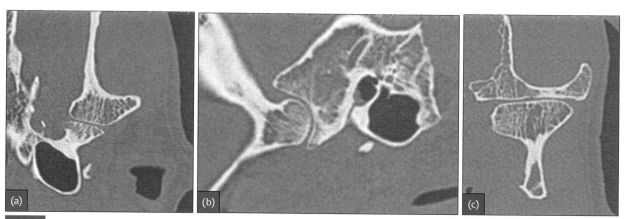

25.14 (a) Dorsal, (b) sagittal and (c) transverse multiplanar reconstructed images of the temporomandibular joint of a dog.

Standard technique

- The animal should be placed in sternal recumbency with the head and neck extended.
- Generally the entire skull is imaged, so the scan margins extend from the rostral aspect of the nose to the level of the axis.
- Both joints should be reconstructed in the same field of view to allow direct comparison; however, for subtle lesions reconstructions can be made of each joint separately with a smaller field of view.
- Reconstruction using bone algorithms with thin slices is recommended; soft tissue algorithm reconstructions may be useful in selected cases.
- Systemic contrast is rarely indicated except in cases of neoplasia or inflammatory disease.

MAGNETIC RESONANCE IMAGING

MRI is the modality of choice for imaging the TMJs in humans, as it also allows assessment of the soft tissue structures. The canine and feline TMJ can be easily identified on most MRI sequences obtained of the head and certain pathology (such as osseous cysts) has been identified (Macready *et al.*, 2010). However, this modality has not been widely used in the clinical investigation of TMJ disorders in veterinary patients.

ULTRASONOGRAPHY

The location of the TMJ is not amenable to ultrasound examination, and this modality has not been used in small animal patients.

OPERATIVE TECHNIQUE 25.1

Approach to the temporomandibular joint

INDICATIONS

Examination of joint; open reduction of dislocation; excision arthroplasty.

POSITIONING

Lateral recumbency with the affected joint uppermost. A sandbag or foam pad under the neck may be helpful.

> **WARNING**
>
> Beware of the eye when positioning towel clips

ASSISTANT

Desirable.

EQUIPMENT EXTRAS

Gelpi self-retaining retractors; small Langenbeck retractors; small periosteal elevator. For excision arthroplasty: a small scalpel blade (size 15 or less); high-speed air drill and 2 mm round burrs; mallet and small osteotome; duckbill rongeurs.

SURGICAL TECHNIQUE

> **WARNING**
>
> The palpebral nerve runs across the face parallel to and dorsal to the zygoma. It should not be a problem unless the incision is made too high.
> The dorsal buccal branch of the facial nerve crosses the masseter muscle horizontally a few millimetres below the zygoma. It should be protected by retraction of the masseter muscle, unless the initial incision is made too low

The TMJ lies ventral to the caudal part of the zygoma. An incision is made following the curve of the caudal third of the zygoma just above its ventral border, curving distally (Figure 25.15). The thin platysma muscle is incised to expose the zygoma and masseter muscle. An incision is made through the origin of the masseter muscle, which attaches to the ventral border of the zygoma. Subperiosteally, the masseter muscle is reflected distally to expose the TMJ joint capsule. This is incised horizontally to expose the mandibular condyle and articular disc (Figure 25.16). Having entered the joint, the capsule is incised latero-medially along its full length at its distal margin to avoid meniscal damage. A small blade is used and the capsule is scraped distally to clear the neck of the condyle and visualize the mandibular notch. The meniscus is preserved.

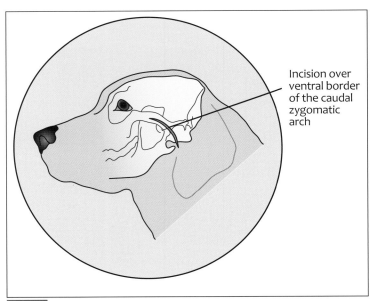

Incision over ventral border of the caudal zygomatic arch

25.15 Local anatomy of the temporomandibular joint (TMJ).

→ OPERATIVE TECHNIQUE 25.1 CONTINUED

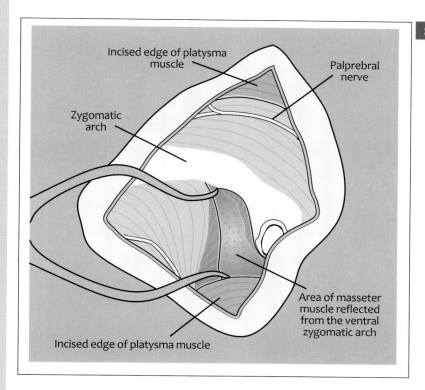

Incised edge of platysma muscle

Palprebral nerve

Zygomatic arch

Area of masseter muscle reflected from the ventral zygomatic arch

Incised edge of platysma muscle

25.16 Surgical approach to the temporomandibular joint (TMJ).

Excision arthroplasty

The air drill and burr are used to make a slightly curved incision from the neck of the condyle to the mandibular notch. The notch is nearly cut through with the burr (Figure 25.17). The incision through the neck of the condyle is completed *gently* using the osteotome and mallet. The rongeurs may be used if necessary to tidy up the osteotomy. The remains of the medial and caudal joint capsule are carefully incised to free and remove the condyle. The meniscus can be left *in situ*. It is important to ensure removal of the entire condyle, whose medial extension is quite extensive.

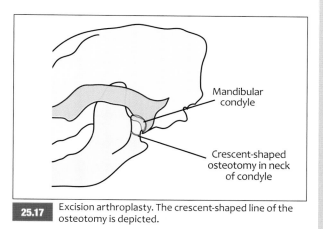

Mandibular condyle

Crescent-shaped osteotomy in neck of condyle

25.17 Excision arthroplasty. The crescent-shaped line of the osteotomy is depicted.

Closure

No attempt is made to close the joint capsule. The masseter muscle is reattached to the dorsal fascia and the platysma muscle and skin are closed.

POSTOPERATIVE CARE

If there is persistent instability after open reduction of a TMJ luxation, a tape muzzle can be applied for 7–10 days to limit jaw movement but to allow lapping of a semi-liquid diet. After excision arthroplasty, jaw movement should be encouraged to maintain range of motion.

Appropriate analgesia should be provided and, within a few days of surgery, normal feeding should be encouraged, including hard food and chews to encourage jaw movement.

OPERATIVE TECHNIQUE 25.2

Zygomatic arch resection

POSITIONING

Lateral recumbency with the affected side uppermost. A sandbag or foam pad placed under the neck may be helpful.

> ### WARNING
>
> - Beware of the eye when placing towel clips
> - The dorsal buccal branch of the facial nerve lies a few millimetres below the ventral edge of the zygoma and should be protected

ASSISTANT

Unscrubbed assistant useful to manipulate the jaw.

EQUIPMENT EXTRAS

Freer periosteal elevator; rongeurs; high-speed air burr or oscillating saw with small saw blade.

SURGICAL TECHNIQUE

If imaging of the jaw in a locked position is available (see Figure 25.11), this is used to identify the area to be resected and to guide the initial incision. A skin incision is made along the middle of the zygomatic arch. The platysma muscle is incised and retracted. The periosteum is incised along the zygomatic arch and the origin of the masseter muscle is detached subperiosteally from the ventral edge of the bone, continuing medially using the blunt end of the Freer elevator. Periosteal elevation will reveal surface landmarks such as suture lines; if a 3D CT reconstruction is available with the jaw in a locked position, the area to be resected can be planned in relation to these landmarks. If imaging of the jaw in a locked position is not available, an unscrubbed assistant can attempt to replicate jaw locking intraoperatively and palpation is used to gauge where the impingement is occurring. At least half of the ventral part of the zygomatic arch is removed in the area of impingement. This can be performed using a high-speed burr, an oscillating saw or rongeurs. Occasionally the resection may need to extend into the maxilla and may need to include the full width of the zygomatic arch. After resection, but before skin closure, attempts are made by the non-scrubbed assistant to induce jaw locking and more bone is removed if necessary.

Closure

The masseter muscle is sutured to the periosteal fascia. The remaining closure is routine.

POSTOPERATIVE CARE

Appropriate analgesia along with soft food is provided for a few days postoperatively.

Index

Page numbers in *italics* refer to Figures.
Page numbers in **bold** indicate Operative Techniques and Imaging Techniques sections.